PREGNANCY
&
CHILDBIRTH
REVISED AND UPDATED

Other Avon Books by
Tracie Hotchner

CHILDBIRTH & MARRIAGE
THE PREGNANCY DIARY
PREGNANCY PURE & SIMPLE

TRACIE HOTCHNER

PREGNANCY & CHILDBIRTH

REVISED AND UPDATED

The Only Book You'll Ever Need

Foreword by Karen Blanchard, M.D., OB/GYN

Interior illustrations by Christine Leahy

AVON BOOKS ◆ NEW YORK

PREGNANCY & CHILDBIRTH (Third Revised Edition) is an original publication of Avon Books. This edition has never before appeared in book form.

AVON BOOKS
A division of
The Hearst Corporation
1350 Avenue of the Americas
New York, New York 10019

Third revised edition copyright © 1997 by Cortona Corp.
Second revised edition copyright © 1990 by Cortona Corp.
Copyright © 1979, 1984 by Tracie Hotchner
Cover art by Doron Ben-Ami
Published by arrangement with Cortona Corporation and the author
Visit our website at **http://AvonBooks.com**
ISBN: 0-380-78039-9

Library of Congress Cataloging in Publication Data:
Hotchner, Tracie.
    Pregnancy and childbirth / Tracie Hotchner.—Rev. ed.
        p.   cm.
    Includes index.
    1. Pregnancy.   2. Childbirth.   I. Title.
RG525.H58   1996   96-23748
618.2—dc20   CIP

Third Avon Books Revised Trade Printing: March 1997
Second Avon Books Revised Trade Printing: April 1990
First Avon Books Revised Trade Printing: May 1984
First Avon Books Trade Printing: May 1979

AVON TRADEMARK REG. U.S. PAT. OFF. AND IN OTHER COUNTRIES, MARCA REGISTRADA, HECHO EN U.S.A.

Printed in the U.S.A.

RA   10   9   8   7   6   5   4   3   2   1

Dedicated to Franklin,
my sweetheart, my husband, my love

Contents

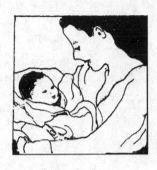

Foreword

by Karen Blanchard, M.D., OB/GYN

Nearly twenty years ago, Tracie Hotchner chose me to be the medical adviser on this book, and I feel privileged to have been involved with it from its beginnings. From the start I learned things that I did not know; I am sure that my colleagues in the medical profession also gained by reading this book, and by listening to their patients who turned to these pages for advice and information. The wise couple and the wise physician recognize that parents-to-be should form a partnership with their physicians—a relationship rich with mutual respect. I hope that doctors and patients will all read this book so that they can work together.

Over the past two decades there have been tremendous changes in the way that expectant couples approach their pregnancies and the manner in which maternity healthcare is provided. The technology that medical practice makes available grows at an ever-accelerating rate and the appropriateness of its application in any individual situation becomes far more than a solely medical decision. This book helps everyone to see what the options are and make informed decisions. The people who should be most grateful for *Pregnancy & Childbirth* are the ones who are going to have the babies . . . it is invaluable for them.

The two decades that have passed since *Pregnancy & Childbirth* was first published have borne out Ms. Hotchner's vision that childbearing couples need all the information they can acquire to make decisions for themselves and for their children-to-be. The author has nurtured this book through several revisions and now has totally reworked the material to keep abreast of changes in the medical field and in the attitudes of expectant couples. Ms. Hotchner has listened to criticism and praise, making changes as needed, always working to make the book a better instrument of its purpose.

This book is written for every person, man or woman, who is approaching the event of childbirth. Whether you only contemplate birth in the imprecise future or whether you are already involved in the process of childbearing, you have to inform yourself in order to participate fully. It is the sole responsibility of the couple themselves to take charge of the care of their unborn child: no one else can do it. *Pregnancy & Childbirth* is unique in childbirth literature: it is a "consumer guide" to provide you with facts on which to base the choices you will make. I commend it both for its medical accuracy and for the easy-to-read style which makes it accessible to expectant couples and those giving them care.

This book is a first step, a source that can advise and guide you throughout your journey to parenthood. There is no attempt to tell you the "right way" to go; this book serves as a road map to broaden your choices so that you can find your own way. You will learn a great deal about the natural process of pregnancy and birthing, about the problems that can complicate the process, and about the medical interventions that can be applied to better the chances of a good outcome. You will learn how you can enhance your own body's abilities to cope with the changes of pregnancy, birthing, and breast-feeding.

Arming yourself with facts and knowledge of what is normal and what is not will give you the confidence to proceed through all the landmarks of a new territory. Committing yourself to taking charge of your own care will enhance your ability to make advantageous use of your other sources of support, such as your healthcare providers, childbirth educators, family, and friends.

The responsibilities of being a parent begin long before you actually hold your newborn in your arms. This book can be your first step on that journey and can sustain you through it. I highly recommend this book for anyone who is involved in the process of becoming a parent. Reading *Pregnancy & Childbirth* will enable them to make decisions about their childbirth and take actions that reflect their lifestyle, family situation, values, and personal physical and emotional needs. I urge you to give yourself that advantage.

Los Angeles, California
October 1996

Acknowledgments

Over the years there have truly been hundreds of people who have made this book better through their generosity with their time, either lending their expertise or sharing personal information. There are really too many of these people to list by now, but I hope you all know who you are, and how much your involvement meant to me, to this book, and therefore to all the expectant couples who come here for guidance.

One new kudo has to go to Maidee Walker, without whose dedicated and super-organized help I could not have achieved the enormous task of rewriting and reorganizing this revised edition. Thanks for your support, and also for your friendship.

And the one person I cannot ever thank sufficiently is Dr. Karen Blanchard. She's been the medical adviser on this book from the beginning, enthusiastically supporting the then-revolutionary idea that expectant couples needed unadulterated facts and full participation in order to assure themselves of an optimal birth.

Karen Blanchard, M.D., received her medical training at Johns Hopkins Medical School and went on to a Fellowship in Maternal-Fetal Medicine at the University of California Medical Center in Los Angeles. She continued her specialization in obstetrics and gynecology with an additional year of research at UCLA as a Walter C. Teagle scholar. Dr. Blanchard specialized in high-risk pregnancies while also serving as an advisor to a home-birth clinic, proving her open-mindedness for a wide array of choices in childbirth. She was a pioneer in the practice of allowing a couple to stay together for cesarean births.

Words of Welcome

Congratulations! You've taken the big step of deciding you're ready to try to get pregnant, or you may have already embarked on that journey with a baby growing inside you. In either case, parenthood is a big decision for a couple to make in this crazy world as we head into the twenty-first century, and this book will be by your side through the whole adventure. With all the things you have to wonder and worry about during this exciting time, I can promise you that this book will give you everything you need to become informed, empowered, and reassured.

Pregnancy & Childbirth is going to become your best friend, as it has been for millions of couples before you. I am honored to know that this book has come to be called "the bible" by many of the new parents who have relied on it over the past twenty years. It is because of so many people's faith in me that you are getting this totally new edition. I have reworked every single page of this book, resulting in a complete revision that now will be relied on by a whole new generation of expectant couples as we cross the threshold of a new millennium.

This book contains absolutely everything you need to know about preparing your body before you get pregnant, taking care of yourself physically and emotionally while the baby grows inside you, learning to protect your relationship during this important passage in your lives, planning for the best possible birth experience, and adjusting to the new baby. When I first set out to write this book many years ago, I gathered every possible scrap of information that existed about childbearing. I have made it my mission to keep on top of changes and evolution in the materity field throughout the years, becoming a consumer advocate, protecting the needs and rights of prospective parents and their babies.

I think that what has given *Pregnancy & Childbirth* staying power, and sets it apart from all the other books, is the high regard I have for expectant couples. Unlike many pregnancy books which talk down to the reader, this book reflects my belief that couples are eager to educate themselves about the pros and cons of every aspect of childbearing and are ready to take responsibility for decisions in partnership with their health-care providers. Parents-to-be like you want to be treated with respect so that they can make intelligent, informed choices along the path to a healthy pregnancy and a safe and joyful birth experience. *Pregnancy & Childbirth* is unique because it celebrates the fact that *you* are unique; this book recognizes that you want thorough, unbiased, up-to-date information in order to have the best possible birth experience.

While browsing the childbirth shelf at your bookstore you may have seen another pregnancy book I wrote called *Pregnancy Pure & Simple* and wondered why. For some expectant couples there is a need for a simpler version of this book—some people have called it "pregnancy light." If this fat book is the encyclopedia, then *Pregnancy Pure & Simple* is sort of the Cliff Notes, for people who don't have the time or desire to read about everything in such depth or detail. You may also see *The Pregnancy Diary* on the shelf, which is just what it says: a week-by-week interactive diary that you fill in with information and your thoughts as the pregnancy progresses. I also wrote *Childbirth & Marriage: The Transition to Parenthood* to help nurture the relationship of the new parents as they evolve into their new roles as parents. Most couples don't understand the enormous effect that a baby is going to have on their marriage. This book gives them support through the rough patches and suggestions on how to make the change work to strengthen you relationship.

As I welcome you to the odyssey of childbirth an amazing thought strikes me: the twenty-first century is around the corner, yet we're *still* making babies the way men and women always have. Despite all our medical gadgets and expertise, no one really understands the miracle of why one particular sperm succeeds at that one micro-moment in time; we haven't even unlocked the mystery of what causes the process of labor to begin. Here we are, smack in the middle of space-age high technology, and we can't even predict precisely when a baby is going to be born. This is not intended to cast aspersions on medical expertise and brilliance, which have saved millions of babies, but rather to marvel at the power of nature compared to mankind's desire to understand . . . to quantify . . . to meddle . . . to control the world around it. As our fascinating and frighteningly fast-paced world rushes headlong into the twenty-first century, it is important to remember that pregnancy and childbirth are a rare and precious occasion to salute the powerful mysteries in life. Don't ever doubt that you are truly in a state of grace when you are "with child," and then bringing that baby out into the light. Rejoice and delight.

East Hampton, New York
November 1996

How to Use This Book

Think of *Pregnancy & Childbirth* as your personal "consumer guide" to pregnancy. It covers every possible aspect of pregnancy and answers questions you might not even have thought to ask. The point of this book is to offer thorough and unbiased information so that prospective parents can make informed decisions throughout the pregnancy experience.

Some people may want to sit down and read straight through the book, but others may be interested in only a few topics at a time.

Don't feel that you have to read everything that's between those covers, although the more you know about all your options, the more you'll be able to get out of this time in your life. But don't feel obligated to read sections of the book that may not interest or apply to you: just look at the table of contents and go right to the section that interests you. It's nice to think of this book as one you can dip into, picking up useful information along the way. I intended the book to be a tool to make things more clear and therefore easier for you. Use the book so it works for you.

Some people will read this book thoroughly before they get pregnant; other people may not turn to it until their sixth month. Each person is an individual and what he or she wants from this book may be quite different. My desire was to research the book so thoroughly, and organize it so logically, that each couple could use it to suit their personal needs and enhance their pregnancy experience. I've made sure that every single thing you can possibly need to know is in here, when and if you want it. Now all that's left to you to do is to take care of yourself, pay attention to your partner, and have a great baby!

CHAPTER ONE

&~&~&~

Before Pregnancy: Getting Yourself Ready

MAKE SURE YOU'RE IN GOOD GENERAL HEALTH

Have a Thorough Physical Checkup

Make an appointment with your family doctor for a complete physical examination. Even if you're feeling fine, it is wise to have a thorough checkup before you conceive. This allows your doctor to catch any health problem you might have (perhaps without realizing it), especially one that might not be as easily treated once you are pregnant.

Your partner should have a good general physical, too. This way you can make sure that he doesn't have any conditions that could interfere with the production or healthiness of his sperm. See page 23 later in this chapter for more about the health of the father-to-be.

Both of you should be tested for sexually transmitted diseases, even if you have no symptoms. STDs (as they are called) are rampant in America and can be dormant for long periods of time or be without symptoms. You owe it to yourselves and your unborn child to do this even if you feel certain you couldn't possibly be at risk.

Visit the OB/GYN Before You Get Pregnant

Before you try to get pregnant, it's wise to have a full examination at your obstetrician's. Have your breasts checked, have a pap smear and

```
CHECK YOUR IMMUNIZATIONS
```

Measles: If you haven't had measles and haven't ever been immunized against them, or are at high risk for hepatitis B, ask your doctor whether you should be immunized now.
Tetanus: A tetanus shot lasts 10 years, so if you haven't had one within that time period, this would be a good time.
Rubella (German measles): Make certain you have had the disease or have had the vaccination. A blood test will tell you are already safe or you need to be immunized now.

blood test, and be tested for vaginal infections. If you did not have a blood test for rubella (German measles) before getting married, you will definitely need such a test now to check your immunity. If you are not immune, the only safe time to be immunized is well in advance of getting pregnant.

Go See Your Dentist

Pregnancy affects your teeth and gums, so it's a good idea to have a checkup and a teeth cleaning beforehand. And if it's determined that you need an significant dental work, it is better to have it done before you get pregnant.

Meet with a Genetic Specialist

You may want to arrange for a genetic screening if you or your partner have any reason to suspect a genetic problem in either of your families. If you feel you may be at risk for any abnormalities, it would be wise to put your minds at rest before becoming pregnant.

Get Into the Best Physical Shape You Can

Develop an exercise routine that fits into your life: something you can manage physically and that you can make time for. Try to get this program rolling before you conceive so that your body gets used to it (since it's best not to strain yourself with exercise you're not accustomed to once you're pregnant).
> **If you're overweight** do not attempt some kind of radical crash diet, because these can put your body into nutritional deficit, which could compromise your pregnancy. Try to go on a *sensible* diet—preferably one monitored by your doctor—so that you are close to your best personal weight when you begin your

pregnancy. This can help you wind up at pretty much that same preferable weight nine months later!

➤ *If you are underweight* you need to get your doctor's advice on how to get your body strong and nutritionally sound so that your baby starts out life with a good foundation.

Put Healthy Things into Your Body

➤ WATER: Think about drinking only purified bottled water: ordinary tap water has been linked to miscarriage and even birth defects (for more on this see pages 118–120 on "Is Your Water Safe?").

➤ GOOD DIET: Get in the habit of eating a well-balanced diet every day, not skipping meals, and trying to eat high-quality protein and other foods and pass up the junk.

➤ "SAFE" VEGETARIANISM: A strict vegetarian diet can affect your fertility. There are natural chemicals in some foods that can affect fertility. Some of these foods are: barley, oats, soybeans, carrots, fennel, and green beans. You might want to consult a knowledgeable nutritionist to adapt your strict vegetarian diet to the nutritional demands of getting pregnant and maintaining a healthy pregnancy.

➤ PRENATAL VITAMINS NOW: Talk to your obstetrician about taking pregnancy vitamin supplements that contain at least 0.4 mg of folic acid *before* you get pregnant. Studies have shown improved fertility and better pregnancies for women who took pregnancy multivitamins beginning before they conceived.

HAZARDS OF PREVIOUS BIRTH CONTROL

Some birth control methods—even after you have stopped using them—can pose a risk to the baby you are going to conceive. You need to know about these risks before you get pregnant so you can protect your body—and the baby you are going to have—from possible harm. In the meantime, the safest method of birth control is the condom (rubber).

Birth Control Pill

Discontinue use for at least 3 months, or two spontaneously recurring menstrual cycles before having unprotected intercourse. If you're on the pill, stop taking it for a full three months before trying to become pregnant. There is a risk of birth defects if you don't give your body a chance to readjust after being on the Pill. It seems that a woman's body needs 60 to 90 days to restore its normal metabolic function—perhaps longer if you've been on the pill for many years. Long-time users of the pill may have to wait many months for the return of periods.

The safest rule of thumb after going off the pill is to wait for two spontaneously occurring menstrual cycles before trying to conceive. Use other contraception during the time you wait for your body to get back to normal.

Women who do not follow these guidelines and get pregnant 60 days or less after stopping the pill have a 1% to 2% chance of babies with abnormalities of bones, heart, eyes and/or ears—all of which form in the first trimester.

The problem for women who have been on the pill is that it causes abnormal nutritional changes that can affect the first 12 weeks of pregnancy. The nutritional change is basically a decrease in the body's absorption, utilization, and availability of the B vitamins: B12, B6, folic acid, riboflavin, and thiamine. These vitamins are needed for the proper formation of bones, heart, eyes, and ears. The pill also causes a drop in levels of vitamin E and in increase in vitamin A, niacin and copper. It can also raise your cholesterol level as much as 35%. Women who are or have recently stopped taking the pill should talk to their doctors about prenatal vitamins.

IUD

Have the IUD removed before attempting pregnancy or as soon as you know you are pregnant. There is a risk of miscarriage or premature birth if an IUD is left in place once you have conceived.

Spermicides

Antispermicidal products like cream, foam or jelly (used with or without a diaphragm or condom) may be linked to birth defects or to miscarriage. Stop using spermicides at least one month before trying to conceive.

Diaphragm

Stop using your diaphragm at least one month before trying to get pregnant. When used with spermicides—which is the only dependable way to use a diaphragm—there is the possibility of causing birth defects or miscarriage.

THINGS TO DO BEFORE CONCEIVING

No Alcoholic Drinks

Alcohol is bad news when you're pregnant. Studies are now showing that alcohol is bad news even in the months *before* you get pregnant. The official recommendation of *how much* alcohol is bad for you has changed throughout the years, with the acceptable amount going down all the time. Experts (who once said a couple of a drinks a day is okay) have been finding damage to the developing baby from even small amounts of alcohol.

It is not logical to believe that there is *any* amount of drinking that is safe. There is the danger that even a few drinks, especially early in pregnancy, could affect your child's personality and ability to concentrate and learn. Alcohol is believed to cause birth defects, mental retardation, and hyperactivity. A few glasses of wine can't be worth compromising your child for life, can they? (If you aren't sure of the answer, or you doubt your ability to give up drinking for the childbearing period, you might consider attending an Alcoholics Anonymous meeting to see if that gives you any help.) For more on the dangers of alcohol once you are pregnant, see the chart on page 170 in Chapter Six.

Absolutely No "Street Drugs"

There is no such thing as a "harmless" drug taken for "recreational" purposes. Anything you put in your body to alter your consciousness is poisonous to the baby inside. Any of those substances are also capable of altering the natural development and physical and emotional health of your baby. People who once thought marijuana was no threat to the developing baby have found out differently (much to the regret of those pot-smoking parents who were ignorant of the risks of their self-indulgence). As long as you're planning on getting pregnant, or are carrying a child, keep in mind all those corny clichés: "Just Say No"; "Get high on life"; "Grow up." Use whatever phrase helps you to realize that pregnancy is serious stuff: you're about to be a parent, and protecting your child has got to become a number one priority, even before he or she is born. See page 168 in Chapter Six for more on "Drugs & Alcohol" during your pregnancy.

Avoid Smoking Before Pregnancy

If you're a smoker, the good news is that what's in the past is in the past: even if you smoked for a long time it has no effect on the baby growing inside you. All that counts now is that you don't put smoke into your body while the baby is in there.

> ➤ *Quitting early in pregnancy,* before the fourth month, is second-best to stopping entirely from the beginning. Continuing to smoke beyond the fourth month increases the chance of a variety of complications of pregnancy and problems for the baby once it is born. If you stop by the fourth month, you're reducing the risk of harm to your baby to the level of a nonsmoker.
> ➤ *The risk of being born too soon or too small* is high for the babies of smokers. Even those mothers who eat well and gain as much weight as nonsmokers give birth to smaller babies— because of carbon monoxide poisoning and reduced oxygen to the infant—which means they are at risk for many other problems.
> ➤ *The babies of smoking mothers* also run the risk of breathing problems later, which can even be fatal. These newborn babies are more likely to have apnea—lapses in their breathing—and are twice as likely to die of SIDS, Sudden Infant Death Syndrome, as babies not exposed to smoke in the womb.

Stop Smoking

They say there's no habit that's harder to break than putting away that pack of cigarettes. You've probably heard that it's easier for an alcoholic or a heroin addict to give up their habits than it is for a smoker to quit cigarettes. Having said this, there are also millions of people who have given up cigarettes—and most of them didn't even have as good a reason to quit as you do, with a baby inside!

If you are a smoker and can walk away from the addiction for your baby's sake, your accomplishment is a gift that you and your baby give to each other. But if you aren't able to quit cold turkey, don't hate yourself for it. Don't just shrug, give up trying, and let the habit take charge. You still have the option of cutting down on your nicotine intake, which at least will reduce the effect on your baby.

The problem with trying to cut down on smoking is that you might just be fooling yourself and managing to take in just as much nicotine. Even if you light up fewer cigarettes per day, you might be compensating by taking more puffs of the cigarette, or taking deeper drags. This can also be true if you switch to a lower tar and nicotine brand, but then smoke more of those cigarettes or drag more deeply on them.

Studies show that smoking while you're pregnant cuts down the oxygen supply to your baby. Smokers also tend to have less appetite, which means you may also be taking in less nutritious food. Both of these results of smoking can cause low birth weight with all its complications and a generally less healthy infant. If you smoke for oral gratification, you could solve the smoking and the nutrition issues by munching on low-fat, high-protein snacks instead of lighting up. For your own health, as well as your baby's, now is the time to put cigarettes out of your life so that you can give your child the best possible start in life.

If you really want to stop, but don't think you can do it alone, there are many organized programs available. Ask your doctor's advice.

WAYS TO SMOKE LESS

— Change to the lowest-tar, lowest-nicotine brand.
— Buy only one pack at a time.
— Smoke cigarettes only halfway down: tar and nicotine are concentrated nearer the filter.
— Keep your cigarettes out of easy reach: make it a conscious effort to go get yourself a cigarette.
— Avoid friends who smoke or places where there's a lot of smoking: it's a contagious habit.
— Keep count of how many cigarettes you smoke a day and gradually cut down the number.
— Tell yourself how wonderful you are for every cigarette you choose *not* to have!

Coping with Withdrawal from Smoking

The worst effects when you stop smoking will last a few days to a few weeks, but take heart that it will lessen with time. Nicotine is a strong addictive substance, and the longer you've been putting it in your body, the harder your task may now be. It's going to be tough to be patient and ride it out, but it will make it easier, to know what a gift of health you've giving to your baby. Be prepared to handle the craving for tobacco, which you'll probably experience intensely for quite a while. This craving is something you should expect and prepare yourself for mentally: mind over matter, distract yourself, reward yourself.

SYMPTOMS OF WITHDRAWAL

— irritability
— anxiety
— tingling or numbness in hands and feet
— light-headedness
— restlessness or problems sleeping
— fatigue, lethargy
— problems with digestive system
— frequent coughing of accumulated secretions

Some people believe that changing your diet temporarily can reduce your nervousness after quitting. They suggest increasing fruit, juice, milk, and green vegetables in your diet and avoiding meat, fish, poultry, and cheese. You might experiment to see if this helps you. Exercising can help, too. Avoiding caffeine is certainly a good idea, because it can make you feel jittery.

Avoid All Medications During Pregnancy

Check with your doctor about any medications you are taking that might interfere with a healthy pregnancy. Unless you and your doctor determine that you absolutely need them, avoid any prescription or over-the-counter medicines. For specifics on which medications are most hazardous during pregnancy, see "Medications to Avoid" on page 177.

Avoid Caffeine

Caffeine has been linked to miscarriage in women who consume a lot of caffeine before and during pregnancy. Caffeine is known to interfere with conception and is linked to birth defects. You can find out more about this dangerous substance on page 76, "Caffeine."

Avoid X-Rays

Avoid X-rays, other than dental, before conceiving. If there appears to be an unavoidable need for X-rays before or during pregnancy, be sure to get a second opinion from *at least* one doctor other than the one recommending an X-ray. Ask whether there is an alternative method of information-gathering, or if the X-rays can be delayed until after the baby is born.

BIRTH DEFECTS: CAN YOU PROTECT YOURSELF AGAINST THEM?

It's important to pay close attention to your health during all your fertile years, not just when you expect to get pregnant. Half the pregnancies in this country are not planned, which makes it even more important to have a thorough physical examination every year. This allows you to clear up any health problems that might jeopardize your pregnancy. Do not wait until after you know you're pregnant to talk to your obstetrician or internist.

It's unwise not to pay attention to your health status during your childbearing years because fetal organs begin to form within three days after your first missed menstrual period. This can be before most women even know they're pregnant. The fetal organs are complete by the 56th day after conception, so the earliest months are the most critical.

It is during the first trimester, or first 12 weeks of fetal development, that most birth defects can occur. This is when the body, arms, legs, and internal organs of the baby are forming. Therefore, it is during this time that your exposure to dangerous substances is most risky.

Unfortunately, many women are not even aware that they are pregnant right at the beginning: this means they may not be being careful about their bodies during the time when it matters most to the developing baby. Do not allow yourself become the woman who discovers she is pregnant and then worries during the whole pregnancy about having a healthy baby because of what she drank, what medications she took, what X-rays or chemicals she was exposed to (pesticides, or toxic materials in the workplace) since conception.

There is no way to guarantee a perfect baby, but there are simple ways to reduce the risk of creating problems for yourself.

Reducing Risk of Birth Defects

From the moment you decide not to use contraception, treat every day as the day your baby may have started growing and be careful about what you put in your body or expose yourself to in the environment.

Stop drinking any alcohol, even wine or beer, from the time that you decide to start a family: there is no known safe level of alcohol consumption, so why take the risk? You can live without a drink—if you drink "to relax," try something healthier. There's also the added benefit of all those empty calories you'll be passing up!

Read "Everyday Dangers" on page 183 to familiarize yourself with everything that can potentially damage the growing fetus. Avoid all of it.

Check with your doctor about whether any medications you now use or have used in the recent past may be dangerous to the fetus. Any medication (or substances like marijuana) used by a women *or man* before conceiving a child have the potential to cause birth defects. This includes topical medicines applied to the skin (such as some acne medications), which you might not stop to think about. See "Medications to Avoid" on page 177.

DETERMINING YOUR DUE DATE

Basic Facts About Your Due Date

The average time from *conception* to full term is 266 days, although it may be as long as 300 days or as short as 240 days. In weeks, the gestation period is 40 weeks, give or take 2 weeks. However, your due date is computed as 280 days from the *first* day of your *last* period. Therefore once you know you want to get pregnant, you'll have an easier time figuring out your due date if you get in the habit of noting on a calendar the day your periods begin.

Once you do get pregnant, this information can cut out some of the guesswork about when your baby will arrive—the Ninth Month Wait is nerve-wracking enough! (However, since only a tiny percentage of babies ever arrive exactly on the day predicted, all these numbers are just a vain attempt at imagining we have some control over when the momentous day will be!)

How Long Will Your Pregnancy Last?

There are various particulars which will not have any influence on the length of your pregnancy: your age, race, the size and number of previous children you might have had. What *does* count in determining how long you'll be pregnant is the history of your periods. The length of a woman's pregnancy tends to follow what her menstrual cycle has been. If you have periods every 21 days, the baby will probably be early. If you have a 28-day cycle the baby may be late. A woman with consistently regular periods is more likely to have her baby on the 280th day of pregnancy than a woman would whose periods have been irregular.

Calculating Your Estimated Due Date (EDD) By "Dates"

The due date is computed as 280 days from the first day of your last period. This is the same thing as saying that the baby takes 9 months and 7 days—280 days—to reach full term. This is called predicting a due date "by dates." The easiest way to figure this out is to:
- take the beginning day of your last period
- add 7 days
- count back 3 months

Listening for the Fetal Heart

Another way to predict the due date is for your health care practitioner to listen for the sound of your baby's heart. The heart sounds can be detected at 18 to 20 weeks with a stethoscope and can be heard at about 10 to 12 weeks by listening with a Doppler device. These methods have a two-week leeway, which makes the estimate of your due date less accurate than the "by dates" system of basing it on menstrual data.

Feeling the Baby to Estimate the Due Date

Although it is not an accurate gauge of your due date, your doctor or midwife can use a method of feeling you externally to find the height of the fundus (the top of your uterus). Generally at about the 20th week of pregnancy, the fundus should reach a woman's navel. This is not a precise method and, in any case, would have to be followed later in pregnancy with an ultrasound to determine the size of the fetus and then estimate its age.

Ultrasound to Determine Due Date

This test (which is described on page 28) can be used to estimate the age of the fetus, usually by measuring the circumference of its head, which corresponds in most babies to their gestational age.

PRENATAL TESTING

The Reasons for Testing

Thousands of babies are born every year with congenital malformations, some of which might have been avoided. There are many pre-pregnancy tests available that can alert a couple to genetic problems that could affect their children. Other tests done in early pregnancy can identify a fetus with severe abnormalities, allowing a woman to arrange for a therapeutic abortion, or to adjust to expecting a baby with a congenital defect. If a couple has reason to fear a specific anomaly with their offspring, a *negative* test will spare them what would otherwise be months of anxiety wondering if their baby will be affected.

Who Needs Genetic Testing?

A couple should seek genetic counseling if either one of them has a disease which has a genetic component—meaning that what they suffer from can be inherited. If they have already produced a child who is affected, they should get tested before getting pregnant again.

Some experts advocate that mothers over the age of 35 should have a genetic screening because age makes them more likely to have a child with chromosomal abnormalities. If you are in this older age group, ask your health-care provider if s/he believes that screening would be beneficial.

Preparing Yourself for Testing

To make the best use of genetic counseling, it is important to have specific knowledge of the health background of both your families. Both of you should ask your immediate family members about their health history and their memories of any relatives who cannot be reached or are deceased.

The March of Dimes provides a free booklet that explains genetic testing and includes a worksheet on which you can make notes about both your medical backgrounds before you go through testing. The paperwork also helps you to organize information that may be relevant about your parents, grandparents, and other relatives. Send a stamped, self-addressed envelope to:

March of Dimes Birth Defects Foundation,
1275 Mamaroneck Avenue, White Plains, New York 10605.

INFECTION YOU CAN PASS TO YOUR NEWBORN

It has been discovered that about one million pregnant women carry a serious bacteria in their genital and intestinal tracts. They may not develop illness themselves but can transmit the microbe to their babies, for whom the bacteria can often be fatal. A Group B strep infection is the most common serious infection in newborns, who get it when the bacteria climb from the mother's vagina to the womb, or during the baby's passage through the infected birth canal at birth.

Microbiologists divide streptococci into groups known by the letters of the alphabet. Before 1940, Group A streptococci were the major cause of serious infections in mothers and newborns. Since 1970, Group B strep have become the leading bacterial infection associated with illness and death among newborns in the U.S. In newborns, Group B strep can cause pneumonia, respiratory distress, meningitis, and bloodstream infection. Such infections are often fatal, or survivors can be left with speech, hearing, and vision problems, as well as mental retardation. Serious Group B strep can also affect adults, causing bloodstream, skin, and other serious infections, particularly among those with diabetes, heart failure, and liver disease.

In an attempt to reduce the incidence of this serious infection in newborns, health officials are recommending that during a pregnant woman's routine prenatal exam about a month before expected delivery she receive cultures of the vaginal and rectal areas. Since not all healthcare providers are aware of this dangerous infection, federal officials are urging pregnant women to ask their providers about being tested and treated. This is one of those potentially serious threats to your baby's life that you can actually head off at the pass.

Officials recommend one of two strategies to prevent Group B strep infections. In both cases, antibiotic treatment is recommended during labor, not before. The first option is treatment with penicillin or other antibiotics during labor to all pregnant women who test positive for Group B streptococci. The other choice is not to do the cultures and just wait until labor, giving antibiotics to any woman who is at risk for transmitting the infection.

RISK FACTORS FOR TRANSMITTING GROUP B STREP

— prolonged rupture of membranes for eighteen hours or more
— premature delivery
— fever of more than 100.3 degrees Fahrenheit in pregnancy
— already had a baby that developed Group B strep

Studies have not yet shown which of these two methods is more effective; however, all treatments pose some threat. Nonetheless, experts believe that the potential benefits of preventing this disease in newborns outweigh the risks of treating mothers with antibiotics.

WHICH INHERITED DISORDERS CAN YOU TEST FOR?

Cooley's Anemia

This inherited blood disease primarily affects Greeks and Italians: most carriers have ancestors from the Mediterranean region. One in 25 people of this ancestry is a carrier and 1 in 25,000 has the severe form of the disease (the odds of having it may sound low, but 4,000 young Americans have Cooley's anemia).

If testing shows that both parents are carriers, the chance that their child will have the severe form of the disease is 1 in 4 (25%), there's a 1 in 4 chance that the child will be perfectly normal, and a 1 in 2 chance (50%) that the child will be a carrier like the parents. (Children who are carriers are usually healthy, with no anemia at all.) The odds remain the same with every pregnancy and the chances do not change regardless of the outcome (good or bad) of any previous children. Genetic testing is important, because if you do get pregnant it will not be possible to detect in utero whether a fetus is affected.

Cooley's anemia is not contagious (it can't be caught from another child who has it); it cannot be outgrown; it cannot develop later in life (a child born without it is at no risk); and the carrier state cannot turn into the severe form of the disease. There is no cure for the disease, although drugs have been approved to remove the excess iron that poisons these children's hearts and livers.

Individuals born with this disease are anemic: they cannot produce a normal amount of hemoglobin. Children with the severe form of the disease would die of anemia if they did not get regular transfusions. This can cause a severe iron overload (along with added absorption of iron from the diet), which can lead to fatal heart and liver disease. The spleen often becomes enlarged and must be removed. The infant appears healthy at birth, but during the first or second year of life becomes pale and listless, has a poor appetite and frequent infections. The bones become thin and brittle, affecting the structure of the skull and facial bones, which causes children with Cooley's anemia to often have a specific appearance.

DES Daughters

Women who were exposed to DES (diethylstilbestrol) when their own mothers were pregnant with them may have anatomical problems that cause complications in pregnancy. If your mother was exposed to DES during pregnancy, you should be tested before getting pregnant to determine whether you have abnormalities in your cervix or uterus. The test consists of injecting dye into the cervix: the dye then fills the uterus and fallopian tubes, showing areas where malformations may have occurred in your own prenatal development. Characteristic of a DES daughter is a short cervix and a T-shaped uterus, which means a 20% chance of miscarriage in the first 20 weeks of pregnancy.

Down's Syndrome (Mongolism)

This condition means there will be varying degrees of physical and mental retardation of the child. A couple may have an increased risk for Down's syndrome because they have already had a previous child with it: the recurrence risk is 1 to 2%. The other high-risk group is women aged 40 to 44, whose offspring also have a 1 to 2% chance of mongolism. Women over 40 produce a dramatically larger percentage of such babies: 1 in 39 births versus 1 in 2,300 births for 20-year-old mothers.

If you have a Down's syndrome baby it is important to have him or her tested, because there are two versions of this condition. Your odds of giving birth to another child with this abnormality depends on which one your child has. The *sporadic variety* recurs in 1% of subsequent births, while the *translocation variety* recurs in 8% of future births. If you have a child with translocation type Down's, both parents should have chromosomal tests. If the mother is a carrier, there is a 12 to 15% chance of recurrence in future pregnancies. If the father is the carrier, the chances of recurrence are only 2 to 4%. If both parents test normal, then the possibility of Down's recurring is the same as for couples who had a child of the sporadic variety: only 1%.

Neural Tube Defects (NTD)

NTDs are defects which involve the central nervous system, development of the neural tube, anencephaly (absence of the rear half of the brain and skull, which is fatal before birth or soon afterward), or *spina bifida* (an open or malformed spine, survivors of which suffer paralysis, deformity, and/or brain damage). These defects occur early in pregnancy, at the end of the first months after conception. At that time the neural tube (which later forms the spinal column) starts to close in a zipper-like fashion. If there is no closure near the bottom of the spinal column, the fetus has spina bifida.

NTDs occur in 1 in 1,000 births: if your family has a history of such a defect, your child is at an increased risk. If you've already had a child with an NTD, the recurrence rate is 4 to 5%; if you've had two children with a defect, the risk rises to 10 to 12%.

Neural tube defects can be detected prenatally because a fetal protein called alpha fetoprotein pours out of the opening of the spinal cord and enters the mother's bloodstream. A blood test is done on the mother to detect signs of this protein: if there are high levels in her blood, she will probably be referred for a sonogram to confirm the findings. If, in turn, these results are suspicious, then amniocentesis can be done to confirm whether there are also high levels of alpha fetoprotein in the amniotic fluid.

Researchers have speculated for years that a pregnant woman's diet might have something to do with NTDs. Spina bifida has been most common to northern Europeans, especially the Irish. In general, NTDs are more likely to occur in babies born to women in a lower socioeconomic class and women who have a poor diet for reasons other than poverty. There was an epidemic of neural tube defects during the Depression, and the incidence has been falling since then.

Research has shown that women who have been taking multivitamin pills at the time of conception have less than half the risk of having a baby with a serious neurological defect compared to women who do not take vitamins. Some authorities are advising all women of childbearing age to take a multivitamin, although other experts are awaiting more research before making this recommendation. Whatever your decision, under no circumstances should you overreact to this information and take large quantities of vitamins at the time of conception or any other time! Although a good quality multivitamin may be advantageous to your baby's health, it is unsafe to take more than the recommended daily amount of any vitamin. Please see page 111 for "Warnings About Vitamins."

Rh Blood Incompatibility

The Rh factor is a genetically determined substance in a person's red blood cells; those people whose cells don't have the factor are

Rh-negative. Rh incompatibility exists in a couple where the woman is Rh-negative and the man is Rh-positive. This happens in about 13% of marriages between Caucasians and 5% of unions between Black Americans.

The danger in pregnancy is if an Rh-negative woman is pregnant with an Rh-positive baby because she runs the risk of becoming "sensitized." Sensitization occurs if the baby's blood cells mix with his mother's blood cells: her blood then develops antibodies which attack and destroy the baby's red blood cells. However, during a first pregnancy it is very rare for sensitization to occur: raised levels of certain hormones suppress the mother's immune system until after delivery. But if, at birth, the Rh factor from the baby's blood enters the mother's bloodstream, it stimulates the production of anti-Rh antibodies. These destroy (or "hemolyze") the baby's Rh-positive cells.

Not every woman who is Rh-negative with an incompatible pregnancy will become sensitized, but there is no way of predicting which women will. Therefore, all such women should receive an injection of Rh immunoglobulin within 72 hours after the delivery of an Rh-positive baby. The vaccine prevents the formation of these destructive antibodies and it should be given after *every* Rh-positive pregnancy. The injection must also be given after any miscarriage or abortion, because blood cells can mix in those circumstances as well.

If a woman does not get the injection, Rh-positive fetal blood cells can enter her bloodstream and may stimulate the mother's immune system to produce anti-Rh antibodies. In future pregnancies these can cross the placenta, enter the fetus, and destroy its red blood cells. This causes hemolytic disease of the newborn, with differing degrees of impact, from mild jaundice or anemia to stillbirth. Babies who develop the disease in utero can often be saved by intrauterine transfusion.

Therefore, once a woman becomes sensitized, all her pregnancies must be carefully watched: once the antibodies have developed, the Rh immunoglobulin will no longer work.

Sickle-Cell Anemia

This is a hereditary disease that primarily affects Blacks: approximately 10% of Black Americans, or 1 in 10, are carriers of the disease. People who have the sickle-cell "trait" are benign carriers: they don't have the disease, but they can pass it on. However, what will happen to their children depends on who they marry. Here's how the odds work:

— *If only one parent has the trait*:
➤ none of the children will have sickle-cell anemia
➤ each child has a 1 in 2 (50%) chance of carrying the trait

— *If one parent has the disease, but the other parent has neither the trait nor the disease:*
➢ all the children will have the trait
➢ none of the children will have the disease itself

— *If both parents have the trait, each child has:*
➢ a 1 in 4 (25%) chance of having sickle-cell anemia
➢ a 1 in 4 (25%) chance of having neither the trait nor the disease
➢ a 1 in 2 (50%) chance of carrying the trait

There is no way to prevent or cure this disease, although several therapeutic procedures are being researched with good results. However, there are simple, inexpensive tests available to learn whether you have the disease or are a carrier. Early diagnosis is important if you do have sickle-cell, but getting the test can also give you peace of mind: 9 out of 10 Black Americans have neither the trait nor the disease. Knowing as a couple what the odds are for risk—and what the disease will be like for your child if the odds are against you—can help you make decisions about childbearing.

A baby with sickle-cell anemia can be diagnosed in utero, but the technique is difficult because it involves taking a blood sample from the fetus. The test can be done, however, if both parents are carriers and would terminate the pregnancy if the fetus tested positive.

Sickle-cell anemia is a disease that is not apparent at birth. It may manifest itself in the first few months, although it usually surfaces between the second and fourth year of the child's life. The disease is more severe if it starts in childhood; the earlier that symptoms begin, the less good the outlook. Many of the children who get the disease early do not survive it: infections (particularly of the respiratory tract) are a frequent cause of death. However, it is not unusual for sufferers to survive to adulthood, at which time the medical crises become less severe and less frequent.

Symptoms of sickle-cell are numerous: irritability without reason, colic, distension of the abdomen, repeated bouts of fever, poor appetite, vomiting, slow weight gain, pale complexion, and jaundice. Some victims have swelling of the feet and/or hands, along with the fever and irritability. Continuous health care is essential to prevent infections. A child with sickle-cell will have to cope with hospitalizations, absences from school, and the inability to take part in strenuous sports.

If a woman with sickle-cell anemia gets pregnant, she may have serious complications. Increased maternal mortality is associated with the disease, and there is also a significant chance that her baby might not survive.

Rubella (German Measles)

Exposure to this disease while you are pregnant can cause miscarriage, birth defects, and stillbirth. If you had German measles as a child (which is not the same as "regular" measles), then you are immune and your baby will not be at risk. If you are married and a blood test was required, it will often indicate whether or not you've already been exposed to German measles. *Every woman who wants to get pregnant should have the blood test to find out if she is safe from rubella: if not, it is easy to get immunized.* (Vaccination against regular measles is not a protection.)

If you are already pregnant and not immune to rubella, stay away from all children you do not know. Children between the ages of 1 and 12 are the main sources of infection: they are supposed to be immunized, but many are not.

GUIDELINES ABOUT RUBELLA

— Get immunized if you are not already immune.
— Do not get pregnant for 3 months after immunization.
— Do not get inoculated while pregnant: the vaccine can harm the fetus.
— If you come into contact with rubella, your doctor can give you a gamma globulin shot to prevent you from getting the disease.
— Do not wait for symptoms: it takes 2 to 3 weeks for the signs of rubella to appear after you have been exposed.
— If a pregnant woman does get rubella, there is only a 1 in 5 chance that her baby will be affected.
— Symptoms are so mild you might not even be aware you've been exposed to German measles. Indications include: a low-grade temperature, a rash spreading from the face down the body, and swollen lymph glands in your neck.

Tay-Sachs Disease

This illness is carried primarily by people of Ashkenazi Jewish ancestry, whose roots go back to Central and Eastern Europe— which is where 90% of U.S. Jews trace their origins. Only 1 in 6,000 births of Jews with this background are born with this crippling disorder, but it is always fatal. The only way the disease can be transmitted is from parent to child; it is present at birth and does not develop later in life.

If two carriers have a child, there is a 1 in 4 (25%) risk that the baby will have the disease. There is the same 1 in 4 (25%) chance that the child will be totally free of the disease, and a 2 in 4 (50%) chance that the child will be a carrier like the parents. The odds remain the same with each pregnancy, regardless of whether other children in the same family have gotten Tay-Sachs or not.

The disease does occur in other ethnic groups, but people of Jewish descent might especially want to be tested before conceiving. In some cases, a couple might even want to be tested before deciding whether to marry and have a family. Even if only one of the partners in a couple is of Jewish descent, it is a good idea for that person to have the test done. If s/he tests positive for Tay-Sachs, then the non-Jewish partner should be tested too, even though only 1 in 900 non-Jews are Tay-Sachs carriers.

The disease is caused by the lack of Hex A, a specific enzyme in the blood. Since the afflicted child cannot manufacture Hex A, various fatty substances accumulate in the cells, particularly the brain cells. The baby gradually loses motor abilities and is increasingly less able to sit up or roll over. It becomes blind, deaf, and eventually mentally retarded. Death usually occurs at age 2 or 3 and almost no affected children live past 4. There is no cure or treatment for this disease at present.

Toxoplasmosis and Cytomegalovirus

Both these illnesses can cause serious birth defects. Cytomegalovirus is one of the ancient viral inhabitants of human beings; toxoplasmosis is fully described on page 22. It is important to get tested for these diseases before getting pregnant, because if you have already had them (which you would probably not know) there is no danger they will recur during pregnancy. However, if you haven't been exposed to the illnesses, you are not immune and should be retested early in your pregnancy to be sure that you have not contracted them while pregnant. Since both sicknesses can cause malformation of the fetal brain, discovering that you have gotten either disease might lead you to consider the option of terminating the pregnancy.

Wilson's Disease

This disease can be identified with prenatal testing and there is a treatment for it. The illness results in defective metabolism of copper in the baby's body, which causes excess copper in the brain, liver, and eyes. Unless treated, Wilson's disease leads to mental derangement and cirrhosis of the liver.

INFECTIOUS DISEASES THAT CAN HARM YOUR BABY

There are a few illnesses which you may have or can get which pose a threat to your baby:

Hepatitis B

This illness is an infection caused by a virus; anyone can get it. You may be a carrier of the virus without having any signs of illness. Hepatitis B can cause severe liver disease in both you and the infant, to whom you can pass it at birth. However, if you have tests done while you are pregnant, your baby can receive treatment when she is born to prevent her from getting the disease.

Herpes simplex Virus (II)

Herpes simplex II is a venereal disease consisting of fluid-filled blisters on any part of the body, although they usually occur around the genital area. Sometimes there is a fever, headache, and painful urination. (Herpes simplex I, which causes cold sores, and herpes zoster, or shingles, are not sexually transmitted nor a danger to the baby.

The way you can get herpes simplex II is from sexual contact with someone who has an active recurrence of herpes. The virus is inactive between flare-ups and can only be passed when there are lesions (blisters). If you are infected, you would ordinarily notice the herpes 3 to 14 days after the physical contact. The danger to the baby is that you can pass the virus through the birth canal if you have active vaginal herpes lesions at the time of birth. A newborn exposed to herpes simplex II can be blinded or die from it. Therefore, if you have the herpes virus you must be examined for recurrent infection as your due date gets closer. And if there are herpetic sores in the genital area at the time of delivery, the baby must be delivered by cesarean section.

You can protect your baby by lessening your chances of having an outbreak of the virus. It is known that mental and physical stress can cause recurrence of herpes. Mothers with a history of herpes simplex II should take extra good care of themselves during pregnancy: eat well, get plenty of sleep, keep clean, and wear loose-fitting cotton underwear.

Some experts believe that your diet may play a role in whether genital herpes flares up. Diet therapy has been suggested as a way to control herpes, although there is no hard proof that following these suggestions will definitely work. However, there are indications that manipulating your diet may prevent an outbreak: it is believed that foods high in arginine promote infection, while foods rich in L-lysine may stop the growth of herpes. Talk to your doctor about supplementing your diet with L-lysine supplement from a health food store. And if you have a history of genital herpes, avoid arginine-rich foods for the last 6 weeks of your pregnancy.

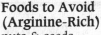

GENITAL HERPES: WHAT TO EAT, WHAT NOT TO

**Foods to Eat
(Lysine-Rich)**
fish
chicken
beef
lamb
milk & dairy products
beans
Brewer's yeast
shellfish
eggs

**Foods to Avoid
(Arginine-Rich)**
nuts & seeds
brown rice
corn
oatmeal
chocolate, carob, cocoa
coconut
raisins
gelatin
buckwheat &
whole wheat flour

     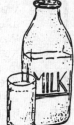

HIV Infection

All women of childbearing age should be tested for HIV infection. The most rapid increase in cases of AIDS (acquired immunodeficiency syndrome) in our population is among women. As the incidence of HIV infection has increased among women of childbearing age, so has the number of infants who have become infected through mother-to-infant transmission. As a result, HIV infection has become the leading cause of death for young children.

However, it has been discovered that the majority of these babies and their families can now be spared this suffering. *Just because a woman discovers she is HIV-positive does not necessarily mean that she has to pass this deadly disease to her unborn child.* An HIV-infected woman's baby may be spared if she is treated with AZT (zidovudine, also known as ZDV) during pregnancy and labor and if her newborn is treated from birth. For more information see page 422 and call the confidential, anonymous AIDS Hotline at 1-800-342-AIDS.

Listeriosis

The listeria bacteria causes a potentially fatal intestinal infection. Pregnant women are especially susceptible to the type of bacteria that causes this disease, so it is important that you follow the instructions below and use caution when preparing food. Although you rarely hear about listeriosis, the bacteria is widespread in the food supply and can cause early miscarriage, premature labor, or stillbirth. If the baby survives listeriosis, there can be damage to the lungs, brain, kidneys, and liver.

WAYS TO PREVENT LISTERIOSIS

— Avoid raw milk or foods made from raw milk.
— Avoid soft cheeses like Brie, Camembert, feta, and blue-veined cheese.
— Wash hands, knives, cutting boards, and counter surfaces after they contact uncooked foods.
— Wash raw vegetables thoroughly.
— Keep uncooked meats separate from vegetables and cooked foods.
— Keep your refrigerator very clean and cold (34–40°F.)
— Leftovers or ready-to-eat foods like hot dogs should be fully reheated until steaming hot.
— Avoid luncheon meats from delicatessen counters or thoroughly reheat them before eating.

Toxoplasmosis

This disease is caused by a parasite that is passed on to humans by eating raw meat or having contact with cat feces. You aren't in danger during pregnancy if you've already been exposed to toxo-

WAYS TO PREVENT TOXOPLASMOSIS

— Don't eat raw or rare meat. Cook it to at least 140°F.
— Wash hands thoroughly after handling raw meat.
— Have your cat(s) tested to see if they have an active infection. If they test positive, ask a friend to keep them during your pregnancy.
— Let someone else clean out the kitty litter box.
— Do not feed rare or raw food to your cats. Infected meat (mice, birds) is how your cats get the disease.
— Avoid other peoples' cats, especially outdoor cats.

plasmosis, which would make you immune to this disease. One third of women, especially those who have eaten rare or raw meat, or have been caring for cats, are immune. A blood test can tell whether you're immune; however, the test is not entirely reliable and must be repeated to confirm its accuracy.

The greatest danger of infecting the fetus is in the last months of pregnancy. The baby can appear normal at birth but may develop symptoms later: it causes neurological problems in the unborn child. The suggestions below can help you protect you against the disease.

GETTING THE MAN'S BODY READY FOR FATHERHOOD

It isn't just the mother-to-be who has to pay attention to how she's taking care of herself during her reproductive years—so does her mate. A woman has to be extremely careful of what she puts in her body or allows around herself, but her partner also has to be aware of ways in which he might be compromising his fertility. A man also needs to know about factors in his environment that affect the *quality* and *health* of the sperm his body produces.

Dangers to a Man's Sperm

If a father-to-be is exposed to certain toxic substances before he impregnates his wife, there may be risks to the fetus. Some of these risks can affect the developing fetus, influence the pregnancy, or affect the child later in life. Being aware of these possible risks helps a man to remove himself from potentially hazardous environments.

Vitamin C

A deficiency of vitamin C can cause birth defects. Take in at least 60 mg a day, which is the recommended minimum. A man's sperm can be damaged and his fertility can be affected if he has less than 60 mg of vitamin C daily.

Exposure to Toxins in the Workplace

A man who wants to father children has to be careful about prolonged contact in his workplace with certain substances that may be harmful to his sperm. Benzene, X-rays, and some art and textile chemicals are known to be hazardous to a man's reproductive system. These substances can cause premature birth, low birth weight, or stillborn infants.

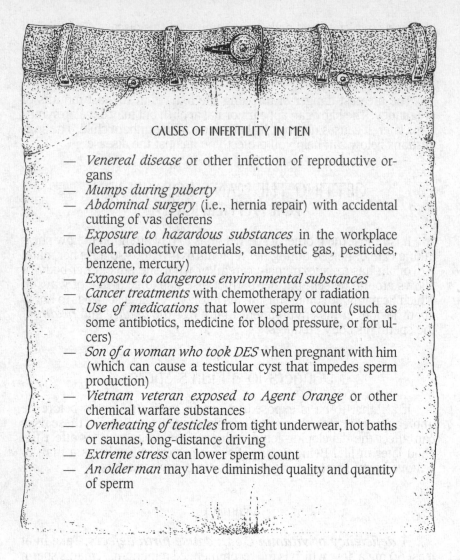

CAUSES OF INFERTILITY IN MEN

— *Venereal disease* or other infection of reproductive organs
— *Mumps during puberty*
— *Abdominal surgery* (i.e., hernia repair) with accidental cutting of vas deferens
— *Exposure to hazardous substances* in the workplace (lead, radioactive materials, anesthetic gas, pesticides, benzene, mercury)
— *Exposure to dangerous environmental substances*
— *Cancer treatments* with chemotherapy or radiation
— *Use of medications* that lower sperm count (such as some antibiotics, medicine for blood pressure, or for ulcers)
— *Son of a woman who took DES* when pregnant with him (which can cause a testicular cyst that impedes sperm production)
— *Vietnam veteran exposed to Agent Orange* or other chemical warfare substances
— *Overheating of testicles* from tight underwear, hot baths or saunas, long-distance driving
— *Extreme stress* can lower sperm count
— *An older man* may have diminished quality and quantity of sperm

Exposure to Electromagnetic Fields

This danger applies to men in jobs such as electricians, welders, and power line repairmen. One study shows these workers are 12 times more likely to have a baby who develops a neuroblastoma.

Regular Exposure to Paint

A painter or other worker who is exposed to paint for long periods can pass on a deadly risk to his unborn children. A father's regular contact with paint increases his child's risk of developing a brain tumor before age ten.

Smoking

A father who smokes before conception may be putting his unborn children in jeopardy. A child's chance of developing leukemia is 40% higher if his or her father smoked before impregnating the mother.

Drinking Alcohol

A man's sperm can be affected if he is a *steady* drinker (more than 2 alcoholic drinks daily) in the month before conception. The result can be a baby at risk: a baby 5 ounces lighter than the average newborn. (For information on the dangers of low-birth-weight babies, see page 67.)

DIFFICULTIES GETTING PREGNANT

This book cannot attempt to cover the whole topic of infertility, which has gotten too complex and is evolving all the time. Infertility is defined as the inability to conceive after a year of regular sexual relations without contraception (or the inability to carry pregnancies to a live birth). If you're having trouble getting pregnant you might want to consult with an obstetrician who is board certified to specialize in infertility, but just for the record here is a chart of some of the factors that cause infertility in women.

POSSIBLE CAUSES OF FEMALE INFERTILITY

— Pelvic inflammatory disease
— Use of an IUD
— Use of medications that diminish fertility
— Post-abortion infection
— Cervical infection treated by cautery or cryosurgery (burning or freezing of the cervix)
— Abdominal surgery resulting in adhesions or accidental cutting of fallopian tubes (i.e., appendicitis or ovarian cysts)
— Exposure to environmental hazards like asbestos, lead, radiation, heavily polluted water, agricultural pesticides
— Cancer treatments like chemotherapy or radiation (as a patient and in some cases as a health-care provider)
— Daughter of a woman who took DES when pregnant with you (see page 14)
— An older woman (technically over 25, which is when fertility starts to decline)

CHAPTER TWO

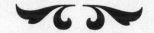

Tests During Pregnancy

Probably the worst thing about pregnancy testing is the way your mind can run wild while you're waiting for the test results. Often a pregnant woman is feeling so vulnerable that the power of suggestion and even her own negative fantasies can be very strong: it doesn't take much for your fears to be triggered that something is wrong with your baby. An expectant father can also be intimidated and worried by prenatal testing and needs reassurance.

Keep in mind that the vast majority of tests during pregnancy are standard procedure: just because you're having a test doesn't mean that anything is wrong. The reason for testing is to eliminate those fears that anything might be abnormal with your baby, as well as to identify problems early in the pregnancy so that appropriate steps can be taken.

Handling the stress of undergoing tests and then awaiting the results is one of the first big challenges of being pregnant, and it often affects both partners. Try to view this time as a chance to learn how to stay calm when you might feel anxious or agitated. Part of becoming a parent is learning how to stay on top of your emotions and not let them run away with you, as well as an opportunity to share your concerns with your partner and begin to function as a team. If you can keep a healthy perspective now, it will be a mental discipline that will serve you in good stead throughout your pregnancy, during labor and delivery, and then once you become parents.

PREGNANCY TESTING

At-Home Pregnancy Tests

The advantage of these products is that you can get immediate results in the privacy of your own home. The only problem is: are the results reliable? At-home pregnancy testing is more accurate than it once was; however, the results are still not completely dependable. If you follow the instructions *very carefully*, the results will be about as accurate as a urine test done in a doctor's office—except that doctors no longer use urine for pregnancy testing because it isn't sufficiently accurate. (The companies which manufacture at-home testing kits are not going to point this out!)

The test works using certain antibodies to detect the hormone HCG (human chorionic gonadotropin) in a woman's urine, which her body produces early in pregnancy. HCG can be detected in your urine or blood once the fertilized egg has implanted in the uterus, which can be as early as six days after conception.

The problem with at-home test kits is that they can be expensive, particularly if you have a lack of confidence in the first results (which many women do) and you want to repeat the test. Another problem is that an incorrect test reading can be dangerous: if you get a result which mistakenly indicates you are *not* pregnant (when you actually are), you might not take appropriate precautions about what you expose yourself to in food, drink, etc.

Blood Test for Pregnancy

The Beta HCG test is a specific blood test for pregnancy which is the most accurate way to know if you are expecting. It can pick up pregnancy as early as 9 days after the fertilized egg has implanted in your uterus. If administered this early (8 to 10 days after conception) the test is about 98% accurate. This means you could have the test only one or two days after a missed period and know whether or not you are pregnant. (The test gives 100% accuracy if you wait four weeks from your last period.)

Such fast results mean that you can start eating right immediately, while avoiding potentially dangerous substances and circumstances right from the very beginning of your pregnancy.

Only a few drops of blood are needed to look for the presence of chorionic gonadotropin (HCG). Unlike a urine test, a blood test can detect the difference between a normal pregnancy and a tubal pregnancy, which is a potentially fatal condition for both the fetus and the mother.

Progestins as a Pregnancy Test

Sometimes a doctor will inject you with progesterone-like hormones as an early pregnancy test. Some doctors inject a woman if her period is late. If the progestogen fails to bring on a bleeding phase the doctor concludes that you must be pregnant. However, a lack of a bleeding phase can be an indication of conditions other than pregnancy, which makes it fairly inaccurate as a pregnancy predictor.

Progestins may cause birth defects. The fetus may be adversely affected by the injection of progestin. *Do not allow a doctor to give you a shot of progestin as a pregnancy test, especially if you want to be pregnant with a healthy baby.*

Pseudo (False) Pregnancy

What does it mean when pregnancy tests register negative, but you are convinced you're pregnant? Sometimes a woman's periods may stop and her body may have the symptoms of pregnancy, but tests indicate she is not. It *is* physiologically possible for thoughts and feelings to stimulate the hypothalamus in your brain, which stimulates the hormones that cause the physical changes of pregnancy.

Pseudo pregnancy is a condition brought on by emotions, the most common reason being a strong desire to be pregnant that can inhibit menstruation. This can set off related changes such as weight gain, enlarged breasts, and a swollen abdomen.

Another possible reason for a false pregnancy can be the opposite emotion, which is a strong *fear* of being pregnant. That anxiety can suppress menstruation, which in turn increases your anxiety. In either case, it might be helpful to consult a psychologist or psychiatrist. Once a woman understands why believing in being pregnant is so important to her, the symptoms usually disappear and menstruation returns.

TESTS DURING PREGNANCY

Ultrasound

Ultrasound works like the radar system of a submarine. A quartz crystal is placed on the woman's abdomen and high-frequency sound waves are beamed toward the fetus. Unlike X-rays (which would be hazardous) ultrasound can depict soft tissue in detail and an image of the fetus in utero.

Ultrasound can be used to investigate fetal development and measure its growth. For example, it might be used in a situation where a cesarean section is planned and therefore the gestational age of the fetus is essential. If there is any question about the reliability of the due date

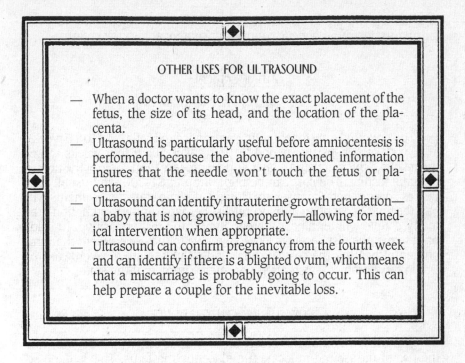

OTHER USES FOR ULTRASOUND

— When a doctor wants to know the exact placement of the fetus, the size of its head, and the location of the placenta.
— Ultrasound is particularly useful before amniocentesis is performed, because the above-mentioned information insures that the needle won't touch the fetus or placenta.
— Ultrasound can identify intrauterine growth retardation—a baby that is not growing properly—allowing for medical intervention when appropriate.
— Ultrasound can confirm pregnancy from the fourth week and can identify if there is a blighted ovum, which means that a miscarriage is probably going to occur. This can help prepare a couple for the inevitable loss.

"by dates" (see page 10) the doctor would do an ultrasound to avoid jeopardizing the infant by removing it before full term.

Blood and Cell Tests

Tests of the fetus's blood and cells can detect around 65 chromosomal and other disorders. Some races or groups of parents are more prone to have babies that are afflicted, although no group of people is immune.

Current research is constantly making breakthroughs in detecting the estimated 3,000 different single-gene defects that can afflict a fetus. Fetal tests can now find many more genetic flaws than used to be possible: for example, prenatal detection is now possible for the classic form of hemophilia and is reasonably reliable for muscular dystrophy.

The new DNA studies are safer for the fetus than some of the earlier techniques and can find important diseases that were never before detectable in the womb. However, only a few laboratories are capable of doing this newer testing and it can be expensive.

What does all this mean for you, personally? It will cost you nothing to find out how this testing might be important for you and your baby. The National Genetics Foundation has a free service for people seeking information about their personal susceptibility to genetic problems in their offspring. To get more information write to them at: 555 West 57th Street, New York, New York 10019. When you fill out the family-health history form they will send you, you then return it for a no-cost analysis of whether you are at risk. If necessary, they will refer you and your partner to one of 54 genetic counseling centers across the country.

Amniocentesis

"WHEN IS 'AMNIO' DONE?"

The preferred time for obtaining amniotic fluid cells is 14 to 16 weeks after your last menstrual period. It then takes about four weeks to get the results, which makes it a later, longer process than some of the newer prenatal testing. The cost can be high, around $1,200, and usually involves some genetic counseling. However, some state governments will pay the entire cost of an amniocentesis, perhaps on the assumption that many couple will terminate a pregnancy if the test is positive. In cold, hard terms, the test becomes less expensive to the government than the burden of bearing the costs of managing a child with a severe case of Down's syndrome, which often becomes a burden of the state.

"HOW IS AMNIOCENTESIS DONE?"

You are awake for the procedure, lying down, which begins with the use of ultrasound to locate the placenta and fetus. This is done so that the needle for the amniocentesis will not be inserted near them. The needle is then inserted through the walls of your abdomen and uterus to extract some fluid. Although it usually does not hurt, you should talk to the doctor about whether you would be more comfortable if he or she first used a local anesthetic at the site where the needle will go in.

The needle that is used is quite long and may look intimidating to you, especially if you are generally squeamish. Depending on your temperament, you may want to close your eyes when they are inserting the needle, although this procedure is not considered difficult by most women.

"ARE THERE ANY RISKS TO AMNIO?"

There is usually no question that the information gained by doing amniocentesis far outweighs the very slim risks. But while the risks in amnio are slight—under 1%—they must be mentioned. The risks to the mother fall in the category of what could *theoretically* happen, although they are highly unlikely. These are: intra-abdominal bleeding, blood-group sensitizing (Rh blood incompatibility), or amnionitis (an infection which could induce labor and thereby abort the fetus). The risks to the fetus, again very slight, are abortion or injury by the needle. However, the fetus instinctively moves way from anything that touches it in utero. Besides, in the rare cases where a needle has touched a fetus, it left a white line on the baby so minuscule it can barely be seen.

ONE WARNING ABOUT AMNIO

It is highly unlikely for anything to go wrong following amniocentesis, but once in a great while the amniotic fluid can leak afterwards. If you notice any fluid leaking after your amnio, call your doctor immediately. He or she will probably have you rest in bed until the leakage stops, which is usually only a few days.

"WHAT DOES AMNIOCENTESIS REVEAL?"

Testing the amniotic fluid can indicate whether the fetus has a chromosomal abnormality like Down's syndrome. However, there is other important information that can be gathered.

INFORMATION GATHERED BY AMNIOCENTESIS

SEX: Skin cells shed by the fetus accumulate in the amniotic fluid: male cells are different from female cells when seen under the microscope.

AGE OF FETUS: Discarded skin cells also indicate fetal age. The maturity of the lungs can also be measured, which is itself an indication of age.

CHROMOSOME COUNT: Discarded cells determine chromosome structure: any deviation from normal usually means fetus is gravely malformed and/or mentally retarded.

CHEMICAL COMPOSITION: Metabolic disorders can be revealed by missing or defective enzymes in the fluid.

BILIRUBIN CONTENT: Helps in determining whether an Rh-incompatible baby needs an intrauterine transfusion.

GASES: Measuring gases dissolved in fluid reveals the amount of oxygen the baby is getting and whether he or she is at risk.

ACIDITY: Inadequate oxygen flow to the fetus can cause acidity of the fluid, another indication of fetal distress.

Amniocentesis can also be performed in cases when a couple is suspected of having a baby with inherited inborn errors of metabolism (which is usually identified because they have already had a child with a metabolic defect).

A third indication for amniocentesis is when the mother is a known carrier of a serious X-chromosome-linked disorder. Diseases that fall into this category are Duchenne's, the most common form of muscular dystrophy, and hemophilia. The diseases themselves are not detectable in utero, but "amnio" can detect the sex of the fetus: a male child has a 50% chance of being affected, whereas a female is at no risk of being affected by either illness.

An additional and vitally important use of amniocentesis is if there are medical reasons to induce labor and it is unclear whether the fetus is sufficiently mature. The amniotic fluid can tell the doctors whether the baby's lungs are sufficiently mature to function on the outside. Premature babies have the greatest likelihood of RDS (respiratory distress syndrome), a severe lung disorder in newborns.

The chart on page 31 shows how much vital information about your baby is revealed in the amniotic fluid.

Alpha-Fetoprotein Testing (AFT)

Alpha-fetoprotein is a simple blood test that can be done on a woman approximately 16 weeks into her pregnancy. This test can detect birth defects as well as give doctors an early warning on other possibly dangerous situations, including the presence of twins or triplets, pseudopregnancy (see page 28), fetal death, and low birth weight. AFT supplies information about the development of the fetal central nervous system and can detect such abnormalities as spina bifida (malformations of the spine), anencephaly (malformations of the brain), and hydrocephalus (water on the brain).

AFP is something of a mystery: its function is unknown, as is the reason why the baby's body stops producing it soon after birth. An analysis of the mother's blood will show the presence of alpha-fetoprotein, or AFP, which the fetus secretes into the amniotic fluid. Traces of the protein cross the placenta into the mother's bloodstream. Small amounts of AFP in the blood are normal, but large amounts (which have been found in 50 of every 1,000 pregnant women) are a warning sign, calling for a repeat of the test.

If a woman has consistently high levels of AFP in her blood, she is given an ultrasound scan. This would immediately show whether she is expecting twins, which would explain the excess. An ultrasound would also indicate if there is a single fetus with an abnormally shaped head, characteristic of anencephaly (a brain abnormality in which the majority of infants are stillborn or die shortly after birth).

However, if ultrasound testing offers no explanation for the high AFP levels, the next step is usually to do an amniocentesis. A high level of AFP in the amniotic fluid is a strong indication that the baby will be born with spina bifida, a neural tube defect in which the spinal cord does not close properly and the AFP apparently pours out into the amniotic fluid. Spina bifida leaves a child paralyzed at birth from below the level of the opening in their spine and often includes brain damage.

AFP testing can also provide information about miscarriages which may have been missed and can indicate false pregnancies. Also, doctors are discovering that *low* AFP levels, which had previously been ignored, also offer important information. Usually, a very low AFP value means that the fetal age has been grossly overestimated. This can be potentially dangerous, because if a baby is believed to be overdue, labor may be mistakenly induced, delivering a premature baby with all the inherent complications.

Chorionic Villi Sampling (CVS)

Chorionic villi sampling is one of the newer prenatal tests which may one day replace amniocentesis. The villi are protrusions on the chorionic membrane, which surrounds the fetus and later becomes the placenta. The procedure is relatively painless: a catheter is guided through the cervix and into the uterus. A small amount of chorionic villi tissue is withdrawn. The sample is not part of the fetus, but contains fetal tissue which can divulge information about genetic abnormalities, including chromosomal, metabolic, and blood-borne conditions. The only significant conditions that cannot be detected from this sampling are neural-tube defects, including spina bifida and anencephaly, but blood serum can be taken from the mother in the 16th week to compensate.

CVS can be done earlier in pregnancy and with more rapid results than amniocentesis, which is usually done around the 15th week of pregnancy and takes about 3 to 4 weeks for results. Instead, CVS is usually done in the 9th or 10th week, and the preliminary findings—including whether Down's syndrome is present—are available in only a day or two. A more thorough analysis that is comparable to that of amniocentesis takes 2 weeks. However, some studies show that there is slightly less accuracy when CVS is used to test for fetal chromosomal abnormalities such as Down's: amnio gives an accurate diagnosis 99.4% of the time, in comparison to CVS's 97.8% accuracy rate.

The obvious advantage of CVS is that it allows a woman to terminate a blighted pregnancy much sooner. If a woman learns through amniocentesis that she is carrying a fetus with Down's syndrome, she is faced with a more complicated, dangerous, and emotionally difficult second-trimester abortion.

CVS does carry a slightly higher risk of miscarriage than that associated with amniocentesis. Other studies show a 1 to 2% miscarriage rate for CVS, while amnio is generally thought to be 0.5 to 0.75% risk. However, CVS may be worth the slightly increased risk of miscarriage for women who are at risk for certain conditions like Tay-Sachs disease or those in their forties with a higher risk of Down's syndrome and limited time to get pregnant again.

Combining Early Amniocentesis and Late CVS

Experimentation is being done at some major medical centers which offer a combination of amnio done earlier than usual and CVS performed later than the norm. In doing CVS into the second trimester of pregnancy, doctors take tissue from the placenta, which is made of fetal tissue and nourishes the fetus, rather than from the chorionic villi. Because these tests are still experimental, there are not yet any studies to indicate the safety of performing amniocentesis as early as 10 weeks of pregnancy, or chorionic villi sampling as late as 20 weeks.

Some obstetricians are doing this test later because their patients want faster results. For example, you might have a routine ultrasound test in your twentieth week of pregnancy that shows something is not quite right with the fetus. You might want a prenatal diagnostic procedure which gives you immediate results, because if the fetus has a serious defect and you choose to terminate the pregnancy, the longer you have to wait to find out, the more difficult it might be. With amniocentesis alone, it can take a week or longer before the fetal cells can be grown in the laboratory in sufficient quantities for diagnosis. With CVS, the cells can be analyzed instantly.

The Emotional Aspect of Prenatal Testing

There are many feelings that you will have as a couple during prenatal testing, emotions that you may not realize or know how to handle. Health professionals—both your own care-giver and the specialists who do the testing—often forget how stressful this process can be for the expectant parent.

Some couples react so negatively to genetic testing before they try to conceive, or to testing during pregnancy, that it can ruin their entire pregnancy experience. It is natural to feel even intense anxiety during the 2- to 3-week wait for amniocentesis results, or even during the shorter wait for results of chorionic villi sampling.

The chart opposite outlines some of the common anxieties that a couple may have and some practical suggestions for how to cope with those emotions. There are also examples of ways that couples frequently try to spare themselves anxiety, but may actually be increasing it while depriving themselves of the pleasurable feelings they could be having.

FEARS, WORRIES, AND ANXIETIES

The Anxiety	Dealing with it
Will the baby be normal?	Get appropriate tests, then let it go.
I drank before knowing I was pregnant.	It takes more than a few drinks to cause defects in most cases.
I ate foods I didn't know were unhealthy early in pregnancy.	Eat extra-well now.
Loss of freedom.	Find a more positive description of motherhood.
Changes in lifestyle.	View change as an adventure, a challenge.
Fear of being an inadequate mother.	Mothering is something learned: there are no grades!
Inability to care for baby.	Everybody has to learn the skills: mistakes are okay.
Self-doubt about being emotionally equipped for motherhood.	You'll grow into it.
Loss of attractiveness.	Believe pregnancy is beautiful and so will those around you.
Labor and delivery.	You'll do the best you can— and that will be good enough.
General angst and anxiety.	Talk out feelings to discover specific concerns.

Being worried is normal!

➢ Being pregnant and facing parenthood mean many reasons to worry for anyone expecting. You're not alone!
➢ Many of your concerns are probably justified: a new baby is a big deal in anyone's life.
➢ Your partner may share many of your concerns.

Dealing with Feelings About Prenatal Testing

➤ *Keep in mind that the odds* are in your favor: the chance of a bad result from testing is very low.

➤ *When you're feeling particularly vulnerable*, remind yourself that amnio and CVS return favorable findings 95 to 99% of the time. (Do *not* let yourself fall into the mind game of "Well, *somebody* has to be the 1%"!)

➤ *Some couples want to wait* until after getting favorable test results before talking about their pregnancy. But experts say it is *not* a good idea to avoid talking about the baby or to stop pregnancy-related preparations like buying maternity clothes or baby products.

Psychologists advise that denying that you are pregnant is shortsighted and counterproductive. Denial can make it more—rather than less—difficult to cope with a bad genetic testing result, if it should happen. Couples who tried to keep their pregnancy a secret and then had to abort a malformed fetus later regretted their secrecy. It is recommended that you not try to keep your pregnancy a secret any more than you would if you were *not* having prenatal diagnosis.

➤ *If you are in a high-risk category* you may want to restrict the people who know about the pregnancy to only your closest friends and relatives until you know the fetus is healthy. You may feel this will spare you the emotional drain of explaining the situation to a lot of people, in the event that test results should indicate terminating the pregnancy. Limiting whom you tell is a personal choice, but be sure you're not doing it because it makes the pregnancy "less real" if fewer people know about it.

➤ *Some couples try not to talk about the baby* until test results are in. Don't assume that by not discussing your pregnancy that you can protect yourself from possible disappointment. Try to accept and enjoy your pregnancy right from the start: get excited, daydream, buy maternity clothes or baby things, allow yourself to experience all the natural reactions.

Couples who thought that by not disclosing their pregnancy they could spare themselves possible pain found that what they had actually done was to deprive themselves of joy.

What to Do About a Bad Prenatal Test Result?

Before you undergo amniocentesis or other prenatal testing, it's important to know what your choices are if you should a positive (bad) test result. You should know before agreeing to any test that there is usually no treatment for genetic flaws found in the fetus, other than the option of aborting it. "Selective" or "therapeutic" abortion, as this is called, is a very personal matter. Therefore before you even decide whether to be tested or not, it's important to discuss with your partner what you would do in the case of a malformed fetus. Would you want to know ahead of time if you are carrying a severely flawed fetus because you feel incapable of raising such a child (or in some cases watching it die in infancy or childhood)? Or is the idea of terminating a blighted pregnancy impossible for you to contemplate?

For some couples, selective abortion can shake the foundation of their self-worth if their feelings of self-esteem are closely bound up with their ability to produce a normal, healthy child. If this seems as if it could be your reaction to such a situation, you could benefit from genetic counseling and getting more information about birth defects ahead of time.

If you do decide to abort a fetus diagnosed as having a serious defect, you will experience many of the grieving emotions of couples who have lost a baby before or after birth (see page 413). Guilt will probably be a predominant reaction. Afterwards you may also find yourselves having emotions similar to those of infertile couples.

Boy or Girl?

Most prospective parents care only that their baby is born healthy, but for others it matters almost as much whether their baby is born a boy or girl. There are the usual reasons that a couple feels strongly about the sex of their unborn child: if they already have one child and wish one of the opposite sex, if they have more than one child of the same sex and want one of the other, or they wish to have only one child and would prefer a certain gender. There are all sorts of personal reasons why a parent may favor one gender over the other, but whatever the reason for your fervent wishes, it's a good idea to try and understand your desires since the outcome of pregnancy is out of your control.

"Why Does Gender Matter So Much to You?"

There are many reasons in a person's history that might make him or her feel zealous about which sex baby they want, although the influences may be unconscious. For example, a woman who was an only child may have always felt her father wanted a boy: her own feelings of inadequacy as a female child might make it appear more desirable to have a male child. In a sense, if she can present her father with a male grandchild, she can give him what she always perceived he wanted (which, in fact, may not have been the case at all).

Another example would be a remarried man who had two sons in his first unhappy marriage. Perhaps to him having a girl child with his second wife represents the start of a whole new life, with no reminders of the first time around. Or there could be an expectant woman who grew up only with sisters and hopes for a baby girl because she fears that she doesn't know enough about boys to be a good mother to one.

It doesn't really matter how foolish or far-fetched the reasons may be that you crave a baby of one sex or the other. Once you begin to understand what is motivating your desire, you can begin to be in control of the situation, rather than feeling that it controls you.

"How Should You Handle Your 'Gender Preference'?"

If you feel adamant about what your baby's gender should be, discuss it with your partner. By talking together (particularly about your own childhood) you may be able to understand some possible reasons for your desires. It doesn't matter whether the reasons behind a fervent desire for a certain sex child make sense or seem rational. What's important is to find out what may be behind your feelings and thereby feel a little less rigid about the issue of your child's gender. If talking about it doesn't relieve your intensity, a professional counselor could be helpful, either for you alone or with your partner.

"What if You Get the 'Wrong' Sex?"

If you are concerned about what sex your baby will be and you get the "wrong" gender, it's important to acknowledge your feelings of disappointment and/or anger. For your own sake and future relationship with the child, do not deny these negative feelings. Do not make a judgment of these negative feelings or belittle them with rationalizations such as, "The baby's healthy and that's all that should matter. I should be grateful instead of being ridiculous about whether it's a boy or girl."

Of course you care that you have a healthy baby and that's the most important thing, but your desire for a child of the other gender is a valid emotion, too. Acknowledge that your feelings are real and you're entitled to them: give them thought and talk about it with your partner or anyone else you can trust.

The important thing, however, is that you do not project these feelings onto the child. Recognize that you are disappointed, but move forward: don't allow your disappointment about the child you dreamed of to interfere with your experience of the child or that child's experience of life. Realize that your disappointment—which is real and understandable—has nothing at all to do with the individual baby who is now a permanent part of your life.

CHAPTER THREE

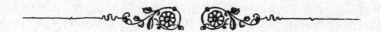

How the Baby Grows

Once you understand how your baby grows inside you, it's easy to see how important it is for you to give her the nutrition she needs.

The Umbilical Cord

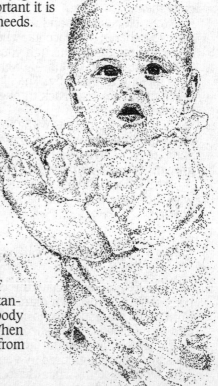

Your baby receives oxygen from your blood, which flows through the placenta into the umbilical cord. Your heart pumps oxygenated blood through the vein in the umbilical cord into the baby's circulation. The "used" blood, from which the baby has taken oxygen, returns through the arteries in the cord into the placenta, which filters the waste products.

The cord is soft and limp: it is slippery and very strong. Because of its slipperiness, the cord rarely gets tangled or knotted. The baby's whole body can move through loops in the cord. When the cord is mature, it varies in length from about 20 inches to 2 feet.

The Placenta

The fetus is attached to you by the umbilical cord, but it receives nourishment from the placenta. It is an organ created by your body to nourish your baby and excrete waste products. The placenta looks like a large, roundish liver: it is 1 inch thick and measures about 8 inches in diameter. One of the reasons you retain fluids during pregnancy is as a safeguard for your expanded blood volume: 330 quarts of blood circulate through the placenta and nourish it every day.

The baby's growth inside your uterus is basically governed by the placenta, which weighs about one-fifth as much as the fetus. The fetus absorbs food and eliminates waste products through this remarkable organ.

By the thirteenth week of pregnancy the placenta is fully formed, and it is fully operational by the fourteenth week. On one side the placenta is attached to your uterus and on the other side to your baby's umbilical cord. It is the baby's lifeline to you: your blood, carrying oxygen and nutrients, reaches the baby through a fine membrane into the placenta. The placenta functions like a sieve, passing oxygen, food, and protective antibodies from you to your baby (although harmful elements can also filter through). The baby gets rid of waste products by filtering them through the placenta into your bloodstream, allowing you to excrete them.

Your bloodstream and the baby's are separate, but they come very close together in the placenta, where materials pass over from one blood system to the other. Through your uterus and the placenta, an amazing 25% of your blood volume—or one-quarter of the blood in your body—goes directly to the baby. The blood from which the baby has already taken oxygen comes back through an artery in the umbilical cord into the placenta.

If there are problems with the placenta and it does not perform properly (due to a cause like malnutrition) this is known as "placental insufficiency." Obviously this condition will have an adverse affect on the growth and well-being of the fetus.

The placenta stops growing entirely between the 34th and 38th weeks of pregnancy: the baby's growth continues, although it slows down.

The Amniotic Fluid

It helps you appreciate the demands that pregnancy puts on your body (and your need for extra nourishment) when you learn that one-third of the amniotic fluid is being replenished every hour by your body and is completely replenished every 6 hours. It is not stagnant liquid, as you might have thought: amniotic fluid is always fresh because it is constantly being produced by your body and being reabsorbed back into your blood system, while the cells of the amniotic membrane are excreting new fluid into the amniotic sac.

The fetus is surrounded by amniotic fluid. The contents of this fluid is interesting: it is filled with salts and other nutrients that the baby absorbs through her skin, as she has been doing throughout your pregnancy. The fluid also contains skin cells shed by the fetus (which is what is examined when amniocentesis is done, see page 30), fetal hairs, specks of vernix (the creamy coating on the fetus), various minerals, sugar, and the products of fetal urine. The baby swallows about a pint of amniotic fluid a day: it is presumed that he voids a similar amount back into the uterus. His stomach begins to secrete gastric juices, enabling his body to absorb those liquids. After the fluid is absorbed, his kidneys filter it, excreting it back into the amniotic sac.

By the 12th week of pregnancy there are about 12 ounces of amniotic fluid; in mid-pregnancy the volume goes up to a pint; at the end of 9 months there is usually a little less than a quart.

Life Inside the Womb

What It Sounds Like to the Baby: Inside your uterus there is constant loud noise. First there is a rhythmical whooshing sound punctuated by stomach rumbles, which are created by air passing through your stomach. Then there is a pulsating noise that keeps exact time with your heart, due to the blood flowing through your uterus. The baby can hear sounds from the outside world, too, but those noises are muted because they have to pass through your body and the amniotic fluid before they reach the baby. Only extremely loud noises can exceed the rhythmical sounds the baby hears at all times inside the uterus.

Tape recordings of these sounds from the womb have been found to have a calming effect on colicky babies after birth. It seems that nature recognizes how important those intrauterine sounds are to a newborn because the maternal instinct is to hold the baby on the left side (no matter whether you are right or left-handed): in that position the baby is near the comforting sound of your heartbeat.

What the Baby Does in There: Fetal activity can be violent: your baby may kick up a storm and can pack quite a punch, too! Some babies seem to get more active at night or when their mothers are lying down for a rest. Sometimes a baby can get active when the parents are making love (which can be disconcerting for you!). It's quite normal for a baby to get hiccups frequently, which can go on for as long as fifteen minutes—short, quick jerks of her trunk and shoulders that you can see as well as feel.

"Parenting" in the Womb

There's a new concept referred to as "prenatal parenting," which has to do with the influence you can have on your unborn baby's development. Traditionally, a baby's birth has been considered the beginning of her emotional and interactive life. People have often not perceived a baby as alive until she takes her first breath and cries. It is clearly true that in the weeks before delivery a baby is not significantly different mentally than she will be at birth. Now modern science makes it clear that a newborn's mental apparatus is not just suddenly "switched on" at birth: studies show that he has been practicing inside the womb for quite some time. The infant in utero has been learning all of the many tasks needed for life on the outside: breathing, sucking, swallowing, touching, smelling, looking, and listening.

It is believed that from at least the 6th month after conception the unborn child can feel, sense, hear, and remember. So there is reason to believe that you can make a connection to your baby before he is born: this "communication" can have important consequences for the baby's development and personality. Feel free to talk to your unborn baby, play music for her, read her stories, and massage her. You may find that if you stroke your abdomen gently when your infant is acting up inside you, she will stop kicking and relax.

There are babies who calm down after birth when they hear music their parents played for them during the last trimester of pregnancy. Other newborns can be soothed by hearing their father's familiar voice, if they talked to their babies while still in the womb. It's up to you how much interaction you want to have with your unborn child: if you don't feel comfortable with it, you certainly shouldn't worry that you're "depriving" your baby! But think about having fun with it. Enjoy some of this exciting information; use it to enhance your pregnancy experience and the adventure of parenting ahead of you.

THE BABY'S GROWTH, WEEK BY WEEK

First Month

Around 4th day   United egg and sperm reach uterus.

1st week   Cells multiply into the blastocyst: growing ball of 100 cells. Outer layer to become the placenta, inner layer will become the embryo.

2nd week   Embryo is 150 cells floating freely in your uterus, nourished by secretions from uterine lining; cells already specialized into what will be their different functions.

3rd week   Preliminary tissues become a tubular, folded structure with beginnings of a heart, brain and spinal cord; deepest cells will form the placenta to nourish the fetus; outer cells around embryo spread out rootlike into uterine lining; other cells will form amniotic sac.

End of 3rd week   Embryo begins to attach to wall of the uterus.

4th week   Whole tiny embryo is forming into the shape of a tadpole.

26th day   Beginnings of arms.

28th day   Basic beginnings of legs, which will be slower in development than arms.

End of 1st month   Embryo complete and is less than $\frac{1}{10}$ inch long, smaller than grain of rice; it would be barely visible to the naked eye.

Second Month

End of 5th week   Foundation laid for what will be brain, spinal cord and nervous system; backbone forming, with 5 to 8 vertebrae laid down; neural tube forms, which is first step in development of central nervous system: one end will become baby's brain, other end the spinal cord; tubular s-shaped heart begins to beat (but located on *outside* of body cavity).

Early 6th week Head starting to form, beginning of brain; beating heart visible but still not in chest cavity: this 2-chamber heart will become a 4-chamber organ later; intestinal tract forming (starts from mouth cavity downward); mouth closed; umbilical cord begins to form with blood vessels through which baby will be nourished; has rudimentary tail (extension of spinal column).

End of 6th week Entire backbone laid down, spinal cord closed over but lower part of back undeveloped; baby grows in curved seahorse shape with long tail (blocks of tissue in back of embryo grow more quickly then those in front); depressions beneath skin where eyes and ears will later be; germ cells appear that will become ovaries or testes; at corners of body are limb buds (first seen in 4th week) which will become arms and legs; by end of week, embryo is ¼ inch long.

6th & 7th weeks Nerve and muscle work together for first time; embryo has reflexes and makes spontaneous movements by 7th week (but mother probably won't feel it until after 16th week).

7th week Chest and abdomen completely formed; lung buds appearing; heart is now inside body and still a simple structure, but has 4 chambers beating strongly enough to circulate blood; mouth can open with lips and tongue visible; face flattening, looks more human with openings for nostrils and eyes perceptible through closed lids; shell-like ears forming but not protruding; inner ear developing, especially middle ear (responsible for hearing and balance); limb buds growing rapidly with paddle shape to arms and legs; hands have beginnings of fingers, toes stubby but big toe has appeared; arms are as long as an exclamation point (!).

End of 7th week Brain and spinal cord almost complete; embryo becomes a primitive, small-scale baby with a lumpy head bent forward on chest; overall length ½ inch (size of a thumbnail).

47th day

First true bone cells replace cartilage: the official transition from embryo to fetus; bones of arms and legs start to harden and get longer; critical joints like knees, hips, shoulders, and elbows are forming.

8th week

Toes and fingers are more pronounced although joined by webs of skin; body has a fishlike shape, head is disproportionately large; face and jaw are fully formed, with teeth and facial muscles still developing; eyes are covered with skin that will later split to form eyelids; heart now pumping forcefully with a regular rhythm; blood vessels visible through the transparent skin; all major organs (heart, brain, lungs, kidneys, liver, intestines) now in place but not fully developed; clitoris or penis begins to appear; ovaries or testicles taking form (but you couldn't tell baby's sex just by looking).

*End of 8th week
(end of 2nd month)*

Baby's physical structure complete with a skeleton made of cartilage that will gradually be replaced by bone cells; by end of this 2nd month baby weighs ⅓ oz. (less than an aspirin tablet) and is 1 inch long.

Third Month

9th week

Physical refinements taking place; baby's face becoming quite human except for jaws, which aren't fully developed; during these 7 days baby will start to open his mouth: once upper and lower jaws fuse at sides baby will be able to suck and chew; the palate to form the roof of the mouth is closing; taste buds and glands that produce saliva appear; vocal cords developing; tooth buds for baby teeth are present; eyes are moving to the front of head: their development is complete except for membrane eyelid; a nose has appeared; fastest growth this week is limbs, hands, and feet; fingers and toes becoming defined, nail beds are forming for eventual nails; chest cavity separates from abdominal cavity by a band of muscle that will become the diaphragm, which plays important part in breathing; heart has completed forming 4 chambers and is beating 117–157 beats per minute; baby is just over 1 inch long; hands are not as big (¼ inch) as whole embryo was 1 month ago.

10th week

Baby's brain developed quickly in past month so head still large in proportion to body; final development of ears: inner portion complete, external parts beginning to grow; stomach and intestines have formed in abdomen, muscle wall of intestinal tract developing; kidneys are moving into their permanent positions; lungs growing inside chest cavity; major blood vessels assuming their final form; umbilical cord fully formed with blood circulating through it; baby has grown to just under 1½ inches.

11th week

Baby now able to swallow and cycle of circulation starts; kidneys have formed and urinary system is operating: baby swallows amniotic fluid and urinates it back into the fluid in which he floats; limbs are still short and skinny, but ankles and wrists have formed; elbows and knees taking shape.

End of 11th week

All baby's essential organs have formed, most beginning to function; from this point organs just continue to grow; liver now producing bile; baby's heart pumping blood to all parts of her body; blood also being pumped through umbilical cord to what is going to become the placenta; baby more clearly recognizable as a tiny human with face becoming more rounded; back of head has enlarged, putting eyes in a more natural position than before; ears have flatter shape and continue to develop; baby's length approximately 2 inches.

12th week

Brain signals and baby's muscles respond and she kicks; not all movements reflex from the spinal cord since brain not yet organized enough to control them (and won't be until after birth); baby becoming more active, but unless the mother is very slender, she can't feel him yet; baby can make stepping movements and curl his toes; brain and muscles coordinate so arms bend and rotate at the wrist and elbow; fingers can close so baby can form tight fist or unclench it; ears completely formed; can make facial expressions like pressing lips together and frowning; already using muscles required for breathing after birth; female external vulva and male penis have gradually molded during 2nd & 3rd months; male scrotum appears, but it's still hard to distinguish baby's sex; umbilical cord starts to circulate blood between baby and group of membranes attached to uterine wall: baby's body begins to depend on those membranes for nourishment; placenta begins to function.

End of 12th week (End of 3rd month) Kidneys fully developed; baby weighs a little more than ½ oz.

Fourth Month

13th week Neck now fully developed, allowing head to move freely on body; face is formed: mouth, nose, and external ears completely developed.

End of 13th week Your baby is properly formed and fills uterine cavity; she is 3 inches long and weighs 1 oz.

14th week Beginning of 2nd trimester: baby will do most of his growing and his organs mature; baby's heart is beating strongly and you may be able to hear it in doctor's office; his heartbeat is almost twice as fast as the mother's; his nervous system begins to function and muscles respond to stimulation from his brain; arms continue development of specialized functions and can grasp, curl, and make fists; baby's movements more vigorous, but the mother probably won't feel them yet; baby develops muscles by energetic exercise, done easily floating in amniotic fluid; baby doubles in weight this week: reaches 2 oz. and 4 inches in length.

15th week Baby able to hear the mother now because the 3 tiny bones of her middle ear are first bones to harden; liquid is a good sound conductor, so through amniotic fluid she can hear the mother's heart beating, stomach rumbling, and voice; some sounds from outside womb also reach her, but brain not developed enough to process that information: auditory centers in brain (which decipher sounds received) not yet fully formed; baby has begun to grow hair: fluff on her head, eyebrows and white eyelashes; *lanugo* (fine downy hair all over baby's face and body) starts to grow: *lanugo* keeps her temperature constant, most will disappear before birth or fall out soon after delivery; baby measures more than 5 inches, weighs 3½ oz.

16th week

Bright light shined on abdomen causes baby to gradually move hands up to shield her eyes; baby moving actively and can even turn somersaults (mother still may not feel it); may begin to suck thumb, which helps develop coordination and has soothing effect; baby can yawn, stretch, and make facial expressions; eyes are large, spaced wide apart and closed.

End of 4th month

Baby will suck if his lips are stroked; if bitter substance introduced into amniotic fluid, he will grimace and stop swallowing; if sweetener is added, he'll drink twice as fast; can swallow and may get hiccups; grows so much he quadruples his weight and doubles his height, reaching 6 inches and 7 oz.

Fifth Month

17th week

Baby's skin is developing and is transparent, appearing red because blood vessels visible through it; *vernix* (creamy white protective coating on skin) begins to develop; hair on head, eyebrows, and eyelashes is filling out; hard nails form on nail beds, with toenails developing later than fingernails; both sexes develop nipples and underlying mammary glands; external genital organs sufficiently developed for baby's sex to be determined by ultrasound; baby measures more than 7 inches long, now weighs more than placenta does.

18th week

Baby can now hear sounds outside mother's body: will raise her hands to cover her ears if a loud sound is made near you; very loud sounds can startle baby enough to make her jump inside you; limbs are fully developed and all joints able to move; she is moving much of the time, testing her reflexes by kicking and punching with well-formed arms and legs; she can twist, turn, and wiggle: mother may feel her movements for the first time; her muscles are almost fully developed, including chest muscles, which begin to make movements similar to those used later on for breathing; *alveoli* (tiny air sacs needed later for breathing) are forming inside her developing lungs; baby measures 8 inches long.

19th week

If the mother hasn't felt baby's movements yet, she'll probably perceive them by this week; buds for permanent teeth begin forming behind those that have already developed for baby teeth; for some babies it isn't until now that they begin to grow hair, eyebrows, and white eyelashes; baby measures 9 inches long.

20th week
(End of 5th month)

Baby's muscles getting stronger every week: active movements definitely discernible now; legs now in proportion to body; movements more sophisticated; kicking, punching, and tumbling will be pretty constant part of mother's life for next 20 weeks!; baby's rapid growth will slow down soon; has reached 10 inches, which is half of what he'll probably measure at birth, and weighs 12 oz.

Sixth Month

21st week

In past few weeks *vernix* has been forming: a greasy coating to protect baby's delicate newly formed skin from months of living in a liquid environment; from this point it protects the skin from increasing concentration of her urine in amniotic fluid; most *vernix* will be dissolved by due date: some remains to lubricate journey down birth canal in labor;

baby reaches 11 inches, weighs under a pound.

22nd week

Baby's body has started to produce white blood cells, essential for combating disease and infection; if baby is a girl, internal organs of reproduction now formed; baby moving vigorously; he may respond to your touch or sounds that reach him; if the mother hasn't felt baby hiccuping yet, she may feel jerking motion inside her now; tongue now fully developed; reaches 12 inches, weighs 1 lb.

23rd week

Skin, which was transparent with blood vessels visible, now becomes opaque; skin extremely wrinkled with loose folds, as though she hasn't "grown into it" yet: this is because there aren't any fat deposits beneath the skin; creases begin to appear on fingertips and palms of hands: by next week fingerprints and toe prints will be visible; heartbeat can be heard through stethoscope or others can put ear directly against the mother's belly.

24th week
(End of 6th month)

Baby's hearing system fully developed: organs of balance in inner ear have developed to full dimensions they'll have for life; baby can hear because water in utero is better conductor of sound than air; as baby reacts to sounds her pulse rate increases; she'll move in rhythm to music she hears; reaches 13 inches and 1 lb., 2 oz.

Seventh Month

25th week

Baby's hands active and muscular coordination developed so she can get her thumb into her mouth; thumb-sucking calms baby and strengthens cheek and jaw muscles; bone centers beginning to harden; body fattening up, growing at faster pace than the head, which has been disproportionately larger until now; body getting long and thin, with fat deposits building up under the skin; she's been hiccuping for some time, but this week has new skill: she can cry!; in past week grew half an inch to 14 inches and weighs 1 lb., 4 oz.

26th week

Recordings of baby's brain waves at beginning of last trimester show she has rapid eye movement (REM) sleep (associated with dreaming in adults), so she may be dreaming now; branches of baby's lungs (the bronchi) are developing; lungs won't be fully formed until after birth, but if born prematurely now there's a good chance her lungs could function; usefulness of placenta begins diminishing this month; amount of amniotic fluid decreases as baby gets bigger.

27th week

Membranes that covered baby's eyes separate and eyelids being to part; he can open eyes and look around for first time (it isn't always dark inside you: bright sunlight or artificial light can filter through uterine wall); eyes almost always blue (true eye color develops a few months after birth); eyebrows and delicate eyelashes fully developed; weighs 2 lbs., but length unchanged at 14 inches.

28th week
(End of 7th month)

If born prematurely now, baby could live independently; lungs (essential for living outside womb) are reaching maturity, but a premature newborn might need medical help to breathe and maintain body temperature; a boy's testicles descend into scrotum; puts on more than a pound this month, for total weight of 2 lbs., 4 oz.

Eighth Month

29th week

Baby can hear even more now: could hear vibrations before, but nerve endings in ears are connected now, enabling him to hear distinct sounds; can hear familiar voices (her heart rate increases when she hears her mother or father); can hear music, but it has to be loud since her ears are plugged by water and *vernix*; after birth, if baby hears music played before birth, he may show recognition by becoming less active while listening; gaining 7 oz. per week and weighs 2 lbs., 11 oz. now; weekly growth in length is under half an inch for total of 15 inches.

30th week

Baby fills almost all the space in the mother's uterus; may be lying with head up or may still have room to do somersaults; from this point baby will probably feel more comfortable with her head settled down in your bony pelvis; brain is growing rapidly; she's practicing opening her eyes and breathing; weighs 3 lbs., 2 oz.

31st week

Baby begins to move less as he runs out of room; probably lying in a curled-up position with knees bent, chin resting on chest, arms and legs crossed; most babies turn into vertex position (head down) during next week (or the doctor or midwife may try to turn him around by manipulating from the outside); air sacs inside lungs become lined with layer of cells that produce *surfactant* (a liquid that prevents the air sacs from collapsing when baby first begins to breathe at birth); measures under 16 inches, weighs 3 lbs., 9 oz.

**32nd week
(End of 8th month)**

Baby likely to have settled into vertex position where he'll stay until birth; a smaller baby has room to bounce between vertex & breech (bottom-down) positions for a few weeks more; mother will know if her baby is vertex: instead of his head pressing on her ribs she'll feel his feet kicking against her rib cage; elbows and knees more visible as they press against uterine wall; growth, especially of brain, is great; gets more plump, giving smoother appearance as wrinkles in skin fill out; both *lanugo* and *vernix* covering his skin begin to disappear; weighs 4 lbs., no significant growth in length.

Ninth Month

33rd week

Lungs almost fully developed, but if born now would probably be placed in incubator; still thin, but perfectly formed with proportions she'll have at birth; still doesn't have enough insulating fat deposits beneath skin to keep warm outside your womb; movements can be vigorous and may cause the mother discomfort if her feet get caught under her ribs; weighs 4 lbs., 7 oz.; measures 1 foot, 4 inches.

34th week

Growth of brain has been enormous in past few weeks; most of body's systems well developed, although lungs may still be immature; he's practicing breathing using his lungs (but with no air available he swallows amniotic fluid into his windpipe, causing frequent hiccups); he practices blinking; hair has grown up to 2 inches long; he responds to familiar voices; weighs 4 lbs., 14 oz.

35th week

Getting rounder every day, losing wrinkled appearance; from now until birth will continuously accumulate fat deposits; skin losing redness, becoming pinker every day; weighs 5 lbs. 5 oz.; measures 1 foot, 5 inches.

**36th week
(End of 9th month)**

Almost ready for birth: would be premature but would do well; in this last trimester baby has gotten antibodies from the mother, natural protection against illness she has had (from measles to the common cold), or diseases she's been immunized against (polio, smallpox); rate of baby's growth slowing, but fat cells being deposited under skin every day to get plump for life on the outside; gains 2 lbs. this month to reach 5 lbs., 12 oz.; measures 1 foot, 6 inches.

37th week

Toenails and fingernails have grown to tips of toes and fingers; muscles of arms and legs strong from vigorous motions; keeps practicing movements of lungs necessary for breathing outside; all organs except lungs are fully mature; baby's head drops into mother's pelvis if she's vertex.

38th week

Reflexes have coordinated so he can blink, close his eyes, turn his head, grasp firmly, and respond to sounds, light, and touch; more *lanugo* falls out, but some may remain at birth on his shoulders, in folds of skin, and backs of his ears: it will fall out soon after birth.

39th week

Baby is now ready to be born; with layer of fat that's been building up under her skin, she's plump enough to be able to regulate her body temperature after birth; skin is soft and smooth, body has filled out; weighs anywhere from 6 to 11 lbs.

Any time now you're going to be a parent . . .

CHAPTER FOUR

❧❧

Eating for Two

Have you ever heard the expression "Your body is a temple"? Well, I'm not sure it was intended to be about *pregnancy*, but it actually does apply. Everything you eat, everything you drink, everything you breathe, everything you touch affects your growing baby. It's a big responsibility, but you might want to consider it the first of the many "sacrifices" and adjustments you have to make as a parent. You may even feel resentful about having to change some of your habits: giving up alcohol or cigarettes, forcing yourself to eat lots of healthy food—giving up skydiving!—but you and your baby will appreciate the results. With the amazing knowledge we have today about how the fetus grows and what can injure it, we should all be grateful that we can protect our babies from the moment they are conceived.

This chapter is full of positive suggestions about all the important things you can eat and do for your body, for your baby's sake. I want to encourage you to eat all the good foods that are important for the baby's growth. And if you haven't started already, why not develop healthy habits for your own well-being, too? Being pregnant is more of a strain on your body than you may realize, and the right foods are what fuels the whole process.

Unfortunately, when you're pregnant there are many potential dangers in your immediate surroundings and in your diet. I apologize ahead of time if the warnings in this chapter alarm you, but it's probably better to hear it from me now, and decide in what ways you want to alter your life, than find out about the hazards when it's too late for you to avoid them! I will pass along the most current information about possible hazards in the environment around you—food, drink, medications, environmental—that might cause harm to your growing baby. Also, this chapter covers the topics about everyday habits, such as smoking and drinking alcohol or caffeine, that are now known to be unhealthy for the developing fetus.

And, yes, I've heard the arguments that many of our mothers indulged in these very substances when pregnant with us. Does that make it right for us to flaunt the scientific evidence that's been gathered for our sake? Don't kid yourself with the rationalization that our mothers drank, smoked, etc., "And *we* didn't turn out so bad, did we?" The truthful answer is who's to say? Who knows how much better off we might be if they had *not* exposed our developing brains to those substances? Some of us may have gotten off for free and others may have been compromised, whether with learning disorders or our central nervous systems or . . .

It's easy for all of us to feel overwhelmed by the seemingly constant (and often changing) data about what is good or bad for us, what causes cancer or doesn't, what raises or lowers cholesterol levels, and whether the "bad" sugar in a soda is better than diet drinks that shorten the life of a laboratory rat. There are those people who want to throw up their hands and say, "*Everything's* bad for you! So what's the point? I'm just going to do what makes me happy." It's a free world and everyone has to make their own informed decisions. But it's one thing to do it to yourself and quite another to be so cavalier about another life growing inside you. Why take chances when you don't have to? There are no guarantees in life, but then again, is your baby really something you want to gamble with when all you have to is give up a few habits and add a few others?

GOOD NUTRITION: EATING RIGHT

Food—and the associated topic of weight gain—are big issues in our society. Most everyone is somewhat obsessed about what they're putting in their mouth and whether they "should" be, judging (and imagining everyone else is, too) by whether they let themselves eat a wedge of chocolate fudge cake. Even if you are one of the fortunate ones who has no problem with eating habits or weight, you still live in a society which celebrates "thin," despises "big and fat": you look at fashion models in magazines and have some expectation that you should look like that, too. And it's not easy to be sure you get three really good meals a days with so little time as Americans have. More two-income couples use fast-food outlets, found at every crossroads, instead living of the home-cooked family-around-the-dinner-table lifestyle.

The point is that food is a loaded issue for most women, and it becomes an issue, even subconsciously, when you get pregnant and get bigger and bigger. Except, of course, when you get pregnant getting big is suddenly considered something positive and eating is encouraged. It does become even more complicated for women with weight problems and/or eating disorders, however, because they may feel that pregnancy gives them the mandate to finally eat whatever they want and get as big as a barn.

"Eating your spinach" is more important now than it ever has been in your life! I don't want to sound like a nagging mother, but when you're growing a baby inside you, the most important thing you can do for *both* of you is to eat a well-balanced diet. Good nutrition is essential to having a healthy baby and can also help you to have a better labor and delivery.

Your Eating Habits Over Your Lifetime

Your baby is affected by what you've been eating your entire life: the good and the bad. The good food you've eaten has made your body the healthiest it can be. But some of the unhealthy things you've eaten— let's call it "nutritional pollution"—can build up in your body. This is especially true of the years closest to when you get pregnant, meaning you shouldn't worry too much about those breakfasts of Cokes and Twinkies back when you were a teenager! It's shortsighted, however, to think of nutrition during pregnancy as something you need to pay attention to only from the moment you actually conceive. If you're lucky enough to read this *before* you get pregnant, you can help yourself have a healthy baby by making an effort to eating well and avoiding pollutants during your fertile years.

What Goes Inside Shows on the Outside

Eating well during pregnancy gives you the added benefit of feeling and looking better than ever. Good nutrition can give you more energy and strength. Your hair and skin will look healthier. All the benefits go double for the baby you're nourishing inside you, with her developing body and mind. When she's born, you'll be able to see the wonderful result of taking good care of yourself during the pregnancy.

Good prenatal nutrition—eating lots of protein and the whole range of well-balanced nutrients—can help prevent prematurity, a low birth-weight baby, and even stillbirth. You don't want the complications of a baby born too small or before he is fully developed (the dangers of prematurity and low birth weight are covered on pages 67). Also, studies have shown that mothers who eat well have fewer complications during pregnancy, labor and delivery. A good diet helps build a strong uterus, which means a good labor with efficient contractions. Eating sensibly can also protect you from infections and anemia. A diet rich in protein also lowers the chance of developing toxemia late in pregnancy (see the section on toxemia in "Complications in Pregnancy and Childbirth," page 419).

"The Baby Takes What She Needs Anyway"

People used to say that it doesn't matter what you eat (or don't eat) when you're pregnant because the baby will take what she needs from your body, anyway. But this is not so: if you aren't putting good food into your body, the growing baby does not have those nutrients to draw from. Eating poorly has a direct negative effect on the fetus: if you short change yourself with a poor diet, you are starving your growing baby. It *is* true that if a woman has a severely limited diet, mother nature will give the baby's body priority over the mother's, especially at crucial stages of the baby's growth. But in a case of malnutrition, what they're talking about is the *survival* of the fetus, not the *quality* or quantity of his development. There's an old saying that "for every baby a tooth is lost": before people knew enough about the importance of rich nutrition during pregnancy, the growing fetus and placenta would take nourishment right out of his mother's teeth, bones, and muscles. This could cause a mother's teeth to fall out: but it's one sacrifice that you really don't need to make to prove your devotion to your baby!

Food for Thought

Your diet can have a direct effect on your baby's intelligence, too. There are two periods during which the baby's brain cells grow rapidly: at 20 weeks and at 36 weeks gestation. The human brain develops most rapidly in the last part of pregnancy, a big growth spurt that takes place about one month before birth. If you are not taking in enough nutritious food, it can mean that cell division in the baby's brain is impaired: by eating poorly you can actually permanently reduce the number of brain cells your baby will have! It can also mean malformed brain cells and impaired connections between the cells, which can result in learning problems and poor motor coordination later.

Some "Food Rules" to Live by for 9 Months

You've heard the saying "you are what you eat." When you're pregnant there's a twist on that: *your baby* is what you eat. By now you should get the message loud and clear:
- Food is serious stuff while you're growing a baby.
- Do not skip meals.
- Do not try to diet now.
- Pay attention to the ingredients of whatever you eat and drink.
- Make an extra effort to eat those foods your growing baby needs.

WEIGHT GAIN

There is no way to have a baby without gaining weight . . . quite a lot of weight! Yet many women still manage to worry about getting bigger and talk about pregnancy as "getting fat." It seems ridiculous to point out that being pregnant means that you are growing a baby inside you and that nature is also preparing your body to breast-feed (even if you choose not to). Everyone knows that. Most people also know that while pregnant women were once limited to gaining 15 pounds, more current research shows that closer to a 25-pound gain is recommended. So how come so many women tend to flip out as their pregnancy proceeds and the scale shows them getting heavier and heavier?

This section addresses this question as well as the issues of how much weight gain is recommended, what makes up that weight, special needs of women who are under- or overweight before pregnancy, and some helpful advice about keeping weight gain under control.

Emotions About Gaining Weight

Weight gain is one of the most emotionally sensitive aspects of being pregnant in our country, where thinness has a high value and being overweight (presumably "over" any weight you see in a fashion magazine) is considered disgusting. Many women are victims of social conditioning to think of "gaining weight" as being "bad" and to view those who are heavy or fat as "ugly."

If, in addition to this social conditioning you have personally had weight problems in your life, being pregnant will probably push "old buttons" for you and cause psychological stress. The first thing you need to do is make a clear distinction in your mind between gaining weight *then* and gaining weight *now*. It will take a conscious effort for you to make this distinction, because for women who had to struggle to shed weight in the past, the fear of getting heavy again can be quite strong.

If you are a woman for whom "gaining weight" are dirty words, you need to fight against this prejudice every time you eat. While you are pregnant, you can try to redefine "fat" so that it is associated with "protection" and view "gaining weight" as a good sign of a normal, healthy baby growing inside. Find a way that will work for you to recondition your response to the topic of food and gaining weight: for example, you might look through this section and find those foods you love that have the important ingredients for pregnancy.

When you eat a baked potato (and you can put some calcium-rich sour cream on it) praise yourself. You are doing something important for your body and your baby. Have some nonfat frozen yogurt, or make a regular yogurt banana shake with added dry milk, ice cubes, and orange juice. Think how much it's helping your baby's bones and teeth to grow strong! View the time that you spend planning, cooking, and eating nutritious foods as affection you're already showing to your child. (Obviously you shouldn't go hog-wild and view this as license to dive into a seven-layer cake saying, "This is for Mummy's little darling"!) What we're talking about here is paying attention to negative attitudes you may have about eating and food and changing your viewpoint. If you don't work to overcome past prejudices, you will not be able to eat properly during pregnancy, or you will be on a merry-go-round of feeling worried, guilty, and resentful about gaining weight.

The Recommended Amount of Weight Gain

The *minimum* amount that a woman is now expected to gain is approximately 24 pounds. Not so very many years ago the medical profession took a different view and tried to keep a woman from gaining more than 15 pounds. As you can see from the chart below, the medical community was battling the natural course of pregnancy in trying to impose this artificial limit and was probably compromising the fetus in those pregnancies. Even with a weight gain of 25 to 35 pounds, most women will have only 5 to 10 pounds to lose after their baby is born.

"How Much of My Gain Is Just Extra Fat?"

I've been encouraging you to eat often and eat well and not get fixated on how much you're gaining, but that doesn't mean you want

WHERE THE PREGNANCY WEIGHT COMES FROM

Fetus	7½ to 8½ lbs.
Amniotic fluid	1 to 2 lbs.
Placenta	1 to 2 lbs.
Mother's blood & body fluid	4 to 8 lbs. increase
Uterine muscles	2 to 3 lbs.
Breasts	2 to 3 lbs. increase
Fat deposits (around internal organs)	2 to 10 lbs.
Total	19½ to 36½ lbs.

to turn into "thunder thighs," either! It's understandable if you're concerned about how much of your weight gain is unnecessary padding. It is possible to keep tabs on your body fat if you want to control the extra weight gain that isn't relevant to your baby—and will have to contend with after the baby is born.

Strangely enough, the way to check on how much superfluous body fat you are accumulating is to measure those thighs of yours! The system is to put a tape measure around your upper thigh early in your pregnancy and then keep a biweekly record of that measurement. If you're not gaining too much fat the circumference should stay about the same throughout most of your pregnancy, although of course later on you have to allow for some fluid retention.

Be sure that you measure the same thigh each time, since most people have one bigger than the other. More important, take care to place your leg in exactly the same position each time before measuring. The measurement will be quite different if you're sitting down one time and standing up the next, which means you'll lose an accurate sense of whether you're putting on superfluous body fat or not.

The Rate and Cause of Weight Gain Is What Counts

If you're gaining weight from nutritious foods and the scale is going up at a steady rate, you're doing fine. Don't get hung up on graphs that show an average rate of weight gain; this is an "ideal" that doesn't necessarily correspond to the reality of how a pregnancy progresses. It isn't reasonable to expect the amount that any one individual gains, or the rate at which she gains it, to follow patterns that are based on statistics. Just because the "average" is considered "normal" does *not* automatically mean that your pregnancy is abnormal if your body doesn't gain according to that exact pattern.

People are individuals and each woman's body behaves uniquely when she is pregnant—the same woman may even gain weight differently in two pregnancies, both of which produce a healthy baby. Don't get too wrapped up in these laws of averages and feel something is "wrong" with you if you don't gain the "right" amount of weight each month.

For example, you may be told that during the first 3 months you should gain only 1½ to 3 pounds. You may also hear the "rule" that weight gain should average about 1 pound every 9 days during your entire pregnancy. This works out to ¾ pound per week, which would bring you to an ideal total of 24 pounds by the end of 280 days. However, nothing is that tidy in life—the pattern of weight gain will be different for every woman and you should view your individual situation as just that.

"When Do the Scales Really Start to Tip?"

From about the 12th week you'll probably notice a substantial change on the scales. If you're been eating sensibly, most of the weight you're gaining is the baby: about 40% of it for most women. Your increased blood volume accounts for about 22% of the gain, your enlarged breasts are responsible for about 8%, and the rest of it is the uterus (10%), amniotic fluid (10%), and placenta (10%).

The second trimester is the peak of weight gain for most women, and you'll put on the most pounds in the fifth and sixth months. Again, it's important to stress that women rarely gain weight in equal weekly or monthly increments. Usually a woman only gains a few pounds in the last trimester. And in the last 2 weeks or so of pregnancy, a woman can even have a weight *loss*—despite the fact that this is the baby's time of greatest weight gain.

Your Appetite Is Going to Increase

By the 4th month of pregnancy your appetite will probably have increased quite a lot, which is nature's way of stimulating you to eat heartily for yourself and your baby. Your energy requirements increase about 15% during pregnancy, so you can see that your hunger is a normal response to the increase in your metabolism.

Because your systems are putting out added effort to build up your body and that of your baby, your protein needs increase by 50%. This translates into a physical need for an extra 300 to 500 calories a day, assuming that you were eating a substantial and well-balanced diet before getting pregnant. Unfortunately, this isn't often the case with today's rushed lifestyles, which means your need for additional "fuel" is even greater.

Check Your Weight Every Week

By making a note of your weight every week you can keep tabs on your baby and perhaps catch a possible problem. If you find you have a *weight loss* or *no gain*, you should go see your doctor and be checked. This can be a sign that something is wrong with the placenta or the baby. A sudden gain after the twenty-fourth week may mean that you have fluid retention (edema) in your tissues related to toxemia. The obstetrician can test for this (see page 419) for information on toxemia).

Restricting Weight Gain Can Be Harmful

It is not good for you, or especially for your baby, to try and restrict your weight to a certain present number. It is during the last 8 weeks of pregnancy that the baby gains 1 ounce a day and her brain develops at the most rapid rate of the pregnancy. So the danger in setting a certain limit on how many pounds you can gain is that you will probably reach your self-imposed limit just as the baby's growth spurt begins. It is at this point that the baby requires more oxygen and nutrients of all types than it has earlier in your pregnancy. If you try to cut down on your salt intake or calories at this point, you compromise the baby's brain-cell growth, as explained below. This reduces the amount of blood that flows through the placenta, carrying oxygen and nutrients.

Do Not Consider a Low-Calorie, Low-Salt Diet

Some doctors may still prescribe a diet low in salt and calories, but it is not nutritionally adequate. Remember that few doctors have training in nutrition, so it is safe to say that restrictions on salt or calories are not in your baby's best interest.

In the last three months of pregnancy a woman needs 2,600 calories daily. And during that period she also needs approximately 90 grams of protein. This is a generous allotment: some doctors say that 75 grams a day is sufficient. However, a low-salt, low-calorie diet causes protein to be utilized in such a way that only one-half of the protein you eat is available to build the baby's body and brain. In other words, if you were taking in 90 grams of protein and were also on a low-calorie, low-salt diet, that protein would be metabolized in such a way that only 45 grams could be used for fetal growth.

Weight Loss at Birth

Let's say you're a fairly large, big-boned woman: even a 40- to 45-pound gain won't leave you with that much to lose once your baby arrives. You are going to lose a dramatic amount of weight as soon as the baby is born. If you're feeling concerned about the amount you are gaining, it's important to keep this in mind. The average weight loss at birth is 13 pounds, made up of the baby, amniotic fluid, and placenta. Then an average 3½ pounds is lost between the first postpartum hour and the 12th day, mostly from water in your body tissues. There is an additional weight loss during the first 6 postpartum weeks, particularly for breast-feeding mothers. This means that there are usually only 5 to 10 pounds of body fat that you'll have to "work at" to lose after that.

Underweight & Overweight Women

If you are underweight when you begin pregnancy, you can gain as much as 40 pounds. If you are *really* thin when you conceive, you probably already have a nutritional "debt." You need to improve your diet as soon as possible, or there is a chance that you'll have problems during labor and delivery, and perhaps with your baby. Whatever diet advice you find here for the average woman, it is that much more important for you to follow it.

If, on the other hand, you are heavier than is right for you, nevertheless you cannot be on a severely restricted diet during pregnancy. This is something you must discuss with your doctor, preferably one who is experienced about nutrition, but it is probably not wise to eat less than 1,800 calories a day. Try to get 6 meals a day, each supplying approximately 20 grams of protein. This will help satisfy your hunger, prevent you from gaining more unnecessary weight, and build a healthy fetus. If you are cutting down on calories, eat frequently so that you prevent blood sugar loss.

NOTE: Make a point of drinking *whole* milk between meals and at any meal that doesn't supply fat. This will help your body make full use of the food you've eaten. Non fat milk is not recommended during pregnancy (see page 87 to read all about milk) and regular milk is worth the extra calories.

Your Obstetrician, Nutrition, and Gaining Weight

It's rare to find a doctor who knows much about nutrition because it isn't taught in medical schools or, if it is, isn't given much attention. In general, doctors are trained to deal with the problems that result from poor nutrition rather than focusing on the importance of diet as an essential foundation for good health.

Because medical thinking used to be to a rigid restriction on weight, some older obstetricians may still demand a limit on weight gain even though this concept is outdated; some doctors can be so strict that their pregnant patients dread prenatal visits because they are lectured and made to feel ashamed about gaining "too much." There are extreme cases where women go so far as to "starve" themselves before the visit to the doctor when they are weighed and then gorge themselves after their appointment. Needless to say, if a doctor treats you like this, do not stay in his/her care. Quite simply *leave* a doctor who puts you on a diet to restrict weight gain during pregnancy or insists on a low-calorie, low-salt diet (which can *cause* toxemia, although it was once thought to be a cure for it).

Some OB/GYNs may reinforce a patient's fears about gaining by cautioning against gaining "too much," without realizing what a loaded emotional issue this can be for many women. The doctor's comments may have the unintentional effect of intensifying the already complicated emotions you may be having. It's up to you to help insure that your doctor doesn't play into any of your doubts or guilt about weight gain. The best way to do this is talk to your healthcare provider about the issues raised here, some of which s/he may not be aware.

Some Friendly Advice About Weight Gain

Don't go hog-wild at the fridge! If you're one of those women who's been on a diet ever since her teens, I hope you won't think that pregnancy is going to be your big chance to eat all those hot fudge sundaes you've been denying yourself over the years! Especially for women who have trouble controlling their weight, pregnancy is a confusing time. You hear all the suggestions about eating often and well, and you might be tempted to say, "All right! I'm going to go for it!" Maybe you figure this is your one chance to let yourself go and not feel criticized (by yourself or others).

Don't make the mistake of thinking that because you're pregnant it's okay to eat things that you usually don't allow yourself. All you'll be doing by eating fattening foods without nutritional value is developing bad habits that will be harder to stop later. For instance, some women begin eating dessert at every meal once they find out they are pregnant, rationalizing that they are "eating for two" and all that food will be put to good use. Sorry to burst your bubble, but this just not true . . . unless you are starting out pregnancy as a skinny beanpole, and *even then*, only if you are also eating well-balanced, nutritious meals before your sweets. You're going to be very sorry for that pecan pie nine months down the road when the baby is born but you still look like you haven't given birth yet!

There is such a thing as gaining too much. I don't want to sound contradictory (since I've been emphasizing the importance of eating well during your childbearing years and of making sure you gain enough during your pregnancy) but gaining *too* much weight is a problem, too. Some studies have shown that there is a relationship between a large weight gain and a higher rate of cesarean delivery. It seems as though the uterine muscles don't function as well if there is excessive fatty tissue. It becomes harder for the baby to descend and for the cervix to dilate.

Another problem with gaining too much weight is that it can be hard to lose a lot of extra pounds once the baby is born. This struggle can contribute to postpartum depression. By the time the baby is born, you're going to be pretty sick of your maternity clothes, but if you've gained a great deal of weight you're not going to fit into anything but those clothes. The sooner you can get into your pre-baby clothes, the better you'll feel—and unnecessary extra weight makes that impossible.

This is not meant to make you panic: you're probably going to get bigger all over when you're pregnant, and that is what nature intended. Just because your hips and thighs are expanding doesn't mean you're gaining too much. In fact, some padding in these areas is essential during pregnancy. One reason for this is that the body has to counterbalance the new weight in front. Another reason for this added fat is nature's way of insuring an "emergency reserve" of fat for the breast-feeding period. Even if you are not going to breast-feed, your body needs extra strength and energy for the emotional and physical demands of the early weeks of having a new baby in the house.

Don't overeat in the first trimester. Some women are so excited when they find out they're pregnant that they eat too much out of eagerness. In the first three months the fetus is so small that pregnancy doesn't really show yet, but some women can't wait to wear maternity clothes! A woman who's particularly thrilled about being pregnant may want to display to the outside world that she's expecting, but if you eat too much in the first trimester, the only growth you can prove is your expanding thighs! Especially if you've had a hard time trying to get pregnant, you may not realize the psychological need to show others— and have proof for yourself—that your dream has finally come true.

The baby probably won't show until after the 16th week, since most women begin to "show" between the 16th and 20th weeks. The pregnant uterus grows upward and reaches the navel around the 20th week: by that time it will be pretty clear to outsiders that there's someone inside! But eating too much is not going to speed up this process, so don't overdo it. Eat sensibly. It's not any more complicated than that.

Avoid sweets and other empty calories. Cakes, cookies, soda pop, and other sugary treats are considered "empty" calories. They have virtually no nutritional value themselves, and they fill you up so you don't have an appetite for foods that are good for you. Products made with refined sugar have the effect of making your blood sugar go up and then rapidly drop back down, which means you'll be hungry again in no time, and perhaps craving more of the same sweet stuff!

If you feel you're gaining too much weight, talk to your healthcare provider about it. The least complicated and most effective way to control weight gain may be to cut out sweets entirely. Substitute other foods for sugary ones, such as fruit, which is sweet and also provides many nutrients. The other advantage is that natural fruit sugar (fructose) doesn't catapult your blood sugar way up and then drop it down fast, the way refined sugar does. A snack of grapes or an apple with cheese can be a midafternoon treat that is good for you and the baby without being fattening.

If you have a sweet tooth and are not comfortable eliminating sugary foods, at least limit them as much as possible in your diet. I'm not trying to take all the fun out of life: if you find that you're absolutely craving a sweet, then go ahead and have it. It makes more sense to have the cookies or the piece of cake than to deny yourself, because usually the craving will boomerang and you'll go out of control later.

Don't eat to cheer yourself up. During pregnancy it is possible that you'll have periods of feeling low (see "Mood Swings" on page

206). Some people tend to eat when they're feeling depressed. If you do feel blue, there are many things you can do instead of stuffing your face! Do nice things to make yourself feel better, but do not start munching. Some of the many small niceties you can do for yourself include: get into a nice warm (but not too hot) bubble bath; curl up in front of a fire or TV with a pile of magazines; go to the movies; get your hair done or have a manicure or pedicure; buy something new for the house. And no matter what you choose to do instead of eating to cheer yourself up, the most important thing is to recognize that you *are* feeling low and to deal with it.

LOW-BIRTH-WEIGHT BABIES

Babies that are born with a low weight at birth are at risk for many problems. You do *not* want to have a low-birth-weight infant: in many cases this is a complication of birth which is avoidable. Maternal malnutrition is the major cause of low-birth-weight babies, which are defined as being 2,500 grams (5½ pounds) or less. A mother who hasn't eaten properly can also retard the growth of the placenta, and low placental weight is related to perinatal mortality.

Babies weighing 5½ pounds or less account for only 8% of births but they represent 75% of neonatal deaths. Low birth weight is the cause of more than 50,000 infant deaths a year, within the first year of life. And 25% of the cases of cerebral palsy occur among the 52,000 cases of *very* low-birth-weight babies (weighing less than 1,500 grams or 3.3 pounds) born each year. Cerebral palsy is a birth disorder of unknown cause that produces permanent damage to motor nerves, resulting in varying degrees of paralysis and other neurological problems.

In a country as wealthy as America there is absolutely no reason for low-birth-weight babies as a result of maternal malnutrition. There are people who can afford protein-rich and well-balanced diets, but are hampered by their own ignorance about the importance of their diet on their baby's development.

People who are in financial difficulties can get assistance in getting good food for themselves and their babies. To find out if you are eligible for food stamps, call your local Department of Health and Human Services. If you are pregnant and on welfare, find out whether you may be eligible for an "unborn child allowance." And to find out about free nutritional supplements for pregnant and lactating women, contact the Maternal and Child Health Service Office in your region.

The most rapid development of the brain takes place in the last trimester of pregnancy and the first month of the baby's life on the outside. An undernourished mother can cause irreversible neurological damage and permanent brain underdevelopment in her baby. Smaller babies are ten times more likely to be mentally retarded than those who weigh 8 pounds or more. There is believed to be a direct relationship between birth weight and intelligence: nearly half of all children underweight at birth had an IQ under 70. Oxygen deprivation, birth injuries, and RDS (respiratory distress syndrome) all primarily affect babies under 5½ pounds.

The point of all this is to encourage you to eat well and gain steadily throughout your pregnancy, hoping to avoid giving birth to an underweight baby. It's been found that women who gain about 35 pounds during pregnancy wind up with babies who weigh an average of 8 pounds. Studies have shown that larger babies are easier to care for, in addition to the other health considerations. A comparison of 5-pound and 8½-pound babies showed that the larger ones were more vigorous, active, mentally alert, and suffered less from colic, diarrhea, anemia, and infections.

WHAT AND HOW TO EAT: EVERYTHING YOU NEED TO KNOW

Have you seen those "daily food guide" lists that they make up for pregnant women, with the required number of servings of each category of food? Who can follow those things, even for a day, much less nine months? It could drive you crazy trying to remember how many of your grain portions you have already satisfied by teatime! Not just that, but considering the pace of most people's lives, it doesn't seem very realistic to expect a woman to measure how many ounces of chicken there are in a portion of caesar salad or whether tomatoes are a fruit or vegetable! Of course, there are always people who feel more certain if they keep a list to organize their intake of foods, but I think that for many women "the official requirements" can be so forbidding that they don't even bother trying to keep tabs on their diet. But for those who would like it, here it is:

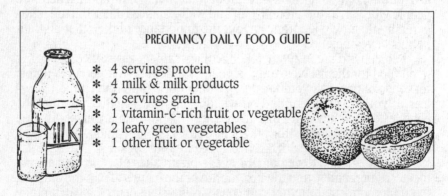

PREGNANCY DAILY FOOD GUIDE

* 4 servings protein
* 4 milk & milk products
* 3 servings grain
* 1 vitamin-C-rich fruit or vegetable
* 2 leafy green vegetables
* 1 other fruit or vegetable

Whether or not you use that list to guide your eating for the next nine months, there are certain important guidelines about your diet to keep in mind. I will go into details in this section, but here are the important basics about nutrition that everyone should follow.

BASIC NUTRITION GUIDELINES

— Eat balanced, sensible meals.
— A minimum gain of 24 pounds, which is gradual and steady.
— Eat 75–100 grams of protein every day.
— 500 calories more than a normal diet, or about 2,600 a day. (Calorie needs will be higher if you are: underweight, under severe emotional stress, had a previous miscarriage or stillbirth, had another baby within a year, or any combination of these conditions.)
— Foods nearer to their natural state have higher food value: fresh is best, frozen next, canned last.
— No restriction on sodium: use iodized salt to taste.
— Daily vitamin supplements of 30–60 mg of elemental iron and 400 to 800 µg (0.2 to 0.4 mg) of folacin.
— In last trimester eat 5 or 6 small meals instead of 3 large ones—for your comfort and easier digestion.
— Your diet before and during pregnancy influences your breast milk, so read that section (page 531) as soon as possible.

How Digestion Works

It's great to eat the right foods, but it's also important to understand how digestion functions and how to make the most of the food you eat.

CHEW FOOD THOROUGHLY

Chewing carefully is the first step in digestion: ptyalin, an enzyme in the saliva, starts breaking down starch into its component sugars. Chewing food completely helps the ptyalin work by mixing it into the food. Many grains and vegetables are made up mostly of starch: cooking breaks down the cell walls and makes starch more digestible. All this help is especially important when you're pregnant, because your digestive tract is somewhat sluggish and needs all the help it can get.

FLUIDS ARE ESSENTIAL

You need to make an effort to drink 6 to 8 glasses of fluid a day (even though that means even *more* trips to the bathroom). Your blood volume increases dramatically when you're pregnant; to meet that need your body has to have additional fluids. Liquids aid the circulation of blood and body fluids and help distribute mineral salts. Fluids also stimulate digestion, preventing constipation and aiding in the assimilation of foods. Protein, for example, requires fluids in order to metabolize. Generous amounts of liquids in your diet also help prevent urinary tract infections, to which pregnant women are more susceptible.

SAFE KITCHEN HABITS

Before we look at the all the foods you should be eating and those to avoid, let's take a moment to note the importance of how those foods are handled. Especially when you're pregnant, your personal health depends on being aware of possible dangers in certain foods and then practicing sanitary habits and safe preparation of *all* types of food, even including fresh produce. Contaminated foods are causing severe illness and even death across America. Food poisoning is a growing problem, not just from well-known high-risk ingredients like raw eggs, ground meat, and poultry, but even from innocent-looking fruits and vegetables "Is *nothing* safe anymore?" you must be wondering, but there's no point in hiding from the facts. These safety tips will be discussed in detail in the section that follows.

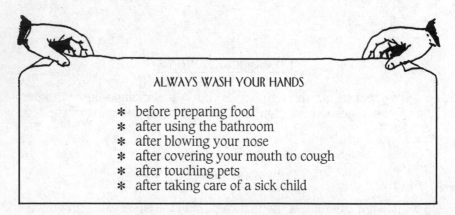

ALWAYS WASH YOUR HANDS

* before preparing food
* after using the bathroom
* after blowing your nose
* after covering your mouth to cough
* after touching pets
* after taking care of a sick child

General Safety Tips About Food

! Check the temperature of your refrigerator and freezer: the refrigerator should be 40°F or colder. The freezer should be 0°F or colder.

! Store raw meats, poultry, and seafood in the coldest part of the fridge.
! Keep foods refrigerated or frozen to minimize bacterial growth.
! If there will be significant time between when you purchase foods and take them home, bring along a cooler to keep cold foods cold.
! Thoroughly wash all fruits and vegetables, including those that will be eaten peeled and the edible leaves of leafy vegetables.
! If possible, use a separate cutting board to prepare foods that are eaten uncooked.
! Keep all cooking utensils, cutting boards, and work surfaces squeaky clean. After use, wash them with warm soapy water or with one of the new kitchen disinfectant cleansers now on the market.
! Keep milk products (even pasteurized milk and soft cheeses) refrigerated and use them promptly.
! Certain foods left out unrefrigerated at picnics or buffets carry a particular risk:
   • ham
   • poultry
   • mayonnaise-based salads (potato, chicken, tuna, egg)
   • cream-filled pastries
! Flavored oil can make you very sick! For example, olive oil with garlic cloves in it can cause botulism. This bacteria is common on root vegetables and botulism thrives when protected from oxygen—as in unrefrigerated oil. Keep any oil with whole flavoring agents (like herbs, peppercorns, etc.) in the refrigerator.

Leftovers or Food Prepared Ahead of Time

My husband's mother raised him to be suspicious of leftovers: he always refers to them as "used food"! But I happen to love leftovers: they are convenient, economical, inspire new dishes, and are often more flavorful the following day. Also, it's so handy to make larger quantities than you need and freeze the rest for a rushed, rainy day. But maybe my mother-in-law knew something from folk wisdom that modern science is now proving true: you need to be especially vigilant about leftover foods because "recycled food" can go bad and make you ill.

Safety Tips About Leftovers

! Don't leave cooked food out on the table for more than 2 hours. Bacteria grow aggressively after that time: refrigerate or freeze leftovers without delay.
! If cooked food has been sitting at room temperature for more than 2 hours, there may be a problem that can't be solved by reheating or freezing.

! Certain bacteria can grow on lukewarm food and they can survive boiling afterward. If microbes have begun to grow on it, then freezing the food will only preserve those toxins!
! If you must serve cooked food over a period of hours, keep it at 140°F or hotter. You can accomplish this by keeping the pot on the stove and serving right from there.
! If there's not enough room in the refrigerator for leftovers, don't put them on the back porch or garage: you can't control the temperature.
! For overflow food at parties or holidays, keep a cooler with ice or a freezer gel pack that maintains 40°F or cooler.
! When cooking foods for later use, do not let them sit out to cool down, which allows bacterial growth. In contradiction of what was once thought, cooked foods should be refrigerated or frozen immediately.
! When reheating foods, make sure they are heated thoroughly, bringing soups or gravies to a full boil.
! Thaw frozen food in the refrigerator or microwave oven, not on the kitchen counter.

Rules for Cooking Large Quantities

! Do not leave food sitting out to cool down: even freshly cooked soup can contain heat-resistant bacteria spores which will multiply in the slowly cooling food.
! Immediately refrigerate or freeze just-cooked food, even if it's steaming hot.
! Do not freeze in a large container: small portions cool down more quickly, reducing the chance for bacteria to grow.

Meat Safety

! Place uncooked meats, poultry or fish in leakproof containers and/or store them on the bottom shelf of the refrigerator.
! Never put cooked meats, poultry, or fish on the same unwashed surface that held raw animal products.
! Never use the same cutting board to cut up raw meat and then to prepare vegetables that won't be cooked. Wash the board thoroughly first.
! To be safe use a plastic cutting board that you reserve only for raw meat and poultry: put it through the dishwasher after each use.
! A clean knife is a safe knife: after using a knife to cut up raw meat, wash it immediately with hot, soapy water.

Ground Meats

! Any kind of meat is especially dangerous once it is ground up.
! Do not take a taste of raw, rare, or even pink ground meat or poultry in any form.
! Hamburgers, meat loaf, ground turkey, and ground chicken should be cooked all the way through until the juices run clear.
! Avoid pink meat or juice.
! When dining out, always order ground meats cooked well done.

Preparing Pork

! Trichinosis from pork is no longer the risk it once was years ago when pigs were fed raw garbage.
! Pork no longer has to be cooked well done: cooked to an internal temperature of 150 degrees, but still juicy and slightly pink, is considered safe from parasites.

Mold on Foods

! Bread and cheese are made from cultivated molds, but molds from spoiling food are unpredictable. It's generally considered safe to eat cheese that has become moldy once you cut away the moldy patch, which usually has an unpleasant taste.
! The safest thing is to throw out any food (jam, tomato paste, sun-dried tomatoes) that has developed mold, whether it's been re-frigerated or not.
! It isn't enough to just scrape off the mold on top of food other than cheese. The fuzz you see on the surface is just the tip of the "iceberg": there is an invisible network of filaments spread into the food.

Salmonella Poisoning

! Most cooks know to be careful about cracked eggs and raw poultry because of the risk that they can carry salmonella. However, this organism has recently flourished because salmonella can now be transmitted from hens to the yolks of intact eggs.
! Tomatoes and cantaloupes, for example, have been linked to large, multistate outbreaks of salmonella poisoning. The skins were contaminated and the produce was not washed before use.

ALPHABETICAL LISTING OF WHAT TO EAT & WHAT TO AVOID

There are a variety of ingredients in foods that are best to avoid, especially when you are pregnant. You should generally be all right if you try to eat foods as fresh as possible and as close as possible to their natural state. The best way to protect yourself from chemicals added to foods is to read what they admit to putting in the package. (The only problem with informing yourself like this is that once you see how many foods are affected, you may worry you'll have to spend your pregnancy in the supermarket aisle reading the small print on packaging!)

Additives & Preservatives

! Many prepared foods and snacks contain additives to keep them "fresh" for longer "shelf life." But what about *your* life and that of your unborn baby? There has been no proof that these additives are safe for your developing baby. The less that's been done to food before you eat or cook it, the safer and more nutritious it is for you and your unborn child.

! BHA and BHT are preservatives found in almost all snack chips, sausage meat, cake mixes, and even some cold cereals and canned foods. These chemicals accumulate in a person's body fat and the safety of their long-term use has not been proven. Therefore eat very little—if any—of foods that have been processed with BHT and BHA.

Antibiotics & Growth Hormones

! Growth hormones and antibiotics used in animal feeds remain in the meat of the animal and you ingest these chemicals when you eat the meats; this may have an effect on your unborn child. DES is a hormone given to cattle to fatten them up. It accumulates in the animals' livers: this means that if you want the nutritional value of eating liver, it may not be worth the risk of ingesting this powerful hormone (although presumably calves' liver would not be much affected since the animal is butchered when young).

! Laws require that cattle cannot be fed DES for 2 weeks before they are slaughtered. But this raises two questions: how can you be sure that this regulation is being observed and/or enforced? And even if meat producers *are* all following the law, how can you know with certainty that after 2 weeks there is no trace of the drug DES?

The safest bet during pregnancy is to buy your meats from a butcher or market that gives notice that their meat is supplied by sources that do not use additives in the feed given to beef cattle or other animals.

Artificial Colors

! Artificial colors are chemically similar to aspirin and should be avoided. Snack foods and drinks are frequently colored with dyes. As a rule of thumb, avoid food products that are vividly false shades of orange, red, or purple. Check *all* food packaging—even things you might not suspect of being "tampered" with—for evidence that they have been treated. And look for foods with packaging labeled "no artificial colors."

! It's not only colorful food that you need to avoid: some processed foods contain colorants to make them seem *less* colorful! Once again, the safest foods are those that are closest to their natural state.

The Dangers of Barbecuing (Grilling)

! Grilling meat, chicken, or fish over hot charcoal, wood, or charcoal "bricks" can be dangerous to your health. Barbecuing produces

---

LOW-RISK GRILLING

— Choose lean meat. Trim excess fat before grilling.

— Precook meat before barbecuing: boil it quickly or cook it in the microwave and pour off the juice (and fat). The meat juices are what contain the harmful substances: precooking destroys up to 90% of them.

— Cover the grill with aluminum foil, punching holes to let the fat drip out.

— Keep a squirt bottle of water by the barbecue to dampen coals that flare up. The dangerous substances are formed on the meat by the fat flaming up.

— Eat meat medium or medium rare, not well done (but don't be confused if this seems to contradict the advice on page 22 to eat meat well done to prevent toxoplasmosis: extended grilling creates these other problems!)

— More carcinogens are created the longer you cook on the grill: strike a balance between "rare" and "well done."

— Some foods like fish can be wrapped in foil to protect them.

— The dangerous compounds form mainly on the outside of the food: after barbecuing remove that outer layer.

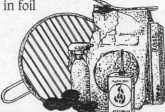

carcinogens, which are substances that can cause cancer. These carcinogens form when fat drips onto the coals. However, there are steps you can take to prevent carcinogens from forming when you use the grill: see the chart on page 75.

The safest methods of cooking your food are stewing (sautéing) on top of the stove, poaching, or microwaving. If you're used to cooking a lot on the grill, you can get ideas for other ways to prepare your food by looking through cookbooks for easy, tasty alternatives to barbecuing. For a change, you might try roasting or baking your food in the oven with lots of herbs and spices to give it flavor.

Caffeine

! Especially when you are trying to conceive and in the first 3 months of pregnancy, eliminate (or at least drastically reduce) your caffeine consumption. In animal studies caffeine caused reproductive problems such as miscarriage, stillbirth, and fetal death. It is believed that caffeine may have disrupted cell division at a stage when constant splitting of the cells was necessary for development of the fetus. High caffeine consumption is considered more than 3 cups of coffee (or the equivalent amount of caffeine) a day.

And even if you take in a lot of caffeine during the months right before you actually get pregnant, it raises your risk of a miscarriage once you have conceived. The most conservative attitude about caffeine is to assume there is *no* amount that is really safe during pregnancy.

WAYS TO CUT DOWN ON CAFFEINE

— Use decaffeinated coffee and tea (but be aware that it still has a little caffeine).
— Do not take any of the pain medications containing aspirin (see the directory on page 172).
— Don't let tea steep very long and do not ever boil it, both of which increase the amount of caffeine.
— Be aware which colas and other sodas have high amounts of caffeine. Switch to another kind.
— After the first trimester, continue trying to keep your coffee intake to a minimum. Even if you drink only 4 cups of coffee a day (or the equivalent in caffeine), it may have an effect on the developing fetus.

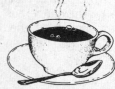

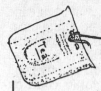

HOW MUCH CAFFEINE IS IN IT?

Milligrams of Caffeine

Coffee (5 oz.)

automatic drip	110–150
percolated	65–125
instant	40–110
decaffeinated	2–5

Tea (5 oz.)

steeped 5 minutes	50–90
steeped 2 minutes	20–45
canned iced tea (12 oz.)	25–35
decaffeinated ¯	0

Chocolate

baking chocolate (1 oz.)	35
cocoa beverage	10
milk chocolate (1 oz.)	6

Soft drinks (12 oz.)

Mountain Dew, Mellow Yellow	53
Coca-Cola, Tab, Shasta cola	45
Sunkist orange	42
(Sunkist diet orange)	0
Pepsi, Dr. Pepper, RC cola	35
Diet-Rite	35
7-Up, Sprite, Fresca, gingerale, root beer	0

Nonprescription medications (1 tablet)

Dexatrim, Dietac	200
No-Doz, Vivarin, Caffedrine	200
Excedrin	130
Anacin, Midol	64
Dristan, Coryban-D	30
plain aspirin (any brand)	0

NOTE: If you are accustomed to taking in a fair amount of caffeine and you do decide to eliminate it from your diet before or during pregnancy, you may experience a headache—a bad enough headache that it can last anywhere up to 7 days. Believe it or not, this is a normal reaction to withdrawal from caffeine! This should give you a pretty good idea of how potent this ingredient is and why fears about its effect on the developing fetus are justified.

WITHDRAWING FROM CAFFEINE

Caffeine is an addictive substance: depending on how much coffee, tea and cola your body is used to, quitting "cold turkey" can be very unpleasant. For this reason it will probably be easier on you to gradually reduce the mount of caffeine in your diet.

> *Switch to a 50–50 coffee blend* or make your own mixture of half-regular, half-decaffeinated coffee.
> *Drink as little carbonated soda as possible*—it fills you up with no nutritional value and colas can even act as diuretics. If you really want a soda, change to a caffeine-free variety.
> *Cut down gradually on the caffeine*, reducing it by a cup or half a cup a day.
> *Eat something at the same time* as you drink the caffeinated beverage to soften the effect on your system.
> *Keep your energy level* up because reducing the caffeine in your system can give you a sense of fatigue. Eating frequent nutritious snacks will keep your blood sugar up and with it a sense of well-being.
> *Get fresh air and exercise every day,* which can help keep your spirits and energy up.
> *If you can't stand no caffeine, don't worry*: you can allow yourself a couple of cups of caffeine a day. Just make sure you keep track and don't go over that amount.

Calcium and What It Means to Your Baby

! Your body needs a great deal of calcium now, primarily to build your baby's bones. Most women are giving their baby more calcium than they're taking in—and if they don't adjust their diet to take in enough calcium, the developing baby will take what she needs from her mother's body. However, both you and your baby will ultimately suffer if your prenatal diet doesn't have enough calcium: your bones and teeth will be weakened and the baby's bone growth will not be adequate.

! During pregnancy it is recommended that a woman increase her normal intake of calcium by 50%, to get it up to 1,200 mg a day. Milk and other dairy products are the best sources of calcium: for example, you can fulfill your calcium requirement by drinking a quart of milk a day, since every cup of it supplies you with 300 mg.

! Avoid calcium tablets. It is not clear how the body absorbs calcium when it is taken in pill form. Therefore, you cannot rely on tablets from a bottle, because your baby's well-being depends on your calcium intake. It is better to get your daily requirement of calcium from real foods, since they supply other essential nutrients at the same time.

However, if you do want to take calcium tablets, they will have the most effect if you take them on an empty stomach. If they are taken with food (or right after it) the calcium will go right through your digestive system without being absorbed.

! Nonfat dry milk is a great addition to your diet. As you can see from the "Calcium Directory" chart following this, there is a great deal of calcium in nonfat dry milk: in only ¼ cup, you get 375 mg. of calcium. You can find ways to add nonfat dry milk to many of the foods you eat, whether it's to a bowl of cereal with liquid milk on it, shakes made of fruit and frozen yogurt or ice cream, or soups, sauces, casseroles, and anything that you bake. Nonfat dry milk is an inexpensive, low-calorie way to give a calcium boost to your diet. (For more information on milk and dairy products, see page 87 later in this chapter.)

! Other vitamins interact with calcium. Vitamin C helps your body absorb calcium. You will notice certain orange juices which are labeled as having "added calcium," for this very reason. So if you're taking a calcium supplement, it helps to take it at the same time as an acidic vitamin C–rich fruit or juice.

Your body needs vitamin D to utilize calcium, so your need for this vitamin doubles during pregnancy, from the normal 200 IUs to 400 IUs a day. But if you are a young pregnant woman— between the ages of 19 and 22—you will need even more vitamin D because your own bones are still growing while the baby's bones are developing. The amount of vitamin D in 5 glasses of milk a day will meet this increased need for the vitamin. Other food sources of vitamin D include: fortified margarine, butter, sardines, canned salmon, egg yolk, and liver.

NOTE: Do not take a vitamin D supplement without your doctor's orders. Overdoses of vitamin D are toxic and can harm your baby. (See "Warnings About Vitamins" page 111.)

Calcium (mg)

Milk (8 oz.)

nonfat *dry* milk (¼ cup)	375
nonfat (skim milk)	300
2%, fortified	295
whole milk	290

Yogurt (8 oz.)

nonfat, plain	450
low fat, plain	415
low fat with fruit	315
whole, plain	275
frozen	200–250

Cheese (1 oz.)

Swiss	280
goat, hard	255
cheddar	210
Edam, Muenster	205
American	200
mozzarella, part skim	185
blue	150
feta	140
cottage cheese, creamed (½ cup)	115
goat, soft	5

Vegetables (1 cup, cooked)

collard greens (frozen, chopped)	355
* spinach (frozen)	280
kale, mustard greens	150
broccoli	135
* chard	100

Fish (4 oz.)

sardines (with bones)	400
salmon (canned with bones)	225
oysters (1 cup)	175
clams	100

Miscellaneous

calcium-enriched orange juice (6 oz.)	225
tofu (soybean curd) (4 oz.)	180
1 medium orange	5
corn muffin	5

NOTE: Spinach, chard, beet greens and parsley are high in calcium *but* they also contain oxalic acid, which binds to calcium and inhibits your body from absorbing the calcium.

NOTE: Do not eat (or drink) anything chocolate at the same time as milk because chocolate reduces the body's ability to absorb calcium.

Cholesterol

Most people don't really understand the issue of cholesterol in food—there's a general tendency to think that cholesterol is something really bad or "dangerous." Actually, whether cholesterol is a problem depends on your own individual metabolism. Some people's bodies have a tendency to over synthesize and assimilate cholesterol—this is an inherited problem. If you inherit it from both parents, heart disease can even start in childhood; if you inherit it from one parent, the problem manifests itself later in life. But the human body can manufacture cholesterol from *any* food source, not just cholesterol-rich food, so limiting the intake of foods that contain cholesterol is not the answer. It just depends on how your individual metabolism works.

Unless tests have indicated that you have an inherited problem, cholesterol is not something you need to worry about during pregnancy. If you have doubts or questions, talk to your general practitioner or internist before getting pregnant and also discuss your cholesterol levels with your obstetrician.

Egg Safety

! Buy only clean, uncracked eggs.
! Keep them refrigerated.
! Use them within five weeks of purchase.
! Avoid eating raw or undercooked egg yolks in any form.
! When preparing *caesar salad, steak tartare*, or other foods calling for raw eggs that won't be cooked before they are eaten, use only pasteurized eggs or an egg substitute (both sold in labeled cartons in the egg section). Other examples: hollandaise sauce, chocolate mousse, eggnog.
! When ordering caesar salad (or other foods mentioned above) in a restaurant, ask if the chef uses raw eggs.

The Dangers of Raw (& Cooked) Fish & Seafood

! Fish used to be considered one of the healthiest foods you could eat, but unfortunately this is no longer true. Water pollution, how fish is handled, and other problems mean that there are hazards to eating fish. The risk is even greater for pregnant women, so it's necessary to follow the following guidelines about safe handling and preparation of any fish.
! Be choosy about where you buy fish. The best place to buy fish, to assure yourself of freshness, is in a shop that specializes in fish and has a high turnover of product. Do not buy from a store where raw and cooked fish are displayed side-by-side and can touch: the bacteria from the raw fish can affect the cooked. Do not buy fish

that is piled high in open display cases or under hot lights, which allows bacteria to grow faster.

! There are ways to tell if fish is fresh. Fish gills should be bright red or pink. Fillets or steaks should have moist flesh with a translucent sheen, as if you can almost see inside. Fish should not have a bad, or fishy, smell. A light mild odor means it is fresh.

! Avoid fish if it has any of the following: discoloration, tears or other blemishes, brownish yellow stickiness, scale loss, or red bruising.

! Fish kept in a hot car can spoil in one hour. If you shop on a warm day, bring along a cooler with ice packs for the ride home.

! Your refrigerator is probably not cold enough to keep fish fresh: most refrigerators hold a temperature of about 40°F. Fill the vegetable bin with ice and bury the still-wrapped fish there, or sandwich the fish between two ice packs.

! Don't let all these warnings make you too anxious: seafood is actually safer than chicken. In fact, seafood is responsible for one illness per 250,000 servings . . . chicken is ten times as risky. And if you exclude all the bivalves that are eaten raw (primarily clams and oysters), that lowers the statistic: fish causes one illness per every 5,000,000 servings!

SAFETY PRECAUTIONS YOU SHOULD TAKE WITH SHELLFISH (MEANING ANY SEAFOOD WITH A SHELL).

! Live shellfish should be refrigerated, not held in water.

! The fact that live crabs and lobsters are in a tank does not guarantee quality. Ask how long they've been in there.

! Whole cracked crabs should be displayed in or on ice.

! Scallops should be translucent: they should not be opaque, even at the edges.

! Do not eat raw oysters or clams no matter how fancy or trustworthy the restaurant. Hepatitis is rampant.

! Any raw bivalve (clam, oyster, mussel, scallop) with an open shell is dead and you cannot eat it.

! If you cook any bivalve and the shell does not open, do not attempt to open and eat it.

CERTAIN FISH IS HIGH-RISK AND YOU MUST BE CAUTIOUS.

! Fish that spend any time *in fresh water* (salmon, snapper, cod) are more likely to be infected with parasites.

! *Swordfish* often contains high levels of methyl mercury, which is considered a "reproductive toxin" and therefore should be avoided by any woman who is even thinking about getting pregnant.

! *Tuna* and *mahimahi* also contain mercury, although at a lower level than swordfish.
! *Whitefish, East Coast salmon*, and *shark* may have high levels of PCBs, which are harmful to the fetus.
! *"Recreationally caught"* fish (meaning that which you catch yourself) often comes from water that is of suspicious quality. This fish also tends to be mishandled: it's not kept sufficiently cold.

WHAT ARE THE SAFEST FISH TO EAT?

! *Flounder* and *sole* are the only two fresh fish that are commonly found which are virtually free of pollutants.
! *Salmon* is one of the most trouble-free fish.
! *Canned* tuna, salmon, and other *fish in a can* are very safe.
! *Processed frozen products* such as fish sticks, breaded fillets, and nuggets are made from white-fleshed fish such as cod, haddock, and pollock and are safe if you keep them frozen.
! *Farmed fish* such as catfish, trout, and salmon have a good record of being free of disease.

LEARN ABOUT SAFE HANDLING AND PREPARATION OF FISH.

! Bacteria multiply rapidly in fish if it is not stored at 32°F or colder, but most home refrigerators are only about 40°F.
! Bring fish home from the store as promptly as possible and store it in the coldest part of your refrigerator or on a bed of ice.
! Fish is highly perishable: you should cook it within one day of buying it.
! Handle raw and cooked fish separately.
! Wash your hands carefully after handling raw fish.
! All utensils and surfaces that the fish has touched should be thoroughly washed and rinsed with hot soapy water.
! Fish and shellfish must be thoroughly cooked, to an internal temperature of 140°F or until it flakes easily (so you're going to have to forget the gourmet style of "rare" or barely cooked tuna and other fish!).
! Thaw frozen seafood in the refrigerator: *not* at room temperature and *not* under warm water, both of which allow bacteria to grow.
! Reheat "cooked ready-to-eat" shrimp as an extra precaution to destroy any bacteria that they might contain.

YOU MUST AVOID CERTAIN FISH.

! Bad news for fans of "raw bars": *never* eat raw clams or oysters (regardless of whether there are *two* "Rs" in the month!). Raw oysters have been singled out by health departments as having the highest health risk of any seafood.

! Beware of shrimp, too: raw shrimp are frequently contaminated with salmonella and frozen "ready-to-eat" shrimp often have high levels of bacterial contamination.

! Avoid fish that come from "hot spots," like the Great Lakes, Santa Monica Bay, Chesapeake Bay, and Puget Sound. For example, women of childbearing age in the Great Lakes region have been cautioned to avoid all fish from that area. Waters with high levels of chemical contaminants can affect the fish which live there: the flesh of fish absorbs and multiplies the contamination of the water in which it lives. Eating fish from this unhealthy water can cause birth defects.

WHAT ABOUT SUSHI?

! Bad news for sushi lovers: most doctors say to make a detour around the sushi bar while you're pregnant. Raw or barely cooked fish can harbor bacteria or parasites.

! However, sushi-related illnesses are usually from raw fish prepared at home. The safest sushi is prepared by expert chefs, who use fish that is blast frozen.

! Avoid eating raw fish like sushi and sashimi *unless* you can be certain that it was *blast frozen* first: frozen at −4°F for at least 5 days, which kills any parasites that might be present.

! Do not eat raw or barely cooked fish you have caught yourself— even the freshest fish from *unpolluted* waters. It can have parasitic worms, which would be destroyed by cooking.

SEAFOOD VITAMINS & MINERALS

Seafood	Per Serving	Function
Crab	90 mg calcium	strengthens bones
Shrimp	1 mg zinc	boosts immune system
Swordfish	10 mg niacin	improves circulation
Clams	14 mg iron	prevents anemia

Grains

Grain products are going to be an important part of your pregnancy diet. Grains supply thiamine, niacin, riboflavin, iron, phosphorus, and zinc. The germ of the grain contains most of the nutrients, yet when grains go through a refining process it is this germ which is removed—so make an effort to eat whole-grain products whenever possible. Whole-grain foods have more value because they contain more magnesium and zinc. Some examples are brown rice, wheat germ, certain cold cereals (such as shredded wheat, wheat flakes, granola, and puffed oats), and hot cereals such as oatmeal and rolled or cracked wheat. Most of the bread companies make whole-grain breads with cracked and whole wheat.

Other foods which fall into the grain category are ready-to-eat cereals (although the sugared ones supply expensive, empty calories), cream of wheat or rice, farina, cornmeal, grits, and rice; all breads, including cornbread, corn or flour tortillas, rolls, bagels, muffins, biscuits, dumplings, and crackers. Waffles and pancakes are also grain products— and you can increase their food value by adding some wheat germ to the batter.

The least nutritious breads you can eat are French and Italian. They are nutritionally inferior even to soft American white sandwich bread, which is enriched. French and Italian breads may taste better, but they are mostly empty calories because they are made with water instead of milk.

Honey

Honey has a number of advantages over sugar for your sweetening needs. First of all, it contains traces of certain nutrients, especially the B vitamins. And since honey is sweeter than sucrose (refined white sugar), you only need about two-thirds as much to get the sweetening power of sugar.

Your system absorbs honey immediately, but it doesn't trigger the same cycle as sucrose does: insulin, low blood sugar, more sugar needed, insulin. And this explains a third advantage of honey, which is that because honey satisfies, you're less likely to eat an excessive amount (as can happen with sugar). With refined sugar, the more you eat, the more you want—the familiar cycle that can result in eating lots of calories with little nutritional value. So whenever possible, substitute honey for sugar— it's a good habit for your own sake.

Iron

! Your body has to create a lot more blood when you're pregnant, and iron is essential to the formation of healthy red blood cells. You're going to have to pay special attention to iron because very few women start their pregnancies with enough iron stored in

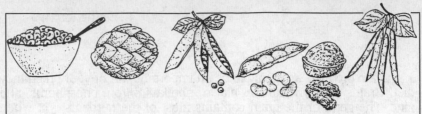

IRON-RICH FOODS

	Milligrams
Cereals (1 cup)	
40% bran flakes	11
raisin bran	9
cream of wheat	8
wheat germ (½ cup)	5
oatmeal or shredded wheat	1
Fish & meat (4 oz.)	
kidney	15
liver (chicken)	10
liver (beef)	9
clams	8
oysters	7
turkey or beef	4
sardines	3
lamb	2
pork or chicken	1
egg (1)	1
Fruit & juices (1 cup)	
apricots (dried)	8
raisins or prune juice	3
tomato or apple juice	1
dried figs (2), prunes (10)	1
Vegetables (½ cup cooked)	
beans (all kinds)	2
artichoke (1)	2
peas, Brussels sprouts	1.5
spinach (raw or cooked)	1.5
Swiss chard	1
potato (white or sweet), raw tomato	.5
romaine lettuce (1 cup raw)	.5
Nuts (¼ cup)	
almonds, cashews	1.5
walnuts	1
Miscellaneous	
Blackstrap molasses (1 T.)	3.5
Brewer's yeast (1 T.)	1.5
Soybean curd (tofu, 4 oz.)	

their bodies to meet the greatly increased need for this trace mineral.

! It is hard to eat enough iron-rich foods to keep up with your body's requirements during pregnancy, when your blood volume becomes so much greater. But even if you do eat a lot of iron-containing foods, what you may not know is that only a small percentage of the iron in that food is actually absorbed by your body, which means there is no sure way to know how much iron you're taking in from your diet.

! The developing fetus will take all the iron he needs from you, no matter how low your iron supply may be. A pregnant woman who is iron deficient (which most women are) may wind up anemic, exhausted, and susceptible to infection. This is why obstetricians recommend an iron supplement of 30 to 60 mg a day, especially during the second half of pregnancy. However, iron pills tend to be constipating; you might want to eat dried fruits such as raisins, prunes, or apricots every day, which can counteract constipation (and supply some added iron at the same time).

! Even though you're taking an iron supplement, you still need to include iron-rich foods in your diet. The chart opposite shows you the foods that are highest in iron. It's also good to know that your body's ability to absorb iron is increased by eating high-acid foods (citrus fruits, tomato, yogurt) and foods high in vitamin C. Furthermore, cooking acidic foods such as tomatoes in a cast-iron pan allows the food to absorb some of the iron from the pot.

NOTE: Drinking tea or coffee with a meal can significantly diminish your body's absorption of the iron in that food.

Milk & Dairy Products

! During pregnancy you need about one quart of milk (4 cups), or the equivalent, every day. Whole milk, skim milk, buttermilk, evaporated and nonfat dry milk, as well as yogurt, are all equal. Remember that a quart of fortified vitamin D milk supplies 400 IUs of vitamin D—as does an equal amount of nonfat dry milk. But if you aren't getting vitamin D from milk, you need other sources of it (see the "Vitamin Directory" on page 112). However, you have to be fairly certain that you aren't getting more than 400 IUs of vitamin D, because too much of it can be harmful. Unlike other vitamins, if you take an excessive amount of A and D, your body cannot excrete them.

! Whole milk is best during pregnancy: the fat in it helps your body absorb milk's calcium most efficiently. Each person has to decide for herself whether she wants to worry about the slightly higher calories in whole milk, or drink skim milk and have less vitamin absorption. However, it is true that a quart of whole milk a day is a lot of calories, so if this fact worries you, it is possible to take supplements instead.

! Milk has a high sodium (salt) content, but do not be concerned by this. Salt is good for you when you're pregnant: your body needs more sodium (see "Salt" on page 96) and your kidneys can efficiently excrete any excess sodium your body cannot use.

! The calcium in milk is what you need: milk products are the best source of this mineral, which is vital to building strong bones and teeth for your baby. The baby's primary teeth begin to form during the 5th month of pregnancy, and her skeleton begins to change from cartilage to bone early in the 6th month. As these important growth stages indicate, all the foods in the milk group are essential in your diet throughout your pregnancy.

! *Some women have lactose intolerance* (milk products don't agree with them). Some adults are not able to consume milk and other dairy products because their bodies cannot digest lactose, a natural sugar present in milk. However, there may still be calcium-rich dairy products that you'll be able to eat without upsetting your system. You can also try Lactaid tablets (or a similar product sold in pharmacies and health food stores), which can be taken along with dairy products to make them more easily digestible.

   You can also concentrate on those dairy products with the least amount of lactose which you may be able to eat, such as natural hard cheese and fermented cheese. There are also reduced amounts of lactose in cultured milk products such as yogurt and buttermilk (but check the carton to find a brand that does not add "milk solids") and some lactose-intolerant people can consume them without a problem.

   Another alternative is to try acidophilus milk, or you can take ordinary milk and add enzyme lactase to it yourself. This enzyme is marketed as Lactaid, which you can find (Lactaid also markets their own liquid milk in some supermarkets).

! What if you just don't like milk? Just because you don't like to drink milk by the glass doesn't mean you can't consume it in your diet. Obviously you can use milk on cold cereal, but you can also "sneak" it into your diet by using milk in preparing hot cereal, soups, or creamed dishes. You can substitute milk for other liquids in baking. You can feel like a kid again by making desserts such as custards and rice pudding with milk! And you can always add nonfat dry milk to blender drinks or any of the above-mentioned foods.

! Instead of milk, there are a variety of milk products you can substitute. For example, two 1-inch cubes of cheddar cheese are equal to 1 cup of milk. Other replacements are hard or semisoft cheese (but *not* including blue cheese, cream cheese or Camembert-type cheeses), cottage cheese, yogurt, and ice milk. Most commercial ice creams do not have genuine milk products in them, so check the labeling (and notice how much fat and calories they're giving you instead!).

Potatoes

You've got to feel sorry for potatoes! They are such a healthy and satisfying food, but they have a mistaken reputation for being fattening. A potato is only slightly higher in calories than an apple, and think how much more filling and nutritious it is! Obviously there are a lot of calories in a baked potato swimming in butter and sour cream, or a plate of greasy French fries, but what we're talking about here is a naked potato. If you have good russet or Yukon Gold potatoes, you'll find they can be delicious without all the fattening stuff. There are so many low-calorie ways to give a potato zip and flavor: usually lots of salt and pepper to start off, and then you can experiment with various herbs or products like Mrs. Dash or other seasonings.

There are many ingredients you can add to a baked or boiled potato to give it flavor and increase the protein and calcium content. And there are such great ways to eat them: try boiled red potatoes eaten alongside a scoop of cottage cheese (mixed with a spoon of low-fat sour cream) and chives. Or bake a potato, split it in half, scoop out the inside, and mix it up with any of the dairy products on the "Calcium Directory" chart on page 80. To avoid taking in excess calories, you might want to try low-fat versions of milk products, which exist in almost every kind of cheese and cream. For example, whip the potato with herbs, Parmesan, and plain yogurt. Or combine cheddar or Swiss cheese and broccoli (or any other vegetable). Of course, you can mix in bits of any leftover meats you might have around, such as ham or chicken, along with some cheese, and then use whipped cream cheese or even just some milk to moisten it.

Potatoes are an especially great food when you're pregnant, but people seem to forget about them. They fulfill so many of your needs. Few people realize that each potato has about 3 grams of protein compared to only a trace in an apple—and, in addition, a potato has twice as much iron, thiamin, and riboflavin, much more niacin, and seven times as much vitamin C as an apple. You should also keep potatoes in mind if you have nausea during your pregnancy, because a baked potato can often be one of the few foods you can tolerate that is also nutritious. So any time during your pregnancy that you can eat a potato, dig right in!

Protein

Protein is the basic material from which most cells are formed, so the protein foods you eat are going to be the building blocks of your baby. You need to try to eat lots of protein every day for your baby to grow big and healthy.

WHAT DOES "COMPLETE PROTEINS" MEAN?

"Complete proteins" are those foods you want to emphasize in your diet. Our bodies cannot fully use the protein in the food we eat, so you need to know which are the most complete proteins so that you can be sure to eat some of them every day.

Proteins are composed of many amino acids, eight of which are considered "essential" amino acids. Another two amino acids are essential during the growing period and the remainder of them our bodies manufacture. Plant and animal foods contain protein, but those in plants are considered "incomplete" proteins because they lack one or more of those essential amino acids. Incomplete plant proteins can be supplemented by adding animal protein; for instance, milk in pea soup, or egg and milk powder in bread. Animal proteins have enough of all the essential amino acids, in a proper ratio, to meet your body's needs.

To get an idea of different foods that all have an equal amount of protein, have a look at this list:

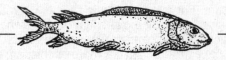

EQUIVALENT AMOUNTS OF PROTEIN

* 1 oz. meat
* 1 oz. poultry
* 1 oz. fish
* 1 egg

* 1 oz. American or Swiss cheese
* 1 oz. (2 Tb.) cottage cheese
* ½ cup dried beans or peas

! The animal proteins supply iron, riboflavin, niacin, vitamins B6 and B12, phosphorus, zinc, and iodine along with the protein. *The best sources of animal protein are:*
  - meat
  - fish
  - milk
  - cheese
  - eggs

! Vegetable proteins are less well-known: people are often unaware of these protein-rich nonmeat and nondairy foods. Vegetable proteins supply iron, thiamine, folacin, vitamins B6 and E, phosphorus, magnesium, and zinc along with the protein.
  - dried beans & peas
  - nuts & nut butters
  - sunflower & sesame seeds
  - tofu

HIGH-PROTEIN IN-BETWEEN MEALS

There are some high-protein snacks you can munch during the day that will supply extra protein while satisfying your hunger. *Some suggestions for high-protein snacks:*
- soy nuts
- peanut butter with celery (or wheat crackers)
- cottage cheese with corn chips
- whole-grain breads or cookies
- nuts and seeds

NOTE: The following nuts are *not* good protein sources because they have too many calories for the amount of protein they provide: pecans, chestnuts, coconuts, filberts, hazelnuts, macadamias, almonds, English walnuts (black walnuts have 40% more protein than English ones).

"PROTEIN USABILITY"—CAN YOUR BODY USE IT?

Our bodies can't fully use the protein in our food, even in "complete proteins." Some foods are more usable than others, which is an important factor to consider when you're deciding which foods to eat to meet the special protein needs of pregnancy. The percentage of protein your body can actually use is the amount your digestive tract absorbs—this is called the "net protein utilization," or NPU. To put it simply, the NPU estimates what proportion of the protein we eat is actually available to our body as fuel.

Research has shown that the protein in eggs most nearly matches the human body's own ideal pattern and therefore is a superb source of usable protein: the white is 100% protein and the yolk is rich in iron. Therefore, egg protein is used as a model for measuring the amino acid patterns in other foods. An example of how the NPU measurement works is that the NPU of peanuts is only 40%, while cheese is 70%.

The chart of "High-Protein Foods" on page 94 should help you get the most food value out of the foods you eat and help meet the high-protein demands of pregnancy.

COMBINING FOODS INCREASES THEIR PROTEIN

When certain foods are eaten in combination, it increases the amount of protein they supply. The high-protein snacks mentioned above are an example. Another example would be having a peanut butter sandwich on wheat bread with a glass of milk. For a complete list on food combinations, see page 101 under "Vegetarian Pregnancy." If you're interested in further suggestions, pick up a copy of the book *Diet for a Small Planet,* by Frances Moore Lappé, and *Recipes for a Small Planet,* by Ellen Ewald. You may notice that Mexican food by its nature already combines many of the combined ingredients in one meal, such as cornmeal, beans, rice, and cheese. Below are some examples:

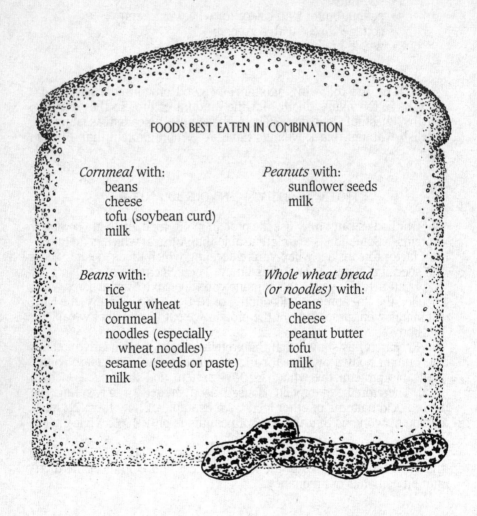

FOODS BEST EATEN IN COMBINATION

Cornmeal with:
    beans
    cheese
    tofu (soybean curd)
    milk

Peanuts with:
    sunflower seeds
    milk

Beans with:
    rice
    bulgur wheat
    cornmeal
    noodles (especially
      wheat noodles)
    sesame (seeds or paste)
    milk

Whole wheat bread (or noodles) with:
    beans
    cheese
    peanut butter
    tofu
    milk

HOW MUCH PROTEIN DO YOU NEED?

During pregnancy you need a minimum of 75 grams of protein a day—and that amount is calculated for an average 120-pound five foot two inch woman. So that means that if there's more of you than that, you'll require more protein, as much as 100 grams daily.

If you look at the "High-Protein Foods" chart on p. 94, you may see that it takes a mathematician to add up the needed grams every day, and it may even seem to you that you'll have to be eating from morning to night to reach that goal of 75 to 100 grams.

Don't panic if you find that it's not possible for you to comfortably consume that many grams of protein each day. You have to trust your own instincts and adapt this "recommended requirement" of 75 grams to suit your own personal needs. Try to be conscious (without driving yourself nuts!) of eating as much complete proteins as you can. But do not feel you have to be a slave to the recommendation: as with every other aspect of your pregnancy, take the information you find here and adapt it to your personality and lifestyle.

HIGH-PROTEIN FOODS

	GRAMS PROTEIN	USABLE GRAMS
Type of flour (1 cup)		
soybean, defatted	65	40
gluten	85	23
peanut, defatted	48	21
soybean, full fat	26	16
whole or cracked wheat	16	10
rye, dark	16	9
oatmeal, barley	11	7
cornmeal, whole ground	10	5
Meat and poultry		
turkey, 3 slices	31	22
pork chop, with fat	29	19
steak, ½ lb. without fat	25	17
hamburger, ¼ lb.	26	17
chicken breast	23	15
lamb chop with fat	20	13
Fish (3½ oz.)		
halibut	22	17
sardines, 3 canned in oil	21	14
swordfish, bass, shrimp	19	15
cod, Pacific herring, haddock	18	14
crab, northern lobster	17	14
squid, 3 sea scallops, sole	15	12
clams, 4 large or 8 small	14	11
oysters, 3	11	9
Dairy products (1 oz. or 1 sq.in.)		
cottage cheese (3 oz.), uncreamed	17	13
cottage cheese (3 oz.), creamed	14	11
milk, nonfat dry solids	10	8
Parmesan cheese	10	7
milk, 1 cup (any kind)	9	7
yogurt, nonfat, 1 cup	8	7
egg, 1 large	6	6
Swiss cheese	8	6
ricotta (¼ cup), cheddar	7	5
ice cream	5	4

HIGH-PROTEIN FOODS

	GRAMS PROTEIN	USABLE GRAMS
Legumes: dried peas and beans (1 cup cooked)		
soybeans or soy grits	17	10
broad beans	13	6
peas, black-eyed peas, lentils	17	10
black beans, kidney beans	17	10
tofu (wet, 3 oz.)	8	5
navy, white, or pea beans; garbanzos	11	4
Grains and cereals		
egg noodles (1 cup)	7	4
bulgur or cracked wheat (⅓ cup)	6	4
barley, millet (⅓ cup)	6	4
spaghetti, all pastas	5	3
oatmeal (⅓ cup)	4	3
rice, any kind	5	3
wheat germ (2 T.)	3	2
bread, 1 slice wheat or rye	2	1
Nuts and seeds (2 T.)		
pine nuts (pignoli)	9	5
pumpkin/squash seeds	8	5
sunflower seeds (3 T.)	7	4
peanuts, peanut butter	8	3
cashews (15), pistachios (3 T.)	9	5
sesame seeds (3 T.), black walnuts	5	3
Vegetables (cooked weight)		
lima beans (½ cup)	8	4
corn (1 ear), broccoli (¾ cup)	4	2
collards (½ cup), mushrooms (12)	3	2
asparagus (6 spears)	3	2
artichoke, 1 large	6	2
cauliflower (1 cup), spinach (½ cup)	3	1.5
potato, medium baking	4	1
Nutritional additives		
egg white, powdered (½ oz.)	11	9
Tiger's milk (¼ cup)	8	6
brewer's yeast (1 T.)	4	2

Salt (Sodium)

DO NOT ELIMINATE SALT FROM YOUR DIET.

Salt is very important to your body when you're carrying a child. A pregnant woman's body fluids expand and her blood volume increases by 40%: salt is the main element in maintaining this dramatic expansion that your body undergoes. If you want to get technical about it, salt is necessary "to maintain the osmotic pressure relationships in the body." This should convince you of the problems created by restricting salt in your diet. What you're doing when you limit the salt your body needs is limiting the blood-volume expansion which the body needs for a healthy pregnancy. The other result of limiting your salt intake can be fatigue and loss of appetite.

The further danger of a low-salt diet is that it can compromise the growth of the placenta and its proper functioning. Salt is necessary in your diet not only to maintain the water balance, but to regulate nerve and muscle irritability. So pick up the salt shaker and salt foods to suit your own taste!

WHAT KIND OF SALT SHOULD YOU USE AND HOW MUCH?

During pregnancy it's important to use *iodized* salt: check the packaging before buying, because many companies now offer a "non-iodized" version. *Do not use the sea salt sold in health food stores.* Oftentimes health food devotees rely on sea salt for cooking, but the problem is that it does not contain iodine, which is necessary to prevent possible thyroid problems during pregnancy.

The best way to figure out how much salt to use is to trust your taste buds: salt your food "to taste" throughout your pregnancy. The taste buds are the body's simplest salt-regulating mechanism, so rely on your tongue to tell you how much is enough.

IS SALT GOOD OR BAD FOR YOU?

The topic of salt in the prenatal diet used to be a controversy: at one time it was (incorrectly) believed that when a pregnant woman ate salt it caused her to retain water, which then caused the swelling associated with toxemia. Therefore, years ago many doctors used to prescribe low-salt diets for women during pregnancy. However, it is now understood that some swelling is a normal part of pregnancy and by itself is not a sign of toxemia (see "Toxemia" on page 419 for more information). It has been learned that a woman's body needs *more* salt—not less—when she is pregnant.

However, there may still be some misguided obstetricians who tell their patients to avoid salt and—even more distressing—some doctors who prescribe "water pills" (diuretics) for pregnant women. This medication is very bad during pregnancy, as it drains your body of important vitamins and minerals and can also interfere with the amniotic fluid. If your doctor should recommend water pills, immediately seek the advice of another obstetrician. ***Do not take diuretics when pregnant!***

AVOID HIGH-SALT FOODS.

Okay, here we go with what may seem like a contradiction: when you see the recommendation to "salt food to taste," that has nothing to do with snack items which are very high in sodium. Putting salt on your baked potato until it tastes good to you is not the same as putting your

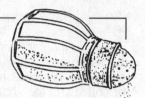

HIGH-SALT FOODS TO AVOID

Cured, prepared & processed meats
* ham
* sausage
* bacon
* hot dogs
* salt pork
* lunch meats
* bologna
* chipped beef

Seasoning salts
* garlic salt
* celery salt
* Lawry's and similar brands
* check labels for other products

Relishes
* pickles
* olives
* pickled vegetables

Salted fish
* smoked salmon (lox)
* smoked sturgeon
* smoked trout
* herring (mackerel) in cream or brine

Prepared meat sauces
* soy sauce
* teriyaki sauce
* catsup
* mustard
* barbecue sauce
* Al and similar products
* Worcestershire sauce

Snack foods
* corn curls & chips
* potato chips
* pretzels
* popcorn
* crackers
* nuts

Soups
* canned soups (check for "low-sodium")
* boxed soup mixes
* soup mix used as a dip for chips (a "double-whammy"!)

face into a bag of potato chips! Yes, the chips may taste good, but that is a different thing than "salting to taste," which relies on your discretion: you have no control over the salt content of prepared foods, which *can* overload your system. These foods put more salt into your body than it needs and can cause excessive water retention. The foods in the chart on page 97 are high in salt and should be avoided or eaten sparingly (notice that *none* of them are very healthy items).

Milk and most dairy products are high in sodium; *however*, they are an essential supply of calcium and protein, so *do not* limit this food group in your diet.

NOTE: *Bicarbonate of soda* (baking soda) is high in salt and should not be used as a digestive during pregnancy.

Sugar Substitutes

A teaspoon of sugar or honey has so little calories that it's really not necessary to use sugar substitutes (unless you're a diabetic). How often have you (or someone you know) put sugar substitute in your iced tea or coffee and then had a nice big dessert? Those little packets of powder have become a habit that many of us have not stopped to think about.

➤ *Sweet'n Low is the most well-known saccharin* product and should be avoided during pregnancy because animal tests have shown it to affect the fetus.
➤ *Equal and Nutrasweet are aspartame sweeteners* which have not been proven to cause problems in the developing fetus and are probably okay in small amounts.
➤ *Try using fruit juice concentrate*, honey, or 100% pure maple syrup (the real stuff) as sweeteners.

Tofu

Tofu, or bean curd, is a high-protein food product derived from soybeans that can contain bacteria. Avoid any tofu that is sold loose, as it often is in fruit and vegetable markets, because high levels of bacteria have been found in loose tofu.

Even packaged tofu can contain low levels of bacteria, so the safest way to protect against such harmful bacteria in this otherwise excellent food product is to cook it to an internal temperature of 160°F. Even with bean curd in a sealed package, to be on the safe side while you are pregnant, do not eat tofu raw.

Vegetables and Fruits

Vegetables and fruits play an important role in your diet when you're expecting. They provide a number of essential vitamins which the body can assimilate most easily in their natural form, rather than as vitamin pills. Fruits and vegetables are also very important for digestion and elimination, which can be problematic when you're pregnant since indigestion and constipation are common complaints.

Vegetables and fruits are usually divided into two groups: "vitamin C rich" and "leafy green," which are segregated below. You may notice that there are vegetables which overlap, such as watercress. You can do yourself and your baby twice as much good by concentrating on those foods which occur in both groups!

VITAMIN C-RICH FRUITS AND VEGETABLES

Fruits
* cantaloupe
  (also high in vitamin A)
* grapefruit
* papaya
* guava
* mango
* orange
* pineapple

Juices
* orange
* grapefruit
* tomato
* pineapple
  (the canned form
  has less vitamin C)

Vegetables
* bok choy
* broccoli
* Brussels sprouts
* cabbage
* cauliflower
* greens (collard, kale,
  mustard, Swiss chard,
  turnip)
* peppers (sweet red,
  green, & chili peppers)
* tomatoes
* watercress

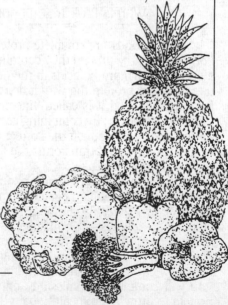

Leafy Green Vegetables

Leafy green vegetables supply vitamins A, E, B6, riboflavin, iron, and magnesium. This food group includes asparagus, bok choy, broccoli, Brussels sprouts, cabbage, dark leafy lettuce (such as romaine, red leaf, chicory, endive, and escarole), scallions, watercress, and greens (such as beet, collard, dandelion, kale, mustard, spinach, Swiss chard, and turnip).

Of course, these foods are also high in fiber and an important part of a pregnant woman's diet because they stimulate sluggish digestion and help prevent constipation and other complaints.

VEGETARIAN PREGNANCY

There's no reason why a pregnant woman can't be just as healthy—or even healthier—on a vegetarian diet than someone who eats meat. A diet without red meat can be perfectly nutritious for you and your baby as long as you sure you're getting enough protein. Any person who is a vegetarian needs to be sure that she is eating a good balance of foods from all the food groups, (other than meat, of course). Many vegetarian diets are not nutritionally sound and don't supply enough protein for general health, much less pregnancy. Please make an extra effort to protect yourself and provide for your growing baby by eating as much high-quality protein as you can every day.

Why Is Protein so Important for Vegetarians?

Animal foods are complete proteins, and when you eat them your body can use the protein they contain. But most plant foods do not have all the essential amino acids in the necessary amounts for your body to use the plant protein the way it does meat. If an amino acid is missing from a plant food it is called "incomplete" because your body cannot utilize it. However, by combining certain foods you can add the missing amino acid(s). If you eat the correct combination of several plant foods at the same meal, it transforms the foods into "complete" proteins that your body then can use.

In order to understand more about amino acids and combining foods to your benefit, you can benefit from reading a classic book called *Diet for a Small Planet*, by Frances Moore Lappé. For easy reference, the chart that follows—"Complementary Plant Protein Sources"—was adapted from that book. Try to keep this chart handy during your entire pregnancy so that you can be certain of eating complete proteins at all times. By eating foods in the combinations listed on the following chart, you will complete the missing amino acids and be taking in enough protein to grow a big, healthy baby.

Are You Getting Enough Protein?

Your main concern should be the quality and quantity of protein you eat. Without enough protein your baby cannot grow adequately and you are more prone to complications during labor. As a vegetarian you have

COMPLEMENTARY PLANT PROTEIN SOURCES

FOOD	AMINO ACIDS DEFICIENT	COMPLEMENTARY PROTEIN
Grains	Isoleucine Lysine	rice + legumes corn + legumes wheat + legumes wheat + peanut + milk wheat + sesame + soybean rice + sesame rice + Brewer's yeast
Legumes	Tryptophan Methionine	legumes + rice beans + wheat beans + corn soybeans + rice + wheat soybeans + corn + milk soybeans + wheat + sesame soybeans + peanuts + sesame soybeans + peanuts + wheat soybeans + sesame + wheat
Nuts and seeds	Isoleucine Lysine	peanuts + sesame + soybeans sesame + beans sesame + soybeans + wheat peanuts + sunflower seeds
Vegetables	Isoleucine Methionine	lima beans, green peas, Brussels sprouts, cauliflower, broccoli + sesame seeds or Brazil nuts or mushrooms greens + millet or converted rice

---

HIGH-PROTEIN SNACKS

* peanut butter on wheat crackers
* any nut butter (peanut, almond, cashew) on celery
* cottage cheese with corn chips
* soy nuts

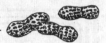

---

to pay special attention to the grams of protein you are taking in during your pregnancy. If you are a "vegan" (a complete vegetarian, who eats no animal products of any kind) you will meet your protein needs differently than if you are a "lacto vegetarian," who eats dairy products, or an "ovo-lacto vegetarian," who eats eggs and dairy. For a chart listing high-protein foods, see pages 94–95.

It's not absolutely necessary for a vegetarian to eat milk and eggs, but she must constantly pay attention to the ingredients of her diet to insure she is getting enough protein.

One way to boost your protein intake is to keep high-protein snacks available whenever possible. That way, whenever you're munching you can feel as though you're making a deposit in your "protein bank"!

DAILY FOOD COMBINATIONS TO ADD

If you are a complete vegetarian:
* 1 cup soybeans and 12 ounces soy milk (or soy yogurt) or
* half cup soybeans and 1 quart soy milk (or soy yogurt) or
* half pound tofu and 1 pint soy milk (or soy yogurt) or
* 1 cup TVP (texturized vegetable protein) and 1 cup soy milk (or soy yogurt)

If you are a lacto-vegetarian or ovo-lacto vegetarian:
* 2 cups cottage cheese
  or
* half cup cottage cheese and 1 quart skim milk (or low-fat yogurt, or buttermilk)

Note: *The food combinations above must be added to your diet every single day of your pregnancy: the body does not store up these ingredients (or any supplements) for a "rainy day."*

HIGH PROTEIN VEGETARIAN FOOD COMBINATIONS

FOOD COMBINATION	GRAMS PROTEIN
3 Tbs. peanut butter 2 slices whole wheat bread	17
4 oz. tofu, 1 cup soybean sprouts 2 Tbs. sesame seeds	19
1 cup lentils 1/2 cup brown rice	18
1 cup split pea soup, 1/2 cup brown rice 1 slice wheat breat	20
1 cup macaroni, 2 oz. cheddar cheese 1 slice wheat bread	24
1 cup Kasha (buckwheat groats) 1 egg, 1 baked potato	19
1 cup egg noodles 1/2 cup creamed cottage cheese	21
1 cup oatmeal, 1 cup skim milk 2 slices wheat bread	19

Ways to Eat Enough Protein Every Day

In addition to your grains and vegetables every day (as shown on the "Vegetarian Food Pyramid" on page 107), you must make a couple of essential additions to your daily diet to assure yourself of getting complete nutrition. What you must add varies depending on how "strict" a vegetarian you are: a lacto vegetarian, an ovo-lacto vegetarian, or a "complete" vegetarian.

Tofu

Tofu, as discussed earlier, is a high-protein food product derived from soybeans that can contain bacteria. Avoid any tofu that is sold loose, as it often is in fruit and vegetable markets, because high levels of bacteria have been found in loose tofu.

Even packaged tofu can contain low levels of bacteria, so the safest way to protect against such harmful bacteria in this otherwise excellent food product is to cook it to an internal temperature of 160°F. So even with bean curd in a sealed package, to be on the safe side while you are pregnant, do not eat tofu raw.

Special Needs of Non-Lacto Vegetarians (Vegans) (No Milk or Dairy)

! If you include no milk or dairy products in your diet, your body requires the following supplements every day:

VEGAN SUPPLEMENTS

* 12 mg calcium
* 400 IU vitamin D

* 4 µg vitamin B12
* 1.5 mg riboflavin

! If you include less than 4 servings of milk or dairy products a day, or if you substitute goat's milk or soybean milk, then your body will need partial supplementation during pregnancy. Talk to your healthcare provider for assistance in determining what quantities of the above 4 supplements are necessary for you personally.
! Make an effort to eat as wide a variety of foods as possible and refer to the chart "Complementary Plant Protein Sources" on page 101 and also look at the information book in the *Diet for a Small Planet* to make sure you're getting complete proteins.

Milk Substitutes for Non-Lacto Vegetarians (Vegans)

Goat's milk and soybean milk are acceptable substitutes for cow's milk, although both are low in vitamin B12. If you want to use soybean curd or milk in place of cow's milk, the following chart gives you a clear comparison of the difference in their nutritional value.

COW'S MILK COMPARED TO SOYBEAN

	CALCIUM	CALORIES	PROTEIN	FAT	IRON
Whole milk (8 oz.)	290 mg	160	8 g	8 g	0.1 mg
Soybean milk (8 oz.)	47	75	8	3	2.5
Soybean curd (tofu) (4 oz.)	155	86	9.5	5	2.5

Possible Deficiencies in a Vegetarian Diet

! *Iodine*—Use iodized salt, not sea salt, which doesn't supply the iodine required by your thyroid gland.
! *Iron*—Generally a vegetarian diet doesn't provide you with the recommended amounts of iron. Enriched grain products will probably increase your intake of iron, but it's likely that you'll need a supplement, too. You should probably have your blood iron levels tested throughout your pregnancy to see how deficient you are. Depending on the results of that iron-level blood test, you will need to take 1 to 3 iron pills (ferrous sulfate or ferrous gluconate, 5 grains) every day, but check with your medical caregiver about this advice first. If your blood is not checked for iron regularly,

THE DANGERS OF SEA SALT

Please put your container of sea salt away during your pregnancy! Many people who patronize health food stores (which usually includes vegetarians) have a special affection for sea salt. However, now while you are pregnant it is preferable to use iodized table salt. During the extra stress of pregnancy your thyroid gland needs the iodine that regular salt provides (see page 96).

you will probably need one tablet 3 times daily, or three 5-grain pills. If you test your iron level only once during pregnancy, do so at about 7 months, because the baby collects more of his iron stores in the last 10 weeks of pregnancy.

It will be easier on your stomach to take the iron tablets with meals. If you find regular pills are hard on your stomach you may find that time-release iron pills are easier on your system. You also should take one 100 mg tablet of vitamin C (ascorbic acid) with each iron pill to help your body absorb the iron. Do not try to take one large daily dose of iron along vitamin C. With one large dose your body won't absorb as much of the iron and you'll lose most of the vitamin C in your urine.

! *Calcium*—Cow's milk and goat's milk are your body's source for calcium. There are plant foods that contain calcium, but the body's ability to assimilate it in this form is limited. A pregnant woman—especially in the last half of pregnancy and during breast-feeding—needs to supplement about 1 gram (15 grains) of calcium every day. (To make up 1 gram, you can take two 500-mg tablets or three 5-grain tablets.) *Calcium gluconate* is the most easily absorbed form of calcium. If you take calcium lactate, you'll need about twice as much for equal absorption!

The baby is calcifying his bones in the last half of pregnancy: if there is no surplus calcium available, the baby will take it from *your* bones. If you're not a lacto-vegetarian, you need 1 gram a day for the second half of your pregnancy and when you are breast-feeding.

! *Vitamin D*—Fortified cow's milk or soy milk supplies vitamin D, but if you aren't getting those, make sure you get a vitamin D supplement. However, do not add more than 400 IUs of vitamin D daily (see page 111 "Warnings About Vitamins").

! *Riboflavin*—Milk is the best source, so a vegans may not have enough of this vitamin in her system. There are only limited amounts of riboflavin in whole-grain and enriched breads and cereals, and in legumes, nuts, and some vegetables.

! *Vitamin B12*—Milk and animal foods supply this nutrient. A deficiency of this vitamin can cause serious complications, so be sure to get a supplement if you don't drink milk.

Vegetarian Daily Food Pyramid

The following food pyramid shows you the "building blocks" that a vegetarian needs for a healthy pregnancy. Vegans (those who don't eat eggs or dairy products) need to pay special attention to the top of the pyramid. Notice the recommended number of servings from each level of the pyramid and learn to incorporate this information into your food choices every day. All vegetarians should make an effort to "build" one of these complete food pyramids each day for the best possible pregnancy, labor, and delivery.

VEGETARIAN FOOD PYRAMID

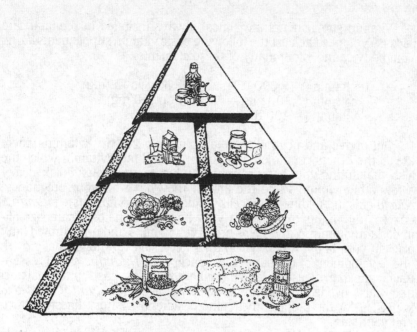

Base of the pyramid (6 to 10 servings)
- Bread
- Cereals
- Pasta
- Rice
- Corn
- Potatoes
- Green peas

Two sides of the second level
- Vegetables (2 to 4 servings)
- Fruits (2 to 4 servings)

Two sides of the upper level
- Milk and milk substitutes (2 to 4)
- Protein (2 to 4)

Top of the pyramid (for vegans)
- Vegetable oil (2 T.)
- Blackstrap molasses (1 T.)
- Brewer's yeast (1 T.)

VITAMINS

Vitamin supplements are almost always included in prenatal care because you need at least the following basic vitamin supplements *daily*. Your body cannot store many of these elements.

- vitamin A (6,000 IU)
- calcium (1,200 mg)
- vitamin D (400 IU)
- folic acid (.8 mg)
- iron (60 mg)

But above and beyond these absolutely necessary vitamins, there are all the others contained in a good prenatal multivitamin which are also vital during your baby's formation. Just to give you a quick idea of a few other vitamins and the impact they have on your pregnancy: *Niacin* aids in building brain cells (as do all the B vitamins). *Vitamin E* governs the amount of oxygen your body uses, helps metabolize all-important vitamin A and helps preserve vitamins and unsaturated fatty acids in your body. *Riboflavin (B2)* is necessary for the normal growth and development of the baby from conception. *Thiamine (B1)* is essential for appetite, digestion, and muscular tone in the gastrointestinal tract and is also needed for fertility, growth, and lactation. *Pantothenic acid* is needed for the proper functioning of adrenal glands, digestive tract, and your skin.

Vitamin C is so important it's a one-man band! It helps your body fight infection, controls poisons produced by bacteria and viruses, strengthens capillary and cell walls, builds a strong placenta, helps absorb iron from the intestines and detoxifies junk foods, and is important in healing wounds. Smokers require larger amounts of vitamin C, about 25 mg per cigarette smoked.

Vitamin C

A new study shows that 200 mg is the amount of vitamin C that the average person's body needs every day. Previously, 60 mg a day was thought to be enough. This study showed that saturating your body with supplements of up to 1,000 mg of vitamin C daily is of no use, since the body cannot absorb more than around 200 mg.

As with all vitamins, the best source is in your diet, not from vitamin tablets. Vitamin C is actually one of the easier nutrients to supply through foods. The following chart shows the foods that are the best dietary sources of this essential nutrient.

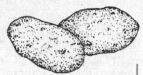

BEST SOURCES OF VITAMIN C

Vegetables (1 cup)	*Milligrams of Vitamin C*
sweet peppers	190
broccoli	98
brussels sprouts	96
kohlrabi	88
pea pods	76
cauliflower	68
potato (with skin)	58
rutabaga	52
kale	54
tomato	50
sweet potato	49

Fruits and Juices (1 Cup)	
guava, fresh juice	330
cranberry juice cocktail	134
orange, fresh juice	124
orange, juice from concentrate	96
grapefruit, fresh juice	94
papaya	86
orange, canned juice	86
strawberries, fresh	84
grapefruit, 1 fruit	82
orange, 1 navel	80
grapefruit, sections with juice	79
kiwi, one fruit	75
grapefruit, canned juice	72
cantaloupe	68
raspberries	62
grape juice, from concentrate	60
tangerine, 1 fruit	52
mango, 1 fruit	46
tomato juice	44
honeydew	42

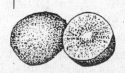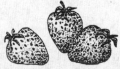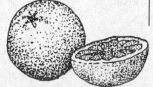

Why Take Vitamins if You Eat Really Well?

Perhaps you don't think you need to take a multivitamin if you are conscientious about eating a well-balanced diet, but only a supplement can assure you of getting the vitamins you need in the quantities necessary for pregnancy. You are right if you believe that food is the best possible source of vitamins—in theory that is true—but in actuality, how much do you know about the food you eat? Unless you're growing it yourself, there's no way to be sure of the freshness of your food and therefore its vitamin content. And if you eat out frequently in restaurants, it's even more difficult to determine how long "fresh" foods have been refrigerated or frozen, both of which reduce the amount of vitamins in foods.

In the modern world there's also the question of how to accomplish a perfectly balanced diet *every single day*: who can be certain of accomplishing that with a busy schedule and eating on the run? In addition, if you have morning sickness there are those days when you're nauseated and lucky if you can get *anything* down! So taking a vitamin supplement is a safeguard that every pregnant woman needs, no matter how well she eats.

No Diet Has Enough Iron & Folic Acid

Regardless of how carefully you plan your pregnancy diet, there's no way to eat enough iron-rich food every day (see pages 85–87 for more about iron). You have to be sure you get 60 mg daily.

Folic acid (also called "folacin") is one of the B vitamins that your body depends on for a successful pregnancy. It is essential for protein synthesis in early pregnancy and for blood formation and the manufacture of new cells.

Your body's need for folacin is doubled (to 0.8 mg) when you're carrying a child. Without a supplement it's common for women to have deficiencies of folic acid, which can result in miscarriage or damage to the unborn child. There are several conditions which can interfere with your body's ability to use folic acid: infection, drinking alcoholic beverages, and certain medications, in particular Dilantin (used to in salt form to treat epilepsy).

WARNING: If you were taking birth control pills until right before you conceived, it is likely that you have a folic acid deficiency going into the pregnancy. Supplements are even more important for women in this situation.

What Is Vitamin "K"?

Until getting pregnant you may not have heard of vitamin K. It is an antihemorrhagic vitamin which is necessary for blood clotting.

WARNINGS ABOUT VITAMINS

Vitamin A
* In excess may cause birth defects
* Is chemically related to a compound in acne medicine that can cause cleft palate, heart defects and brain abnormalities
* Do not take more than 6,000 IUs daily

Vitamin B6 (Pyridoxine)
* Can cause nerve problems in mother
* Do not take more than 200 mg a day

Vitamin C
* This vitamin is an active metabolic agent: the full effect of large doses on the infant isn't known
* May impair fetal bone development
* Can cause scurvy in the newborn
* Do not take more than 1 gram (1,000 mg) a day

Vitamin D
* Can cause mental retardation in baby
* Can cause heart or bone defects in baby
* Do not take more than 400 IUs daily

Vitamin E
* Raises blood pressure if you're not used to it
* Women with high blood pressure or a rheumatic heart condition should restrict intake to under 150 IUs daily
* For all other women, do not take more than 800 IUs daily

Vitamin K
* Can cause jaundice in newborn, which may damage baby's nervous system
* Available by prescription only

Vitamin K doesn't come directly from food, it is synthesized by stomach bacteria. Deficiencies are rare because intestinal bacteria manufacture it for the baby, but the continued use of antibiotics may upset the normal bacterial environment of the intestines and interfere with the natural production of vitamin K.

The newborn's intestines do not contain the K-producing bacteria at birth—it takes a few days before the bacteria are available to manufacture vitamin K. A vitamin K injection is usually given to babies when they are born to guard against the possibility of hemorrhage.

If Vitamins Are Good, More Must Be Better?

Do not make the mistake of thinking that the more vitamins you take, the better it will be for your baby. Just the opposite is true. Vitamins are powerful elements—we know that when we see the problems from a deficiency—but any vitamin taken in excess may be the cause of birth defects.

Especially with vitamins A and D there is a danger of taking too much: unlike other vitamins, your body cannot excrete A and D if they are taken in excessive amounts. *Any* vitamin can be harmful or dangerous if taken in large dosages.

VITAMIN DIRECTORY

VITAMIN A

Foods
* fortified whole milk
* fortified margarine
* butter
* egg yolk
* fish liver oils
* liver and kidney
* deep green and yellow vegetables (cooked vegetables provide A more readily than raw ones)

Daily requirement
* 6,000 IU during pregnancy
* 8,000 IU when breast-feeding

What it does
* builds resistance to infection
* functions in vision
* helps formation of tooth enamel, hair, and fingernails
* necessary for proper growth and function of the thyroid gland

VITAMIN DIRECTORY (*cont.*)

VITAMIN B
(includes all vitamins B1 through B12, including niacin)

Foods
* Brewer's yeast:
  • purchase at a health food store
  • start out with a teaspoon in juice and build up to one tablespoon
  • do not use live yeast
* bread
* whole grains
* wheat germ
* liver

What it does
* prevents nervousness
* helps skin problems
* provides energy
* prevents constipation

B1 (THIAMINE)

Foods
* pork and pork products
* liver, heart, and kidney
* peas and beans
* wheat germ

Daily requirement
* 1.2 mg in pregnancy
* 1.5 mg while breast-feeding

What it does
* essential for appetite and digestion
* needed for fertility, growth, and breast-feeding
* needed during illness and infection

B2 (RIBOFLAVIN)

Foods
* milk—each quart contains 2 mg

Daily requirement
* 5 to 10 mg

What it does
* necessary for normal growth and development of the baby from conception

VITAMIN DIRECTORY (*cont.*)

NIACIN

Foods	✳ liver
	✳ beef
	✳ poultry
	✳ tuna
	✳ milk
	✳ peanuts and almonds
	✳ brown rice
	✳ wheat
	✳ peas
Daily requirement	✳ 20 to 50 mg
What it does	✳ prevents infections and bleeding of gums

B6 (PYRIDOXINE)

Foods	✳ yeast
	✳ liver
	✳ wheat germ
	✳ whole-grain bread
	✳ cereal
	✳ green beans and leafy green vegetables
	✳ bananas
	✳ meat and fish
	✳ nuts
	✳ potatoes
Daily requirement	✳ 2 to 20 mg
What it does	✳ essential for the metabolism of fats
	✳ produces antibodies that fight disease

B12 (COBALAMIN)

Foods	✳ yeast	✳ meat and fish
	✳ liver	✳ eggs
	✳ wheat germ	✳ milk
	✳ whole grains	✳ oysters
	✳ kidneys	
Daily requirement	✳ 8 to 15 mg	
What it does	✳ essential for development of red blood cells	

VITAMIN DIRECTORY (*cont.*)

VITAMIN C

Foods
* citrus fruits
* cantaloupe
* strawberries
* green and red bell peppers
* broccoli
* cauliflower
* tomatoes
* potatoes
  (Overcooking or cooking vegetables in too much water destroys the vitamin C. Ascorbic acid [synthetic] is identical to natural vitamin C.)

Daily requirement
* 80 mg minimum
* do not exceed 1 gram
* stress, alcohol, smoking, the pill, and aspirin all interfere with absorption and levels in the body
* smokers require larger amounts, about 25 mg per cigarette
* ascorbic acid (synthetic) is identical to natural vitamin C

What it does
* helps the body resist infection

CALCIUM

Foods
* milk
* stone-ground grains
* vitamin C helps in absorption

Daily requirement
* 1,200 mg
* pregnant women give more calcium to the baby than they're taking in
* for better absorption take calcium gluconate or calcium lactate pills on an empty stomach with sour milk, yogurt, or an acid fruit or juice

What it does
* builds baby's bones and teeth

VITAMIN DIRECTORY (*cont.*)

VITAMIN D

Foods	* vitamin D-fortified milk * fish liver oils * mackerel, salmon, tuna, sardines, and herring * another source is sunshine
Daily requirement	* 400 IU * varies with exposure to the sun and your complexion: dark-skinned people need more sun to manufacture vitamin D
What it does	* helps absorption of calcium from the blood into tissue and bone cells

VITAMIN E

Foods	* whole grains * peanuts * corn * eggs
Daily requirement	* 30 mg
What it does	* governs the amount of oxygen the body uses * promotes healing

FOLIC ACID

Foods	* liver * leafy green vegetables * broccoli and asparagus * peanuts
Daily requirement	* 800 micrograms (0.8 mg) (The body does not store folic acid so 0.8 mg *must* be taken every day.)
What it does	* essential for blood formation and formation of new cells

IODINE

Foods	* iodized salt
Daily requirement	* season food to taste with iodized salt
What it does	* helps thyroid gland function properly, regulating your metabolism

VITAMIN DIRECTORY (*cont.*)

IRON

Foods	✳ liver (or liver pills, if you hate liver) ✳ fish and meat ✳ egg yolks ✳ raisins ✳ dark molasses
Daily requirement	✳ 30 to 60 mg ✳ many young women are iron-deficient before pregnancy ✳ more iron is needed in the second half of pregnancy
What it does	✳ iron is the main component of blood hemoglobin that carries oxygen to the baby and your cells ✳ the baby draws on your supply to store iron in its liver to carry it through its milk diet during the first four to six months of independent life

VITAMIN K

Foods	✳ vitamin K doesn't come directly from food—it's synthesized by stomach bacteria
Daily requirement	✳ for baby: a vitamin K injection is usually given to babies at birth to guard against hemorrhage
What it does	✳ necessary for normal blood clotting

ZINC

Foods	✳ seafood ✳ liver ✳ beets ✳ barley ✳ carrots ✳ cabbage
Daily requirement	✳ minimum 15 mg
What it does	✳ promotes healthy function of organs ✳ promotes wound healing

Is Your Water Safe?

It's a sad comment on what we've done to our world when a person can't safely take a drink of water nowadays! But that's the way it is. When you're pregnant, you don't really have the choice of feeling cynical and saying, "Oh well, since *everything's* bad for me, I'll just 'live dangerously' and pour myself a glass of water!" When you're carrying a child, the things said jokingly may be closer to the truth than you might want to admit. I do not want to make you afraid of putting anything in your mouth, but there *are* potential hazards in your water supply that you need to know about. Before you get pregnant—and of course during pregnancy—you have to protect yourself from contaminated water. (And if you're planning on feeding your baby with powdered formula later on, you might want to use bottled water to mix it.)

Ordinary tap water all over the United States can contain organic chemicals, mutagens and/or carcinogens (substances that cause cancer). In some areas, industrial chemicals can have been discharged into the surface water supply, or pesticides like DDT may have gone into the soil and from there into the underground water supply. You can have your tap water tested to see whether your own water has been polluted. However, the most widespread danger in water from the tap is lead. Even at fairly low levels, lead can cause serious developmental problems in the fetus and health problems later for an infant who drinks the contaminated water.

WHERE'S THE LEAD COMING FROM?

There are a variety of ways that lead can get into your household water. It isn't always easy to discover the source of the lead: you may require the advice of a home inspector. Some of the sources of lead are:

! *If you have public water* it may pass through lead pipe service lines from the town's water mains.

! *If you have an older house* the problem can be in your pipes, which may have lead or solder with a high lead content.

! *Lead can build up overnight* while the water sits in your indoor plumbing, waiting for you to turn on the tap.

! *New faucets frequently contain lead*, which contaminates the water during early usage. If you have a new house or new sinks, the manufacturer should be able to provide data on the amount of lead their product leaks.

! *If you have well water* the lead can come from the pump. See more on well water in this section.

! *A brand-new house* has as much chance of having contaminated water as does one that is a hundred years old.

IS THERE A "SAFE" LEVEL OF LEAD IN WATER?

It is your own decision whether there is an amount of lead in your water that you find acceptable. Considering the dangers of lead, it would appear to be a little like drinking alcohol: it causes serious damage to the baby, but maybe you can get away with some small amount (as yet undetermined). The Environmental Protection Agency (EPA) has stated that lead at less than 15 parts per billion of lead in water can be considered safe. Yet consumer groups and environmental watchdogs believe that 10 parts per billion, or even 5 parts per billion, is a "safer" amount, and many pediatricians tend to agree with this.

GET YOUR OWN WATER TESTED

It seems logical that the only way to be sure about lead or other contamination in your water system is to have it tested. You can call the EPA toll free at 1-800-426-4791 for the name of state-certified laboratories near you, and brochures with more information. The cost of a test for lead can be anywhere from $20 to $70 or more, depending on the individual lab. The laboratory should be able to tell you what other water contaminants they can assess.

If you are living in a brand-new house or apartment that has been inspected for a "certificate of occupancy" this does not mean that your water has gotten a clean bill of health. The testing done when a house is built or purchased is not sufficient: these tests ordinarily look for bacteria, not lead or other toxic materials in the water supply.

WELL WATER CAN BE DANGEROUS

The U.S. government has advised that people with new submersible pumps with lead-alloy parts should drink bottled water. Lab tests have shown that these pumps, especially when they are new, are likely to leak high quantities of lead. As a precaution you and your family should drink only bottled water, at least until your home water supply is tested.

Millions of Americans use well water: anyone in their fertile years or with small children is advised to have their water tested. If your water comes from your own well (or is serviced by public water from a well) the pump may be putting lead into the water. Some submersible well pumps are made of lead alloys which can leak the toxic metal into your household water.

First you have to find out whether lead that may be in your water is coming from the well rather than from the indoor plumbing (pipes and faucets). The best way to test is to take a water sample directly from the containment tank at midmorning. The way you do this is by letting the tap run for 30 seconds before collecting the water sample.

WAYS TO PROTECT YOURSELF FROM LEAD IN THE WATER

! "First draw" water means from a tap where the water has rested overnight. This is the water that is often the most contaminated, but testing should show whether in your case the lead occurs consistently only in the "first draw" water. In this case, the advice is usually to run any faucet for a full minute (count 60 seconds!) before using the water.
! Run any faucet for 60 full seconds if it has not been used for many hours.
! Keep a pitcher of "safe" water in the refrigerator for drinking and cooking so that no one will use "first draw" water.
! Consider replacing a well pump that contains lead alloys.
! If the lead level of your water is high and can't be traced to other parts of the plumbing in your house, it's easy to find a plastic or stainless steel pump as a replacement.

HOW TO GET THE LEAD OUT OF YOUR WATER

There are a variety of filters available that can remove most of the lead from drinking water. The cost ranges from $100 to $1,000. Evaluations of water filters have shown that the most effective ones are the reverse-osmosis type, which are expensive. If your lead level is low, simple filters and distillers, including countertop models or those that attach to faucets, may be sufficient.

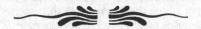

CHAPTER FIVE

The Changes in Your Body

There are so many physical changes you go through when you're pregnant, and so many ways that the baby seems to take charge of your body. Some days you may even feel you are at his mercy—when he kicks you in the ribs and you have to make constant trips to the bathroom and all you want to do is sleep or eat salty pretzels! If it makes you feel any better, you're not alone: everybody has at least some of the physical symptoms that are covered in this chapter. You'll find all the moans and groans of pregnancy here, along with all the known remedies you can try for relief, listed alphabetically for easy access.

With these enormous changes taking place in your body it's no wonder that you may be experiencing any number of discomforts. Most of the listings that follow are normal—and a small price to pay for the little bundle of joy who will be the pot at the end of that rainbow! Although minor problems can be dealt with, that doesn't mean that you should just *assume* that the discomforts are natural. Pregnancy is a normal, healthy state that should be reasonably pleasant for a healthy woman. Pain, extreme fatigue, or distress are signals to check in with a doctor. *Do not simply dismiss discomforts!* This chapter helps you understand and cope with lesser complaints, but you shouldn't hesitate to call your doctor if you have any doubts or further questions.

At the end of this chapter, you will find a chart "Danger Signs During Pregnancy," which outlines the symptoms that something may be going wrong in your pregnancy. *Notify your doctor or midwife right away if you have any of these symptoms.* By seeking professional help immediately you may be able to avoid serious problems for yourself or the baby.

ABDOMINAL PAIN

Most women experience some pain in their abdomen. It's probably caused by stretching of the muscles and ligaments that support the uterus. The discomfort may be in the form of cramps or sharp stabbing pains. It can be brief or may last for several hours.

NOTE: Since abdominal pain can also be a sign of problems, if you have any doubts you should call your doctor or midwife and describe the symptoms.

Helpful Hints About Abdominal Pain

➤ Sitting in a comfortable chair or lying down should help.
➤ If the pain is intermittent (it comes and goes, or it isn't persistent) it is probably muscles stretching.
➤ There's no need to worry if you have no fever, bleeding, or unusual symptoms.
➤ Be sure to mention the pain when you next have a prenatal checkup.

ALLERGIES

Pregnancy is a major stress on the body that can aggravate allergic conditions you already have. In some women, being pregnant causes them to develop allergic reactions for the first time. Preventing allergic reactions is the best way to deal with them—if you can determine what you're reacting to, avoid it if you can! (Of course, if your problem is the pollen season, or your beloved cat, there's not much you can do to prevent contact.) See the section on "Stuffy Nose" (page 145) for more advice.

In case you've never had allergies before, here are some of the things that your body may be reacting to:

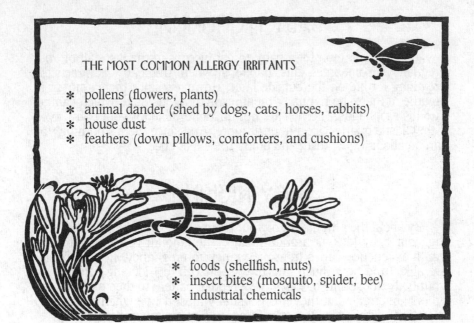

THE MOST COMMON ALLERGY IRRITANTS

* pollens (flowers, plants)
* animal dander (shed by dogs, cats, horses, rabbits)
* house dust
* feathers (down pillows, comforters, and cushions)

* foods (shellfish, nuts)
* insect bites (mosquito, spider, bee)
* industrial chemicals

Helpful Hints About Allergies

➢ If you have severe allergies, consult your doctor early in pregnancy about managing them. An asthma attack or an anaphylactic reaction is dangerous because it can deprive your baby of oxygen.

➢ If appropriate to your climate, use air conditioning in your house and car to help filter the air.

➢ Keep your house as dust-free as possible with frequent vacuuming.

➢ Keep an electric air filter running all the time in the rooms you're in most.

➢ Do not smoke or spend time in rooms with smoke. Whatever your allergies, smoking or being in a smoke-filled room can make the allergic reaction worse. If there are smokers around you (at home or work), keep an air filter running to remove the second hand smoke.

➢ Stay indoors when pollen counts are high.

➢ Use hypoallergenic bed pillows and bedding.

➢ Do not take any cold or allergy medicine such as Contac or Allerest: they contain antihistamines.

➢ Always consult a doctor before taking any medication.

➢ Nose sprays and drops are not safe during pregnancy; only those made of saline (salt water) can be used.

➢ If you lose a lot of fluids due to sneezing or a runny nose, drink plenty of fluids to compensate.

BABY HICCUPING

It's quite common for a baby to get hiccups in the last half of your pregnancy. Sometimes this happens when the baby is practicing breathing for life on the outside later. However, since there's no air to breathe in there, he naturally breathes in amniotic fluid, which can get into his esophagus. Hiccups are not uncomfortable for your baby, even if they last a quarter of an hour or more. And since there's nothing you can do about it, just relax and enjoy the experience.

BABY KICKING

By about the fifth month of your pregnancy, you'll probably be feeling your baby kicking around inside. The amount of movement that you'll experience varies from pregnancy to pregnancy: no two babies are alike, and how much and how soon you feel kicking depends on your body, too. Some babies have a regular pattern to their exercise and others are erratic, but the fetus is usually most active when the mother is resting—either at night, or before you first get up in the morning.

Helpful Hints About Kicking

➤ Try shifting your position if the kicking is uncomfortable for you.
➤ Think of the baby's kicking as a sign of her good health, getting her ready for life on the outside.
➤ CALL YOUR DOCTOR if—after the thirtieth week of pregnancy— the baby suddenly moves around a lot less during any 24-hour period.

BACKACHE

Lower backache is often the result from walking and sitting improperly. The uterus is moored by two sets of ligaments: the round ligaments insert into the groin on the left and right, in front of the birth canal; the uterosacral ligaments attach just below the small of your back to each side of the bony structure of the pelvis. Another cause of backache, especially later in pregnancy, is the increased weight you're carrying in front. The way you walk, sit, and stand can aggravate or help avoid backache.

Leg & Lower Back Pain (Sciatica)

You may have felt pain in your lower back, buttocks and/or running down one or both legs. This is because as your uterus gets larger it can put pressure on the sciatic nerve in your back. The pain will usually pass as the growing baby changes position, although for some unlucky women it can bother them until the baby is born.

➤ Applying a heating pad to the area can give you relief.
➤ Get off your feet as much you can; rest whenever possible.
➤ Find a masseuse who is familiar with the pregnant body and can give you therapeutic massage therapy.
➤ If the pain is severe your doctor may suggest bed rest for a few days or recommend special exercises.

Helpful Hints About Backache

➤ *Don't stand in one place or position too long.* If you cannot move around, then try putting one foot forward with all your weight on it and then switching to the other leg.
➤ *Lean forward when standing* at a kitchen counter, ironing board, worktable, etc. Bend your knees slightly and support your weight on your hands or elbows.
➤ *When you lie down put a small pillow under your side at waist level.* This is a "side relaxation position," which keeps your shoulders and hips in proper alignment while you're sleeping.
➤ *Put a footstool under your feet while you're sitting.* To relieve backache your knees should be at a slightly higher level than your hips. (If you don't have a footstool, use a box or blocks of wood.)
➤ *Walk and sit properly to prevent backache.* Make a mental note to tuck in your buttocks and abdomen every time you rise from sitting; good posture when you walk (with your hips tucked well in) is also insurance against lower backache.
➤ *Doing the "pelvic rock" relieves backache.* Kneel on all fours with your elbows straight, legs slightly apart. Inhale as you curl your back up and tuck your head under; exhale as you relax your back. Do this exercise 20 times before you lie down to take a rest or sleep; it aids circulation while you're lying down.

BLEEDING & SPOTTING

It is normal to have pink-stained or red-streaked mucus that occurs right after intercourse or after a vaginal examination by your doctor. If you have brownish-tinged mucus or spotting that occurs 48 hours after intercourse or vaginal exam, that is normal too. *But if you have any doubts, or if you have signs of more bleeding than described above, call your doctor.* Bleeding is one of the symptoms of miscarriage; the sooner your doctor knows about it, the greater the chance of averting a problem.

BODY CHANGES

There are many changes that your body will go through when you get pregnant: some of these changes will last only as long as the pregnancy itself, but some will be with you forever. As you can see, you shouldn't go buying a lot of new shoes right before you get pregnant or even during pregnancy, because they probably won't fit afterwards.

Permanent Changes to Your Body:

- Area around nipples may darken and get broader.
- Shoe size can increase by half a size.
- A dark line appears downward from your belly button.
- Your genitals may darken.
- Stretch marks may appear on your abdomen, thighs, and breasts.
- Your rib cage increases in size to give the lungs more space: you may need a larger bra or blouse size.

Temporary Changes to Your Body:

- Your blood volume increases by 25%, so your heart has to work harder.
- All the ligaments in your body stretch.
- Your breasts get larger and the veins more prominent.
- Your lungs work more effectively.
- Your digestive system uses food more efficiently.

BREASTS

Your breasts will swell during pregnancy, sometimes as much as three cup sizes! This is because the milk glands are beginning to develop. It is normal for your breasts to tingle, throb, or hurt. The veins often become more prominent because of the increased blood supply to the breasts. The areola (the area around the nipple) may darken and become broader due to hormonal changes. The increased color around your nipples (and the line on your abdomen down from your belly button) do not go away right after pregnancy.

Nipple secretion is common later in pregnancy. The sticky, yellowish watery secretion is colostrum, which will be your baby's first food. Colostrum comes in before your milk supply begins. As your due date gets near, the secretion takes on an opaque, whitish look which resembles milk. If you want to, you can gently express the colostrum from your nipples.

Helpful Hints About Your Breasts

➤ A lack of support *during pregnancy* is what causes breasts to sag—most of the weight gained by the breasts comes in the early months.

➤ Breast-feeding is often blamed for sagging bosoms, but they actually result from insufficient support in the first and second trimesters.

➤ Wear a support bra all through pregnancy. If your breasts get *very* large, it's a good idea to wear a bra even when you're sleeping.

➤ Lumpy breasts are quite common during pregnancy. Don't be alarmed.

➤ However, if a lump feels suspicious in any way (it is hard or stationary or causes dimpling of the overlying skin) bring it to your doctor's attention.

➤ In some cases your doctor may want to screen for breast cancer.

➤ Screening can be done with diaphanography, which illuminates the breast with light. This causes no harm to the fetus.

➤ If the lump seems suspicious, a biopsy of the breast may be necessary: this is not dangerous to the fetus.

CONSTIPATION

Constipation is a common complaint of pregnancy, when the mother's bowels are sluggish. The is the pressure of the uterus on the bowels. Also, the increased level of progesterone in your system relaxes all smooth muscles, which makes the bowels less efficient. However, being "normal" does not mean having a daily bowel movement—during pregnancy it may be sufficient for a woman to have a bowel movement every second or third day. Constipation is actually the passing of hard stool, not, as many people think, having infrequent bowel movements (unless they also happen to be hard). As long as the stools are not watery, loose, or bloody there is no need to be concerned.

Helpful Hints About Constipation

➤ Eat plenty of fresh fruit, which has a laxative effect as well as being nourishing. Apples have the greatest laxative action, along with dried fruits such as prunes, figs, dates and raisins. It is especially helpful eaten at night.

➤ Green vegetables add roughage to your diet, which stimulates the intestines. Raw or lightly cooked vegetables with the skin left on are best for digestion.

➤ Plenty of fluids are very helpful. Also, your body requires more liquids now, so drink at least 6 to 8 glasses of fluids every day.

➤ A cup of hot water (with lemon juice or rind) in the morning and before going to bed is helpful for some people.

➤ Fiber from whole-grain breads, bran muffins, and cereal helps stimulate your intestines.

➤ Exercise, even if it's only walking, helps constipation.

➤ Licorice candy has a mild cathartic action which sometimes gives relief.

➤ Natural fiber laxatives that mix with liquid (such as Metamucil and Peridiem) have none of the drawbacks of chemical laxatives and can be used as often as you want. Some people find they work well if taken before bed, others prefer taking them in the morning. Experiment to see which works best for you.

➤ Regularity is important. Regular bowel movements also help control intestinal gas. Try to establish a set time to move your bowels: train yourself to go to the bathroom right after breakfast, for example.

➤ Some people find it easier to move their bowels if their feet are elevated while sitting on the toilet (which releases the anus). You might want to try using a footstool or box.

CONTRACTIONS OF THE UTERUS (BRAXTON-HICKS)

Periodic contractions of your uterus, which may begin near the end of your second trimester, are called "Braxton-Hicks" contractions. These contractions serve two purposes: they circulate blood to the placental site, and more important, they exercise and strengthen your uterus for labor. These contractions may also be responsible for early effacement (thinning out) and dilation (opening up) of your cervix before labor actually begins.

These contractions begin with a tightening feeling in the top of your uterus and gradually spread downward until the whole uterus is hard—and then it relaxes. If you feel an isolated lump or knob, that's probably just the baby stretching out her legs. To tell whether you're having a Braxton-Hicks contraction, feel your entire uterus with both your hands to know whether the entire uterus is involved. You might want to take advantage of these contractions later in pregnancy to practice the breathing from your childbirth education classes.

DAIRY INTOLERANCE

Milk and milk products are highly recommended for women during pregnancy because of the calcium they contain. Some people are "lactose intolerant," meaning they have difficulty in digesting the milk sugar lactose. However, if you cannot tolerate milk, or if you just dislike the taste of it, there are many ways you can get calcium (see page 88).

Helpful Hints About Dairy Intolerance

➤ Natural cheeses, especially fermented cheeses, have very little lactose. Try eating those.
➤ Cultured milk products such as yogurt and buttermilk (brands without added milk solids) have reduced amounts of lactose.
➤ Many people with lactose intolerance are able to tolerate other dairy products, such as Lactaid brand milk, which have 70% of the lactose converted to a more easily digestible form.

DIZZINESS, FEELING FAINT

Dizziness is most common in the second trimester, when your enlarged uterus presses on major blood vessels, causing a drop in your blood pressure. Hormonal changes cause a relaxation of the blood vessels, so blood pools in the legs, the furthest point from your head. Also, low blood sugar from going too long without food can be another reason for feeling dizzy.

The size and position of the baby determine how dizzy you might feel, or the extent of fainting, or feeling as though you might. Fainting is quite rare and, even if it happens, will not harm your baby.

NOTE: Report any dizziness to your doctor, who can decide whether or not it may be a sign of a problem.

Helpful Hints About Dizziness

➤ When you're changing positions, always get up gradually, especially from a sitting or lying position. Faintness is often caused by standing or sitting up too quickly.
➤ Generally make a point of moving slowly: you want to avoid creating blood pressure changes.
➤ Eat more frequent, smaller meals.
➤ Carry snacks with natural sugar, such as fruit, fruit rolls (check the ingredients), or raisins to raise your blood sugar.
➤ If you're in a crowded or warm environment that makes you

feel woozy, open a window and sit near it or get out into the fresh air.

➤ Wear clothes that are loose around the neck and waist. Avoid restrictive clothing that forms tight bands, which might cut off circulation.

➤ If you feel light-headed, or think you're going to faint, lie down with your feet elevated, or sit with your head down between your knees until the dizziness passes.

EYESIGHT

During pregnancy there may be changes in your vision and/or the comfort of your contact lenses. You may not see as well; your vision may seem less sharp. These changes are temporary and are probably related to fluid retention. Hard contact lenses can even become so uncomfortable that you can't wear them. Ask your ophthalmologist if you would be a candidate for soft lenses and consider switching for now, or just using your glasses until after the baby is born.

WARNING: Some vision problems are a sign of serious problems during pregnancy. If you experience blurring, dimming, double vision, or spots in front of your eyes that lasts for more than two hours, contact your doctor immediately!

FATIGUE

You're most likely to feel fatigued early in pregnancy, when you may feel as though you need several hours of extra sleep a day. The reason for feeling tired or low energy is that your body is making the necessary adjustments to pregnancy, the way it did to your growth during adolescence (when sleep requirements are also high). You may also have less energy in the first trimester, while the placenta is being formed, because it is not complete until the end of the third month.

Fatigue can increase in the first trimester from a deficiency in iron or protein. Make sure that you are filling all your nutritional requirements. Common signs of fatigue are: impatience, irritability, inability to concentrate, and loss of interest in sexual activity.

Helpful Hints About Fatigue

➤ Don't fight the fatigue! If you're usually an active, energetic person, you may be disconcerted by your diminished energy level. Just accept it: think of it as your baby asserting his needs (now is a good time to get used to having your life disrupted!).

➤ Listen to what your body is telling you: slow down, take it easy, pace yourself. Overexertion when you feel fatigued can harm your baby.

➤ Go to bed earlier. You should get as many hours of sleep as you need so you wake up feeling rested.
➤ Take naps: even if you can't take a long nap, just 5 or 10 minutes with your feet up and your eyes closed can be refreshing.
➤ Let other people relieve you of some of your chores and obligations, or just choose which ones you'll have to skip for now.
➤ Don't feel guilty about sleeping more! It's the old American work ethic making you worry that you're being "lazy," but your body *needs* the rest. When your body was going through changes as a teenager, you didn't feel guilty about sleeping a lot—so don't now!
➤ Be aware of the side effects of feeling fatigued so that you aren't confused by your behavior during the first trimester.
➤ If you continue to feel fatigued after careful resting, tell your doctor. It may be a sign of anemia.

FOOD: AVERSIONS & CRAVINGS

Food cravings are the cartoon joke of pregnancy—you've heard about pickles, ice cream, and all that. It was once believed that when a person had food cravings, they were steering her toward foods that her body needed. But the truth is, these signals are not reliable: since when does a pregnant body *absolutely need* a hot fudge sundae? As much as you might wish it to be true, cravings are *not* the body's natural way of making up for a nutritional imbalance. If it were true, pregnant women would go around craving liver to make up for their iron deficiencies!

It is true that your taste for certain foods may change while you're pregnant. It's also true that a mineral deficiency can trigger food cravings, but the item you crave may not be what's missing in your diet. Most food cravings disappear by the fourth month. If you do feel overcome by cravings, concentrate on eating balanced meals and try getting lots of tomato juice and fish—both are good sources of trace elements that just might be missing from your diet.

This brings up another point about food cravings: they may not be about food at all. If you find yourself communicating cravings to your partner at awkward times, like late at night, the cravings may be an attention-getting device. What you are craving may not be food: you may not realize that what you desire is time or attention or affection or support from your mate. If this might be true, find a quiet time that you two can talk about this. It's already difficult for a man to deal with the physical and emotional changes that a woman goes through during pregnancy—don't make it any harder for both of you by setting up situations with food cravings whereby he has to prove his devotion by going on midnight missions to find a store that carries your favorite frozen chocolate cheesecake!

Helpful Hints About Food Cravings

➤ If the food you crave is nutritious, eat it.
➤ If you crave something that you know isn't good for you or your baby, try to find a replacement that will satisfy you.
➤ Beware of the salty pregnancy cravings such as pickles, potato chips, pretzels, and other snacks—they will make you retain water.
➤ If you have an aversion to a food, there's no reason to force yourself to eat it, but if you can't face foods from an entire food group (such as red meat and chicken), then figure out which nutrients they supply and compensate with other foods.

GAS PAINS

Intestinal gas is a common complaint of pregnancy. The stomach and intestines may distend and you will get a bloated feeling. You may have discomfort if the gas gets trapped, or if you find yourself having to pass gas.

Helpful Hints About Gas

➤ Milk of magnesia after each meal increases intestinal activity, which may reduce gas.
➤ Avoid gas-producing foods such as beans, corn, onions, cabbage, parsnips, fried foods, sweet desserts, and candy.
➤ Pureeing vegetables can make them more digestible and may give you relief.
➤ Regular bowel movements reduce gas. (See suggestions under "Constipation" on page 127.)

GROIN PAINS

Groin pains are mild, achy sensations in one or both sides of your abdomen. They are probably due to the stretching of ligaments that support the uterus. Gentle exercises that emphasize stretching may help.

GUM (PERIODONTAL) DISEASE

Gum disease in pregnancy has recently been linked to premature, low-birth-weight babies. Infection in your gums may increase by seven times your risk of delivering a premature baby of low birth weight. Untreated periodontal disease is thought to be the cause of a large number of premature births for which there is no other explanation. An infection in the mouth can interfere with the baby's development and lead to premature birth. The bacteria do not to attack the fetus directly, but they appear to release toxins into the bloodstream that reach the placenta and interfere with fetal development. In addition, the infection stimulates the body to produce inflammatory chemicals (similar to those used to induce abortion) that can cause the cervix to dilate and set off uterine contractions.

It is known that any infection in one's body (like pneumonia or urinary tract infection) can increase the chance of premature birth. Doctors know that preterm births can be cut in half if common reproductive tract infections, like bacterial vaginosis and chlamydia, are treated. When you have periodontal disease there is a risk—even from brushing your teeth or eating an apple—of releasing bacteria and their toxins into your bloodstream.

Helpful Hints About Gum Disease

➤ Plan a prenatal visit to a periodontist (a dentist who specializes in gums).
➤ You can avoid gum disease by nightly flossing and regular thorough teeth cleaning by a dentist, periodontist or dental hygienist.
➤ If you already have infection in your gums, a periodontist has to scrape pockets of disease from the roots and surface of your teeth. Sometimes infected gum tissue has to be removed.
➤ Your dentist may prescribe treatment with an antibiotic like Augmentin.
➤ If left untreated, periodontal disease is a threat to you as well as your unborn child: after years of neglect, periodontal infection gradually erodes the bones in the jaw, which causes the teeth to loosen and fall out.

HAIR & NAILS

The changes in your body due to hormones will lead to increased growth of your nails and hair. Your hair may change in other ways: it can become more or less oily, as your skin can. Your hair may also seem to have more or less body.

Helpful Hints About Hair

➤ If your hair gets oily, try changing your shampoo or wash it more often, scrubbing your scalp vigorously.
➤ If your hair is drier now, wash it less frequently and use a moisturizing conditioner.

➤ *Do not use hair dye when pregnant.* Permanent hair dyes can enter the bloodstream and it is not known what effect this might have for your baby.
➤ Check with your doctor about non-permanent dyes such as cellophanes.

HEADACHES

It isn't unusual to have headaches when you're pregnant. They are caused by the changes your body is going through. Hormones may cause congestion of the mucous membranes, making sinus headaches common.

Do not take aspirin! Aspirin may be harmful to your baby during development and can cause complications during labor. Avoid all over-the-counter medications, since many contain aspirin and acetaminophen: read all labels carefully (see page 172, "Aspirin Directory"). It also is unsafe to take aspirin substitutes such as Tylenol and Anacin, because they have been used only since the 1970s: the long-term effects of these drugs on the fetus are not known. *Do not take ibuprofen* (brand names Advil, Nuprin), because it can cause problems in the unborn baby and complications during labor. Although you should not take aspirin or headache medications, there are many non-drug remedies for headaches.

NOTE: No medication should be taken without your doctor's approval.

Helpful Hints for Headaches

➤ Tension is the most common cause of all headaches.
— Try to avoid getting tied up in knots.
— If you do get tense, lying down in a quiet room will probably help.
— Put a cool wet washcloth over your forehead and eyes, or behind your neck.
➤ If you feel there's ongoing tension in your life, you might want to try yoga or meditation, which are effective in relieving tension.
➤ Sinus headaches can be relieved by applying hot and/or cold compresses to the aching area around your brow. Experiment to see which works best for you.
➤ Get sufficient rest. Lack of sleep can cause headaches.
➤ Being in crowded, overheated, or unventilated environments can set off a headache. Get outside for fresh air and "breathing room."
➤ Eat regularly. Low blood sugar can cause headaches.
➤ If the headaches are persistent, severe, or are accompanied by problems with your vision, inform your doctor.

HEARTBURN & INDIGESTION

Heartburn is a burning sensation you feel in your chest, but it actually has nothing to do with the heart. There are two principle causes of heartburn. It is caused when digestive fluid backs up from the stomach and irritates the lining of the esophagus. The increased amount of progesterone in your system relaxes the smooth muscle tissue everywhere in your body: one of these is the cardiac sphincter of the stomach, which separates the esophagus from the stomach. This allows stomach fluids to reenter the esophagus. These stomach secretions are also pushed up into the lower portion of the esophagus when your uterus gets larger and pushes your stomach upward. The esophagus is not protected by the same mucous lining as the stomach, so the acid fluids burn.

Since the movements of the smooth muscles are slowed down in pregnancy, the stomach secretes less hydrochloric acid and pepsin. During digestion these are the substances that start the breakdown in your stomach of the food proteins. Therefore, food remains longer than usual in the stomach, with the smooth muscle between the stomach and esophagus more relaxed. There is a positive side to these changes in digestion which cause heartburn: food moves more slowly through your system, which allows the nutrients from the food to be absorbed more efficiently.

Helpful Hints for Heartburn

➤ Avoid greasy or spicy foods.
➤ Avoid large meals, especially right before going to bed.
➤ Sleep with your head elevated: this keeps the stomach acid from flowing back up into your esophagus at night.
➤ Avoid alcohol, which is not recommended during pregnancy anyway.
➤ Do not take bicarbonate of soda (baking soda), which has a high salt content and causes water retention and swelling.
➤ Sip milk (warm, if you prefer), which coats and soothes the stomach. Buttermilk works best for some people, and also provides protein and calcium.
➤ Suck on antacid tablets or take liquid antacid, which is many times more effective than tablets. Check to make sure the antacid does not contain acetaminophen.
➤ Milk of magnesia is soothing after meals and whenever heartburn occurs.
➤ Chewing gum after meals lessens heartburn for some people.
➤ Near the end of pregnancy, when the baby's head settles into your pelvis ("engagement" or "lightening"), this will take pressure off your stomach and should ease heartburn.

HEMORRHOIDS & RECTAL BLEEDING

Hemorrhoids are the result of increased pressure on the veins in your anus, which is the equivalent of varicose veins in your legs. Hemorrhoids can be itchy, painful, and can cause bleeding. Rectal bleeding is often the result of cracks in the anus caused by constipation, but it is sometimes a sign of a more serious condition.

NOTE: Always consult a physician for a proper diagnosis about rectal bleeding.

Helpful Hints About Hemorrhoids

➤ Don't let yourself get constipated, because straining and pushing worsens hemorrhoids. Use suppositories if necessary, or see "Constipation" on page 127.

➤ Do the Kegel exercise (on page 161) to stimulate circulation to your rectum.

➤ It may be possible to clear up hemorrhoids by taking 25 mg of vitamin B6 at each meal for several days. This can be followed by 10 mg at every meal to prevent a recurrence. But as with any remedy, check first with a doctor.

➤ Sit only on hard surfaces once you have hemorrhoids: sinking into a soft chair cuts off circulation in the lower colon. If you have to sit for many hours, use a wooden chair or put a board on your seat.

➤ Sit in a modified yoga position whenever possible once you have hemorrhoids. Sit tailor-fashion on the floor, legs crossed and let your belly fall forward, taking weight off your pelvis and back.

➤ A cold compress soaked in witch hazel (keep a bottle in the fridge) placed over the anus can be comforting.

➤ Put petroleum jelly on a tissue, lie with your hips on a pillow and *gently* push the hemorrhoid back into the rectum with the tissue. Keep the muscles tight around the rectum and stay this way with your hips elevated for 10 minutes.

ITCHY STOMACH

Pregnant stomachs often feel itchy and can become even more itchy as your pregnancy progresses. This is because the skin is stretching, which can cause dryness. Keeping your stomach well moisturized with cream may help, but it probably won't entirely eliminate the itchiness. Try to avoid scratching, which will only make you feel more itchy. Aveeno baths may help (Aveeno is an oatmeal-like substance sold in most pharmacies).

MUSCLE CRAMPS

Cramping muscles are due to the slowing of your blood circulation. Another cause of cramping can be the sudden contraction of one of the two round ligaments that moor your uterus in front. Shooting pains down your legs can be due to pressure of the baby's head on certain nerves. Cold weather seems to set off cramps in some women.

Helpful Hints About Cramping

➤ A heating pad, hot-water bottle, and massage all give relief.
➤ Elevating your legs can prevent cramps.
➤ Increase your intake of calcium:
   — Put dried milk powder or bonemeal into a glass of milk before bedtime.
   — Or have a glass of milk before bed with 10 to 25 mg of vitamin B6 and two tablets of calcium with magnesium (which helps absorption).
   — Or take calcium lactate in 10-grain (650 mg) tablets with 100 mg vitamin C as follows: three tablets on an empty stomach before breakfast and two later in the day on an empty stomach.
➤ Increase your intake of potassium by eating an orange, a banana, or half a grapefruit before meals or as a snack.
➤ To relieve leg cramps: with your legs stretched out in front of you sit or lie down and force your toes back toward your face, pushing down at the same time on your knee to straighten your leg.

NAUSEA ("MORNING SICKNESS")

Nausea is the most common complaint of the first three months of pregnancy. One-third of pregnant women are afflicted with digestive disturbance or vomiting, but it usually stops by the end of the first trimester. Nausea is caused by the higher level of estrogen in your system, which influences the stomach cells and causes irritation as acids accumulate. Another reason for nausea is the rapid expansion of the uterus. Improvement will be gradual: the nausea and/or vomiting (see page 154) will not just suddenly stop one day. You'll find you have more good days than bad ones, until there are fewer and fewer days of nausea, and then it will finally disappear.

Early morning is usually the worst time of day because stomach acids have accumulated during the night and your blood sugar is low after hours without food. You don't want to have to leap out of bed in the morning: plan ahead to wake up earlier than you need so you can move more slowly in the morning and give yourself time to try some of the "before rising" remedies below. There is a wide variety of ways to prevent nausea and to cope with it: you'll have to experiment to see which works best for you. It's important to try to *avoid* getting nauseated, because it's harder to eat once you feel ill—yet an empty stomach can *cause* nausea!

If you're having trouble keeping anything down, fluids are more important to your body than solids over a short period of time. Drink plenty of fluids, especially if you're losing them through vomiting. Ginger ale and regular (*non-diet*) caffeine-free colas are rich in carbohydrates, and the carbonation can make you feel better, too. Most women tolerate icy-cold liquids best. A good midafternoon supplement when you're feeling nauseated is some sherbet or shaved ice.

Medications: If you absolutely cannot keep any food down, your doctor may prescribe medication. However, be very cautious about any antinausea drugs, since so many have been found dangerous. Together with your medical provider you have to weigh any risks in the medication against the benefit of essential nutrients for your baby, which are lost if you can't keep anything down.

Helpful Hints About Nausea

- To prevent a drop in blood sugar, eat some protein and a little natural starch or sugar immediately before going to bed—such as milk, or juice with fruit, or cheese and crackers.
- A light, sweet snack before bed (such as toast and jelly or fruit bar cookies) works for some people.
- Before going to sleep, put crackers, popcorn, or dry toast by your bedside: before you even raise your head off the pillow in the morning, nibble something. Remain lying down for 20 minutes before rising.
- At breakfast, avoid foods containing fats (butter, bacon, cream cheese) and don't take acidic foods (fruits and fruit juice) on an empty stomach: eat them at the *end* of breakfast.
- Vitamin B6 (pyridoxine) may have antinauseant properties. Ask your doctor about taking 10 to 25 mg of B6 with meals or throughout the day to see if it gives you relief. Under no circumstances exceed 200 mg of B6 a day (see "Warnings About Vitamins," page 111).
- Yogurt, as a source of B vitamins, can be helpful.
- A high-carbohydrate diet is often recommended: start with nibbling crackers before rising and staying on a diet high in carbohydrates (starches such as pasta, bread, and potatoes) as long as the nausea persists.
- A high-protein diet, which keeps the blood sugar high, works for many people. Even though it's hard to face substantial food when you're nauseated, to eat protein you have to force yourself

to eat dairy products, eggs, fish, chicken, and/or red meat (see "High Protein Foods" on page 94).

➤ Never let your stomach get empty:
 — Keep snacks nearby so you can always keep something in your stomach.
 — Have 5 or 6 smaller meals instead of 3 large ones.
 — Nibble on appealing, nutritious foods between meals.

➤ A mid-morning snack of a banana can help.

➤ Keep "emergency snacks" (such as saltines, graham crackers, zwieback, or a banana) handy in your purse or glove compartment so you aren't caught off-guard by a wave of nausea. This is especially important for women who work outside the home or are out a lot.

➤ Strictly avoid coffee or sweets. Some people like to suck mints or hard candy, but this can have the reverse effect: sugar can stimulate your digestive juices, which can irritate an empty stomach.

➤ Avoid greasy or spicy foods.

➤ Apricot nectar helps some people.

➤ A baked potato sprinkled with salt is easy to eat if you're nauseated and can't face the idea of food. Potatoes have a surprising amount of vitamins, minerals, and even some protein (see "Potatoes," page 89).

➤ Try drinking either very hot or very cold liquids: experiment to see whether the extreme temperatures make you feel better.

➤ Emotional and physical fatigue can both increase morning sickness; get extra sleep and give yourself lots of time to relax.

➤ Herbal tea can help: try peppermint, spearmint, chamomile, or peach leaf. At a health food store you might find red raspberry leaf tea, which is said to relieve nausea and vomiting. Use tea bags or brew 1 teaspoon of herb to a cup of boiling water.

➤ Ginger is an old home remedy for gastrointestinal disturbance: it is reported to be a safe and effective remedy for morning sickness. You can find it in capsule form in health food stores.

Seasickness Wrist Bands

These bands were developed for motion sickness based on the principles of the Chinese science of acupressure. They can be a marvelous solution for nausea during pregnancy because they have no undesirable side effects. They consist of stretchy material that slips over your wrist with a small button on the inside that you line up on the underside of your wrist. This button presses on the point used in acupressure that corresponds to motion sickness. They come with instructions, but often you have to move them around to find the exact place on your own wrist that responds. You will probably find there is a spot where you get a reaction quite quickly. I have tried them for seasickness and find that if I place them *incorrectly*, I feel a little dizzy and nauseated right away, which means that proper placement would eliminate those symptoms. These wrist bands are sold in many drug stores, but if you can't find them there, then try a store specializing in water sports or boating.

NOSEBLEEDS

Nosebleeds occur during pregnancy as a result of the increased blood volume. You may also experience nasal congestion, which can be caused by the increased hormone levels in your body. Stuffiness will usually last until after you deliver. You may develop a postnasal drip, which can occasionally lead to nighttime coughing.

Helpful Hints About Nosebleeds

- ➤ Put a little petroleum jelly in each nostril to stop the bleeding.
- ➤ Eat citrus fruit and other sources of vitamin C (see "Best Sources of Vitamin C" on page 109) because vitamin C deficiency can be a cause of nosebleeds.
- ➤ You can make your own pregnancy-safe nose drops by putting a 25% solution of menthol into white oil (available at your pharmacy). Using an eye dropper, put a few drops in each nostril; tip your head back so the menthol runs into your throat, then spit it out. Do this in the morning and evening to stop nosebleeds.
- ➤ *Do not use nose drops or spray.* The side effects can be harmful to the baby. Besides, nose drops can actually make nosebleeds worse.

OVERHEATING

Your metabolic rate increases 20% during pregnancy, which means you're going to feel warmer, even in the winter, when everyone around you is chilly. You may perspire more, which is the body's way of cooling you off and ridding your body of waste products.

Helpful Hints About Overheating

- ➤ Wear layers of clothing so that you can peel them off when you start to feel too warm.
- ➤ Bathe or shower more often and choose an effective antiperspirant.
- ➤ Drink fluids freely to replace those you're losing through perspiration.

PINS & NEEDLES (TINGLING)

You may experience a tingling feeling of pins and needles in your hands and feet. This may give you the impression that your circulation is being cut off, but it is not. No one really knows what causes pins and needles during pregnancy, or how to prevent it. However, for your peace of mind it's nice to know is that it isn't an indication of anything serious.

Helpful Hints About Pins & Needles

➤ Changing your position or moving around may help.
➤ If you experience swelling of your hands, there's a chance you may be developing "carpal tunnel syndrome."
  — This condition places pressure on a nerve in the wrist, causing a burning sensation that may radiate up the arm.
  — The symptoms may increase at night because fluids have accumulated all day in your hands, increasing the swelling.
  — Ask your doctor whether you could be developing this condition and ask about possible treatment.

SALIVA, EXCESS

Excessive salivation (also known as pytalism) can sometimes accompany morning sickness (nausea) and also occurs in the first trimester. What happens is that your mouth floods with foul-tasting saliva, more than can be swallowed: you have to spit it out constantly. This is a rare condition, but if it does occur, it begins two to three weeks after your first missed period and can persist throughout pregnancy. There isn't really a satisfactory treatment, but you can experiment with some of the remedies for nausea earlier in this chapter and see if they help.

Helpful Hints About Excess Saliva

➤ Foods containing starch may aggravate this condition; you might want to eliminate many of the vegetable foods containing starch from your diet.
➤ Rinsing your mouth with strong mouthwash or sucking peppermint candies may give relief.
➤ Mild sedatives may help, but *you must check with your doctor* about this, as with all prescribed medications.

SHORTNESS OF BREATH

Feeling short of breath can sometimes accompany dizziness and faintness (see page 129). A pregnant woman's respiration is deeper: you take in more air than before because you are oxygenating the baby's blood as well as your own. Your lungs have more space because the rib cage increases in size, which allows you to take in more air and use it more efficiently. Your total lung capacity remains the same, but there is a greater amount of air going in and out. This increase in the size of your rib cage is permanent: you may need a larger bra or blouse size, even after you lose every pound you gained during pregnancy.

Helpful Hints About Shortness of Breath

➤ Take 3 or 4 deep breaths before getting up from a sitting or lying position.
➤ It's not unusual to be conscious of the need to breathe: move around or take a walk to alleviate that feeling.
➤ Shortness of breath can get worse in the last weeks of pregnancy. Your expanding uterus is largest then and presses on the diaphragm. If it gets too uncomfortable you can sleep propped with pillows in a semisitting position.
➤ If you're having trouble sleeping, you can take pressure off your rib cage and lungs by propping 2 pillows behind you, one of them lengthwise to raise your shoulders.

SKIN PROBLEMS

Most women's skin is affected in some way by pregnancy. It's important not to pick at or fuss with these skin conditions; if you do it will tend to leave a lasting mark. Don't worry: most of these problems will disappear after the baby is born (with the exception of stretch marks and, in some women, darkening of the genitalia).

Pimples

➤ If in the past your skin has broken out before your period, you will probably get pimples now, because similar hormones are affecting the oil glands under your skin.
➤ Keep your skin as clean as possible: use an antibacterial soap followed by an astringent or toner.
➤ Avoid using makeup. Don't use foundation when you're at home. If you want to use any at all, use a light, water-based product that won't aggravate your skin's oiliness.

➤ Drink plenty of water.
➤ Ask your doctor about trying a supplement of 25–50 mg of vitamin B6.

Bumps on Your Skin

Bumps are probably caused by hormonal influences on your blood cells and nerves. They will disappear after the baby is born.

Tiny Red Marks

These spots are caused by distended blood vessels that rise to the surface of your skin. They will be another effect of pregnancy that will disappear after the baby arrives.

Brown Spots

Brownish spots (in black women the spots are white) on your face, neck, and abdomen are often called the "mask of pregnancy," or "pregnancy cap." The spots will usually be gone within a month after delivery.

➤ These marks may be an indication of a folic acid deficiency.
➤ By taking 5 mg of folic acid per meal you may be able to restore normal skin within two to three weeks, but before trying anything check first with your doctor.
➤ If the problem is severe, you might want to consult a dermatologist (a doctor who specializes in skin problems).

Dark Nipples & Genitalia

In many women the area around the nipple (the aerola) darkens around the third month, which is due to hormonal changes in your body. Brown spots may also appear on the secondary aerola (the surrounding skin). Some women's external genitalia may get darker and a dark line may develop between the umbilicus (belly button) and the bottom of the abdomen. The darkening may be permanent.

Stretch Marks

Almost 90% of pregnant women develop stretch marks, but some experts say stretch marks are preventable. These specialists contend that healthy tissues are elastic and that stretch marks are scar tissue, which is what occurs whenever the skin lacks normal elasticity. Stretch marks are most common on the abdomen, but thighs and breasts can also be affected. Most of these pale, reddish streaks either disappear after delivery or turn a silvery color. The marks are most pronounced in brunettes, although redheads have the most sensitive skin and should take extra care of it during pregnancy.

To help alleviate stretch marks:
— Get adequate protein in your diet.
— Take vitamin C and vitamin E supplements (with your doctor's approval).
— It may help keep your skin supple to have an oil bath and daily applications of cream, cocoa butter, or oil.
— Lubricating your stomach, thighs, hips, and breasts will not prevent stretch marks, but it will probably minimize them.

Skin Eruptions

To add insult to injury, right on top of the stretch marks on their stomachs, some women get an itchy, rashlike skin eruption. Some get this rashy eruption on their arms, thighs, or buttocks. It may be uncomfortable, but it poses no threat to you or the baby, and it will disappear after delivery. If it's really bothering you, a dermatologist can give you medication for the symptoms.

SLEEP PROBLEMS

Sleep is affected in some way for all pregnant women. As your stomach grows bigger you may find it increasingly difficult to get comfortable. This can often be worst in the final weeks, when the baby seems to be more active at night and you are the biggest and most uncomfortable. Sleeplessness may be nature's way of preparing you for the first weeks of the baby's life when the hungry newcomer is not going to let you sleep through the night!

Helpful Hints for Sleep Problems

➤ Do not fight sleeplessness: insomniacs often say that resistance makes it even harder to fall asleep. You can read or do sewing in bed, or go to another room and lie on a couch listening to music or TV (unless your mate can sleep through the noise in the bedroom).
➤ Give up your previous ideas about sleep: if you think of yourself as "needing" a certain number of hours of sleep, then not getting them can distress you. Instead, think of these months as a time when everything is in flux: accept the changes instead of fighting them (which just magnifies the problem).

➤ A cup of hot cocoa or malted milk before bed can be soothing. Milk is a relaxant. Chamomile tea (or herbal teas such as "Sleepytime" with chamomile in them) can be relaxing. Make the drink as hot as possible for the most benefit.

➤ Take a hot bath (but not too hot!) right before bed. Hot water is so effective at relieving physical and mental tension that it can knock you right out: watch out that you don't fall asleep in the tub!

➤ Do not sleep on your back (which puts all your weight on your internal organs and can aggravate hemorrhoids).

➤ Sleep on your side with one leg crossed over and a pillow between your legs (or under the "crossover" leg) to improve circulation.

➤ Try to adjust your usual sleeping position until you find one that suits you.

➤ Your bed should be large—in late pregnancy, even a double bed might not be big enough for comfort.

➤ Invest in a queen-size or king-size bed if at all possible: later on a larger bed will make it easier to breast-feed comfortably in bed.

➤ You may need a softer surface, one that has more "give" than a hard mattress, especially in the later stages of pregnancy. Try a contoured foam mattress pad: "egg carton" and other types of pads are available from hospital supply stores. You can get one for just your half of the bed.

➤ Sleep apart from your mate if you're having trouble sleeping and it's interfering with his rest. (But this may not be necessary if you have a larger bed and a reading light on your side.)

➤ Shortness of breath can cause sleeplessness at the very end of pregnancy. Take the pressure off your rib cage and lungs by propping two pillows behind you, one of them lengthwise to raise your shoulders.

➤ Sleeping pills are not a good idea unless you aren't able to get any rest at all. Consult with a doctor about this, but under no circumstances should you take a sleeping pill very often, because you will develop a dependence on them.

STUFFY NOSE

Nasal stuffiness is a normal side effect of pregnancy. If you already have allergies, they can be aggravated (see page 122). You may also find that a stuffy or runny nose, watery eyes, or other allergic reactions happen to you for the first time when you're pregnant. Antihistamines and decongestants are usually the remedy to dry up a person's symptoms, but these medications can be harmful to your unborn child. *Do not use over-the-counter cold or allergy medicines.*

Helpful Hints for Stuffiness

➢ Breathe steam by taking a steam bath or steam shower.
➢ Stand in a hot shower, breathing deeply.
➢ Put a few drops of eucalyptus oil into a pot of very hot water. Lean over the pot with a towel draped over your head and breathe deeply, allowing the steam to help clear your blocked sinuses.
➢ Use a cool mist humidifier or vaporizer, especially while you sleep. These machines should be kept clean because bacteria and mold can grow in them.
➢ Cover your nose with a hot washcloth to soothe your sinuses.
➢ Massage your sinuses using finger pressure: in firm, gentle, circular motions rub on the bony ridge at your eyebrows, underneath your eyes, and alongside your nose.
➢ Drink hot liquids, chicken broth in particular, if you have a cold. Warm liquids make it easier to cough and clear your throat and chest.
➢ Do not take any kind of antihistamine or cold remedy designed for decongestion (Dristan, Contac, Allerest, Coricidin). None of them is safe during pregnancy.
➢ Use only saltwater (saline) nose sprays.

SWEATING

Your thyroid gland becomes more active when you're pregnant, which can cause you to sweat more. You also manufacture more heat when you're pregnant, so your body has to sweat more to maintain your body temperature. Sweat is also the body's way of disposing of additional waste material in your system from the baby. If you develop an irritation or rash from sweating, powder yourself with cornstarch or a medicated powder. If you find yourself sweating more at night, put a towel on your pillow or a beach towel underneath you.

SWELLING (EDEMA)

Swelling (or edema) is a natural condition of pregnancy that affects almost all women. It may cause you some discomfort, but swelling is normal: it's particularly common late in the day, in warm weather, or after you've been sitting down or standing up for long periods. This swelling is a result of the rise in female hormones during pregnancy—particularly the estrogens manufactured by the placenta—which cause fluid retention. These are the same hormones that cause water buildup and swelling in the days before your period and in women on the pill.

There is a normal increase in fluid in all the cells of your body. Even in women with no signs of edema, the total amount of water weight they gain can be as much as 15 pounds! All this is even more true for women carrying twins: with a larger placenta, more hormones are manufactured and therefore more fluid is retained. Studies have shown that women with edema have slightly larger babies—and fewer premature babies—than those without. Women who are heavier tend to gain more water weight during pregnancy, while thin women tend to gain more fat. Your body has many reasons to need more fluid during pregnancy. It is a safeguard for the expanded blood volume, and the body retains fluids to protect you from going into shock during birth from the unavoidable blood loss.

A doctor should not try to tamper with the normal edema of pregnancy by telling you to eliminate salt from your diet or prescribing water pills (diuretics), which can harm you and the baby. You need to make sure that your obstetrician is not influenced by the old belief (since proven incorrect) that by eliminating edema a doctor could eliminate toxemia (see page 419).

Water pills (diuretics) are harmful during pregnancy. They cause a potassium deficiency, which can then cause listlessness, fatigue, mental depression, insomnia, constipation, and harm to the kidneys. Diuretics can cause deficiencies of 35 nutrients—anything your body needs that dissolves in water. Diuretics can also lead to many problems of the placenta and the formation of the fetus.

However, although some swelling is well and fine, *severe* swelling is another story: it can be a sign that you have kidney problems or other complications.

NOTE: Report to your doctor right away if you have anything more than mild edema, or if the swelling persists for more than a day.

Helpful Hints About Swelling

➢ Vitamin C increases urine production and can be even more effective in removing excess fluids than a diuretic. See "Vitamin C" on page 108 for amounts.
➢ Vitamin B6 is a very effective diuretic, particularly when used along with vitamin C. Vitamin B6 can sometimes upset the stomach, so always take it with food or milk. See Vitamin B6 on page 114.
➢ A diet high in protein (up to 150 grams a day) can help rid your system of extra fluids. Carbohydrates, on the other hand, encourage fluid retention, so try decreasing them in your diet at the same time.
➢ Apple cider vinegar can act as a harmless diuretic. If you have a temporary flare-up of edema (due to having eaten salty food, for example), try a teaspoon or two before meals to see whether it helps rid your body of excess retained fluid.
➢ Frequent, low-key exercise, such as swimming or walking, helps reduce swelling.
➢ Avoid high-salt foods (see page 97 for a list of salty foods), but

don't cut salt out of your diet. Instead, increase your protein intake and salt foods to taste.

➤ Avoid tight clothes that constrict you at the wrist, ankles, or waist. Wear loose things that feel comfortable.

➤ Remove rings if your fingers get puffy. If your hands have already swollen and the rings won't come off, first soak your hand in cold water, then soap your hand and finger, with the finger pointing up, and try to slide it off gently.

➤ Change positions when you're sitting or standing to help circulation. Avoid standing still in one position.

➤ Remedies for tired feet and ankles: if they feel tight and burn, soak them in cold water. Roll or rotate your ankles. The pelvic rock (see page 162) improves circulation in your legs, which decreases swelling.

➤ Swollen breasts can tingle, throb, or just plain hurt! The milk glands are developing and there is an increased blood supply to the breasts, which makes the veins more prominent. A cold compress should help.

➤ Swelling of the vaginal area can be painful: a cold compress (try a cold can of soda wrapped in a dish towel) held against the area can give relief.

➤ Drink 8 to 10 big glasses of liquid a day.

TEETH & GUMS

There used to be a saying, "For every child a tooth is lost," but with today's dental care this is obviously not true. Although your mouth *can* be affected by pregnancy, your teeth are inert once they are formed; they don't undergo remodeling the way bone can. If a mother's diet doesn't provide the necessary calcium for her baby's development, it is true that calcium will be taken from her body, but it would be from her bones, not her teeth.

Pregnancy can affect your teeth and gums through changes in estrogen and progesterone levels exaggerating the way your periodontal tissue (the gums) respond to plaque. You are more susceptible to gum problems, especially in the upper jaw, most of all during your eighth month. Bleeding gums may occur because the increased blood volume puts pressure on the capillaries.

The hormonal changes of pregnancy can also decrease your body's immune response to bacteria: they can enter your bloodstream from teeth that have cavities or gum problems. Since blood-borne infections can cross the placenta and reach the baby, any source of infection should be eliminated.

Helpful Hints About Teeth & Gums

➤ A good diet helps prevent tooth and gum problems. You should be protected by getting sufficient calcium, high-quality protein, and a good supply of vitamins C, B, and D.
➤ Brush regularly and floss every night before bed. To further reduce bacteria, brush your tongue when you brush your teeth.
➤ See the dentist at least once during your pregnancy and have your teeth professionally cleaned at least once, but preferably twice, during pregnancy.

URINATING FREQUENTLY

In the first months of pregnancy the hormonal changes in your body can send you to the bathroom more often. The hormones affect your adrenal glands, which change the fluid balance in your body. Also, your kidneys work more effectively during pregnancy: they clear the waste products from the body more rapidly. The amount of urine you produce increases in the first trimester, but the amount of urine diminishes as the pregnancy goes on (to a level below normal for a nonpregnant woman).

Another reason for the frequent need to urinate is that the growing uterus presses on your bladder. At the end of pregnancy when lightening (also called "engagement") occurs, there will be an increase in your frequent urination. Engagement is when your baby's presenting part (usually the head) settles into the pelvic cavity. Although this will give your lungs more room to breathe, it will also put additional pressure on your bladder. In a first pregnancy this can happen 2 to 4 weeks before delivery; in later pregnancies, lightening may not occur until labor begins.

Helpful Hints About Frequent Urination

➤ Do not restrict your fluid intake to limit frequent "pit stops": your body needs additional fluids when it is working for two.
➤ Increased urination at night is caused by water retained in your ankles during the day, which moves through your kidneys when you lie down.
➤ You can cut down midnight trips to bathroom by not drinking any liquids after 7 P.M.

URINARY TRACT INFECTION (UTI)

Urinary infections are more common during pregnancy, when your body is more susceptible to any kind of bacteria. Cystitis is the most common bladder infection: you have urge to urinate every few minutes, but can only pass a few drops, perhaps with a burning sensation. Pyelitis is a kidney infection in which the normal path of urine elimination is blocked and waste material backs up into your body. Symptoms are similar to those of cystitis, but may be accompanied by a high temperature, chills, and blood in the urine.

Helpful Hints About UTI

- ➤ One way to prevent a UTI is to drink plenty of fluids, especially water, to keep your system flushed.
- ➤ Wear cotton underwear (or at least those with a cotton crotch) and avoid tight underpants, leggings, or tight-fitting pants.
- ➤ Keep the vaginal area scrupulously clean, washing with unperfumed soap. Always wipe from front to back after using the toilet.
- ➤ At the first sign of a UTI, notify your doctor. S/he will prescribe one of the antibiotics approved for use during pregnancy.

VAGINAL CHANGES

The vagina goes through many changes during pregnancy, some of which are temporary, while others stay with you afterward.

Vaginal Bleeding

Bleeding during pregnancy is a danger signal, although in the first trimester there's not necessarily any cause for alarm. Some women have scanty, short periods even once they're pregnant. It may also be due to "implantation bleeding": approximately 7 days after conception the group of cells that will become the embryo attach to the uterine wall, and some bleeding may accompany that.

NOTE: However, you must notify your doctor immediately if you have any bleeding during pregnancy.

Vaginal Color Change

The color of your vagina may deepen. The tissues at the entrance to your vagina and inside it take on a dusky, purplish color instead of the usual pink. This is known as "Chadwick's sign." The color may deepen as the pregnancy advances and is more striking in women who have had more than one baby.

Vaginal Discharge

Probably the most noticeable change in your vagina is the increase in discharge, due to the (normal) excess activity of the mucus-secreting glands of the cervix. There is often an accompanying increase in the vaginal odor, which can be unpleasant for you and perhaps distasteful to your partner during sex. Keep the genital area clean and dry, but don't overdo washing with soap, which can be drying and irritating.

Douching

Douching gives only short-lived relief for vaginal discharge, since it is the secretions themselves that have a strong odor. Douching will not lessen vaginal discharge, although it may temporarily lessen the odor. Some doctors feel it is safe to douche, but others are opposed. Consult with your own obstetrician first. Use a douche bag, not a bulb syringe, with the source of water kept low (less than 2 feet off the ground). The nozzle must be inserted no more than 2 inches within the vaginal entrance. The water must flow out freely: do not hold the lips of the vagina together.

NOTE: You may not douche: 1) in the last 4 weeks of pregnancy; 2) if your membranes have ruptured, or 3) if you have had vaginal bleeding at any time during the pregnancy.

VAGINAL INFECTIONS

Bacterial Vaginosis

This common, easy-to-cure infection is hazardous during pregnancy.

➤ Bacterial vaginosis affects one-quarter of all pregnancies, yet many women who are infected do not know they have it.
➤ This infection is different from yeast infections and more threatening to your baby's health.
➤ This very common vaginal syndrome can be a serious health problem during pregnancy, yet many healthcare providers do not even test for it.

SYMPTOMS

➤ A fishy odor is the most common sign of bacterial vaginosis.
➤ Vaginal irritation can accompany the odor.
➤ Excessive moisture or discharge.

WHAT CAUSES IT

> When a variety of unwanted bacteria invade the vagina they displace the microbes that ordinarily live there.
> Douching increases the risk of infection.
> Multiple sexual partners increase your risk, although the infection is also common among monogamous women.
> Black women tend to have a higher percentage of infection, which could help to explain the high risk of infant mortality among blacks.

WHAT ARE THE RISKS?

> This infection causes 6% of all premature births, which makes it a major underlying cause of infant mortality; premature babies run a high risk of dying in their first weeks of life.
> The risk of having a preterm birth for a woman with bacterial vaginosis is the same as the risk for an expectant woman associated with smoking cigarettes.

WHAT TO DO

> Request a test if you suspect you might be infected.
> It is simple for an obstetrician to check for this infection, which then can be easily eliminated with standard antibiotics.

During pregnancy the vagina offers a chemically hospitable environment for certain infections, in particular a yeast-like fungus called *Candida albicans*. Sexual partners pass this irritation on to each other, and in the man it can cause burning on urination. Your doctor can do vaginal smears and cultures to determine if you have such an infection: it is readily curable and does not cause a systemic illness. Although vaginal infections tend to recur during pregnancy, they subside after delivery.

Softening of the Vaginal Tissues

You will probably notice that the tissues of your vagina soften as your pregnancy progresses. Your vagina will become increasingly elastic, readying itself to stretch for the baby. Adequate vitamin C in your diet is important to keep the vaginal tissues elastic.

Vaginal Swelling

Increased blood supply to the vagina can have the effect of causing uncomfortable swelling. You may want to try a cold compress (such as a cold can of soda wrapped in a dish towel) for relief. However, this increased circulation may also have a positive sexual effect for some women: you may become more rapidly and intensely aroused during sex. Some women become orgasmic for the first time in their lives when they're pregnant, or they become multiorgasmic. This increased blood supply to the vagina is one of the physical changes of pregnancy you can be grateful for because some of this increase will remain with you after delivery.

Vaginal Varicose Veins

The lips of your vagina can develop varicose veins like your legs (see below). Try sleeping with your bottom raised up on a pillow. Wear a sanitary pad pressed firmly against the swollen part of your vulva. If the problem is severe enough, you can talk to your doctor about getting a "maternity garment" that compresses the vulva by putting pressure on the perineal area. These vascular support garments require a doctor's prescription and are available through companies such as the Jobst Institute (800-537-1063).

Varicose Veins

There are combined causes for varicose veins: the increased blood volume and blood flow during pregnancy place pressure on the veins on the pelvic and leg veins, causing them to bulge. Your enlarging uterus places pressure on the pelvic veins, and later in pregnancy the baby's head also presses down. Varicose veins are hereditary. The increased pressure in your circulatory system will recede dramatically after the baby's birth, but varicose veins do get worse with subsequent pregnancies, so do everything you can to keep the condition under control. Hemorrhoids are a form of varicose veins.

Helpful Hints About Varicose Veins

➤ Exercise regularly. A long, brisk walk every day can help.
➤ Elevate your legs when you're lying or sitting down: preferably raise them above the level of your heart.
➤ Wear support panty-hose or elastic support stockings (but do not wear stockings with elastic tops or girdles with elastic bands on the legs: they cut off circulation). Put them on before you get out of bed in the morning and take them off before you go to sleep.
➤ Vitamins C and E may help prevent or control varicose veins but there is disagreement about this. Consult with your doctor; do not undertake any vitamin therapy on your own.

➤ Put wood blocks or old books under the foot of your bed or between the mattress and box springs. This will elevate your feet a couple of inches above your had: at night, gravity will be working in favor of your legs. It may take awhile for you (and your mate) to get used to this new slant on your sleep!

➤ When you're sitting, elevate your legs. Do not sit with your legs constantly down. Raise them up to reduce pressure.

➤ Don't gain too much weight: excessive weight gain causes the veins to dilate.

➤ Don't stand around or sit still for long periods of time: try to keep moving around.

VOMITING

Vomiting, like nausea, diminishes as your pregnancy progresses. However, it is not predictable: you may have vomiting in the morning, in the evening, or at irregular times. You may also have a stretch with none at all and then it may begin again. As with nausea, vomiting won't stop all at once, it will taper off. There is *no* conclusive evidence that vomiting is influenced by emotional factors (as some people may suggest to you). The hormonal changes your body is going through may be intense and/or you may be more sensitive to them than other women. If you have been vomiting fairly often, do not be concerned if there are flecks or streaks of blood in the vomit: repeated vomiting may rupture a tiny blood vessel in the throat or esophagus, which will soon clot or heal by itself.

Severe and unremitting vomiting (called *hyperemesis gravidarum*) is a rare complication that must be controlled in the hospital with medication. This illness occurs most frequently in women with abnormally high hormone levels, which happens when there are multiple births or abnormalities in the placenta. While there is reason to believe that this disorder results from a hormonal imbalance, there is also reason to believe that emotions play some part because it is seen most frequently in women under emotional stress.

Helpful Hints About Vomiting

➤ Vitamin B6 can help control vomiting: discuss this with your doctor. Once vomiting has begun, at least 250 mg a day is recommended; if vomiting is severe, some doctors give injections of 300 mg (or more) of vitamin B6.

➤ The danger with repeated vomiting is dehydration and loss of calories. Be sure you let your doctor know how much you are vomiting. If you can't keep anything down for a stretch of time, you may have to be hospitalized for intravenous feeding so that your baby's health isn't compromised.

SYMPTOMS OF SERIOUS PROBLEMS

Most of the complaints covered in this chapter happen to many women and are fairly easy to cope with or are transitory. However, there are serious complications of pregnancy with symptoms you need to be aware of; if you show any of these symptoms, you should tell your medical practitioner right away. The possible cause for these symptoms is in parentheses.

DANGER SIGNS DURING PREGNANCY

* *Pain or burning on urination* (urinary tract infection [UTI]; sexually transmitted disease)
* *Vaginal spotting or bleeding* (premature labor; miscarriage; placenta previa or abruptio)
* *Leaking or gushing fluid from vagina*, less significant near due date (rupture of membranes)
* *Blister or sore in vaginal area* (herpes, sexually transmitted disease)
* *Itching or irritating discharge* (vaginal infection; sexually transmitted disease)
* *Uterine contractions*, more than 4 or 5 in 1 hour not near your due date (threatened miscarriage)
* *Severe nausea or vomiting*, several times in 1 hour or over several days (hyperemesis gravidarum; infection)
* *Severe abdominal pain* (ectopic pregnancy; placenta abruptio; premature labor)
* *Chills & fever over 100°F* not accompanied by a common cold (infection)
* *Dizziness or light-headedness* (toxemia)
* *Severe headache* that doesn't let up, especially in second half of pregnancy (toxemia)
* *Swelling of face, eyes, fingers or toes*, especially if the puffiness is sudden (toxemia)
* *Sudden weight gain* (toxemia)
* *Visual problems:* dimness, blurring, spots, flashes, blind spots (toxemia)
* *Noticeably reduced fetal movement* (fetal distress)
* *Absence of fetal movement for 24 hours* from 30th week of pregnancy and beyond (fetal death)
* *A hot, reddened painful area behind your knee* or on your calf (phlebitis or blood clot)

CHAPTER SIX

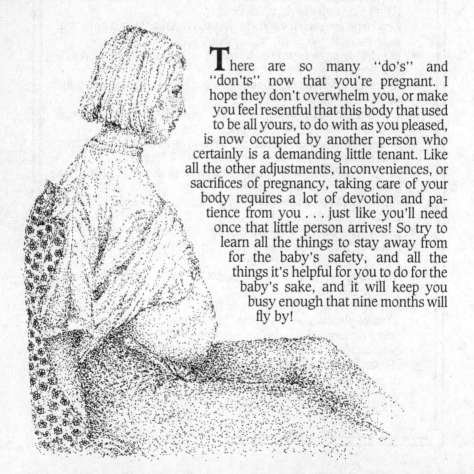

Taking Care of Your Body

There are so many "do's" and "don'ts" now that you're pregnant. I hope they don't overwhelm you, or make you feel resentful that this body that used to be all yours, to do with as you pleased, is now occupied by another person who certainly is a demanding little tenant. Like all the other adjustments, inconveniences, or sacrifices of pregnancy, taking care of your body requires a lot of devotion and patience from you . . . just like you'll need once that little person arrives! So try to learn all the things to stay away from for the baby's safety, and all the things it's helpful for you to do for the baby's sake, and it will keep you busy enough that nine months will fly by!

EXERCISE

Labor and delivery are physically demanding and stressful; a lot is required from your body in giving birth, which will probably be more comfortable for you if you have good muscle tone. Pregnancy is a kind of aerobic activity in itself: your heart generally beats faster, there's about 50% more blood plasma circulating, and your body is carrying extra weight. Be prepared for the fact that your body is not capable of the level of exercise that you might have been used to before! For example, jogging one mile now can take as much effort as it did to go three miles before you were pregnant. So cut yourself some slack in your expectations of yourself, especially if you're a high-performance, high-achiever kind of person.

Exercising while you're expecting is also good for you emotionally, which can be a real bonus when you consider those pregnancy mood swings! Keeping active can be as important for your mind as it is for you physically: exercising causes increased circulation, which can relax a lot of tension. The increase in oxygen in your system from exercising can even make you feel a bit "high." And by making the effort to keep fit, you can counteract the pregnant woman's tendency to feel clumsy or "fat," particularly in the last trimester, when it's not uncommon to feel like a beached whale!

Before singing the praises of exercise, it's important to know that there are medical conditions which would rule out exercise. This is one of the reasons to always check with your obstetrician before starting any kind of exercise program. But you should be aware of the high-risk circumstances in which exercise of any kind should be avoided:

REASONS TO AVOID EXERCISE

— Pregnancy-induced high blood pressure (hypertension)
— Preterm rupture of the membranes
— Preterm labor (in this pregnancy or a previous one)
— Bleeding in the second or third trimesters
— Evidence of intrauterine growth retardation
— Indications of a weakened cervix

Doctors' New Attitudes About Exercise

The medical community used to put limitations on how women could exercise: they used to tell women to keep their heart rate under 140 beats per minute and to limit themselves to 15 minute sessions. But newer reports by the American College of Obstetricians and Gynecologists eliminate many of those previous restrictions. Doctors now agree that mild to moderate prenatal exercise is known to make your postpartum recovery easier, helping you to return more quickly to your pre-pregnancy level of strength and flexibility. Put more simply: if you keep your body in good shape, you'll probably get back into shape faster and more easily after the baby is born.

However, each woman is an individual and you should not exercise without first checking with your healthcare provider. Ask a doctor before you undertake *any* exercise, even "pregnancy-safe" exercises you read about, or see demonstrated in a gym or on a video.

"How Much Can I Exercise?"

The phrase about exercise "no pain, no gain" is not relevant during pregnancy. In fact, it can be dangerous. If you feel any pain while exercising, your body is telling you to stop.

Moderate activity 3 to 5 times a week is considered a safe and healthy exercise plan. Exercising regularly is best so that your body isn't stressed by sudden or infrequent demands on it. About 15 minutes of strenuous exercise each time is a good yardstick, with a full workout of aerobics lasting no more than 30 minutes (which should include 10 minutes to stretch and warm up and another 5 minutes at the end to cool down and stretch again). An important reason not to extend exercise much beyond half an hour is because during prolonged exercise, some blood flow is diverted away from the uterus to your limbs, which deprives the baby of oxygen. Also, high internal temperatures have been linked to some types of birth defects, so you want to avoid getting too heated up.

Monitor your level of exertion, the length of time you spend doing the activity and the temperature around you when you're exercising. If you were exercising before pregnancy, you can continue at your same *perceived* level of exertion—which means that you can feel or experience the same amount of exercise, but now you have to keep in mind that the weight of the baby changes your ability and capacity.

"How Can I Tell If I'm Exerting Myself Too Much?"

There are three ways to determine whether you've pushed yourself too much during exercise. First, you should be able to carry on a conversation comfortably while you're working out. Secondly, it's fine to perspire, but if you are pouring with sweat you've gone too far: your body can't take it. And thirdly, if your pulse is still over 100 after a 5-minute cool-down, you've done too much. But the best guideline of the three is that you should be able to comfortably talk while exercising.

Never exercise to the point of fatigue. A little bit of exercise several times a day is better for you than exercising a lot all at once. The basic fact you need to know is that a pregnant woman does not have resiliency. A woman who isn't pregnant can restore her energy by lying down for half an hour. But when she is pregnant, it can take that woman *half a day* to recover from the fatigue. Another reason it's unhealthy to exercise to the point of exhaustion is that your body accumulates lactic acid: this is called "acidosis" and it is not good for the baby. But even though strenuous exercise does divert blood from the internal organs (which includes the uterus) to the muscles, most studies suggest that as long as you don't exercise to the point of exhaustion, the fetus will get an adequate supply of blood and oxygen.

Beware any activity that raises your body temperature significantly. Hyperthermia, or overheating, has the potential to cause birth defects during the first trimester and can lead to premature birth in the last trimester. For example, treadmills and stair machines can elevate your body temperature and heart rate. The safest advice is to avoid vigorous exercise when it's hot and humid: exercise at cooler times of the day and wear light clothing in a natural fiber that can "breathe." Also, drinking plenty of fluids, preferably water, during exercise is another way to keep from getting too hot.

"What's the Best Way to Do Exercise?"

Stretch: Always stretch out your muscles and joints slowly before starting any exercise, even walking. Exercise should always be slow, rhythmic, and regular. If you exercise only sporadically it can be a shock to your body and possibly cause injury. Play music while you exercise, especially with a beat that encourages you to exercise rhythmically and also increases your enjoyment.

Position: Avoid lying flat on your back while exercising, especially in the first trimester, because it causes your heart to pump less blood, which then can reduce blood flow to baby. Lying flat is also a problem after the fourth month, when the uterus could compress blood vessels that are nourishing the fetus. This seems logical since if you lie flat on your back for a long time during labor it can compromise oxygen flow to the baby and cause fetal distress.

Discomfort: For exercises on the floor you might want to use pillows for comfort. When you're lying on your back you might want to have at least one pillow under your knees; another pillow under your head and a small pillow for the small of your back should take care of any discomfort.

What about eating?: In general, eat an adequate diet: simply being pregnant requires 300 extra calories a day and exercise demands even more. Drink plenty of water before and during exercise and be sure to drink fluids afterwards to replenish any you may lose through perspiration. It is not good to exercise on an empty stomach. Before exerting yourself eat a light snack about half an hour beforehand, or a bit longer if it's more comfortable for you.

Breathing: A deep cleansing breath before starting each new exercise is a good habit to get into: inhale deeply through your nose and exhale through your mouth. It's important to remember to breathe deeply throughout the time you're exercising. This is true for anyone who exercises, but it's especially true for a pregnant woman, whose body needs additional oxygen for her baby. When you breathe, *exhale* through your mouth during the most difficult parts of any exercise and *inhale* through your nose as you relax your muscles. It's so easy to forget to breathe deeply, or even to hold your breath without realizing it: remind yourself that you need that additional oxygen for your muscles and for the baby.

Getting up: To sit up from a lying position, roll over on your side and use your arms to push yourself up sideways. This way your abdomen won't have to work (and stretch out of shape) to raise you up.

"What If I've Never Exercised Before Now?"

If you haven't been active person before, there's no reason to think you're going to change dramatically now. In fact, if you haven't built up your strength and stamina over time, it's considered a poor idea to put strain on your body when you're pregnant.

If you do want to get your body moving but aren't accustomed to aerobic exercise, then it's probably wise to limit yourself to nothing more vigorous than brisk walking. Taking a 20- to 30-minute walk on a regular basis is good for your general health, in particular your digestion, circulation, psyche, and your figure.

NOTE: Don't force yourself to walk more than your body can comfortably handle: for some women the cartilage in the pelvis softens so much that walking any distance becomes difficult. Follow your instincts and listen to the signals your body gives you.

Avoid Stomach Exercises

Avoid any exercise that pulls on abdominal muscles. Sit-ups are a prime example: unless you are conditioned to them you should not do sit-ups during your pregnancy (and even if you are fit, you should quit as soon as sit-ups become uncomfortable). The longitudinal muscles of the abdomen (the ones that run up and down) are designed to part in the middle to allow room for the expanding uterus. But if you sit straight up from a prone position it encourages those muscles to part even further. Even though you'd think that stomach exercises would help strengthen your belly, experts say that doing sit-up-type exercises when pregnant can slow recovery of abdominal tone after delivery.

There is a way to tell which movements are not good for your stomach. Once your uterus is big enough that you appear to be definitely pregnant, lie down on your back and try to sit up straight. You'll see a longitudinal ridge that forms at the midline of your stomach . . . now that you've seen it, lie right back down! You want to avoid any action that raises this ridge. Leg raises while lying on your back are equally harmful.

RECOMMENDED EXERCISES DURING PREGNANCY

— **Walking**: It's best at a quick pace for about 30 minutes.

— **A stationary bicycle**: Recommended because your center of gravity changes dramatically as your pregnancy progresses, but without the danger of falling! Just pay attention to your posture and don't lean over the handlebars in a way that could give you a backache.

— **Swimming**: Probably the best all-around sport when you're pregnant because it uses many muscles while rarely producing strain or stress on the joints.

— **Pregnancy exercise classes**: Calisthenics designed specifically for pregnant women, which are best done under supervision so that you don't strain your body without realizing it.

SOME GOOD EXERCISES FOR PREGNANCY

Whatever exercise you do during pregnancy, be protective of your joints. This is true for anyone who exercises, but your body is going through changes that affect the joints so you want to be extra careful not to make rapid jerky movements—try to move smoothly, without rushing. In any exercise you do, maintain muscle control of the "down" (or less strenuous) motion as well as the more active phase of the motion: this is a principle of isometric exercise and will protect your joints and muscles from shock as well as increasing the usefulness of the exercise.

The Kegel Exercise

This exercise is the most important one of all during pregnancy: if you do nothing else, at least learn how to do "Kegels"! It is not a strenuous exercise—in fact, you can do it anywhere, anytime, without anyone even knowing—but it's important to do it often to prepare your body for labor and delivery. Kegels strengthen your pelvic floor muscles for childbirth; the exercise also gives you enough control to be able to totally relax those same muscles, which is also very important for delivery. By doing Kegels throughout pregnancy, you will help the vagina regain its previous shape and muscle tone more quickly after birth.

The pelvic floor muscles are the same ones used to stop the flow of urine. You can get a feel of these muscles when you're urinating: practice by stopping the flow of urine. Once you get the feel of these muscles, you can practice contracting them regularly during the day. Some people pick a frequent reminder—like a red light if you drive a lot, or every time they see a stop sign—to remind them to do their Kegels. Once you recognize where these muscles are, you should exercise them every single day.

The best way to get a mental picture of the Kegel exercise is to think of an internal elevator going up inside you: contract the pelvic floor muscles a small amount at a time, imagining an elevator going up one floor after another, counting up to the tenth "floor." Then release the muscular tension little by little, counting backward slowly, floor by floor. Try to develop enough control so that you don't release the muscles completely until the "elevator" is back down to the "first floor"—but not before (releasing the contracted muscle is more difficult). Another way to visualize Kegels is to contract the muscles in a wavelike, front-to-back rhythm, including the anus in the exercise. Release in reverse.

Kegels are easiest to do sitting down, but once you get the hang of it, you can do them standing up or even walking. You can also do them lying down on your back with your knees bent and your feet on the floor about a foot apart. You can do Kegels when you're in bed or in the bathtub. And a really pleasant way to do Kegels is during lovemaking. When your partner's penis is inside you is a really good time to practice: suddenly tighten your pelvic floor muscles. Hold that tension for as long as you can, for a count of up to ten. As time goes on, your mate can feel how those muscles are developing by how much pressure he feels. It is a lovely addition to lovemaking!

Try to do about 25 Kegels every day, at various times. This may seem like a lot, but once you get into the habit, Kegels will be something you'll do without any big mental effort. And don't stop once the baby is born. In fact, doing them right after the baby is born can do you a lot of good. If you've had an episiotomy, Kegels can help pull the stitches together and begin healing and strengthening those muscles. You might not be able to feel yourself doing the exercise in the first 24 hours after the baby is born, but they are doing you good!

Pelvic Rock

Although it might sound like the name of New Age music, the pelvic rock is a useful exercise! Pelvic rock relieves backache, strengthens your abdominal muscles and also brings the baby forward (taking her weight off your back, which improves your circulation).

Doing the Pelvic Rock

Kneel on all fours like a cat.
— Keep your elbows straight, legs slightly apart, and your back straight. Make sure your arms and thighs are perpendicular to your body and to the floor.

— Curl your back up, arching like a cat, while inhaling and tucking your head under.
— Do not use your backbone to pull the arch up, which might increase lower backache instead of relieving it. Make sure you use the lower abdominal muscles to push the arch up.
— While exhaling, let your back relax slowly.

Relaxation Exercises

You may not think of relaxation as an exercise, but it's probably the most important one you can learn during pregnancy. Practice the technique at least twice a day, before a nap and at bedtime. Once you get the hang of it you'll probably be asleep before you even have time to finish the relaxation routine. The reason it's so important to learn this exercise is because it trains you how to lie down and relax immediately, removing one of the problems of early motherhood, which is how to take catnaps.

The instructions that follow are similar to the relaxation you'll be taught in childbirth education classes, which trains you how to prevent the spread of tension during labor from the working muscle (the uterus) to nearby inactive muscles. This will let the uterine muscles have the maximum effectiveness with the least possible discomfort to you. Relaxation exercises enable you to recognize the reactions of your own body so that you'll be able to interpret sensations of muscle tension, fatigue, and release. Tension can build up when you're pregnant; there are some easy exercises you can do anywhere in order to relax.

LEARNING TO RELAX

1) Get as comfortable as you can. Add pillows under your knee and foot so you don't cut off circulation.
2) Tighten (contract the muscles) your right arm; release it. You should feel all the tightness/tension leave. That should feel good.
3) Tighten and then release your left arm.
4) Contract and then release the muscles of the right leg.
5) Repeat with left leg.
6) Now tighten the right arm and right leg at the same time; release them.
7) Do the same on the left side.
8) Contract the opposite arm and leg on both sides.
9) Contract the right hand and release; contract the left hand and release.
10) Scrunch up your face, then let it go slack.
11) Tighten the pelvic floor (Kegel exercise); release it slowly.
12) Check yourself for relaxation. Your body should be like a rag doll's: your hands should be loose and open; your neck, face, and shoulders relaxed.

13) Your jaw should be loose: a lot of tension accumulates around the mouth. Open your mouth very wide, stretching the entire area, then release it. Your tongue should be loose and resting against your teeth.

14) Your eyes should be relaxed: not scrunched shut, not wide open.

Tension-Releasing Exercises

— **Neck Stretch**: Rotate your head slowly in a circle. First stretch to the left, then let your head drop gently to the front, then stretch to the right, then back. After a couple of turns in one direction, reverse and make a circle going the other way.

— **Shoulder Roll**: This is designed to loosen your shoulders and upper back. First press your shoulders forward (as if they could meet in front). Then pull your shoulders up to your ears; now drop them down again. Next push your shoulders back, pulling your shoulder blades together in back and lifting your chest.

— **Stretch and Flop Over**: Stand with your feet apart, knees slightly bent, and let your head hang down. Let all your weight hang down with your arms loose; touch the floor if you can.

— **Back Roll**: This is a good substitute for massage. Lie flat on your back with your knees up to your chest (or later in pregnancy, as far up as they'll go). Let your hands rest on your knees. Now roll from side to side, with your hands to guide your legs—you can let your hand pull one leg over, leading the rest of the body. This massages your back muscles, where you have tension.

Abdominal Exercises

To strengthen your abdominal (stomach) muscles, there are several exercises that don't use the longitudinal muscles the way sit-ups do (and which you want to avoid during pregnancy).

➢ **Opposite Arm and Leg Reach**: Lie on your back, lift your head, and with rounded shoulders reach your right arm toward your left toe. Your leg should be straight and about a foot off the ground, with the foot flexed. (Reminder: never point your toes while exercising or you might get leg cramps.) You should feel a stretch: hold it, then lower and relax. Switch legs. There is another way to do this exercise, which is to lie flat on your back with your knees up and your feet flat on the floor. One hand reaches to the opposite knee, your head raising each time you make the motion. (Reminder: be sure to inhale as you lie back down and exhale as you stretch up and across.)

➤ **Leg Raise**: Lie on your back with your knees bent. Bring one knee up to your chest and straighten the leg toward the ceiling, flexing your foot. Slowly lower it (while exhaling), keeping your leg straight out. This exercise is good for circulation in your legs as well as for your abdominal muscles.

Other Exercises

➤ **Tailor-Sitting**: This is also called "knee press" and strengthens your inner thighs and perineum (the area between your vagina and anus), which is important for labor and delivery. This exercise is quite easy and you can even do it when you're sitting around with friends (pregnant or not, they can join you!). Sit on the floor and pull your feet, with the soles together, as near your body as is comfortable. With your back straight, press your knees gently to the floor 6 times, using your hands. (NOTE: *Do not bounce* the knees up and down as you may have done in exercise classes pre-pregnancy.)

➤ **Hip Roll**: This helps take bulk off your thighs. Sitting up with your legs straight out in front of you, shift your weight and roll from side to side, massaging the other thigh on each side as you roll over.

➤ **Lower Back Strengthener**: The pelvic rock is the best lower back exercise, but here is another: get on all fours like a cat. Pull one knee in toward your nose while tucking your head under to meet the knee. Then straighten out your head and, at the same time, extend the leg straight out behind you. Keep the motion slow and smooth.

What Not to Do When Exercising

— Avoid intense exercise: it's too much for your body now.
— Never exercise to the point of fatigue: you can't bounce back easily from physical exertion.
— If you feel any pain during exercise—STOP! Follow your body's signals and use common sense.
— Avoid lying flat on your back, which cuts off blood flow to the baby.
— Avoid prolonged periods of standing still, which also compromises circulation.
— Never point your toes when exercising or stretching to prevent leg cramps. Always flex your foot (keep it perpendicular to your leg).
— Don't take up a new sport; your body can't handle it now (although it's okay to continue any sport if you've been doing regularly so that your body is conditioned to it).

— Avoid activities that raise body temperature. Overheating can cause birth defects in the first trimester and can cause premature labor in the last trimester.
— Avoid treadmills and stair machines, which can elevate your body temperature and heart-rate. Misuse of these machines can cause miscarriage or premature labor.
— Avoid any exercise that pulls on abdominal muscles, which are separating to make room for the growing uterus. Stomach exercises now will slow recovery of abdominal tone after birth.
— Avoid any exercise with potential for even mild abdominal trauma (such as sit-ups).
— Avoid jarring motions and any exercise that requires excessive twisting of your joints.
— Stop if you feel any pain while exercising. Trust your body's signals and use common sense.
— Be prepared for body changes that can throw off your balance, especially in the last trimester.

Exercises to Avoid During Pregnancy

— **Jogging** is a hard exercise for the pregnant body: it is not good for your breasts, especially now that they're larger, and it also jars your lower back and knees.
— **Weight-bearing sports** such as backpacking are not a good idea; they put too much strain on you.
— **Scuba-diving** can restrict your circulation. Decompression sickness (which can happen to anyone) is dangerous for the fetus.
— **Horseback riding** (unless you're an accomplished rider) can mean a fall because your center of gravity is changing all the time.

WARNING! STOP EXERCISING IF YOU HAVE:

* Pain of any kind
* Bleeding
* Dizziness, light-headedness
* Shortness of breath or severe breathlessness

* Loss of muscle control
* Heart palpitations
* Uterine contractions
* Headache

— ***Downhill skiing*** (unless you're already a serious skier) can cause you to fall because your center of balance is off, especially later in pregnancy.

— ***Snow skiing above 10,000 feet*** can deprive you and the baby of all-important oxygen.

— ***Diving or jumping into water*** could force water into your vagina.

— ***Water-skiing*** is another sport where balance is necessary and should be avoided by all but expert skiers. A fall could force water into your vagina.

— ***Mountain biking*** often puts you in risky conditions such as narrow bumpy paths, biking on wet roads, etc., where you are in danger of falling.

— ***Bicycling*** is another sport that demands balance and yours is constantly changing as you get bigger in front. Also, any racing-type bicycle is a bad idea because you can get a back- ache from leaning over the handlebars. You can always con- tinue cycling on a stationary bike.

— ***Tennis in the last trimester*** is not recommended because as you get bigger your body cannot handle sudden moves; you also lose a sense of balance.

— ***Calisthenics not specifically for pregnancy***, whether in a gym class or video, should be avoided because they are not geared to the needs of a pregnant body.

SAFETY TIPS: EXERCISE FOR DIABETICS

— 133 beats per minute is the highest your heart rate should go.

— Have a snack, preferably with a glass of milk, before exercising.

— Don't exercise when the temperature is in the eighties or above, especially if the humidity is high.

— If you are insulin-dependent, you'll want to avoid in- jecting into the parts of your body you're exercising (for example, your legs if you're walking).

— If you're on insulin, your doctor will recommend not reducing your insulin intake before exercise.

DRUGS & ALCOHOL
WHEN YOU'RE PREGNANT

There are two categories of drugs—prescribed medications, and "street" or "recreational" drugs—but it is dangerous to use any substance while you are pregnant. The baby's growing tissues are extremely sensitive, and her body doesn't yet have functioning mechanisms for neutralizing drugs and eliminating them from her body. These mechanisms remain incomplete for at least 4 weeks following a full-term birth, so the baby is completely vulnerable to any substance that you put into your body for any reason.

If and when your doctor says that it is necessary for you to take medication during pregnancy, talk to him/her about limiting the use of any drug to the smallest effective dose for the briefest possible time period. If any doctor tells you that a medical condition you may have requires medication, discuss the side effects of that drug and ask what the effect would be if you were not to take the medication at all. If any drug is prescribed to you, before you make the decision to take it get as much information about it as you possibly can and talk to the doctor about any risk to the baby compared to the benefit to you.

The first three months of the baby's development is when there is the greatest risk of injury from drug exposure. The critical period of major organ development in the embryo occurs from the fourth to the eighth weeks (see "The Baby's Growth," page 43). If you take any drugs during this crucial stage of the baby's growth, it can cause permanent birth defects. It is considered hazardous to use any drug during that first trimester. During the second and third trimesters, drugs may impair the normal development of your baby's brain, nervous system, and external genital organs.

Alcohol: Spirits, Wine & Beer

Alcohol is dangerous to your growing baby: it can damage the nerve cells of the developing brain. Experts *used* to say that you could have a certain number of drinks during pregnancy, but now they have found that there is no "safe" amount of alcohol when you are pregnant. Although much is known about alcoholic mothers and the devastating effects on their babies (known as Fetal Alcohol Syndrome, or FAS), researchers do not know the smallest amount of alcohol that can produce a birth defect. It is known that even moderate drinking while pregnant can retard the baby's growth inside you and can cause "neurobehavioral deficits," which can include problems with learning skills, attention, memory, and problem-solving. Mental handicaps and hyperactivity are the most debilitating aspects of FAS, but more subtle versions of these cognitive-behavioral problems can result from the mother drinking smaller amounts.

There are other reasons to avoid alcohol: it interferes with your body's absorption and utilization of important nutrients. Alcohol actually robs your body of the good things you're taking in because it uses those nutrients for its own metabolism: the food and vitamins you're taking in for the baby get used instead by your body to cope with the alcohol. Also, alcohol has the indirect effect of lowering your appetite, which means you're substituting the empty calories of alcohol for real nutrition. And "binge drinking" is a serious problem, too: even one day or night of excessive consumption, especially in the first trimester, can leave your baby damaged for life.

Abstaining from alcohol during your entire pregnancy is a favor you can do your baby that will last a lifetime.

Cocaine & "Crack"

There is an entire generation of babies who are being damaged for life because their mothers used cocaine—even briefly—during their pregnancies. Many mothers-to-be underestimate the dangers of cocaine: the same woman who won't take an aspirin because it might harm her baby may think it's harmless to snort a few lines of cocaine. But she is poisoning her unborn infant: cocaine is brutal on the developing baby, causing a painful withdrawal at birth, followed by developmental and neurological problems as the child grows up. It can cause early onset of labor as well as miscarriage due to sudden separation of the placenta.

If you expose your baby to cocaine, he is more likely to die before birth or to be at risk when born prematurely, with a smaller-than-normal head and brain. Lasting damage can include: retarded growth, stiff limbs, hyperirritability, learning disabilities, a tendency to stop breathing (with a risk of Sudden Infant Death Syndrome ten times greater than normal), and in extreme cases, malformed genital and urinary organs, a missing small intestine, strokes, and seizures. The point is this: if cocaine attracts you, isn't it worthwhile to stay far away from it during your childbearing years?

Research shows that a single cocaine "hit" can cause permanent damage to the growing baby. While a single dose of cocaine and its metabolites clear out of the adult body within 48 hours, the unborn baby inside that adult remains exposed for 4 or 5 days. Cocaine is fat soluble, which means it can penetrate the placenta, the baby's source of nourishment. The baby's body converts a significant amount of the cocaine into "norcocaine," a water-soluble substance that does not leave the womb and is even more potent than cocaine. Norcocaine is excreted into the amniotic fluid which the fetus swallows, exposing himself again to the drug. Researchers believe that if a baby is exposed to any amount of cocaine, he cannot escape its damaging effects.

If you used cocaine during the early part of your pregnancy (perhaps before you even knew you were pregnant), you should seriously consider discussing this fact with your medical caregiver. Some doctors or midwives may not venture an opinion about how to handle the situation, while other professionals believe that any use of cocaine during the first

DANGERS OF ALCOHOL & STREET DRUGS

Liquor, wine, beer
— No amount of alcohol is safe: avoid it entirely during pregnancy.
— More than 2 oz./day of hard liquor can permanently harm your developing baby.
— Alcohol causes physical defects, learning disabilities, and emotional problems.
— Excessive drinking *even one time* can cause "fetal alcohol syndrome": physical abnormalities and behavioral problems for the child's lifetime.

Amphetamines
("uppers," "speed")
— These drugs are dangerous stimulants to the baby's nervous system.
— Has long-term effects on the child.

Cocaine, crack
— Can kill your baby.
— Can cause a baby to be born addicted, suffering a painful withdrawal at birth.
— Causes long-term problems in development and behavior.

Heroin, morphine
— Can cause fetal addiction, meaning an agonizing withdrawal for the newborn.
— Baby may need a blood transfusion.

LSD, psychedelics
— Increases the risk of miscarriage.
— May cause chromosomal damage to the unborn child.

Marijuana, hash
— Smoking even small amounts of grass can cause fertility problems.
— Can cause complications of pregnancy and low-birth-weight babies.
— Can cause stillbirth and early infant death.

Tranquilizers
(Quaaludes, downers)
— May cause deformities in first trimester.

trimester is so detrimental to the developing fetus that they recommend aborting such a pregnancy.

Marijuana ("Grass") & Hashish

Marijuana was once thought to be fairly harmless, but studies have shown that it has some of the same dangerous effects on the fetus as cocaine does. Smoking even a moderate amount of grass can have serious consequences to your developing baby. Studies were done on pregnant monkeys, using small amounts of THC, the active chemical in marijuana. The effects on the pregnancies and babies included: delayed conception (infertility), problems during pregnancy, stillbirth, early infant death, and smaller than normal babies, who are at risk (like any low-birth-weight infant) for health and developmental problems.

It is known that THC builds up in the germ cells of the ovaries and testes of people who smoke grass. Though damage to the man may be temporary, because he constantly produces new sperm, the effect on a woman can be lasting. You are born with a certain number of eggs: if those eggs are injured, there is no way to undo the damage. Therefore it is advisable for prospective parents to stop smoking marijuana long before becoming pregnant, although no one knows how long before conception you should stop to insure a healthy baby.

Marijuana interferes with cell division, meaning it affects the fetus when it is first forming. Grass also interferes with your body's immune system, so your white blood cells become less capable of fighting viruses and other illness. A marijuana smoker may be more susceptible to viral infections, at least one of which—rubella—is known to cause birth defects.

Aspirin

For yourself and your baby you don't want to make the dangerous mistake of taking any aspirin products during pregnancy. Doctors have been advising for years that pregnant women shouldn't use aspirin because it is linked to unusual bleeding problems, including newborn brain hemorrhage. But mothers-to-be don't seem to understand that aspirin is a serious health problem because they continue taking it, sometimes not even aware that the products they're consuming have aspirin in them. For example, many ointments that you apply to your skin for pain relief contain aspirin, which can be absorbed through the body tissues. (There is a list of these below in the chart "Ointments Containing Aspirin.")

Many people don't know which over-the-counter and prescription pain medicines contain aspirin. The chart below lists the vast majority of these medications, which should protect you from unintentionally taking aspirin. Although the list comprises common brand-name prescription and over-the-counter products that contain aspirin, there are also many generic or store brand-name preparations, so you should check the ingredients of anything you're thinking of taking.

AN ASPIRIN DIRECTORY

Advil (ibuprofen); Alka-Seltzer; Alka-Seltzer Plus cold medicine; Anacin (and Anacin Maximum Strength); Anaprox; APC; APC with Butalbital; APC with Codeine; Arthritis Pain Formula (by Anacin); Arthritis Strength Bufferin; Ascodeen-30; Ascriptin; Aspergum; Aspirin suppositories
Bayer Aspirin; Bayer Children's Chewable Aspirin; Bayer Children's cold tablets; Bayer Timed-Release aspirin; BC Powders; Buff-A comp; Buffadyne; Bufferin; Butalbital
Cama Inlay-Tabs; Cetased, Improved; Cheracol capsules; Clinoril; Congesprin; Cope; Coricidin D decongestant tablets; Coricidin for children; Coricidin Medilets for children; Coricidin
Darvon with A.S.A.; Darvon-N with A.S.A.; Dristan decongestant; Duragesic
Ecotrin; Empirin; Empirin with Codeine; Emprazil; Emprazil-C; En Tab; Equagesic; Excedrin; Extra-Strength Bufferin
Feldene; Fiorinal; Fiorinal with Codeine; 4-Way Cold Tablets
Gemnisyn; Goody's Headache Powders
Indocin
Measurin; Midol; Momentum Muscular Backache Formula; Monacet with Codeine; Motrin
Naprosyn; Norgesic; Norgesic Forte; Norwich aspirin; Nuprin; Aleve
Pabirin buffered tablets; Panalgesic; Percodan and Percodan-Demi tablets; Percogesic; Persistin
Quiet World Analgesic/Sleeping aid
Robaxisal tablets
SK-65 Compound; St. Joseph Aspirin for Children; Sine-Aid; Sine-Off Sinus Medicine tablets— aspirin formula; Supac; Stendin; Stero-Darvon with A.S.A.; Synalgos (and Synalgos-DC) capsules
Tolectin; Triaminicin tablets
Vanquish; Verin; Viro-Med tablets
Zomax; Zorpin

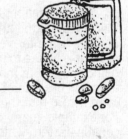

In newborns and their mothers, aspirin can lead to uncontrolled bleeding and circulation problems for the baby. Aspirin has a significant effect on blood platelets, the microscopic discs that are essential to clotting. If the function of these platelets is impaired, bleeding can become very difficult to stop. Although it's good to avoid aspirin throughout your pregnancy, it's particularly important that you not take it anywhere near your due date. If you know you've taken aspirin within 5 days of when your labor begins, it would be foolish and dangerous to keep it a secret:

OINTMENTS CONTAINING ASPIRIN

Absorbent Rub; Absorbine (Arthritic and Jr.); Act-On Rub; Analbalm; Analgesic Balm; Antiphlogistine; Arthralgen; Aspercreme; Banalog; Baumodyne; Ben-Gay (all kinds); Braska; Counterpain Rub; Dencorub; Doan's Rub; Emul-O-Balm; End-Ake; Exocaine (Plus or tube); Heet; Icy Hot; Infra-Rub; Lini-Balm; Mentholatum & Deep Heating; Minit-Rub; Musterole (all kinds); Neurabaum; Oil-O-Sol; Omega Oil; Panalgesic; Rid-A-Pain; Rumarub; Sloan's; Soltice (all kinds); SPD; Stimurub; Surin; Yager's Liniment; Zemo (all kinds)

be sure to tell the doctor, who will keep a special eye out for you during childbirth and may want to have the newborn specially evaluated for aspirin-related bleeding problems.

If you are planning on circumcising your baby boy and you took aspirin within the 5-day interval before delivery, it is significant for the baby's health. Tell the pediatrician, who might recommend waiting several days longer than normal for the circumcision, to avoid bleeding-related complications.

WHEN THE MOTHER GETS SICK

When you're pregnant it's easy to get worried if you get even the most common illness. There's the fear about whether your malady can harm the baby, or whether there is danger in the medicines you might have to take. Another problem is that some illnesses seem to linger longer when you're pregnant, which can make the discomfort or worry even greater.

Here are some suggestions about ways to avoid getting sick in the first place. This advice is basically about keeping scrupulously clean as a protection from possible contamination. Although some of these warnings may seem like overkill to you now, "an ounce of prevention" is a valid cliché. There are a number of ways you can protect yourself that are well worth the trouble to avoid getting sick now, when you can least afford it.

WAYS TO AVOID GETTING SICK

Don't Get Run Down

By taking very good care of your body, you can keep your resistance up. We've all seen how people who let themselves get run down are susceptible to whatever germs are around. The obvious ways to protect and insure your good health are to eat a good diet, get plenty of sleep, moderate exercise, and pace yourself, listening to your body's cues about how much it can realistically do. Perhaps most vitally important to physical well-being is to avoid getting stressed out. Protect and nurture your mental and spiritual self and your body will not break down on you.

Stay Away from People When They're Sick

This may sound obvious, but before you were pregnant wouldn't you often spend time around people who had colds or stomach bugs without giving it a second thought? You can't do that now because those people may be contagious and you can't afford to get sick right now. Stay away from crowded spaces where people are coughing and sneezing, especially in the months when so many people have colds. This means convention halls, subways, buses, etc. I'm not suggesting that you become a recluse, or go out in public wearing a gas mask. You have to use common sense, but you shouldn't take this advice too lightly. There are cities in Asia with extreme crowding where it's not uncommon to see people walking around wearing the kind of masks you see on doctor in an operating room—either to protect themselves from other people's illness or because they are sick and don't want to infect their fellow citizens.

If you find yourself in the company of someone who's had a stomach flu, is coughing, or has a runny nose, at the very least limit your physical contact with them. Also, someone you're spending time with might have a sick family member at home, whose germs can also pass to you. It may sound self-evident, but everyone needs reminding about basic hygiene in these situations. Your hands are the greatest carrier of germs: if you shake hands with someone who has covered their own mouth when coughing, you then carry those germs right into your own system when you touch your own mouth or eyes. The same is true in public when you hold a handrail, for example—you are picking up whatever germs other people's hands have deposited there.

How to Avoid Germs

— Don't kiss people, especially on the lips.
— Don't share food or drinks.
— Wash your hands whenever it crosses your mind: after shaking hands with anyone (sick or not), or after spending

time in crowded public places when you've touched surfaces.
— Keep your fingers out of your mouth, nose and eyes—most people touch their faces without realizing it. Use a fresh tissue for your nose and eyes and a toothpick for anything lodged in your teeth.
— Don't share a toothbrush, Water Pik, or bathroom cup.
— Use disinfectant spray on telephones in your home or put a tissue over phones you use elsewhere.
— Limit time spent around children (see below).

Children Are Major Carriers of Illness

Children spend time around other children and their illnesses pass quickly from one to the other and then home to their parents and siblings. Find polite ways to avoid spending time around other people's children, whether they're school-age or are in daycare environments. If you're around children with symptoms such as coughs or runny noses, avoid kissing them on the face, and wash your hands after playing with them. All during your pregnancy do not sip out of children's drinks or finish up food from their plates (kid's leftovers are such a temptation!).

If your own child or one you've spent time around develops any kind of rash, avoid close physical contact because he may be carrying one of several common childhood diseases such as German measles (rubella), chicken pox (varicella), or "fifth" disease or CMV (cytomegalovirus). Unless you are certain that you are already immune to all of these illnesses, see your doctor right away to be tested.

➤ *Chicken pox (varicella) is a common childhood illness*. If you're exposed to chicken pox it's unlikely to cause any problem because most women of childbearing age in America today had the disease as a child (which would make you immune now). To find out whether you had chicken pox, ask your mother or try to find your own childhood health records. Otherwise, your obstetrician can run a test to see whether you have already been exposed. If you are part of the small 10% who are not immune, your doctor may want take the precaution of giving you a shot of VZIG (varicella-zoster immune globulin), which has to be done within four days of being exposed to the disease. It isn't certain whether the baby is protected by this injection, but it will lessen the complications for you since this illness can be quite severe in adults who contract it. If you are infected early or late in pregnancy it can be harmful to the developing baby, but the possibility of this happening is statistically slim.

➤ *Mumps is also rare during pregnancy* because most of us had it as children or were immunized against it. Once again, check with your parents or your childhood pediatrician (if s/he's still in practice) to learn whether you are immune. But if not, even if you are exposed to mumps you probably won't come down with it because it isn't highly contagious.

> ***Hepatitis A*** *is very common among children under five*: one in three of them gets it. It's usually a mild disease with no symptoms (not to be confused with hepatitis B, a contagious liver disease) and isn't passed on to the developing baby. Hepatitis A is passed through feces; to avoid any infection during pregnancy the best protection is to wash your hands religiously any time you change a diaper or help a child on the toilet and, of course, before you eat.

Avoid Airplane Travel Whenever Possible

Haven't you noticed how you (or people you know) have gotten a cold or flu after a long airplane flight? This is because all the germs that passengers cough and sneeze into the cabin are recirculated in the same pressurized air and blown right in your face through the air vents. There are everyday colds and coughs, but people who have been traveling may also have been exposed to more complicated illnesses abroad, so you want to avoid having any contact with them.

Be Vigilant About Safe Food Preparation

See page 70 for important safety tips about how to purchase, store, and prepare foods in ways that protect you from possible food poisoning.

Avoid any restaurant where you have suspicions about the cleanliness of the kitchen, bathrooms, hygiene habits of the food preparers, or the freshness of the ingredients.

Getting a Cold or the Flu

Many women find that a cold lasts longer when they're pregnant, so if you do get one you want to keep it from becoming severe. We all know the "rules" about colds: get plenty of rest, plenty of liquids (especially warm ones, such as chicken soup), and keep a fever down. You can do this without aspirin by taking cool showers or baths, putting an ice pack on your pulse points such as the wrists and back of the neck, drinking cold liquids, or spraying yourself with a product such as Sea Breeze that contains some rubbing alcohol. Pamper yourself and make sure you keep eating, even if you don't really feel like it. The old saying "starve a fever" does not apply when there's a baby growing inside you.

But don't ignore the symptoms if a cold or flu gets bad. Call your doctor if your fever gets to 102°, if you're coughing up phlegm that is yellow or green, if you are having trouble eating or sleeping, or if the cold goes on for more than a week. In any of these cases, the doctor has to make a judgment call about whether the possible small risk from medication may be worth it for your health.

Stomach Bug

Most stomach flus that include vomiting or diarrhea last about 24 hours, so your suffering will probably be short. There's no harm to the baby if you aren't able to eat solids for a day or two, as long as you don't get dehydrated, which is usually the only risk when you've lost a lot of fluids. Take in as much clear liquids as you possibly can: the best are water, seltzer, weak tea (preferably decaffeinated), diluted nonacidic fruit juices, and clear broth. Small frequent sips is the best thing for your body, if you can manage it. If not, sucking on ice chips may be tolerable. Avoid milk and cola, which is commonly believed to be helpful but may actually make your stomach worse.

Of course, you may want to call your doctor for any further suggestions or reassurance.

NOTE: Always Consult with a Medical Care-Giver Before Taking or Stopping Any Medication (Prescription or *Over-the-Counter*).

MEDICATIONS TO AVOID

Accutane (isotretinoin)	— An acne drug that causes severe, often lethal birth defects.
Ace inhibitors	— Given for high blood pressure.
	— Causes deformities in first trimester.
	— In second and third trimesters can cause fetal death.
	— If you've been on an ace inhibitor, talk to your doctor about an alternative medication.
	— *Do not just stop taking the medicine*: that could be dangerous for you and the baby.
Aerosol ribavirin	— Used to treat severe lung infections in small children.
	— For pregnant health-care workers who handle it, breathing the mist can cause birth defects.
Anabolic steroids	— Used for bodybuilding and sports to build muscle.
	— Should be avoided before and during pregnancy.

MEDICATIONS TO AVOID (*cont.*)

Anesthetic gases
— Hospital personnel and doctors may be exposed to the gases in the operating room.
— Suspected to be the cause of high rates of sterility, miscarriage, and birth defects among these people.

Antibiotics
— Some antibiotics can cross the placenta and cause birth defects or even fetal death.
— Check with your doctor before taking any antibiotic to be certain it cannot harm your developing baby.

Anticonvulsants
(Dilantin, etc.)
— Can cause abnormalities such as cleft lip and cleft palate.
— If it would be dangerous to your health to stop the anticonvulsant, folic acid may counteract possible birth defects.
— Be sure you discuss this with your doctor before changing your medicines.

Antidepressants
— See Prozac.

Antihistamines
— Cause malformations in the baby.
— "Dries you up," but can also affect the amniotic fluid.
— Ask about antihistamines designed for safe use during pregnancy.

Antimetabolites
(antitumor drugs)
— Medications such as Aminopterin can cause malformations of the fetus.

Antinausea pills
— Have caused malformations in the offspring of test animals.
— Avoid if possible, but talk to your doctor if nausea prevents proper eating.

Aspirin
— Affects your blood-clotting mechanism: can be fatal to you during labor and delivery.
— Can cause miscarriage when taken in large amounts.

Aspirin (*cont.*) — Frequent use toward the end of pregnancy may cause hemorrhage in newborn.
— See "Aspirin Directory" on page 172.

Birth control pill — Can cause fetal malformations.
— See page 3 for more on the pill.

Blood pressure drugs — See "Ace inhibitors" and "Reserpine."

Cancer chemotherapy — Pregnant nurses who handle these drugs during their first trimester have high risk of miscarriage.
— Healthcare professionals who are pregnant or trying to conceive should avoid exposure to these medications.

Cortisone (corticosteroids) — Can cause fetal abnormalitics or stillbirth.

Cough syrup — Especially dangerous early in pregnancy.
Even over-the-counter brands may affect baby's development.

Diet pills (dextroamphetamines) — Can cause heart defects and blood vessel malformations.

Diuretics (water pills) — Causes blood disorders or jaundice in the newborn.

Haldol (haloperidol) — A tranquilizer used in treating schizophrenia.
— Can permanently alter the baby's brain chemistry: however, this might decrease the baby's chance of developing schizophrenia later in life, since the illness runs in families.
— Discuss with your doctor the risk versus benefit to the baby of taking Haldol.

Iodides (expectorants) — Can cause a goiter in the unborn baby.

Nose sprays & drops — Can be strong enough to contract blood vessels in the placenta, reducing oxygen and nutrition carried to the fetus.

MEDICATIONS TO AVOID (*cont.*)

Phenacetin	— Causes possible damage to the baby's developing kidneys.
Progestins	— Linked to birth defects, particularly genital defects in female babies.
Prozac (fluoxetine)	— Most widely prescribed antidepressant in the U.S.
	— New studies suggest possible increased risk of premature delivery and minor newborn health problems. However, five previous studies showed no ill effects.
	— The manufacturer recommends avoiding during pregnancy because of lack of conclusive data about effects on unborn children.
	— Do not abruptly stop this medication during pregnancy; consult with the doctor who prescribed it.
Reserpine	— Drugs to lower blood pressure can cause blood disorders and jaundice in newborns.
Sulfa drugs	— Taken late in pregnancy, can disturb the baby's liver function and produce a form of jaundice associated with brain damage.
Tegison (etretinate)	— Used to treat severe cases of psoriasis.
	— Even after this drug is discontinued, it stays in a person's body for 2 years.
	— Tegison can continue to cause severe birth defects long after you stop taking it.
Thyroid medications	— Can cause goiter in the infant.
Tranquilizers	— Taken in the first trimester may cause fetal deformities.
	— Check with your doctor about tranquilizers that may be designed for safe use during pregnancy.
Vitamins	— Can be dangerous in excess quantities.
	— See "Warnings About Vitamins" on page 111.

SMOKING WHILE YOU'RE PREGNANT

For your health, as well as the baby's inside you, please stop smoking now. Give your child the best possible start in life by not contaminating his world with the products of your cigarette smoking. If you are around second-hand smoke, it can have as many ill effects on the baby as if you were smoking yourself, so stay out of situations where you'll be around cigarette smoke. Fewer workplaces allow smoking anymore, but social occasions may still arise where you may have to move your seat or leave for your health's sake.

We all know how unhealthy smoking is for us, and for the people around us, so it's no surprise that it's harmful to a developing baby inside a smoking mother. When a woman smokes, she is cutting down the oxygen supply to her baby: she's cheating her baby of the very thing he needs in order to grow. Studies have shown that lead in the blood vessels of infants is in proportion to the levels of lead in their mothers' blood from smoking. The toxic ingredients that are inhaled with cigarette smoke—carbon monoxide and cyanide—retard fetal growth. Smoking is linked to low-birth-weight infants, which are less hardy. Another reason for low-birth-weight babies is that their smoking mothers gain less weight when they are pregnant. They smoke more and eat less.

New studies show that when fathers smoked around nonsmoking women during their pregnancy, their baby's risk of dying from crib death (or SIDS, Sudden Infant Death Syndrome) was tripled. This effect on the babies' risk of SIDS was almost as great as if the mother herself had smoked during pregnancy.

Each cigarette you smoke has a direct effect on your baby, so if you find that you can't stop smoking "cold turkey," you'll still be doing the baby a favor by reducing the number of cigarettes you smoke and how strong they are. For some suggestions on how to stop smoking, or at least cut down, see the chart on page 7.

Newly Discovered Dangers from Smoking

The risk of ectopic pregnancy is now believed to be higher for women who smoke, and their risk of miscarriage may be much higher if *their mothers* smoked while pregnant with them. These conclusions are drawn from a study of 15,000 women in England; the results suggest that smoking causes long-term, multigenerational damage to a woman's fertility.

The study discovered that chemical extracts of cigarette smoke inhibit the "beating" activity of the cilia, which are the tiny hairlike fibers that line the fallopian tubes. It is the motion of the cilia which helps move fertilized eggs along the fallopian tubes and into the uterus.

Ectopic pregnancy occurs when the fertilized egg implants in your tube, which can burst if it goes undetected, threatening your life. Not only do you lose the pregnancy, but it also affects your future fertility if you lose a fallopian tube. Smoking women run a higher risk of ectopic pregnancy than nonsmokers.

It now seems as though there is a "smoking grandmother" factor to your reproductive health. If your mother smoked, it may be the cause of problems when it comes to getting pregnant yourself. The study concluded that if your mother smoked when she was pregnant with you, your fertility may be damaged. It appears that tobacco smoke may disrupt the hormonal balance in pregnant women, which may disrupt the growth of a female child's reproductive organs (and her chance later in life for a successful pregnancy).

If you do not smoke—but your mother did—the risk of miscarriage may be 30% higher than normal. If you smoke and your mother also did when she was pregnant with you, the risk of miscarrying is 60% higher.

Smoking After Childbirth Linked to Infant Death

Many mothers-to-be stop smoking during pregnancy to protect their babies from retarded growth and other harmful effects of prenatal exposure to tobacco smoke. But they often start smoking again after they become mothers, assuming there is little or no risk once the baby is born. This is not true: tobacco smoke may be deadly to infants. Nursing mothers who smoke (and caregivers or other relatives who expose babies to cigarette smoke) may double the infant's risk of dying from Sudden Infant Death Syndrome (SIDS, or what used to be called "crib death"). SIDS is a particular threat when mothers smoke during the months of breast-feeding, and when parents and others smoke in the same room as the baby.

Breast-fed babies have a lower incidence of crib death, but if a nursing mother also smokes during that same time period, it cancels out the protection against SIDS that breast-feeding would otherwise provide. See pages 525–528 for more information on SIDS.

HAZARDS TO AVOID DURING PREGNANCY

All the warnings you've already heard have probably made you a little worried . . . now I'm sorry to have to present you with this long list of the dangers lurking everywhere! I know it must seem that there's no "safe zone" now that you're expecting—as though you're in jeopardy the minute you step foot outside your house—but at the same time you'll see that there may be hazards around every corner *inside* your house, too! But "forewarned is forearmed": it seems better for you to know about possible hazards and then decide on a case-by-case basis what applies to you. The truth is that many of the dangers listed here are somewhat specialized, so it's unlikely that you will personally encounter a great many of them.

! ! ▮ ! ! ▮ ! ! ▼ / ! ! ▮ ! ▮ ▮ ! ! ▮ ! ! ▼ / ! ! ▮ ! !

THE EVERYDAY DANGERS AROUND YOU (ALPHABETICAL)

Aerosol sprays
— Inhaling the fumes can be harmful to the developing baby.
— Use pump sprays instead of aerosol.

Air pollution
— Car exhaust fumes are dangerous for the baby (see "Carbon monoxide").
— Avoid walking or jogging near traffic.
— When driving in heavy traffic, keep your windows closed and vent on "recirculate."

Anesthetic gases
— Health personnel in operating rooms encounter high levels of these gases.
— They have abnormally high rates of sterility, miscarriage, and birth defects.
— Suspected cause for health professionals is their exposure to these gases.

Cadmium
— It is a component of tobacco smoke, wastes from electroplating plants, and is released by tires burning or wearing down.
— Retards fetal growth and linked to fetal deformities.

Caffeine
— Exists even in decaffeinated coffee and tea.
— Stimulates fetal nervous system.
— Refer to pages 76–78 for more information.

Carbon monoxide
— Avoid driving in traffic jams or in an enclosed space (tunnel, parking garage).
— Extended exposure can cause low birth weight or infant mortality.
— Vehicle fumes also contain lead, a poisonous gas.

! ! ▮ ! ! ▮ ! ! ▮ ! ▼ ▼ ! / ! ! ▮ ! ! ▮ ▮ ! ! ▮ ! ▼ ▼ / ! ! ▮ ! ! ▮

THE EVERYDAY DANGERS AROUND YOU (ALPHABETICAL)

Cat litter box
— Soiled kitty litter carries toxo-plasmosis.
— See page 22 for more on this disease which can damage the unborn child.
— Have someone else clean the litter box.

Chemotherapy drugs
— High risk of miscarriage for nurses who handle certain cancer medications in their 1st trimester.
— Fetal loss linked to on-the-job exposure to three drugs: cyclophosphamide, doxorubicin, and vincristine.
— All three stop cancer by disrupting cell growth and killing actively growing cells.

Cleaning products
— Avoid strong-smelling household cleaning products.
— When you're around cleaning agents make sure there is enough ventilation.

Computer chips
— Women exposed to chemicals used in making chips are at risk.
— Studies show a high miscarriage rate in factories where chips are made.

Fish
— Can be contaminated by water they live in.
— See pages 81–84 for further information.

Food additives
— Artificial colors and preservatives are dangerous for the developing baby.
— Meat growth hormones and antibiotics used in meat production are also unsafe.
— See page 74 for more details.

Garden chemicals
— Wear gloves when handling plant products.
— Wash your hands after gardening.

THE EVERYDAY DANGERS AROUND YOU (ALPHABETICAL)

Garden chemicals (*cont.*)	— Do not breathe fumes of strong-smelling garden or lawn chemicals.
Gasoline	— Gas vapors can cause cancer and birth defects.
	— Do not fill your own gas tank during pregnancy: vapor retrieval hoses can be defective and expose you to fumes.
	— Notice warning signs at gas stations!
Hot tubs/Jacuzzis	— High temperatures (over 106° F) can cause brain damage in the unborn baby.
	— Keep water below 104° F.
	— Get out after 10 minutes and cool off, then go back in if you don't feel light-headed.
Lead in paint	(see "Paints")
Lead in water	(see "Water")
Lecithin	— A fat-emulsifying substance sold in health food stores, often as a diet aid.
	— Beware during childbearing years: may damage the developing fetus.
Mercury	— May occur as *mercurous chloride* in medical or industrial compounds.
	— Overexposure can cause brain damage, blindness, or cerebral palsy.
Microwave ovens	— There are questions about whether leaking microwaves can harm your unborn child.
	— As a precaution, use a meter to learn if your microwave has a leak.
Paints	— Paint may contain lead or toxic vapors.

THE EVERYDAY DANGERS AROUND YOU (ALPHABETICAL)

Paints (*cont.*)	— Avoid old furniture being refinished or old paint being sanded.
	— Avoid latex paints being sanded.
PCBs	— Cancer-causing chemicals banned since 1979, but still present in the food chain.
	— Water supply in some areas still affected.
	— PCBs cause birth defects.
	— Avoid fresh-water, bottom-feeding fish such as flounder, sole, and catfish.
	— See pages 81–84 for more on fish.
Pesticides	— Excessive contact with almost any pesticide can harm the unborn child.
	— Stay away whether it's farming chemicals or weed killer for your lawn!
Photographic chemicals	— Darkroom chemicals in high doses are dangerous to the unborn child.
	— Completely avoid these organic and metallic chemicals in the first trimester.
	— You can work in the darkroom in the second and third trimesters, but take precautions.
	— Wear goggles, impermeable gloves, and be sure there's adequate ventilation.
Meat, raw or rare	— This can cause toxoplasmosis.
	— See page 22 for more on this disease.
Solvents	— Substances such as turpentine and toluene can be hazardous during pregnancy.
	— High concentrations can be encountered in industrial arts or crafts.
	— Avoid long exposure to the fumes.

THE EVERYDAY DANGERS AROUND YOU (ALPHABETICAL)

Tobacco smoke
— Toxic substances in tobacco smoke can stunt the baby's growth.
— The danger exists if you're the smoker or are inhaling secondary smoke.
— See page 181–182 for more on smoking.

Toxic ingredients
— Carefully read the label of any product you use during pregnancy.
— You must not inhale products such as cleaning fluid, contact cement, volatile paint, lacquer thinner, some glues, some household cleaning products such as oven cleaner, etc.

Uranium wastes
— Radioactive material from mining was used for Colorado roads and house foundations.
— Cinder-blocks made of this radioactive substance were used for house building in many other states.

Vaginal products
— Avoid feminine hygiene douches and gels containing povidone-iodine.
— During pregnancy this can cause thyroid defects in baby.

Water
— Chemicals and lead are present in the public water supply and well water.
— Consider using bottled water in your childbearing years, since even a small amount of lead can cause birth defects.
— New and old faucets can leak lead.
— See pages 118–120 for information on ways to reduce risks.

❗❗❗❗❗❗❗❗❗❗❗❗❗❗❗❗❗❗❗❗❗❗❗❗❗❗

THE EVERYDAY DANGERS AROUND YOU (ALPHABETICAL)

X-rays
— Strictly avoid X-rays unless absolutely necessary.
— Always tell doctors and technicians that you are pregnant before any testing.
— Dental X-rays are safe if you wear a lead apron.

❗❗❗❗❗❗❗❗❗❗❗❗❗❗❗❗❗❗❗❗❗❗❗❗❗❗

NOTE: If you have questions about these or any other medications and your doctor does not have the answers, contact the March of Dimes. There may be a local office listed in your area, but the national office is at 1275 Mamaroneck Avenue, White Plains, New York 10605.

DOMESTIC VIOLENCE DURING PREGNANCY

You may be as shocked as I was to discover that pregnant women are frequently victims of physical and emotional abuse by their partners. You'd think that being pregnant would be some kind of protection against being harmed—that no man would raise a hand to a woman when she is carrying his child—but sadly, just the opposite is true: pregnancy is actually considered an increased risk factor for battering. In some relationships abuse takes place for the first time during pregnancy—it may come as a complete shock to the woman. But if you are someone whose mate has abused her before pregnancy, be on alert for more of the same now, because unfortunately, a pregnant woman can bring out the worst in some batterers.

The concept of widespread domestic violence in America may be hard for many of us to believe. Our society is in denial that battering happens to such a large part of the female population. Domestic violence is the dirty secret which has yet to come out in the open in America. Our denial mechanism is powerful about this national epidemic of wife abuse, so it's no wonder we can't make room for the fact that battering so often involves pregnant women.

Those women who suffer at the hands of the man they live with often live in shame and fear, unwilling to disclose anything about the hell they live in. Often the women who are victims of emotional and physical abuse are in denial about what is happening to them, which may be a small part of why they remain with their abusers.

Statistics don't tell the whole story because many incidents of abuse are not reported. If a woman is already afraid of her spouse she'll be unlikely to report the incident to the police for fear of her partner's retaliation for "ratting" on him and also because she feels humiliated to admit having been the object of abuse. Most women don't press charges against their abusers. If a woman is physically injured by her partner she may also be afraid to seek medical treatment for fear of her husband's angry reaction to being exposed—a man who has injured his wife will often become even more abusive if she tries to get medical attention because he's worried that a doctor will discover his mistreatment. A victim of domestic violence may also keep her situation hidden from possible rescuers because of her own embarrassment at how the healthcare provider might judge her for being in such a degrading position.

And of course it isn't just the pregnant woman who is in danger of being hurt, it is her unborn child, too. The March of Dimes reports that nearly 40 percent of fetal deaths from miscarriage may be the result of the mother having been beaten or kicked sufficiently to cause her to lose her baby. Often a beating can bring on premature labor, resulting in a low-birth-weight baby who is high-risk for complications after birth. It is a disturbing and frightening thought that a woman who is pregnant—who is physically and emotionally at her most vulnerable and defenseless—is potentially in danger in her own home.

Pregnancy and Spousal Abuse

Although we'd all like to believe that no man would never raise a hand to the woman carrying his child, or ever kick or beat her in the belly, just the opposite is true. Sadly, hundreds of babies die before they are ever born because—there's really no delicate way to put this—their fathers kicked the crap out of their mothers and caused miscarriages. You do not want to become part of that statistic.

No one knows for sure why spousal abuse happens more frequently when a woman is pregnant, but it's possible to make an educated guess. Perhaps it is a woman's vulnerability and neediness when she is expecting that opens the door for a man to display abusive behavior which he hadn't felt free to exhibit before. To understand domestic violence you have to know that it is about power and control—a man displays mental and physical abuse to exert dominance over "his woman." Where pregnancy is concerned there may be additional motivations for the abuse. Some possible reasons are:

➢ Jealousy that a woman is able to be pregnant and he can't carry the child.
➢ Resentment that the woman suddenly gets so much attention.

> Anger that he has to take a backseat to the "main event" of the pregnancy when he is accustomed to commanding center stage.
> Fear that he will become less important once the baby arrives.

It is estimated that 25 percent of all women, pregnant or not, suffer abuse at the hands of the man nearest and dearest to them. That "one in four" statistic becomes even more chilling when a woman becomes pregnant—because then her chances of being abused rise to 40 percent.

If your mate has displayed frightening or threatening behavior before, there's a good chance it will worsen once you're pregnant. If he has already inflicted physical or sexual abuse in the past you'll need to be on high alert during your pregnancy to protect yourself and your baby from the man in your life.

Don't think "It can't happen to me," or "He'll stop once I'm pregnant"—I wish I could assure you that this was true but the facts show otherwise. You can protect yourself and your unborn baby better if you are aware of the increased risk you now have of being hurt by your partner. Depending on how serious the circumstances in your personal situation, you may have to make plans to seek a safer place to live—at least during your pregnancy.

The terrible connection between pregnancy and spousal abuse is something every woman should know about: for herself, for the sake of children she already has, and on behalf of other women she cares about. All of us have become more aware of domestic violence since the publicity surrounding the terrible death of Nicole Brown Simpson. There are stories in the media every day about women who are brutalized or killed by the man in their lives. But even with all that publicity, information about spousal abuse remains a well-kept secret, a horror which remains unspoken for most of its victims. Keeping this terrible secret often magnifies the fear and feelings of helplessness for the woman who is suffering.

Domestic violence is not a phenomenon that's happening in only a few publicized cases: it is all around us. If you want to know where spousal abuse is happening, look around you: at the woman driving in front of you at car pool . . . at the woman next to you in gym class . . . at the lady behind you in the supermarket line . . . at your female superior at work . . . at the bank teller or waitress serving you . . . at the performer entertaining you, or the nurse or female doctor giving you care. One in four of those women is living in fear of the man in her life—and she is probably too frightened to tell anyone. There's always the chance that as you read this you might be one of these women, too, in which case this section of the book is not just a warning of a possible danger from your partner but may be information which will literally save your life.

Spousal abuse knows no boundaries—it doesn't matter what race a woman is, what her income level is or how much education she's had. Domestic violence is everywhere you look, even though you may not see it. There won't necessarily be any telltale marks—abusers are clever, they learn to inflict physical damage where it won't show in public. Similarly, psychological abuse can be a hidden terror, too. Mental abuse can go on for a long time without its being apparent to anyone else . . . until a woman has a breakdown or summons the courage and strength to get out.

Perhaps the most chilling fact about wife abuse is that the violence in the home will probably escalate in severity and get worse over time: this increase is especially true if the first incidence goes unreported to the authorities. For this reason it's tremendously important to recognize the warning signs of an abusive partner so that you can respond appropriately. What is it that would make a man strike his pregnant wife, or heap mental abuse on her? Most batterers' behavior is based on a need for power and control, and apparently the more they have, the more they want. If a man gets away with his initial attempts at abuse it gives him a psychological advantage: he has begun the process of rendering his woman frightened and powerless.

How Can You Tell if Your Mate Is a Potential Abuser?

In order to recognize the pattern of behavior in an abusive man it helps to understand that emotional abuse can also be a precursor to physical abuse, so it's essential to be sensitive to the telltale signs of a batterer. The following lists should help you to know whether you're in good hands during your pregnancy—or whether your husband's hands might turn on you.

EARLY SIGNS OF AN ABUSIVE PARTNER

— He tracks all of your time.
— He calls the house or your job frequently to check up on your whereabouts.
— He constantly accuses you of being unfaithful.
— He discourages you from having relationships with family and friends.
— He prevents you from working or going to school.
— He criticizes you for little things or blames you for everything that goes wrong.
— He gets angry easily when using alcohol or drugs.
— He controls your finances and forces you to account for the money you spend.
— He makes fun of you or humiliates you in front of others.

Comparing these signs to your own partner can be a trauma in itself. It can be really hard to face the possibility that the father of your child is—or might become—a batterer. You have to summon the clear-headedness to be as objective as possible when applying these criteria to your own mate to determine whether he could be a danger to you. If you find that "the shoe fits" don't delude yourself by excusing potentially violent characteristics, even if they are being exhibited by a man you love. You aren't doing yourself—or the child you are going to have—any favor by trying to justify your mate's behavior. You hear women say defensively, "He's just being protective of me," or "It's just jealousy—it's kind of sweet." The characteristics mentioned above are warning signs of behavior that eventually might turn violent. If a man displays many of these traits there is the possibility that his controlling conduct can develop into physical or sexual abuse.

The following is a list of the kind of behavior that indicates a man has already escalated into the dangerous, violent zone. If any of these are true of your partner, you should read the final part of this section on strategies to develop so that you are prepared for a frightening episode and know how to handle it.

BEHAVIOR OF A DANGEROUS MAN

— He destroys your property, especially things with sentimental value.
— He threatens to harm you or your children.
— He hits, punches, kicks or bites you or your children.
— He uses—or threatens to use—a weapon against you.
— He forces you to have sex against your will.

Being Prepared for a Violent Incident

Women can't always avoid incidents of violence but there is a variety of reactions to abusive behavior which can make you feel you have some control over the situation. The table below suggests strategies which may help you in a domestic crisis, and can help you to see how carefully an exit must be planned.

SAFETY PREPARATIONS FOR A VIOLENT INCIDENT

➤ *Practice how to get out of the house safely.*
— Consider which doors, windows, elevators, stairwells or fire escapes are the quickest exit.
— Get in the habit of leaving your purse and car keys in an accessible spot.
— Keep an extra set of car keys hidden in case your spouse confiscates your keys.
➤ *You may not be able to get to a phone.*
— You may be cornered by your spouse or be afraid of triggering a reaction if you try to dial the phone.
— Teach your older children how to dial 911.

— If your children are not able to make this judgment on their own, pick a code word you can use to trigger them to call the police.

— Choose one or two close friends or relatives you can call for help, people to whom you have told your code word as a signal to call 911 for help.

➤ *Decide ahead of time where you can go if you need to leave.*

— Once you're in a very threatening situation you may not be able to think clearly and make the best decision about how to escape or where to go.

— Plan ahead for where you would be able to go if you're in jeopardy at home with your partner.

— Even if your mate swears there will not be a "next time" make a contingency plan for that eventuality.

— Ask a close friend or relative whether—in a domestic crisis— you could stay with them for a while. Figure out how to get access if they are often out of the house. You need the peace of mind of knowing there is refuge.

— Think of a back-up destination just in case.

— If your children are old enough, explain these plan-ahead strategies to them so they can cooperate if it comes down to leaving quickly.

➤ *Be aware of the warning signs of abusive behavior.*

— Develop an awareness of how your mate acts and reacts prior to getting "worked up."

— Awareness allows you to perceive whether a situation is dangerous and remove yourself if need be.

— Make an effort to avoid potentially abusive situations, knowing that once you're pregnant your condition may make him even more prone to acting up.

— Trust your instincts and judgment about whether a situation is becoming very serious and do whatever is necessary to protect yourself and your unborn baby

— Use whatever tactics you know will work to calm him down and head off a major confrontation. Within reason, give him what he wants if your intuition tells you that will defuse the situation.

— If you anticipate an argument, move to an area of your living space where you can't get trapped.

— Avoid rooms without an access to an outside door, such as the bathroom, garage, kitchen, or anywhere near weapons.

➤ *Alert people close to you about the possibility of trouble.*

— You may feel humiliated to admit this private information to anyone, but if you can overcome this embarrassment it will actually be less stressful in the long run.

— You are not alone: it is estimated that one in four women is suffering as you are. There's a chance that the person you tell about your situation may have one of her own which she's never talked about.

— People who care about you need to know that you may be in jeopardy.
— If you won't choose confidantes for your own safety, then do it for your unborn baby, who runs a high risk of premature birth (and therefore death) if her father attacks you.
— Make the choice to tell selected people about your mate's potential for violence. This allows you to be free to tell the truth about the situation you're living in
— If there's anyone who lives within hearing distance of your home, ask them to call the police if they hear suspicious noises coming from your house.

Why Don't You Just Leave Him?

"Why don't you just leave?" is a question often asked of abuse victims by people who do not understand the cycle of fear that battering creates. Women are often unable to leave their abusers because their sense of self-worth and self-preservation have been so eroded by the mental and/or physical abuse that they don't have the self-confidence or courage to go. Another misconception is that the victims of domestic violence are somehow responsible for what is done to them. Make no mistake: a woman does not "ask" for spousal abuse through her behavior any more than a rape victim is "asking" for it based on how she dresses or dances.

Once the abusive pattern has begun in a relationship, a woman can feel powerless against her tormentor. She often cannot imagine any way out of the hell she is living in—terrified of her abuser, she believes she is alone in her suffering. Her abuser often convinces her that no one would believe her anyway.

A Few Last Thoughts on "DV" and Pregnancy

This section on domestic violence during pregnancy does not pretend to be a comprehensive examination of the problem, but rather a wake-up call for all of us. This warning is meant for women who have suffered abuse in the past, those who might be at risk without realizing it and equally to all the people who make up the support system of an expectant couple. It may be up to extended family or even strangers to come to the aid of a woman who is in danger from her partner. A woman who is suffering at her husband's hands may be in denial about her own jeopardy. Such a woman may even feel powerless to protect the baby she is carrying—but that does not mean that others should turn a blind eye in such a situation.

Some people might say that it should be a community responsibility to reach out to any woman who may not be able to ask for help, or does not recognize the danger she and her unborn child are facing from an abusive man. No woman, especially a pregnant one, should have to put up with mental or physical abuse just because she cannot find a way out. Those people who make up the circle around an expectant woman need to be alert to signs of a dangerous expectant father or a fearful mother-to-be. She and her baby deserve a better beginning than that,

CHAPTER SEVEN

Taking Care of Your Mind (and Your Partner's)

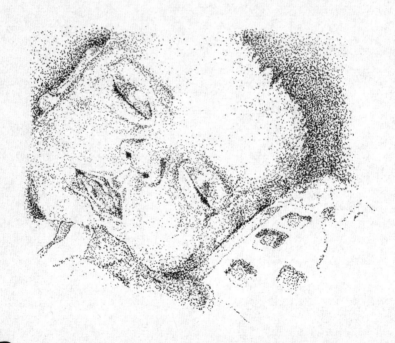

Pregnancy is a life crisis. Everything is changing; change is disorienting and can be frightening. However, this momentous time in your life can also be enriching and thrilling for the new insights and outlooks it gives you.

Try to think of pregnancy as a crisis similar to puberty, as simply a period of personal growth. Think back on how you felt as an adolescent: it was a time of ''becoming,'' when you were teetering between being a

196

girl and becoming a woman. If you were like most young woman, you felt anxious, awkward, self-conscious, and like a stranger in your changing body. You might have felt angry and confused by the swift changes you couldn't control. The rest of the time you probably felt adventuresome, attractive, and on the brink of great things. At times you may have experienced all these feelings at once and your system would get overloaded by so much input. The "circuit breaker" was a fit of tears or anger or withdrawal. Or simple bewilderment. Pregnancy throws you into a similar state.

The physical changes that are a natural part of being pregnant are also going to bring about an emotional imbalance. You are in limbo; it is a time of *becoming*. It is an *identity crisis*. You are going from Woman to Mother; some women may be going from Girl to Mother because they have always associated "really growing up" with having a baby. Either way, all aspects of your life are spotlighted: your personal direction, your relationship with the baby's father, your adequacy as a person (and potential mother), the world's condition, and your own mortality! Making a baby means you are "replacing" yourself, which forces you to think about how far you have gone along life's road.

Once you can sort out all the confusion caused by pregnancy, the result is *emotional growth*. You will probably be more in touch with yourself and have a better understanding of where you have been and where you are headed. There are women, however, who go through these nine months trying to avoid facing the psychological aspect of having a baby. The issues raised by being pregnant are weighty and difficult: some are hard to wrestle with, and others leave you certain that you have no answers at all. It might be possible to avoid all this, just as it would be possible to have the baby and ignore her! If you sail through pregnancy as if nothing were different—as if the only change is that your belly is getting bigger and bigger—you will probably get hit with all the feelings somewhere along the way, as if by a boomerang. Instead of denying that pregnancy makes a difference, you'll be better off accepting that pregnancy involves *all* of you: your mind as well as your body.

The period of personal growth that began with pregnancy doesn't end with the delivery of your baby. The reality of being a parent is going to extend this unsettled period in your life. You will probably feel out of balance during the early weeks, and sometimes months, of your child's life. One sure thing is that you will never be the same as before you had your baby!

You'll want to get the most out of this important time in your life. This chapter will let you know some what to expect and give you some pointers for the emotional journey you'll be taking in pregnancy.

Absentmindedness

Absentmindedness often happens to pregnant women, and it can give you the creepy feeling that you're losing your mind unless you know that it's normal. You may find that you forget appointments, mix up information, or can't remember where you put things. It can make you feel like a senile little old lady—or someone whose sanity is slipping! Don't worry: it's just that your attention is focused on yourself and the pregnancy and taken away from other things. Don't get upset by it. Just knowing that it is normal may help you accept the fact that you forget to take a certain book to your office—*three* times in a row!

Absentmindedness may even get worse in the last couple of weeks of pregnancy. All your concentration will be on when the baby will arrive and what labor and delivery will be like. You may not only forget things, you may just generally walk around in a daze.

"Dropsies"

Another strange thing that can happen to pregnant women is that they keep dropping objects. Some women also experience "dropsies" when they're about to get their period, and for a similar reason. This temporary clumsiness is a result of fluid retention and the effect of pregnancy hormones on the joints of your fingers, which can make them feel loose. These can combine with the loss of concentration, so that you aren't able to get a good grip on things. You may have to force yourself to pay extra careful attention to what you're doing with your hands, or to just avoid handling breakable objects as much as possible.

ACCEPTING THE PREGNANCY

Accepting the pregnancy is the first and most important psychological task you have. That may sound obvious, but there are women who glide through the early months of pregnancy giving it as little thought as possible (which is especially easy before you begin to "show"). It's important for you and the baby's father to begin to think about the reality of having a baby. Until now your thoughts about a baby and parenthood have probably all been in soft focus, a pastel picture of the loving threesome.

Conflicting feelings are sure to surface once you recognize what parenthood is going to mean. Don't worry that something is wrong with you for feeling this way: it is *good* to have conflicting feelings! It means you are coming to terms with the situation and can figure things out ahead of time. You don't want the horrible shock of waiting to face all this until the last possible moment: once the baby is in residence! There will be so many practical things to deal with that you'll be glad that you've done some emotional homework.

Emotional turmoil is something positive: you are adjusting to being pregnant and becoming a mother. Don't imagine that having second thoughts or fears (discussed on page 202) means that you've made a mistake. You need to toss pregnancy around in your head the way one wrestles with any big life decision. We've all been taught that once a woman is pregnant, she should walk around with a saint-like expression and attitude. Baloney! Being pregnant isn't all fun. Neither is being a parent. Accepting those realities leaves you freer to enjoy the good parts.

TALK ABOUT WHAT YOU'RE FEELING

> ➤ ***Communicate what you are feeling and thinking*** during your pregnancy. Talk to your mate. Talk to your friends. Talk to older women (whether your mother is included among them depends on your relationship with her, as discussed on page 207 ''The Grandparents and Others'').
>
>   It's not unusual for pregnant women to feel isolated nowadays. Many women are postponing motherhood until their thirties or even forties and some are deciding against it altogether. This means you might be the only pregnant person you know (the first—or last—in your circle to have a baby). Also, most couples live far away or are cut off from their extended families. It can be lonely. If that is true for you, find someone to talk to. The baby's father is the logical first choice: it can bring you closer together as he learns what you're thinking and shares some of his feelings with you.
>
> ➤ ***Talk to your mate:*** You are both going through a lot of emotional flip-flops. Keep your channels of communication open. If you don't share your feelings with each other, they can create a distance between you, instead of being a way for you to understand and get closer to one another. Do not make the mistake of thinking, ''He's got enough to worry about right now, so I won't bother him with this. It's too silly.'' What *is* silly is trying to deny or belittle your feelings. Unacknowledged feelings have a way of becoming a problem, which they won't if you communicate them. It is far better to tell your mate you don't think you're spending enough time together and have him explain why he disagrees and thinks you're being unreasonable than to harbor that feeling. Your resentment can accumulate until you feel angry and hurt, and then you will explode. He then feels unjustly attacked, which he *has* been, because without any prior discussion, how could he possibly know what you've been feeling? Then you will have created a much more complicated problem.
>
> ➤ ***Your childbirth education teacher*** is an excellent person to talk to. You may choose a teacher fairly early in your pregnancy and make plans to start classes in your seventh month. But there is no reason why you can't call her up before that just to discuss something that may be bothering you. Some teachers will even invite you to do that when you first contact them. Childbirth instructors, for the most part, are sensitive, caring women who

have dedicated a good part of their lives to helping other women through childbirth. They make fast, intense bonds with many of the women and couples they have trained, precisely because pregnancy is a time in people's lives when they need support. These teachers are aware of and sensitive to the needs and problems you may be encountering. Don't let their expertise and kindness go to waste if there is something bothering you.

➤ **Talk to your friends**, even if they don't have children. They may be interested in what you're going through, although not ideal confidantes. Imagine trying to discuss a difficult love affair, for example, with someone who has never been in love or made love. It may be like talking to a friendly person who nods and looks sympathetic but unfortunately speaks only Tibetan. Still, a friend is a friend, and you need yours now.

Some friends who have opted for a child-free lifestyle may not be able to give you the kind of support you need. Because of social and family pressures on them to procreate, they may feel defensive about their decision not to. Others may have ambivalent feelings about their decision not to have children (perhaps a mate who refuses—or a career which would not allow them enough time to be the kind of parents they would want to be). These women might feel confused and threatened by your pregnancy—talking intimately with you about it might make it worse. But many friends who have decided against being parents themselves may be interested in helping you deal with your fears and conflicts.

➤ **Early bird classes** are rare, unfortunately, but some communities have them. They are discussion groups designed for prospective parents anywhere from the fourth month of pregnancy on. Some of the group time may be spent discussing practical issues such as breast-feeding and baby care, but usually the primary purpose is as an outlet for the psychological changes of pregnancy. Early bird classes are usually organized by the people who are in charge of childbirth/education classes; ask around in your community. If you're really energetic, you might want to put together such a group yourself.

➤ **Communicate with yourself: start keeping a journal**. Get a notebook and think of it as a place to let go of feelings and ideas that you may not want to share with anyone else. If you make a habit of writing in your journal—even one sentence a day—it will not only serve as an outlet but will help you focus on yourself. Writing in a diary at any time in your life can give you information and insights about yourself that you otherwise wouldn't take the time to recognize. A pregnancy journal is also a very special remembrance of this time in your life. You will no doubt cherish the notebook long after you've forgotten the daily hopes and fears, ups and downs, of pregnancy. (This is why I made *The Pregnancy Diary* for you!)

DREAMS

Dreams can be vivid and sometimes disturbing. Do not be frightened by your dreams. As with dreams at any time, they can seem real—and you can be more impressionable about such things when you're pregnant. Dreams have an important function at this time in your life. Think of them as messages, information about yourself that you have no other way of finding out. Dreams are things to discuss, ideas to recognize. No matter how real they seem, don't get carried away thinking of them as realities.

➤ *Dreams of mistreating the baby* or not caring for him properly are common. They represent a realistic, legitimate fear: you probably don't know much about baby care and are worried about doing a good job. Try to see these dreams for what they are. If you dream that you haven't fed the baby and he shrivels up, don't start worrying that something is already wrong with your baby before delivery or that you want to harm him. The dream is not an omen—it simply reveals your underlying concern about "doing right" by your child, about your abilities as a parent.

➤ *Dreams of losing the baby* may have a meaning similar to the preceding kind of dream. The theme of losing the baby, however, may not necessarily be about losing the newborn. It may be your concern about losing the baby from your *uterus*—where you have had him all to yourself, closed and safe.

➤ *Nightmares about the baby dying* come from an understandable concern for your baby's health and perfection. If you have dreams like this near the end of your pregnancy, they may be a defense mechanism. Everybody worries at one time or another that something will be wrong or go wrong with their baby—dreams like these may be a psychological preparation for a possible unwanted outcome.

➤ *Nightmares*, in general, may be a way of expressing *hostility* toward your unborn child. She is going to overtake your life, disrupt your privacy and comfortable routines. Nightmares can express feelings you may not be able to, or may not be consciously aware of. Again, don't make the mistake of taking dreams and nightmares literally and then feeling guilty or frightened. You may be more superstitious when you're pregnant, so don't let that tendency carry you away.

THE EIGHTH MONTH

The eighth month may be the most uncomfortable for you physically. The baby has almost reached maximum size and hasn't yet settled down into your pelvis ("engagement" or "lightening"). Your veins may be swollen; you may be short of breath, have less mobility, or have an embarrassingly leaky bladder. You'll probably feel pretty sick of your maternity clothes and fairly fed up with being pregnant. Impatience and anxiety about when the baby will arrive can start to nag at you.

➤ *You must prepare* for the physical separation from your baby, as well as the labor and delivery. You may dream about "losing" your baby (see above), or of having her delivered in some bizarre, frightening way. It is natural to be anxious about the Great Unknown of what your baby's journey into the world will be like—how childbirth will feel and how you will handle it. Dreams or daydreams are ways to express those concerns.

➤ *You need a lot of assurance* at this time from your mate. You need to be reassured that he will support you through labor and delivery in whatever way you've agreed upon (even if it's in spirit only). Your mate may need some reassurance and comforting for similar concerns he may be having—so don't depend on him for all your assurance. Seek outside support, too. Turn to friends, relatives, your childbirth teacher, your midwife or doctor. This can be a tough time—you're sad that your pregnancy is over, but eager to be done with it; you're excited about meeting your baby face-to-face, but sad about losing her from inside you. You may be fearful about being a good mother. You need outside support and should make sure you get it.

➤ *Do nice things* for yourself. Get a pedicure. Go out to a lovely dinner. Take a drive. Go to the movies or to a concert. Do things to lift your spirits (if they need elevating) or just take your mind off yourself. Enjoy these last few weeks of precious time you have to yourself or as a couple.

➤ *Practice breathing exercises* from childbirth classes *every day* even though your motivation may be low. Daily practice is essential to comfort and ease when the real thing happens. You may be getting Braxton-Hicks contractions (see page 128 for more information), which are not only accomplishing effacement of your cervix but are an excellent opportunity to practice your breathing exercises.

FEARS

Fears of one kind or another have probably bothered you at some time during your pregnancy. You may have worried about some medication you took before you knew you were pregnant. You've probably been afraid of losing your freedom. Fear is nothing to be ashamed of— fear of the unknown is healthy. You dispel fear by getting information, by getting an understanding of what is happening.

"I'm Feeling Scared."

The first thing you need to do is admit that you're feeling frightened. One problem with feelings that you do *not* acknowledge is that these hidden feelings can come out in behavior you don't understand. If you deny your feelings there is a chance they will surface as some physical complaint (since you wouldn't pay attention to them when they were "only" in your head!). Accept whatever you are feeling; do not discount your feelings or your mate's. Never say, for example, "I feel scared, but there's no reason to be." Don't place judgment on your feelings, or on the feelings your mate is having. Listen. Deal with the feelings: get reassurance.

"Will My Baby Be Normal?"

This is a fear you may have during your pregnancy. Everybody worries that their baby won't be perfect: that something has already gone wrong long before delivery. Only a tiny percentage of babies have any problems (but if you're a true worrier, you'll be concerned that *someone* has to be in that small group and it may be *you!*). It is much more likely that you will be in the huge majority and have a healthy baby. As you should with all fears, don't try to deny that you are worried: recognize the fear and then put it out of your mind. Worrying won't change anything. If you are superstitious (which is a trait that can get exaggerated during pregnancy), you may worry that too much worrying can *cause* something to go wrong with the baby. The only ill effect is a loss of sleep for the mother!

"Will I Be Able to Take Care of a Baby?"

Once he is born, this is a common and legitimate fear. Most Americans today grow up with no knowledge of childbirth and early child care. Most Americans girls play with dolls and then do some baby-sitting. This isn't a culture where there are babies around all the time so that you can learn by watching how to dress, diaper, feed, burp, calm, or amuse a newborn. Many women in this country don't have female relatives around when they're pregnant or after birth, so there is no trusted, experienced person to ease you into child care by leading the way. It is frightening and overwhelming to be faced with a teeny, fragile newborn who is at the same time capable of raising hell if he doesn't get fed/burped/changed/soothed right this *instant!* As with all fears, the way to lessen them is to get information. So read books (Spock is still the tops), talk to people who have had babies *recently*, and try to spend time around any babies you can, just to get used to them. If you get accustomed to seeing how a little baby's face gets all scrunched up and red when he is having a good cry, it won't be such a shock when *your* little angel starts wailing and looks like he's going to burst!

"I'm Worried About My Freedom and Independence."

This is another concern for prospective parents. Of the many fears you may have, this is one to spend time thinking about: you *are* going to lose your freedom, it's that simple. One thing you can do is redefine what freedom means. If you cling to previous ideas that freedom means being able to go *wherever* you want exactly *when* you want, then you are going to experience frustration and anger—having a child in your life makes that kind of freedom close to impossible. Even if you can afford full-time help, your schedule will still be secondary to breast-feeding, caring for a sick child, etc. Having a child means having to think about her health, education, and welfare a great deal of the time (more or less constantly!). Even when you're away from your baby, your "freedom" is compromised by having had to arrange for someone else to be with the child and to organize all her paraphernalia for the substitute; and then while you're away, you think about whether everything is all right at home.

What you lose when you become a parent is the spontaneity (or impulsiveness) of movement. Once you have a baby it's hard to make a move without considering the child. This is as true when you have a toddler and you want to walk into another room (risking total destruction of the first room if you don't think about the child!) as it is of planning a business trip. The conclusion of all this is not to fear your loss of freedom but to anticipate it. Spend some time now deciding what your priorities are and which activities—to do with business or pleasure—are the important ones for you. Once the baby arrives you will have less time for yourself. If you have decided ahead of time what you are *not* willing to give up, as well as what *is* expendable, you are less likely to experience the baby as "taking away" your freedom.

"I Hate the Way I Look."

Loss of attractiveness is something many women worry about. It is not merely a question of vanity, nor does it have only to do with American ideas about Thin Is Beautiful (although that may be part of it). Your body image changes when you are pregnant. It helps to understand how this affects you emotionally. If you once again recall adolescence, you will remember that your body-image changes in puberty had a powerful effect on you. Developing breasts, pubic hair, your first menstrual periods, stronger body odor—you had many things to adjust to. Pregnancy presents you with its own set of physical changes that demand your adaptation. Just as with puberty, pregnancy changes the way you look—the new shape of your body and therefore different clothes. Every woman has some idea about her body image: her stature, coloring, and the makeup and clothes she chooses. The way you look is tied up with the way you feel about yourself, who you are, how others perceive you. When you are pregnant, your body image changes, and this can be disconcerting to some women. They have to revise the way they "see" themselves, and they have to get used to being "seen" differently by the outside world.

When women are afraid of losing their attractiveness during pregnancy it is usually their *sexual appeal* that they are concerned about. A large part of most people's identity has to do with which gender they are and how the opposite gender reacts to them. The feedback they get from other people reinforces their feelings about themselves—it is "stroking" from the outside world. If that feedback diminishes or is greatly changed, it can be disorienting.

I will exaggerate a little to dramatize what being pregnant can *feel* like to women who are used to getting a response to the way they look. A strikingly attractive woman, wearing a stylish outfit that accentuates her sleek figure and her graceful walk, comes into a restaurant. The captain rushes over and leads her to a table. Heads turn. Conversations undergo a slight pause. Men admire her, women admire her. Cut. The same woman comes to the same restaurant, only now she is six months pregnant. Her maternity dress billows around her as she waddles in, albeit gracefully. The captain takes her to a table; she has to go so slowly that he turns around to see if she's following. His is the only head that turns. To this woman, being ignored in public is like being hit with a wet washcloth. She may experience this change as mass rejection; she is no longer attractive, at least not the way she was before.

If you are feeling any loss of attractiveness, seek out reassurance. The most obvious place to go is to your mate, but start with yourself. Try to view what is happening to your body as a wondrous transformation. If you stop thinking of your bulging belly as fat, you will begin to see it as globelike, shining, and uniquely beautiful. A pregnant belly is a sensual, sensuous object; have you noticed how people want to stroke it? Once you have begun to perceive your changing body more positively, encourage your mate to do the same. If you want to hear nice things about yourself, don't go around saying "Ugh, I'm getting huge": you rob your mate of the chance to say, "You look fabulous," and you will most likely color the way he views your changing body. He has some adjustments to make, too, and if you say, "Oooh, come feel how big our baby is getting," your chance of getting a positive response is greatly improved.

"I'm Going Crazy with Nightmarish Ideas."

Phobias and obsessions may overtake you during pregnancy. You may get a car phobia and suddenly be very nervous about driving. You may find that you are suddenly superstitious and obsessed with dreams and symbols. Phobias and obsessions are one way to express some of the fears you may be having (discussed earlier in this chapter). Pregnancy is an intense time in your life and you may experience many things more intensely. Don't worry, you aren't going crazy (no matter what other people say!).

Questions about your changing body and psyche, about labor and delivery, and about your baby may nag at you. Read, ask, listen. That's the whole point of this book. And never precede a question with, "I know this doesn't matter, but . . ." or "This sounds stupid, but . . ." *No question is stupid: it is only stupid not to question.*

MOOD SWINGS

Moodiness, known also as "emotional lability," affects all pregnant women at one time or another. You may have a wide range of rapidly shifting moods in response to situations that wouldn't generally trigger such extreme reactions. You may have unexplained crying, emotional outbursts, and attacks of anxiety.

> *Hormonal changes* have to be considered along with the body-image changes and identity crisis that may be affecting you. Progesterone is produced in large amounts during most of your pregnancy and has a depressant effect on the central nervous system. It can feel as if you're walking around in a fog. Some women are more sensitive to these hormonal changes. They are similar to the shift in the estrogen-progesterone balance which makes some women short-tempered and/or weepy before a period. If that has happened to you, be prepared now.

> *Ambivalence* about being pregnant and about the baby may be a cause of shifts in your moods. As I've said before in this chapter, acknowledge your feelings, do not try to suppress them. It is *okay* to have mixed feelings about pregnancy and parenthood. Only a fool imagines that once a baby arrives, everything's going to be just as it was before. It's all going to be changed—and in ways that you have no way of knowing yet. Thinking ahead may make you wonder if you've done the right thing—at the right time—with the right mate. It is fine to have those feelings. Do not, however, expect that you can *resolve* your ambivalence and reach a place where you no longer feel any conflict. Accept ambivalent feelings at times about your child(ren) as a natural, honest part of being a parent.

> *Depression, anxiety, confusion* are going to occur in even the most positive pregnancies. Try to roll with it and not make a big deal out of it. You will only prolong these periods if you feel the need to figure them out—"*Why* was I depressed on Wednesday? Nothing *seemed* to be wrong." If your instinct is that you *can't* figure out why, then leave it at that. Obviously if there are real problems in your life causing depression, you should deal with them and get help wherever you can. If you expect to have times of feeling low and realize they are a normal part of pregnancy, they will pass more readily.

> *If you are 100 percent happy*, with none of these mood swings or other effects, *beware*. Look over your shoulder a lot

because there may be a boomerang headed your way, carrying all the feelings you have suppressed or ignored. You may be denying a deep hostility or resentment toward your pregnancy. Many women are ambivalent about having a baby before they get pregnant. Others don't realize their ambivalence until well into the pregnancy when they begin to give it serious thought. These feelings may be so powerful that they are frightening, so you swallow them down and go through your pregnancy on an even keel, without the normal dips and turns. The result can be that these feelings will hit you like a ton of bricks one day, before the baby's birth or after. Unless you recognize these feelings for what they are, you could wind up taking it out on the child. Of course there may be women who genuinely are totally, 100 percent happy during their pregnancy—which is wonderful.

MOTHERHOOD

The process of "becoming a mother" is an awesome task. You may develop an identity for yourself as a mother that is separate from that of your own mother. You may accept those qualities you respected and valued in your mother and reject those aspects of her mothering that you disagreed with. This is a complex task full of guilt and conflict. You may feel some identity confusion with your own mother and other women until you sort this out. And unless you *do* go out of your way to consciously reexamine how you feel about what kind of mothering you (and your siblings, if any) had, you will unconsciously repeat it. What you saw around you growing up has become "fact" for you: whether a baby is picked up when she cries, whether a baby is chubby or thin, whether a baby is bundled with three layers in the carriage. You might automatically repeat what you saw and will socialize your child(ren) in the exact same way unless you stop to look at your feelings about mothering.

THE GRANDPARENTS AND OTHERS

Parents, in-laws, and other people can be a source of comfort and support during pregnancy and/or a meddlesome aggravation. Whichever the case in your life, you should be aware that whatever relationship is established with these people during pregnancy will probably continue during the early part of the baby's life. If you live far from the baby's grandparents, then the only decision you have to make is whether you want your mother or your mate's mother to be there after the baby is born. That decision depends on how well you get along with those women and whether you want them to be the one(s) to help you through the first weeks.

But if you live within visiting distance of your parents or in-laws (or other people who have similar roles in your life), then during your pregnancy you must set the stage for how much involvement—or lack of the same—you want them to have later. It is great to have an extra pair of hands around during those first few weeks but your helper should be doing housework and cooking, freeing you to get to know your baby. Some grandparents will shun such "menial tasks" and want to take charge of the baby . . . which is not what you need. So try to honestly evaluate how it will be—even discuss it with your parents and in-laws if they are open enough to have a direct talk about it.

If you *know* you don't want any of them closely involved during the first weeks, then don't let them get too involved in the day-to-day aspects of your pregnancy, because then they may *assume* they are going to have an active role in the early postpartum period.

YOU AND YOUR PARTNER

Your relationship with your mate may have to weather some difficult times during your pregnancy. Nine months is a short time in which to make the rapid shift from being "just Alec and Cynthia" to being "Cynthia and Alec, parents of Neil." You have to change your whole view of the world now that you are about to become Mommy and Daddy.

> *A sense of permanency* is one effect that pregnancy has—it can be like a seal on your marriage (or whatever other arrangement you may have). Now that there's going to be a baby, it's no longer so easy to leave. Regardless of how good a relationship may be, this new bond may feel a little tight at first! Get used to the idea by talking to each other about it—agree ahead of time that neither of you will take the other's comments as a personal insult or rejection. (When discussing the sense of permanence a baby implies—don't let this spill over into the other areas of insecurity that can exist during pregnancy.)

> *There is a need to depend on someone* during pregnancy. Don't deny that pregnancy makes a difference, just admit it. Let your partner know how you are feeling and the ways in which you especially need each other right now. This baby may be the first time that you realize the extent to which you and your mate are truly tied together. This merger may feel like a trap—you may feel stifled by the *idea* of your diminished independence if that has been important to you. The effect on your relationship may be that you fight the need to lean on your mate; you may even pull away from each other. Once you understand what's going on, you probably won't feel the need to withdraw.

> *Evaluating each other* as prospective parents can be a source of conflict. Although in the past you may each have had daydreams about what kind of mama or papa your mate would be, now it is nearly a reality. You are evaluating "the father" in

your mate and he is judging "the mother" in you. As mentioned earlier in this chapter, *you* are evaluating *yourself* along the same lines, so being judged by your mate only compounds the confusion you may already be feeling.

Don't be surprised if you start criticizing little things about the baby's father—or if he does the same with you. This process of facing the reality of parenthood frequently causes tension in a couple. You may also find that you make unusual demands to test his loyalty and devotion to you. If these sorts of petty grievances do crop up, try to recognize them for what they are . . . and point it out to each other. As with many of the psychological changes you have to work through during pregnancy, if you do not understand why they are occurring—and "call" each other on them—then the friction and conflict can become problems in themselves.

STRESS FACTORS

When you are pregnant you can be more sensitive to outside stresses. Any sort of problem—your health or that of relatives, your financial situation, marital discord, having to move, changing or ending a job—can be more difficult to cope with now. You should be aware that stress may hit you harder and you may not bounce back from it as easily as you did before you were pregnant.

A baby's activity inside you increases when you're under emotional stress. Studies have shown that maternal emotional upsets lasting for long periods resulted in a prolonged increase in fetal activity: up to ten times the normal level. Some mothers find that when they are really tired their baby's movements increase then, too.

There may be a relationship between emotional stress during pregnancy and general restlessness in the newborn. A mother's anxiety in pregnancy has been linked to a newborn baby who cries more, particularly before feedings. These studies may be the flip side of the traditional saying that "a happy pregnancy makes for a happy baby." But please don't think that because you're under emotional pressure you will definitely have a fussy baby. By the same token, an easy pregnancy won't guarantee you an easy baby!

Stress during your pregnancy can get in the way of the natural bonding process at birth. If you are under stress, it may delay your preparation for the infant and therefore your bond with the baby. During pregnancy a foundation is laid for mother–infant bonding.

Stressful Events That Can Delay Bonding

➢ moving to a new geographic area
➢ martial infidelity
➢ death of a close friend or relative

As a *reaction* to stress you may experience one or more of the following symptoms, which suggest a conscious rejection of the pregnancy, especially if they persist beyond the first trimester:

➤ preoccupation with your physical appearance or a negative perception of yourself

➤ excessive physical complaints

➤ excessive emotional withdrawal or mood swings

➤ absence of emotional response to fetal movement

➤ lack of preparatory behavior in the last trimester (making plans and getting the baby's room and clothes ready)

If you are aware of some of these symptoms in yourself and know you are under stress, try to seek out professional help while you are pregnant. That way you can cope with the problems before the baby is born and save yourselves heartache later.

THE BABY'S FATHER

Many books and caregivers virtually ignore the baby's father. Aside from the physical carrying of the child, which of course he cannot experience, a man is as deeply affected as the mother by pregnancy and birth. The health of the family depends partly on a man's successful transition to parenthood, yet there are few support systems to help prepare him. He is often left out of the pregnancy experience, yet expected to deal with a woman who may be complaining and demanding, to cope with new financial burdens, and to struggle with his feelings about becoming a father. There is rarely any help for him. All the attention is focused on the baby's mother; the father's needs might as well not exist. This can cause justifiable resentment, followed by anger and withdrawal.

The coming of a child can mobilize a man's personal strengths or highlight his weaknesses. He needs to be encouraged to participate in the new threesome. The traditional concept of male virility did not allow a man to experience the loving side of himself. In the past a man was excluded from almost every aspect of pregnancy, birth, and early child care. That has changed now—or at least men now have the option to get more involved without risking their male identity. This is a difficult and exciting time for parents, but you need each other in order for it to bring out the best in both of you.

Fears

Fears are common for fathers-to-be, but it may not be socially acceptable for a man to admit to them. Encourage your mate to open up. One fear a man will certainly have in common with his mate concerns the *baby's normalcy*; the same advice given to mothers (see page 202) applies to fathers.

➤ **Finances**, insurance, and other money issues are often considered the man's area of expertise. A child *can* mean a real change in your finances, but some men may focus too heavily on the financial aspect instead of dealing with fears about their own abilities. A man can share his wife's fears about being able to care properly for the baby, but he may express this fear by concentrating on finances, just as a woman may express her need for additional attention by having food cravings.

➤ **A loss of independence** is a common fear for men, particularly as a pregnant woman may lean on him more. The woman does need to depend more on her mate during pregnancy, and this can frighten a man; it threatens his sense of independence, plus he may be unsure of whether he can give her the support she needs. His anxieties may become more concrete in the third trimester, when the woman needs his help more because she is less able to help herself.

➤ **Sex** is an area where a man may feel fearful. Some men feel a drop in sex drive and activity during pregnancy. They are afraid that they will hurt the fetus during sex regardless of whether medical facts contradict that. It does not matter whether there is proof that sex cannot hurt the baby; what matters is that his paternal drive is developing. Do not be worried about this decrease in sex drive: generally it comes from protective feelings toward the baby—and a chance to put the baby's needs before his own. (For more information about sex during pregnancy, see Chapter 8.)

Envy and Jealousy

Envy can affect a man without his knowing it: it may come out in disguised ways. The unconscious longing to experience pregnancy and birth may show up in a burst of creativity or an increased drive to accomplish. These may be ways of sublimating the desire to be pregnant.

A man may also feel jealous of a woman's new closeness with her mother during pregnancy. He may feel shut out, fearful that she doesn't love or trust *him* enough. If his wife does have a renewed closeness with her mother (or other female friend, or relative), be aware that this may hurt her partner's feelings.

Nurturant Feelings

Her mate's nurturant feelings may not even be noticed by a woman, but many men do feel more protective and gentle during pregnancy. A prospective father has to learn to "mother" a woman—doing additional tasks, taking care of her in new ways. He may even become the prime mothering figure for her if her parents are far away.

➤ *This may be a chance for a man to try out being nurturant* in anticipation of the baby's arrival.

➤ *Nurturance also comes from a need to be more involved* and identified with the woman in order to begin a paternal tie to the coming infant.

➤ *When a man's motherliness is awakened* during pregnancy he is better able to respond to his baby—and he can get great pleasure from his nurturance if the woman, and later the baby, are receptive. Dr. Erik Erikson has said, "Each sex can transcend itself to feel and represent the concerns of the other . . . so real men can partake of motherliness."

➤ *Identifying with feminine aspects of themselves* can be frightening to some men. This identification can be so worrisome it causes impotence. A man may throw himself into supermasculine (macho) endeavors in order to counteract this fear.

➤ *A man has few socially acceptable ways* of expressing to others and himself that he will soon be a parent. Instead of (or in addition to) increased nurturance, a man may take on extra chores or ready the house for the baby's arrival to express this desire to be nurturing.

➤ *The paternal role* is something a man has to prepare himself for and may be worried about. If his relationship with his own father has been good, he will probably be more relaxed about developing as a father. If his relationship with his father was bad, however, a man may distrust his own abilities to father.

Try to talk about what you liked or disliked about your father and the way you interrelated. This will help you formulate your own image of what a good father should be. A man is reidentifying himself as a model for his child when he thinks about his own childhood and/or feelings of his possible inadequacy as a father himself. He will need support in thinking this through and asserting the best aspects of his personality.

➤ *Pregnancy syndrome* (also called the Couvade syndrome) is any symptom developed by a man which disappears after the birth of his child. The symptoms include: nausea, dizziness, heartburn, headache, abdominal cramps, constipation, diarrhea, food cravings, marked changes in appetite or weight during the prenatal period. These symptoms are not a psychiatric disorder but a way for a man to express identification and involvement with the pregnancy. However, they *are* a manifestation of deep psychological stress in anticipation of the birth. *Anxiety, envy*, and *hostility* can be expressed by pregnancy symptoms. A man may be feeling left out; he may be worrying whether his mate and the baby will be okay; he may be concerned that the woman will be even *more* withdrawn from him after the baby arrives.

Couvade syndrome can also be seen as a man's inner psychological reorganization in preparation for fatherhood. It can happen long-distance if the parents are separated. These pregnancy symptoms usually disappear right after the delivery of a healthy baby.

Withdrawing

A man's reluctance to participate during labor and delivery can be detrimental to both partners. By supporting his mate through pregnancy and delivery a man is preparing himself for fatherhood. If he is present at his baby's birth, a man's paternal feelings can be aroused and the "bonding" that takes place will then encourage his later participation in child care. You get out of being a parent what you put in: men don't get much chance to "put in." By asserting his involvement with his mate and then with his newborn a man can claim the place that has been denied all men for too long. Both partners must be aggressive in protecting the father's rights and responsibilities.

But a woman should not view a man's disinterest as a personal insult or as a sign of a rift in their relationship. Pregnancy and child-rearing are areas where women are often several steps ahead of men, if only because the sexes are raised with such different attitudes about this. A woman has to be patient for her mate to catch up with her: she can hold out a loving hand and encourage him along the way, or she can pout and withdraw and regard his lack of interest as an attack on her or the baby.

In order to involve a man during pregnancy you might ask him to read this book or others. You should be careful not to project an attitude (which women can do without even realizing it) of superior knowledge or sensitivity. Men feel excluded and uninformed as it is; if you are uppity in any way, it can reinforce his feeling of inadequacy and drive him away. If you want to go to childbirth education classes (see page 259) and your mate does not want to attend, ask him to come to one class. After that, if he is still against it, tell him you'll use a friend as coach. Choose a class that is oriented to couples (not just to women) and has a relaxed atmosphere. You might ask any couples you know who have been through prepared childbirth classes how the men liked the teacher and pick an instructor who gets a good "review" from other men.

If a man feels truly uncomfortable about participating in the labor and delivery, don't push it. Stick to your word and *do* choose a friend or relative to be your labor coach. A man may simply not be very interested in the birth process and it may take him weeks or months to really get turned on to the child. Let it happen at whatever his natural pace is or your enthusiasm or criticism may put him off even more.

However, there are two reasons for a man's adamant refusal to be involved that you may be able to alter:

1. *Fear of hospitals* is a reason some men are reluctant to be there during childbirth. Many people are afraid of hospitals—just on the general principle that they are places of sickness and death

(which they are, primarily), or else because they had a bad experience in a hospital. Familiarize yourselves with the hospital you plan to deliver in, if you are having a hospital birth. Take the official tour, more than once, perhaps. Just getting used to the place may help alleviate his fears.

2. **Fear of inadequacy** is another reason some men choose to avoid staying with their mate at this crucial time in her life. Some men are quite squeamish and are afraid they won't handle themselves well during the messy parts of labor and delivery. Other men are more concerned about not being able to meet a woman's emotional/psychological needs during the rigors of childbirth. In both cases all that is needed is some gentle encouragement. Men who imagine that they will "faint seeing the blood" should talk to other men who have stayed by their mates' sides and been so involved that they hardly noticed whether there was blood or not. Men who may not feel equal to the emotional demands should be assured that their simple presence—even if they barely say a word or give more than a gentle pat—may make a woman feel more secure and relaxed.

Running Away

Running away, either figuratively or literally, is a response some men have to pregnancy. They find excuses: longer working hours, sports events they "must" participate in during nonworking time, business trips, and the like. These men feel so overwhelmed by the external and internal demands of pending parenthood that they run away from these responsibilities and personal confrontations.

One danger is that this creates a vicious cycle: the woman feels ignored or abandoned and either makes outright demands on her husband to give her more time and attention or exhibits extravagant emotions to get his attention. Either tactic simply drives a man like this farther away. His autonomy is threatened. He is being called upon to *give*: this makes him feel suffocated or angry or inadequate.

It is not unlikely for a man like this to have an affair as a way of proving his independence to himself and asserting his denial of what is happening at home. Unless either or both partners can recognize his running away for what it is—and get help in the way of professional mediator—*the marriage may break up*. This is not just idle dramatics: marriages *do* break up during pregnancy or soon after a baby is born. In cases like this, such an outcome may be avoidable if the couple seeks help.

<u>Work</u>

Work can take on new importance for a man when he is an expectant parent. He may throw himself into work for a variety of reasons. It may be his unconscious desire to procreate. It may be his awareness of duties as a provider and the additional income needed to support a child. And it may be a way to avoid facing the pregnancy. Impending fatherhood may so overwhelm him that he puts a great deal of energy into an area where he feels competent, safe, and ultimately rewarded—none of which he may feel about pregnancy and childbirth.

Whatever the reason that a man throws himself into work, do not make the shortsighted and self-centered mistake of regarding this as rejection or neglect of you. A man has to face and resolve his feelings about this crucial time in his life as best he can. Work is one area where a man may express some of these complicated and unfamiliar feelings.

Best of all, concentrate on the *quality* of time you spend together, not the *quantity*. Diminished time together will be a fact of life once the baby is born. Don't forget that *your* time will be more limited then, so don't get hung up now about your mate's long hours at work. Begin to view your time together as special time, to be utilized in ways that give both of you pleasure, relaxation, and stimulation.

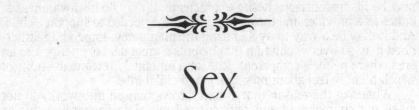

CHAPTER EIGHT

Sex

SEX DURING PREGNANCY

Sex is what got you here in the first place! Ironically sex during pregnancy can be touchy and anxiety-ridden. It doesn't have to be. Your sexual relationship has the potential to be more communicative and rewarding than ever before. In order to take advantage of this special time, you and your mate have to understand the ways in which your sex life may change during pregnancy, and then you have to *talk to each other* about it. If you both can overcome any reticence you may have about discussing or experimenting, pregnancy may give a new breadth to your sex life that can continue after the baby is born.

Anxieties About Sex

➤ *The most common fear* is that sex will *harm the fetus*. Some people are afraid they will "infect" the passage. The fact is that intercourse does not introduce infection to the baby, who is safely protected by an intact bag of fluid on the other side of a closed cervix. Another fear is of crushing the baby. Nature has provided excellent cushioning for the fetus: a woman can even fall without harming her baby. If either partner remains fearful about hurting the baby, then talk to your doctor or midwife about it.

➤ *Some people's anxiety comes out as guilt:* they are afraid that their increased sex drive during pregnancy can lead to abnormal sexual behavior later in their child. They are "projecting": the parent feels guilty and perhaps overwhelmed about new eroticism and projects a judgment onto the baby, imagining that there must be a punishment (a sexually deranged child) to compensate for so much pleasure. Enjoy yourself—you deserve it. Pregnancy has so many *unpleasant* side effects that the very least you deserve is a good time in bed!

➢ **The baby's reaction** to its parents' lovemaking can make some people anxious. A fetus does respond to sound waves and to his mother's movements (some of them sleep when their mother is active, and when she is napping or bathing, they wake up). After lovemaking some babies kick or squirm; this can give the impression that the baby is watching. Some parents are worried by this feeling that a third person is in the room (especially when it is an impressionable child!). Don't worry. The baby cannot see what you are doing. Some men actually have fantasies that the baby not only can see but might bite their penis.

➢ **A fear of miscarriage** may affect either partner. Sex and orgasms have not been shown to have any bad effects on pregnancy, but if a couple is afraid, they are not going to enjoy intercourse. A woman may be so concerned about a possible miscarriage, particularly in the first trimester, that she would rather give her mate oral and/or genital pleasure but abstain herself. A good way to deal with this anxiety is to concentrate on massaging and caressing and especially talking things over. It is important to stay in touch emotionally as well as physically. Eventually the anxiety should subside if you take things slowly. The partner who is fearful needs validation first of all: he or she needs to know that the other person accepts the fear even if it isn't rational. Then you can ease past it.

➢ **The role of sex in bringing on labor** makes some people anxious. Some doctors routinely prohibit sex during the last six weeks of pregnancy (without giving a reason—see page 230), which may reinforce some people's fears. However, labor will *not* start just because of coitus or nipple stimulation. It is true that if conditions are ripe for labor to begin, lovemaking can facilitate the progress of labor. Hormonal activity resulting from sex is the same as that during labor—and the sex hormones seem to enhance labor's progress.

Research hasn't determined what factors or hormonal balance cause labor to begin. Uterine contractions alone—which can be initiated by medical induction—do not cause cervical dilation. Similarly, uterine contractions resulting from orgasm are not linked to dilation. If you are already in labor, however, sexual stimulation can increase your contractions. Stimulation of the nipple has a direct physiological effect on the uterus, causing it to contract. This effect is the same whether it is from lovemaking or from the baby sucking later on—studies show that a breast pump stimulates uterine contractions during labor.

Bleeding After Sex

If bleeding accompanies intercourse it may not be serious, but you should consult your doctor to rule out the possibility of miscarriage or other problems.

In the first trimester, bleeding may be caused simply by a deep thrust by the man that brings his penis up against the cervix (the mouth of the uterus). The cervix is softer than usual during pregnancy, and there is so much extra blood in the vessels that pressure may cause a small amount of bleeding. This is nothing to worry about; such bruises, which are like a nosebleed, heal quickly. This bleeding can be eliminated by avoiding deep penetration.

Shallow penetration may solve the problems of pain or vaginal spotting after intercourse, but it is still worth the peace of mind to have any bleeding checked out by the doctor.

A Woman's Body Image

This subject was discussed in the preceding chapter, which suggested ways in which the changes in your body might be causing changes in your head. Perhaps the most significant way in which a woman's changing body image affects her is in the area of sexuality.

➤ *The strangeness of your new body* shape may make it hard for you to accept this new image of yourself. You may lose confidence in your ability to attract your mate.

➤ *You may recall times* in your life when you were heavy and think of this as the undesirable body you had before. It is important to recognize if "old tapes" are playing in your head, touching on negative feelings about yourself and your body you had in the past.

➤ *Your fear may be that you are becoming fat*, which is a dirty word in America. We are conditioned to believe that if a woman is fat, she is undesirable. And fat (undesirable) women are ignored or abandoned by men. Thus the change in your body image may be making you worried, unconsciously, that your mate is going to leave you. If this anxiety is preying on you, it will certainly affect your ideas, conscious or not, about lovemaking—whether sex will help you "hold on to" your mate or drive him away (since you are unconsciously operating on the assumption that he is so disgusted by your new body that he is going to leave).

➤ *Your mate may have less interest in sex* and you may translate his lack of turned-on-ness as displeasure with you physically. There are many reasons why a man's sex drive diminishes during pregnancy.

➤ *Your mate may find your body ugly*, with the big belly and perhaps stretch marks. What may happen is that *you* will then feel ugly and be angry at the baby for making you that way. Try instead to focus your attention and your mate's on the positive aspect of your new body.

➤ *In the last trimester* you may get disgusted with your body. You may be sick of being pregnant and your awkward size. However, most men are *not* negatively affected by a woman's body at its most pregnant—and it may be your fear of this (or a projection of *your* disgust onto your mate) that is upsetting you as much as the body changes themselves.

➤ *Certain body changes may be confusing and anxiety provoking* for you. Early in pregnancy your breasts will increase in size and in the same way that breasts do when they are sexually stimulated. Then during sex they may become slightly more enlarged. See the section on "Increased Sex Drive" on page 222, which covers a woman's possible guilt or anxiety about the increased eroticism that is part of her new body image.

➤ *Take positive actions* to counteract your negative feelings about your body-image change. As with any of the irrational worries that may bother you during pregnancy, it does not matter whether they "make sense" or not. They are your feelings and they are real. If your body-image change makes you feel insecure, then get reinforcement to bolster your ego. Your need for affection and reassurance increases—so get those needs met.

Find the beauty in the fullness of your new shape, because it is there. Share with your mate the changes that your body is going through and marvel at the transformation. Your belly can be a new part of you for both of you to enjoy. A pregnant belly is sensuous. The tight roundness feels good to run your hands over. And it is exciting later in the pregnancy to lie naked together and watch the baby move.

Some woman *like their bodies better* when they are pregnant. They find their new body image more positive than prepregnancy. They enjoy the new roundness and mystery, the feeling of ripening and creating. Try to see it that way yourself.

Communication About Sex

Communication about sex can be difficult—most of us are raised *not* to discuss it—but it is essential during pregnancy. A lack of communication at this time can draw partners apart, when the honesty of shared feelings is so crucial to meeting their own and each other's needs.

➤ *You have to be willing to discuss* the fact that *your mate may be turned off* to your changing body shape and odor. Unless you can both discuss it as objectively as possible, the man may simply withdraw.

➤ *You may be disgusted* with your body. It is important to talk this out with your partner in order to resolve some of these feelings so that they don't control your sex life.

➤ *The "dependency period"* is roughly ten weeks before and after birth: this is a time when a pregnant woman feels the most vulnerable and needs the most support. However, although she may need reassurance during these sensitive weeks, she may often be giving off rejection signals. Unless a man and woman have learned to really talk to one another, the man is not going to realize that this is a "mixed message," and what the woman *really* needs and wants the most is stroking. Sex is especially beneficial during this time because it helps alleviate tension, which can build up as the due date nears. Also, when other kinds of communication fail, sex is a way of talking to each other without words, forming bonds that words might not be able to.

➤ *Sex can express unacknowledged feelings* (which have been cautioned against in many sections of this book). Withholding and aggression can crop up in the sexual part of your relationship when they aren't acknowledged or resolved by other kinds of communication. The feelings of pregnancy are intense and changeable—the first step in handling them is to consciously acknowledge them. Refusing sex can be a way of expressing unmet needs or fears. Unless you realize that, the needs and fears will remain unresolved, and in addition, you will have a problem with your sexual relationship. Also, having intercourse when you don't want to can produce morning sickness. During pregnancy your mind and body (the psyche and the soma—thus the word *psychosomatic*) are particularly tuned into each other, so you have to pay special attention to your thoughts and feelings.

➤ *A man may wind up having an extramarital foray* if the two of you have not nurtured an atmosphere of open communication. A prospective father may have an affair if he does not feel free to express *and* listen to the confusing, powerful emotions of this time in your lives.

➤ *Gentle reassurance is* what both of you need from each other. You are both faced with a lot of new information and sensations during pregnancy, and you need to support one another. If you talk about these personal, frightening feelings, the communication can create a stronger, deeper, more trusting relationship.

A Decrease in the Man's Desire for Sex

Sexual appetites can go through some dramatic changes during pregnancy, and the partners won't necessarily be feeling their interest increase or diminish at the same time. A decrease in sexual desire affects men and women for different reasons. There are several reasons for a decline in sexual interest for the man:

> *Fear of hurting the fetus*, mentioned at the beginning of this chapter under "Anxieties About Sex," is a major reason. Although it *is not possible* to hurt the baby during sex, some men will feel better if a doctor reassures them of this. However, the man's weight should never rest entirely on the woman without the support of his arms. Some men will still avoid sex—the rational facts cannot dispel their emotional response.
> *Unwillingness to impose* on the woman, who may be tired or feeling some of the discomforts of pregnancy, is a reason some men back off sex.
> *The "mistress/mother conflict"* is behind a decrease in sexual desire in many men, who may not even realize it. A man can have mixed feelings about the growing motherliness of the "girl" he married. His interest in you sexually may decrease as your belly grows because you become associated with his mother in his mind. This throws him into a conflict with the sexual taboo against a man sleeping with his mother. A man is usually not even aware that this is what is influencing him.
> *See the section on the man's feelings,* later in this chapter, which covers many of the sexual reactions a man may have to a pregnant woman, some of which cause him to withdraw from sexual activity.

A Woman's Decreased Sex Drive

> *Fatigue, nausea,* and some of the other physical discomforts of pregnancy don't make a woman feel very sexy. However, although there are physical deterrents to sex, it is often emotions—guilt, conflict—that have more effect on a woman's desire for sex or lack of it.
> *A woman may feel a conflict between her sexuality and her developing role as a mother.* In making the transition to "mother" demanded by pregnancy, a woman may have some trouble integrating her sexual self (which she probably associates with her prepregnancy identity: a more self-centered, self-gratifying existence) and her maternal self (which in its purest, least realistic form has to do with being concerned with the child's well-being ahead of, or even instead of, her own). Until a woman has resolved some of this identity crisis in developing her mothering role, her interest in sex may dwindle. Some women have a hard time connecting the image of "mother" with the idea of sexual desire and activity. It is important to sort this out to restore a healthy sex life, and also to pave the way for breast-feeding. Breast-feeding can stir up some of the same

conflicts: sexual pleasure (which many women get from breast-feeding) versus breasts as the means by which to nourish a child.

➤ *In the third trimester* a woman can lose interest in sex because all of her physical and mental energies are going into fixing up the house for the baby and getting ready for labor and delivery.

➤ *If a woman who is uninterested* in sex makes love just to please her mate, it can cause worse problems than abstaining. A man will feel her unspoken reserve and lack of enjoyment and *take it as a rejection of him.* A woman who makes love without wanting to is setting up barriers. If you don't want to make love, it is important you tell your partner that your disinterest is caused by the anxieties and pressures of the pregnancy. These are times when both of you are very sensitive, so you must each guard against situations where you can take things the wrong way.

➤ *You can stimulate* your sex drive in a number of ways. Plan a purposely sexy evening of a candlelit dinner with wine and romantic music. You can read a sexy book together, or see an X-rated movie. Buy an outrageous negligee and surprise your mate with it. Or he can surprise you by wearing a raincoat with nothing underneath. Sure, I'm kidding, but kidding-on-the-square. Enjoy yourselves. Laugh. Play out fantasies. Experiment. Each of you ask the other what his or her secret sexual fantasy is. Tease each other; fulfill each other.

Increased Sex Drive

An increased desire for sex can grow. You may feel mentally and physically free because you don't have to worry about birth control. However, a major reason why many women feel an increased desire for sex is because a pregnant woman's body state is the same as a state of sexual arousal. The hormonal changes are the same as during arousal. The breasts and genital tissue are engorged with extra blood; there is increased vaginal lubrication and increased steroid and estrogen production. When sexually aroused a pregnant woman feels yet a further increase. She may get *vaginal sensations* in the night which are the equivalent of a man's "wet dream." Breasts are supersensitive to any arousal because the already engorged tissues become even more engorged (although the tenderness that may accompany engorgement will pass as the body accommodates to it).

Even women who usually have a low sex drive can feel a new urge. It can be frightening and feel all-consuming. *Talk about it with your mate.* Some women become very erotic and are obsessed with strange sexual fantasies. Some become preoccupied with sex and are then afraid that their increased sexual appetite will frighten their partner. Don't hide these feelings—share them with your mate.

The second trimester is the time when most women feel this increased eroticism. Some women reach orgasm for the first time in this period, and other women experience multiorgasmic capabilities. This is because of the increased blood flow to the pelvis, which means a woman becomes aroused more rapidly and more intensely.

The Man's Feelings About Sex

➤ *The underlying change* is that a *woman is being transformed* right before his eyes. She can feel the changes going on inside and out, but he can only guess at them. A man has to make a mental and physical adjustment to a "new" woman—a woman who is different in many ways from the lady he has known.

➤ *A man may be overwhelmed* by the "earth mother" aspect of your changing image: your superfeminine body, heavier scent, extra lubrication, and increased engorgement. It may be frightening to him. Give him a chance to adjust slowly.

➤ *A man may become impotent* because of changes in your vagina. Because of your *engorgement* he may feel there's no room for him inside you; because of your *lubrication* he may feel there is too much room. Either feeling can make him lose his erection. This womanliness—this difference in you—may make him feel temporarily pressured and inadequate.

➤ *Similarly, a man may feel inadequate* because you are now having rapid orgasms and he is going at the same rate he always was. Also, if you have become orgasmic—or multiorgasmic— for the first time, a man has to adjust to this, both physically and mentally. He may worry that he cannot meet your increased sexual needs or capacities.

➤ *A man may turn to a nonpregnant woman* rather than trying to make love to his transformed mate. As with all these changes you will both be best able to cope with them by keeping your lines of communication open.

➤ *Even if a man does not literally leave he may feel kicked out* by the fetus and withdraw emotionally. A man needs to feel that all your attention is not focused inward, that the baby is not getting all your love and energy. If he feels left out now, it will only be worse once the baby is born. Postpartum there will be times you will have *no choice* but to give your attention to the baby, instead of your husband.

➤ *A man may feel guilty* receiving sexual gratification when a woman doesn't want any for herself. There are times when a pregnant woman is not interested in being aroused herself but wants to give pleasure to her mate. One example of this is a woman who is afraid that sex may cause a miscarriage. The man may be picking up signals that the woman does not really want to be giving him oral and/or genital stimulation, that she is doing it out of a sense of "duty." He must talk to her about this so that he doesn't have to feel guilty or in her "debt." Things must be straightened out so that a woman is participating sexually because she *wants* to.

➢ *New forms of sexual behavior* are not easy to get used to. We are all creatures of habit; change can be disorienting or frightening. Our attitudes toward sex are formed by what we learned in childhood and adolescence. For instance, some people may not be able to enjoy mutual masturbation (discussed on the following pages) because it feels regressive, unclean, something children do (and perhaps should not). Try out new sexual alternatives at your own pace and make an effort to talk together if either of you feels uncomfortable. If you still can't enjoy yourself, then try something else. The whole point is to share enjoyment—it's not a test or contest.

Exotic new postures may be embarrassing at first. A man may be afraid of failing (consciously or not). He may fear that his penis is not big enough or his erection not hard enough for any positions other than ones he already knows and has tried. Once again, loving, gentle reassurance will get you through these awkward or funny moments.

POSITIONS FOR LOVEMAKING

Positions for lovemaking have to be adjusted to your pregnant body; as the fetus grows you have to try new ways to be comfortable during intercourse. For conservative people this experimentation with new positions and alternate modes of sex can be threatening. It may make them feel guilty or they may try to avoid sex altogether.

➢ *Take it a little at a time* and go back to positions you are comfortable with: protect yourselves from tension in your sex life. These new explorations can give you increased pleasure, both during the pregnancy and in your continuing lives together.

If either of you feels hung up about new positions or other changes in your sexual relationship, think of it this way: sex is good for you and your baby. Intercourse is good exercise for the pelvic floor muscles. You need these muscles to be in prime condition for labor and delivery. So the message to these people is: make love as much as you can. If you continue to feel guilty due to how good it feels, you can rationalize that it's for your own good!

➢ *The man on top but lying partly sideways* is one position which will carry you through most of pregnancy. This way most of his weight is off of you.

➢ *The woman-on-top position* is comfortable for many people, especially because the woman can control how deep the penetration is.

➤ *Side positions*—either front-to-back or front-to-front—are excellent during pregnancy. There is no pressure on your belly, which can now be caressed as a new erogenous zone. Side positions can give you both a whole new perspective on lovemaking, freeing your hands for exploration and letting you see each other in a new light. A side position with the man behind so that you can fit together like a "spoon" is good for the end of the pregnancy when the woman's belly is largest.

ORGASM

➤ *Orgasm is one of the areas of change in sex* during pregnancy because there is an increased blood flow to the genitals, which increases sexuality.
➤ *Some women experience orgasm for the first time* when they are pregnant. Although this is exciting and pleasurable, it also involves some mental readjustments. If you have not had an orgasm before now, you may have resigned yourself to never having one. Discovering the thrill of orgasm for the first time will mean changing your mindset about yourself sexually.
➤ *If you become multiorgasmic for the first time* you may feel overwhelmed and perhaps frightened by your new capacities and sexual appetite. Until now you may have always assumed that sex involved a period of arousal in which there was foreplay, then increasing sexual tension and excitement which reached a peak and a climax—and that was it. Then you'd lie in postcoital bliss, feeling drowsy and loving.

Now you discover there is more! Your orgasm may go on longer than experienced before, or you may have an additional orgasm(s) on the heels of the first one, or you may still feel aroused after the first orgasm and want to continue energetic lovemaking. You have discovered that there is not just *one* peak, but perhaps several. Although some of this heightened sexual capacity may stay with you after pregnancy, much of it is temporary. After the baby's birth your sexual appetite will return to what it was prepregnancy. So don't worry—be happy!

Problems Having an Orgasm

➤ *Orgasmic problems* for a pregnant woman are not uncommon. For example, in reading this section, if you do *not* feel an increased orgasmic capacity you may wonder if there's something wrong with you. You may begin to worry about having orgasms. There is no better way to insure *not* having an orgasm than to be focused on wanting one (it is just the same as when a man is worried about erections—the more he worries, the more likely he is to be impotent). The best treatment is to create a relaxed, nondemanding space in which you feel loved and cared for. Make a conscious decision to have sex *without* orgasms— just for the pleasure of caressing and kissing. Take away the orientation toward a goal—remove the element of "achieving"— and you not only will enjoy sex again but will probably have an orgasm before you know it. Just remember that a strong desire for an orgasm can inhibit it. If you are having trouble reaching orgasm, you can get more tense and make it even harder for yourself to relax, enjoy, and climax. Some of the reasons you may be having orgasmic problems are:

➤ *You may generally have trouble relaxing* because of anxiety about the impending birth. You may be worrying about labor and whether you will be an adequate mother. Try giving each other massages as an introduction to lovemaking. It can relax you and relieve any pressures you might be feeling about your sexuality and orgasmic capabilities.

➤ *When you are pregnant your life is out of control* and you know it. The pregnancy and baby have taken over. The fear of a loss of control can lead to generalized tension in some women. For them orgasm may equal "letting go." They are so anxious about this feeling of their life being out of control that sex and orgasm are areas where they can express their fear and "hold on" by not climaxing.

➤ *Some women's genitals remain engorged* even after an orgasm in late pregnancy. This may mean that lovemaking leaves them in a state of continued sexual tension; a sense of lingering semiarousal. Orgasm occasionally fails to relieve this tension. Some women compulsively seek orgasmic release, but don't get it regardless of how many orgasms they have. If you have this feeling of continual sexual tension, you should know that it is because of an increased blood flow to your genitals, which can take quite a while to subside. The more you are stimulated, the longer this tension will remain.

➤ *Uterine spasms after orgasm* may occur in the third trimester instead of the rhythmic contractions you are accustomed to with orgasm. Near term some women may have regularly recurring contractions for as long as half an hour after orgasm. Pain and abdominal cramping are also possible, although usually in women who are having their first baby. This residual vasocongestion can become chronic. In a woman who is pregnant for the first time, the postorgasm resolution can be 10 to 15 minutes longer than prepregnancy. If this is not your first baby, you may find that it takes your body 30 to 45 minutes longer than before you were pregnant for your body to return to a relaxed state.

➤ *The rate of orgasms often declines* in the last trimester. So if you find you are less orgasmic as your due date nears, be assured it is normal.

➤ **Early labor contractions are similar** in rhythm and intensity to the uterine contractions of an orgasm. People often liken labor contractions to bad menstrual cramps—but labor is a lot more fun to anticipate (and easier to tolerate) if you look at it in this rosier light!

➤ **If you were wondering how the contractions of orgasm affect the fetus**—they do cause a slight change in the fetal heart rate. This change does no harm. Think of it as giving your baby a nice ride in your contracting uterus.

CHANGES IN VAGINAL SECRETIONS

There are increased secretions when you are pregnant. These secretions may have a strong odor, which can be a turnoff to you or your mate. Douching will not stop the secretions or their smell (see "Douching" on page 151).

The change in the odor or taste of this extra lubrication is caused by the increased blood supply to your genitals during pregnancy. One way to change the scent is to massage the area with a scented body oil, perhaps the same one you may be using for massages. Health food stores and some drugstores sell body oils scented with lemon, spices, or other scents.

SEX IN THE THIRD TRIMESTER

➤ **This can be the most awkward time sexually**. Your belly is big and it may be cumbersome. You get tired more easily; ordinary physical movements can be more difficult. This doesn't leave you with much enthusiasm for sex or much energy once you are making love.

➤ **Certain positions** may be more comfortable, particularly rear-entry positions with the woman standing and bending over or on her side and the man behind.

➤ **You may want to avoid maximum penetration positions** not only because they may be uncomfortable but because they may also cause anxiety.

➤ **Mutual masturbation** can be very satisfying in the last trimester. It can open communication between you and your mate and can lead you into sexual experimentation, which will add new richness to your sexual relationship.

➤ **In the latter part of pregnancy many women feel the need for increased affection.** Hugging and kissing not specifically related to sexual intercourse can meet this need. It can also be lovely just to lie together and cuddle: touching, caressing, massaging, and just looking at each other without talking. These kinds of "nonsexual" (i.e., nonpenetrating and perhaps non-orgasmic) encounters can be intensely romantic and bring you closer together.

ALTERNATIVES TO INTERCOURSE

Massage

Massage is both an alternative to sexual intercourse and a lovely way to initiate lovemaking. You can say things with your hands, through stroking, that are beyond words. Massage creates a whole new avenue of communication and expression. It is also a wonderful way to rid your body of tension and really relax.

Once you become proficient at erotic massage, you will be giving your mate reassurance, pleasure, and love. If you have never given (or gotten!) a massage before, first get a nice oil. Any vegetable oil (olive, safflower, etc.) is fine, but it is more fun to get a pleasantly scented oil from a drugstore or a health food store. First of all, the person to be massaged should have a warm shower or bath, to get extra clean and relax the body. Then place towels over the bed—or wherever you've chosen to give the massage—and have your mate lie down, naked. Cover him with two or three towels: they will keep him warm, feeling cozy and protected. Start with his hands. Coat the palms of your hands with some oil and then rub them together so that your hands and the oil are warmed. Then firmly caress his hand, pulling gently on each finger as you massage it. When you feel comfortable with your technique on each of his hands, move to his feet and do the same thing.

If you feel awkward giving a massage, you might want to buy any of the books now available that describe sensual massage with drawings or photographs. Basically you want to firmly and smoothly caress your mate's body, which can be as pleasurable and gratifying to you as it is to him. Using your hands skillfully shows your desire and love for your partner (even if your vagina doesn't want his penis right then, or vice versa).

Obviously all these suggestions apply equally whether the pregnant woman is receiving or giving the massage. The reason that I describe the man receiving a massage is only because so much attention is paid during pregnancy to what the woman wants and needs. I wanted to balance the scales a little and remind both of you that the man deserves loving care, too!

Masturbation

Masturbation has an important place in your sex lives during pregnancy, but either of you may have hang-ups that you need to overcome first. Some women may feel guilty about their increased erotic needs. Once you read the earlier section of this chapter that explains the increased sex drive in a pregnant woman, you should be able to accept and enjoy this heightened eroticism.

Masturbation is an excellent way to relieve sexual tension, particularly in the second trimester. Your mate may not be around, he may not be in the mood for sex, or you may have had intercourse with him and still feel aroused. If you have always thought of masturbation as evil or dirty, try to recognize this as the attitude of those of your parents' generation, who were frightened or disgusted by sexual impulses and expression. Masturbating can be a very pleasant alternative or supplement to sex that you share with your mate.

> ➤ *Although many women find they have orgasms more easily* during pregnancy, there are some who have a *fear of "letting go" sexually* when they are pregnant. They hold back the experience of orgasm, which in some women evokes the image of letting go or of releasing the fetus. Masturbation may be a way to overcome this feeling because it may give you a feeling of being more fully in control of the sexual situation. If you have difficulty reaching a climax during sexual intercourse, you might try masturbating—by yourself or with your mate—as a way of gradually overcoming the fear of letting go which may be inhibiting you.
> ➤ *Mutual masturbation* is an excellent alternative to intercourse during pregnancy. It relieves tension and can encourage you to explore new sexual avenues together. Mutual masturbation, and variations on it, can be a way to share a sexual experience when one of you does not want to have intercourse because of anxieties or discomfort.
> ➤ *Using a vibrator* either when you are masturbating alone or together can add a fun and exciting dimension. Remember, pregnancy is a time for change. So if you haven't tried a vibrator before, you can make up for lost time now—and discover what you've been missing! And there's no harm to the baby from the minimal vibration or the noise.
> ➤ *As with intercourse, if you have spotting, pain, or reasons to suspect you might miscarry*, abstain from orgasm with masturbation. The uterine contractions from an orgasm with masturbation can be even more intense than those from sexual intercourse.

WHEN SEX ISN'T ALLOWED

Being forced to give up sex can be a big strain on a relationship. Some women do withdraw emotionally during pregnancy, and if this is coupled with a ban on sex by your obstetrician, it can drive the man elsewhere to get his emotional and physical needs met. Sex is an important outlet for many feelings (anger, anxiety, or insecurity) that you may not be conscious of during pregnancy; sex is also a way to express love and affection. If this avenue of communication is shut off, it can upset a couple who are already riding on the roller coaster of pregnancy.

Some doctors routinely demand that a couple abstain from sex for the last 6 weeks of a pregnancy. Most of these doctors do not give a reason for this decree. Don't just follow these orders without asking for reasons *why* you can't make love. You don't need any more strains on your relationship than are absolutely necessary, and a long, forced abstinence can be damaging.

There are many people who make love right up to delivery time. There are many doctors who put no restrictions on a couple's sex life. If your doctor's orders to abstain seem too rigid, then discuss it. Consult another doctor if you are not fully convinced of the reasoning.

WARNINGS ABOUT SEX DURING PREGNANCY

— Blowing air into the vagina can be dangerous. This is the only sexual activity that has been documented as potentially harmful. By doing this you can detach the placenta from the uterine wall and cause an air embolism. (This does not rule out cunnilingus.)

— The man's entire weight should never be on the woman. He should support himself at least partially with his arms if he is on top, or he should lie slightly sideways.

— Great pressure should never be put on the uterus.

— Reasons for no sex at any time:
  • vaginal or abdominal pain
  • uterine bleeding
  • membranes have ruptured
  • you have been warned or think miscarriage might occur

SEX AFTER THE BABY IS BORN

Your body has many changes to undergo after birth, all of which can affect your sex life. Your hormones must readjust to prepregnancy levels. Your blood supply and the fluid content in your body must be reduced. Your uterus and vagina have to return to their normal size. Your perineum has to recover from any tears or bruises or from an episiotomy. And your milk supply has to be either established or repressed. All that has to take place while you are also getting accustomed to being a parent and having a new little person in the house. Recognize what a tremendous upheaval you are going through internally and externally and give yourself time to cope with it all.

When and How to Resume Sex After Birth

Although there are many doctors who suggest a four- to six-week wait after delivery, many couples do not wait that long. There are several reasons to start having sex again as soon as possible after the baby is born. Some couples stop having sex six weeks before birth and then wait for six weeks afterward: that is *three months* without sex. Even if these couples use alternatives to intercourse, this "celibacy" may not be necessary. The frustration this causes in a relationship can surface in many ways and create needless problems. The six weeks before and after childbirth are a time when sex can be an important and helpful bond.

➤ *A six-week wait* is too conservative for many women. Having sex again sooner is better for them—they start having sex two to three weeks after childbirth and feel great.

➤ *If you had no lacerations* and no episiotomy, there are may be no medical reason you can't start making love within three weeks if you feel the desire. Check with your doctor, but if he won't let you and you feel his recommendation is too conservative, then ask another doctor.

➤ *A good way to judge* whether your body is ready for sex is to wait for it to recover from the delivery. Recovery is generally complete when the *lochia disappears*, which means that the placental site has healed. You can also wait until *your episiotomy incision has healed*. There is a potential risk of infection until then. Again, check with a doctor if you have any doubts.

Reasons for Rapid Resumption of Sex

➤ *Sex reduces tensions*. It is one of the few nonverbal (and nonhostile!) ways that are available to you and your mate as an outlet for tension.

➢ **Sex reaffirms your desirability**. Many women come to doubt their attractiveness while they are pregnant, particularly in the last trimester. By resuming sex you begin to rebuild a positive self-image in this area.

➢ **The hormonal climate** of sexual activity speeds the uterus to its prepregnant state in the same way breast-feeding does. It releases hormones that help return your body to normal—and you to *feeling* normal.

Low Interest in Sex Postpartum for the Woman

➢ **Lowered estrogen levels**, mentioned elsewhere in this section, account for some of a woman's possible disinterest in sex.

➢ **A woman's physical and emotional energies** are often so used up by the baby that there is a delay in the return of her sexual interest.

➢ **Low sexual interest** may also come from the trauma of having your life turned upside down, with the arrival of the newborn and his constant needs. This upheaval may give you the feeling that your own needs are not being met. *You* may want to be nurtured by your mate without the expectation of sexual intercourse attached to it.

➢ **Sexual activities** without intercourse seem to be a good solution for some people. "Pleasuring" is most satisfying to a woman who isn't ready yet for sexual intercourse. Sensual exchanges that include stroking, massaging, and stimulation for the fun of it (rather than as a warm-up for intercourse) can get you through this transitional time. They can also set the foundation for when your normal sex drive returns.

Decreased Sexual Drive in the Man

➢ **A man may be turned off** sexually from watching the birth. A woman in labor may be frighteningly different from her usual "feminine" self—the noises she makes, her facial contortions, the uninhibited positions she is in during birth. These can be overwhelming images for a man to fit into his conception of his partner.

➢ **It may be hard for a man** to believe that his wife's body will ever return to a size that is appropriate for his penis. It can be helpful to a man to try and appreciate the wondrous nature of the vagina, and to realize that it can stretch and shrink back to its normal size just as a penis changes in size.

➢ **A man's acceptance** of the changes in a woman's vagina during labor and delivery can help her deal with the fear *she* may be having: "Will I ever be the same again?" It will help you both readjust to sex if you realize that the vagina is designed to make room for the passage of a baby and then return to its prepregnancy size.

➢ *It can take time* for a man to get used to the idea that the lovely, dark, warm place that has always been there just for him also has a fantastic and practical function as an exit for the baby! Making love may be difficult until a man gets used to this new concept. Some women may have the same difficulty relating to this new view of her own body.

➢ *If a man "knows" ahead of time* that his sexual attitudes are going to be negatively affected by the birth, then it may be better for him not to be there. If he is certain that he'll feel this way, then he will probably create that feeling for himself. His negative attitude may make it hard for the woman to open up and relax, which is necessary during labor and delivery. Instead of reducing anxiety—which is a main reason for having a mate present—a man with this outlook may increase the tension for his mate.

Anxieties May Interfere with Postpartum Sex

➢ *The fear of getting pregnant* again may bother some people. It is something you haven't had to worry about for a while, and resuming birth control can be worrisome and/or annoying.

➢ *You may be worried* about being "all together again" internally and be cautious about sex play for this reason. Generally it is safe to assume that when the lochia has stopped, the uterus has healed. Lochia is the menstrual-like flow of the uterine lining that lasts for a week or two after delivery (see page 480). Some women may still be fearful after the lochia has stopped; they need to proceed slowly with resuming sex.

➢ *Your mate may be worried about hurting you*. You probably will be tender at first and it may upset him to think he is causing you any pain.

➢ *Fear that the baby will cry* when you are in the middle of lovemaking is a common concern. It is hard to adjust to a new presence in the house, and you may not feel as free as before since you're listening for the baby.

➢ *Fear that the baby will get infected* from love play is something you should not worry about unless the father is genuinely ill—with strep throat, for instance. A child adapts to the flora of both parents; there is no reason not to make love and then breast-feed the baby, for example.

The Baby's Influence on Sex

➢ *The child can be felt as an intruder*, ruining your privacy. You may be worried that she will need attention during intimate moments or quiet times with your mate. The baby will undoubtedly intrude on you at awkward moments, whether it's right in the middle of passionate lovemaking or when you are playing cards together. *The important thing is to get back to these intimate moments after the interruption.* Learn to be somewhat flexible and to not allow the baby's needs to put an end to whatever you were doing—do not let it be more than an interruption.

➤ *Another solution* is to take advantage of other times together with your mate. Just remember: it's your house and your life. Don't let the baby take away your options. By giving up control of your life for the child's needs you're starting bad habits.

➤ *A woman can get absorbed* in her baby. You can be so satisfied with your attachment to the baby that you have little need for other emotional ties. However, your mate's emotional needs are the same as—if not greater than—they were before the baby's birth. He is unlikely to be getting the same kind of "sexual" satisfaction from the baby that you are.

➤ *Physical contact* with the baby can be very satisfying to a woman—sometimes to the exclusion of her mate. Your desire to hold, touch, and caress may be satisfied by your contact with the baby. The intimacy of mothering can decrease your interest in lovemaking.

➤ *The baby can demand a woman's energy full-time*, especially if she is home all day. By the time your mate comes home and you have put the baby down for the night, you may *need time and space for yourself.* Your mate, quite naturally, wants to spend time with you. The baby's demands on you have come first and tired you out, which can leave the man feeling neglected and not needed.

Breast-Feeding and Sex

Lactation alters your estrogen levels. Your hormones are suppressed, but many women feel a higher sexual interest than prepregnancy. At one time this suppression of hormones was believed to be effective for contraceptive purposes, but it *simply is not reliable.* Some women ovulate despite the fact that breast-feeding supposedly suppresses ovulation.

Increased Sexual Stimulation During Breast-Feeding

➤ *Some women* find that nursing puts them more in touch with themselves and their bodies, which can heighten their sexuality.

➤ *The hormone oxytocin*, which is produced during sucking, is a sexual stimulant. Often the sucking of the baby can produce sexual stimulation, up to and sometimes including orgasm.

Women who become aroused to this point may feel guilt and have fears about a perverted sexual interest in the baby. Relax. Nursing feels good. It causes hormones that are sexually arousing to be released into your system. That's all there is to it.

Women who find nursing very sexual—to the point of orgasm, for instance—can direct this eroticism toward their mate. You can enjoy this sensuality with your mate rather than regard it as something he is excluded from, even though it began during breast-feeding.

Many nursing women experience heightened sexual pleasure and more intense or frequent orgasms when they make love. The hormones enlarge your veins and promote growth of new blood vessels in your pelvis. This raises the potential of your vagina and clitoris to respond to stimulation.

Decrease in Sexuality While Nursing

➤ **Nursing does inhibit** vaginal lubrication, although it doesn't prevent sexual responsiveness. Use unscented K-Y Jelly or a similar product if you have this problem.

➤ **The lowered estrogen** levels that can accompany lactation account for decreased lubrication. It can also mean a lowered interest in sex. It is quite normal not to want sex, or not to be easily turned on. If you're aware of this it can prevent your mate from feeling rejected or confused.

➤ **Some women who do not choose to breast-feed** may be unwilling to experience the possible sexual stimulation from suckling, or the conflict between baby and husband.

➤ **Some breast-feeding women** have painful cramps during intercourse. This might mean they will want to postpone sex until their bodies have balanced their hormone levels.

➤ **Breasts themselves can be symbolic** of a tug-of-war a woman may feel. You may be uptight about your mate sharing the "baby's" breasts—later on you may want your breasts to be for your mate and not for the baby any longer. The larger issue is whether a woman can love both her baby and her mate without feeling a conflict in her devotion to either of them. A man can often feel neglected in favor of the baby, and be sexually jealous when the baby is fed.

Conflict Between Mothering and Sex

Some women may feel a clash between their self-image as a mother and that of a sexy, abandoned lovemaking partner. This is part of the ongoing identity crisis common during pregnancy.

It is important that you sit down and discuss this conflict as calmly as possible with your partner. If you do not face and resolve this question, it may cause harm to your relationship. You may want to seek professional counseling.

Physical Changes and Sex

Even when your mind has returned to its normal level of eroticism, your physical responses to sexual stimuli may take longer. You may find your reactions to sex are less strong than they were before pregnancy. There are reasons for this: your vaginal walls are thin and lubrication can be sparse for several months postpartum. This means your body will not respond sexually in the accustomed manner. You may feel much better after your first period.

> *Your diaphragm* has to be refitted after childbirth, when you will probably need a larger size. When your partner first tries to enter you, it may be difficult and painful.
> *Exhaustion* may leave you too tired for sex. It takes your body a full six weeks to recover from childbirth. On top of that you have the new demands of your baby to cope with. Try to explain this to your mate: sometimes men have a hard time really understanding what this exhaustion feels like. Your mate may feel you are using tiredness as an "excuse." If so, let him spend a day alone with the baby! Don't suggest this in a hostile way, but simply let him get an idea of how you may be feeling.
> *Hormones* play a large part in sexual readjustment. Estrogen levels are low after birth and will remain low if you are breast-feeding. Some women take longer postpartum to return to a hormonal balance. This requires patience on both your parts. A woman may need extra fondling, kissing, and other foreplay to become aroused. Don't worry—you will be functioning normally before long.
>
> Low estrogen levels may be one reason for low sexual interest. Hormone imbalance is also the reason for insufficient lubrication, and breast-feeding will prolong this condition. Use unscented K-Y Jelly or have a doctor prescribe estrogen cream until your vaginal lubrication returns to normal.

Pain During Sex

> *Pain during postpartum intercourse* is something many women do not expect. Unless you are prepared for it, you may be shocked by the intensity of pain. Even women who have had cesarean deliveries can have this discomfort. This can occur at the vaginal opening or inside the vagina; there can be irritation, even with the use of jelly.

Do not go too far in the beginning. Take it easy so you don't "psych yourself out."

It is a good idea to have the woman on top during love-making. That way she can control the entrance of her mate's penis. If she is still somewhat dry, she'll want to be especially careful and have him enter her very gradually.

➤ *Your mate can go in gently and stay inside you without moving much*. Build up your sexual stamina gradually. Be patient with yourself and communicate to your mate what you are feeling and what you do or don't want to do sexually each step along the way.

➤ *Your perineum may be sore and stiff* after childbirth. There may be tears and bruises that have to heal. If you don't let your mate know and just grit your teeth, you will come to dread even the thought of intercourse. A coldness and touchiness can then build up between you. Your mate may feel rejected. Give yourself a chance to return to normal—attempt sex gradually and with lubricating jelly, if necessary. But let your mate know how you're feeling and why.

➤ *An episiotomy can make sex especially difficult*. (See the section on "Episiotomy" on page 385 for more information.) A warm bath right before lovemaking may help. Do not use Vaseline or other non-water-soluble lubricants. They can keep the air out and allow bacteria to grow in the episiotomy site. A good position after an episiotomy or with a sore perineum is for both of you to lie on your sides with your mate behind you, "spoon" fashion.

Physical Interruptions to Sex

➤ *Leaking milk* can interrupt your sex life. Be prepared for leakage at unpredictable times. Many women lose breast milk in uncontrolled spurts when they are sexually aroused and during orgasm.

If the baby cries in another room, your breast milk may start to flow, which can elicit the conflicted feelings about mate and baby discussed earlier in this chapter.

If either partner is fastidious, this leaking milk may be a turn-off. You may feel disgusted with your body and its secretions. There's not much to do about it except take a bath or shower together after making love and clean up the spilt milk without worrying about it too much!

➤ *Lochia*, the postpartum vaginal discharge, may also leak during sex. If you are accustomed to lovemaking when you have your period, then this is virtually the same thing. If you have always avoided sex at that time, you may have a negative reaction to lochia. However, the flow should not be as great as from a menstrual period, especially if you are taking it easy postpartum. You may feel disgusted by your body and these secretions. It may help you to think of it as your body cleaning itself out after pregnancy and birth—think of it as a *good thing*, as the road to the return of your normal body and its functions.

CHAPTER NINE

Choices in Childbirth

You have many options about where you will give birth and who will attend you. In order to decide what is the right setting for you—and what technical aids and attendants you do or do not want—you need to know the pros and cons of the available choices in childbirth. Your community may not offer all the possible options but *you can change that*. This chapter not only describes the choices that exist but it also suggests ways in which you can broaden the opportunities if they are limited where you live.

Time is short. You're about to get pregnant or you already are, so you have to move quickly if you want to bring about change. Consumer pressure and protest are the most effective tools you have. Forming a consumer group, writing letters, and even picketing all bring results. The area in which these tactics are most powerful is *within the hospital*. Because hospitals are profit-making institutions they *need your business*: they have to at least listen to you if they hope to get you or keep you as a customer. However, if you live in a "one hospital town," the monopoly principle applies—if you have no "hospital down the block" to turn to as a threat, then you haven't got much leverage. The same is true on a lesser scale for doctors. Chapter 10, "Choosing a Doctor and a Hospital," goes into this in depth.

239

In terms of out-of-hospital choices you do not have the same kind of consumer power. If options for where to give birth do not exist, you cannot just *create* them. Obviously if you decide to have your baby at home you have the power to make that choice. But if your community has no midwife who can attend you at home, or if the existing medical facilities won't offer you emergency backup care, then your freedom of birth choice has been limited by the community. If no doctors in your area offer deliveries in their office, your only option is to ask one or two if they would—although you're unlikely to find one who is willing. However, as more couples question and challenge the medical establishment—and if that status quo is inflexible in the face of consumer demands—more out-of-hospital alternatives will surface.

GETTING WHAT YOU WANT IN A CHILDBIRTH EXPERIENCE

> *Ask, don't demand*. Simply by asking for anything you are questioning authority. You are calling into question the expertise and years of experience of professionals. Except in rare cases this is threatening to them. When people feel threatened, they get on the defensive: they become hostile, belligerent, and indignant. Once they feel like that, the *last* thing they're going to do is change their routine and grant your request!

It doesn't matter whether what you want is "right"—morally, legally, or medically. If you think in those terms, you will go in with a chip on your shoulder and a superior attitude . . . and lessen your chances of getting what you want. Keep your objective in mind. Remember that you have limited time and that you want to change what may be a long-standing system. You have to go about getting what you want in the most expedient way. This may be one of the few times in life when the means justify the ends; i.e., it is to your ultimate benefit to adopt whatever attitude will get you results.

> *Give reasons for what you want*. Learn as much as you possibly can ahead of time. The powers-that-be are more likely to listen—to really pay attention—if you make a convincing case for your request. Imagine the possible arguments they'll give you so that you'll be prepared with answers. If you know both the pros and cons of what you want and what is currently offered, then you may have some effect. Your "reason" doesn't need to be based on facts: emotional reasons for requesting certain procedures or eliminating others can be very persuasive.

> *Request options ahead of time* even if you're not sure you're going to want them later.

> *Home birth*: Arrange for a doctor and/or hospital that will give you emergency backup care, even though you don't anticipate needing them. If you haven't cleared the way ahead of time and

you later need to be transferred to a medical setting, you may find yourself out in the cold (more on this in Chapter 11, "Home Birth").

➤ **Hospital birth**: Arrange with your doctor in advance to dismiss certain routine procedures (whether it's an enema or having the baby taken away immediately after birth) or to secure other options (rooming-in, early discharge) even if you haven't yet decided whether that will be what you ultimately want. If these instructions are not written on your chart, you may not have the option when the time comes.

HOME BIRTH VS. THE HOSPITAL

Many people all over America have dedicated themselves to making childbirth a safer, more enriching, and meaningful episode in our individual and collective lives. Many of them disagree about where childbirth should take place and what the priorities are in the situation. The intention of this book is to present the pros and cons of *all* options, to illuminate all the gray areas. There can be many variations and modifications on a home birth, as you will see in Chapter 11. A hospital birth can run the gamut from nearly like a home birth to totally high-tech. Try to gather as much information as you can and make an evaluation based on physical and emotional considerations.

Choices in Childbirth:

ALTERNATIVE BIRTHING ROOM

Called an alternative birth center in some hospitals, the alternative birthing room is a homelike environment within the hospital in which a woman can deliver almost as if she were at home—except that she has the medical facilities down the hall should she or her baby need them. Many people believe this to be the ideal compromise between a technological, depersonalized hospital birth (which cannot offer the emotional experience of a home birth) and a birth at home (which cannot offer the medical backup of a hospital). An ABC, as it is sometimes called, would be the perfect choice for a woman who wants a completely natural childbirth but would not be comfortable having her baby at home.

➤ **Only women who are defined as "low-risk"** have the option of using an ABC. "Low-risk" means that prior to labor there are no indications of any potential problems. The chart of factors that would put you in the "high-risk" category—thereby excluding you from a birthing room or a home birth—can be found in Chapter 11, "Home Birth."

➤ *A birthing room approximates a home setting* as much as possible. Most of them are carpeted, have plants and pictures and a large bed so that your partner can lie down beside you. There is often a rocking chair, which laboring women can find comfortable, and a beanbag chair, which can be put on top of the bed. It molds to your contours and gives you support during second-stage labor. The beanbag also raises your bottom off the bed so that the baby's shoulders can be delivered more easily. Sometimes there is furniture for other people whom you may have invited to attend.

➤ *An ABC emphasizes the normalcy* of birth. You labor and deliver in bed, without the usual transfer from one bed to another for birth. Also you are not usually covered in sterile drapes, which is routine in hospitals.

➤ *There are no routine drugs or medical intervention.* Although it is possible to have an enema, shave, and/or IV in a birthing room, they are not required as they are in many normal labor/delivery areas. You can learn more about these routines in the following chapter, "Choosing a Doctor and a Hospital." You can then discuss these things with your doctor *beforehand*. They will be options for you when you are in labor, but they will not be forced on you in the ABC. The same is true for fetal monitoring. There is no routine use of fetal monitors in a birthing room, but your doctor might possibly need more information about your baby's condition during labor. He then has the option of attaching a monitor until he is satisfied that all is well.

➤ *Eating and/or drinking* are usually optional in a birthing room. You can discuss this with your doctor ahead of time and then see how you feel during labor.

➤ *A couple determines who attends* the birth. Siblings are usually allowed as long as there is an adult whose sole responsibility it is to look after the child. If you want to have friends be with you for your birth, that is your option, although birthing rooms usually aren't very large, so you might be limited in numbers because of that.

➤ *You can choose the position for labor* and delivery that suits you best. You can be on your hands and knees, although many doctors don't feel comfortable with this as a *delivery* position. You can walk around. You can squat. You can deliver from a side-lying position.

➤ *You can wear what you want* in most birthing rooms. This may not sound like much, but to many women it is comforting to be able to wear something familiar rather than a hospital-issue gown. Your own clothes can give you a feeling of being more connected to "real life" or more in control of the situation; you probably aren't going to be wearing much anyway.

➤ *You can leave the hospital within 6 to 24 hours.* This is known as "early discharge," and as long as everything is normal with you and the baby after birth, you can go home. Among the benefits of early discharge (page 311) are that you save money, you can return to familiar surroundings and begin integrating the new baby into your life right away, and you are not subjected to the hospital routines that can interfere with breast-feeding and your initial relationship with the baby.

➤ **The cost is lower** than for an ordinary hospital delivery and average three-day stay, which is the routine at most places. You use less (if any) drugs and equipment in a birthing room and usually stay only a short time after delivery: the cost can be one-half to one-third of the average hospital charges for childbirth.

➤ **Alternative birthing rooms (ABCs)** began in a limited number of hospitals across the country. They were often installed because of a trend within the community back to home birth: prospective parents who were angered and frustrated by a non-responsive hospital chose the "unknowns" of home birth. Most medical professionals are frightened by home birth and most hospitals could not afford to lose customers—thus ABCs were both a philosophic and economic response to people's rejection of hospital birth.

Ironically, however, many hospitals have come so far in their family-centered attitudes that their alternative birthing rooms have become obsolete. What happened was that some hospitals with 4,000 to 5,000 births a year discovered that the birthing room was used for only a handful of deliveries each month. These hospitals, which had been allowing women to labor and deliver in the labor rooms, stopped promoting or enhancing their ABCs. Instead, they concentrated on upgrading the quality of the labor and delivery (L&D) areas, redesigning them as multipurpose birthing rooms. Nowadays ABC is more of a concept, not necessarily a specific place.

The new L&D rooms allow a full range of birth experiences, from a totally unmedicated natural birth to the most complex, medically intensive care. This trend is an improvement in health care because it removes the rigid demarcation between high-and low-risk birth. By allowing flexibility for a full range of possibilities in birth, it eliminates the sharp line that was drawn between two kinds of birthing: one that required medical intervention and one that would not permit it.

➤ **You can encourage your local hospital to put in an ABC.** Start an organization and call it "Concerned Citizens." Ask local people to join: psychologists, pediatricians, OB/GYNs, childbirth educators, and anybody else you can contact who has some prestige in your community (bank presidents, clergymen, local government officials). Through childbirth education classes you can contact a lot of prospective parents and get their names. Contact the hospital where you would like to give birth *if* they had an alternative birthing room. Make an appointment with the director of obstetrics and gynecology and go with two or three representatives of your group. Ask if they've read Drs. Klaus and Kennell's book, *Maternal-Infant Bonding,* a medical study which can be viewed as an argument for what a birthing room offers.

If the hospital is at all up-to-date, they will probably tell you that they have already been thinking about putting in an ABC. It is to your benefit that they already know about birthing rooms, so you won't have to educate them or have so many prejudices to overcome. However, do not be lulled by the statement that a hospital has been "thinking" about it—talk is cheap. Your effort as a group of "concerned citizens" is what can make the difference between words and action. Follow up your visit with letters restating the importance of going ahead with an ABC as soon as possible. Point out that valuable public recognition will be paid to their hospital for being the first in the community to adopt such a progressive stand on childbirth. Emphasize that although the ABC may not be the choice of every expectant couple, the hospital will attract couples who would otherwise refuse to deliver there.

There are two major reasons why a hospital may hesitate to open an ABC. The first one is economic. They have to take over floor space that is in the OB/GYN area. This may mean converting an existing labor room or part of a recovery area, which could mean lost revenue. Decorating the birthing room is a minimal cost, but a cost all the same. Then the hospital only gets a patient for an average of 12 hours, usually with no medication costs: yet they have to maintain costly medical/technical options anyway.

The other problem is one of staffing considerations. Some hospitals staff their ABC entirely with certified nurse-midwives, who might also give prenatal care to the hospital's clinic patients. A CNM's training is specifically for attending normal childbirth, so one of her strengths is to be able to give constant support, helping insure the normalcy of the labor and delivery. But hospitals that do not employ CNMs may have to reorganize their maternity floor staff so that an obstetric nurse can be assigned full-time to any woman using the alternative birthing room. In most ordinary maternity areas each nurse has several laboring women to look after and she goes from one to another. Therefore the ABC requires more staff to be available—whenever the birthing room is not being used the hospital is "overstaffed." Thus until the ABC is publicized and becomes popular it may be unprofitable.

ANALGESIA (PAIN MEDICATION)

An analgesic is any drug that relieves pain; this includes tranquilizers, barbiturates, and narcotics. Any woman giving birth in a hospital has the choice to request analgesia. Women giving birth in out-of-hospital settings are almost never given the option of drugs. The emphasis at home is on the naturalness and normalcy of childbirth, and also analgesia during labor can have side effects that are less controllable outside the hospital.

Any drug taken during labor and delivery reaches your baby. *Any drug.* If someone tells you otherwise, they are either lying or misinformed. Even a minimal dosage of a painkilling drug has a much greater impact on your baby, whose body is not yet able to rapidly eliminate the drug from his system.

There are many instances in which the benefit of an analgesia to the mother is more important than the potential harm to the fetus. A small amount of a tranquilizer may relax a woman who is becoming so anxious that her tension could impede the progress of labor. A small amount of a narcotic might help a woman through a particularly difficult part of labor so that she doesn't need more powerful analgesics or anesthesia. It is also true that the right kind of loving support and encouragement can be at least as effective, if not more so, than drugs. However, there are many instances in which that kind of attention is not available in a hospital.

In Chapter 12, pages 402–404, there is a chart on the effects of drugs commonly used during labor. Be sure that you and your mate have read that section and discussed it with your doctor *beforehand* so that you are all in some kind of agreement about what analgesia should be administered if it becomes necessary. However, you will not know *until you are in labor* just how you will feel and how you will cope with it. Do not hobble yourself by making ironclad decisions that will limit your freedom later. You may think, "I can't get through it without painkillers," or you may think, "I will refuse any drug no matter what!" If you do that, you are making a decision based on incomplete information. It is fine to have an opinion ahead of time, but for your own sake and your baby's, try to keep an open mind.

GENERAL ANESTHESIA

General anesthesia is rarely used in uncomplicated childbirth. A general anesthetic is harder to recover from for both you and the baby. There are times when it is used for cesarean sections, but it is very rarely used for a vaginal delivery.

Besides the physical hazards of general anesthesia, there is also the problem that you neither experience the birth in any way nor do you have any contact with your baby until many hours after her birth. This is a loss for both of you, since you miss the "sensitive period" following birth in which maternal-infant bonding most readily takes place.

There are a few cases of women who are so terrified by the idea of childbirth that they do not feel they can handle it at all. They want to be "knocked out and know nothing," awakening to find a child has been born. Whether it is because of a woman's social conditioning, or a personally traumatic experience, it is vital to discover what is causing her such terror. Her fear must be affecting other areas of her life as well—it will certainly have an influence on her relationship with her baby. After investigating why a woman is this afraid, some determination can be made as to whether or not general anesthesia is best for her.

LOCAL ANESTHESIA

A local anesthetic during childbirth allows a woman to be fully awake for her baby's birth, although she is numb in the area that has been anesthetized.

A local may be used on a woman who has had childbirth training but feels the need for additional help for any of a number of reasons: her pain threshold is low; she didn't fully believe the training would work; she didn't practice enough; her labor is very long and she cannot maintain control, etc.

The chart including information about anesthesia during labor (page 402–404) tells you the various local anesthetics, how they are administered, and what their effects are.

PAIN RELIEF FROM "ALTERNATIVE MEDICINE"

Hypnosis

Even though hypnosis may have the reputation of being a magician's trick, when managed by a qualified health professional for medical purposes it has proven successful. If you're interested in learning self-hypnosis for childbirth, the first thing you need to do is put yourself in good hands—you don't want to fool around with "fringe" elements with something so important. Ask your doctor for recommendations of practitioners of hypnosis. Mental health providers such as psychologists or psychiatrists have often been trained in hypnosis techniques, so you can call the local chapter of the American Medical Association (AMA) to locate someone to assist you.

Hypnosis has been used in the past for surgery with the intention of reducing bleeding, lessening anxiety and pain, and speeding up the recovery process. It has also been successfully employed to aid in stopping smoking or other addictions and to overcome a variety of emotional problems. The power of suggestion, the strength of "mind over matter," is a big part of what you learn in childbirth training—being taught self-hypnosis can give you that much more ability to relax your body and mind. In some women it has allowed them to perceive no pain at all, even during an unmedicated episiotomy or cesarean.

Hypnosis is a technique that you have to be taught and have to practice, many weeks and preferably months before labor begins. Don't think of it as the parlor trick of some powerful hypnotist who "puts you under" and takes control of you: self-hypnosis is a technique that allows you achieve a high level of suggestibility, but it requires dedication and practice. Not all people are hypnotizable—it's estimated that only 25% of those who try, or one in four, are susceptible to successful hypnotization.

Acupuncture

Acupuncture is the ancient Chinese method of placing needles just under the skin at points that correspond to the area of pain or other physical problems. It has been used in China for centuries to eliminate pain, even to the point of conducting pain-free surgeries with no other aid than the needles. You may have already had the good fortune to find a talented acupuncturist who has given you relief if you have had the misfortune to suffer from symptoms that traditional Western medicine has been unable to conquer (or if you are wary of "modern medicine"). If so, it will not take any convincing to consider having your acupuncturist present during labor and delivery. Of course, you have to make sure that s/he and your doctor are willing to cooperate with each other, which may take some convincing, depending on your medical doctor's open-mindedness to alternative medicine and your acupuncturist's willingness to wear a beeper as your due date approaches.

If acupuncture is new to you, but you are curious about trying it for childbirth, you might consider making an appointment beforehand if you're fortunate enough to have one in your area. This allows you to talk about the treatment beforehand and learn whether it appeals to you as a possible substitute for pain relievers or anesthesia. It might be good idea to have an acupuncture treatment ahead of time so that you can experience it and dispel any worries about how painful it might be. The the very thin needles are placed just below the skin and are a minor discomfort (particularly compared to most labor and delivery).

Acupressure and Massage

Acupressure is a technique which involves putting direct pressure on the same points on the body as defined for needles in acupuncture. The success of pain relief with acupressure depends on the skill of the practitioner, although even in expert hands it rarely has the same effectiveness as acupuncture.

Massage, a heating pad, or pressure applied against your lower back during back labor are all ways to reduce your level of discomfort during labor. Your partner or a friend can massage tight areas of your shoulder, neck, back, and legs, but a professional masseuse will have more strength in her hands and be more knowledgeable both about anatomy in general and where you are holding tension which can cause pain. If you know a masseuse and think you'd like to have her there during labor, talk to her and your doctor about it in advance of your due date.

TENS (Transcutaneous Electrical Nerve Stimulation)

You can look at the TENS box as modern medicine's answer to acupuncture because it works along the same premises. TENS has been used by people at home to manage chronic pain from causes like nerve damage and arthritis, especially in cases where other methods haven't given relief. It's being used in some hospitals for childbirth and other appropriate situations. Increasing numbers of hospitals are making TENS boxes available for maternity patients. You might want to talk to your doctor ahead of time about the possibility of using it. If you're interested, it might be a good idea to experiment with the TENS on Braxton-Hicks contractions so that you can get the hang of it before labor begins.

The box is the size of a transistor radio and is attached by wires to four electrodes that stick painlessly on your skin. When you turn on the TENS, you feel a tingling sensation, an electrical stimulation of the nerve pathways that is supposed to block "pain messages" to your brain. You control the intensity of the stimulation with a dial so that you can turn it up during a contraction and back down in between. It doesn't have an effect on the baby, which is a benefit that can't be claimed by the usual medical methods of pain management.

Herbal Medicines

Herbs are serious ingredients to put into your body: just because they come from nature and are not made in a factory doesn't mean they are harmless. In fact, some herbs are potent and form the basis for various prescription medications which are made in laboratories.

Some herbal teas have been used in other cultures to terminate pregnancy: they can cause miscarriage as well as less dramatic conditions such as intestinal problems and heart palpitations. Therefore do not use herbal teas during pregnancy or labor no matter who tells you they're "harmless." The other problem with herbal cures is that they can vary in potency and can also contain ingredients which can be toxic or cause an allergic reaction.

CESAREAN DELIVERY WITH YOUR MATE PRESENT

This is an option that was once very rare but is now offered across the country. Due to a liberalization of U.S. hospital policies, fathers are frequently present in the delivery room, and prolonged contact between mother and infant is usually delayed only a few hours at most. This constitutes a dramatic and rapid change: in 1979, approximately 35% of the hospitals in this country allowed fathers to attend cesarean deliveries; 1984, 80% did. A couple may have many reasons for wanting to be together for a cesarean.

> ➤ ***Probably the most important reason*** is that *you want your mate to support you* through what is a frightening process. No matter how safe cesareans have become, and despite the fact that you may have already had an uncomplicated cesarean, it is still major surgery. There are a number of preparatory procedures, then there is the insertion and administration of the local anesthetic that numbs you from the waist down, and then there is the cutting, and afterward the sewing. In the midst of all the attendants with sterile masks and the bright lights your baby is born. You can be more focused on your baby's birth and enjoy that thrill more if your mate is with you for comfort and support during the medical/surgical aspects of a cesarean. Cesareans are described in depth starting on page 430.
> ➤ ***Your partner may want to see and share*** the moment of his baby's birth. Paternal-infant bonding is as important as the mother's early attachment to the baby.
> ➤ ***If a couple is together,*** it emphasizes the personal, emotional aspect of a cesarean. Often when a woman has a baby by cesarean section she is most aware of the surgical attendants and apparatus. There may be a tense quiet in the operating room, or the nurses and doctors may be chatting among themselves. A woman can feel isolated and disconnected from the excitement and joy that are part of a baby's birth. If a couple is together, the birth of their child can have its appropriate emotional importance.

Preparing for a Man's Presence at a Cesarean

If you know you are going to have a cesarean and you would like your mate to stay with you there can be hurdles to overcome.

> ➤ ***If you*** live near a hospital that already allows couples to stay together for cesareans, then you're in luck. Ask your doctor

whether he has admitting privileges at the hospital and whether he is willing to allow your mate to be with you. If not, call the department of obstetrics and gynecology at the hospital and they will give you the names of doctors who have done cesareans with the mate present. Then you can interview them and take your pick.

➤ *Next you must find an anesthesiologist* who will give his or her permission to have your mate present. Your doctor may know of one who is open-minded and flexible. It might be best for your doctor to contact the anesthesiologist so that they can talk about it between themselves as colleagues.

➤ *Once you have found a doctor* with whom you feel comfortable, one who respects your desires, then either the doctor or you and your mate have to approach the hospital. If your doctor has a long-standing reputation—i.e., he has some "clout" within the institution—it is possible that they will grant your request. If he does not have that kind of influence, and only a few doctors do, then the director of the department of OB/GYN has to be persuaded. It may be an uphill battle. Be prepared for getting the runaround: inconsistent replies and irrational arguments. You have to be patient and eloquent in order to make this childbirth choice possible. What you have on your side is that several of the most prestigious university hospitals in the country have had successful test programs in which they allowed fathers into cesareans; many have adopted it as official hospital policy. Two examples are Yale University and Harvard University, through its affiliate, Boston Lying-In Hospital.

Arguments You'll Hear

➤ *The first argument* you will hear is that having the father present increases the chance of infection. Statistics prove that the infection rate was unchanged in the test programs. A father is scrubbed, gowned, and masked just like everyone else in the room. If you are told that each additional person in a sterile area potentially introduces infection, point out that frequently there are students, interns, and residents in an operating room.

➤ *You will be asked* (perhaps with disdain) why a man would want to watch his mate's abdomen being cut. Explain that the usual procedure is to have the father seated at her head with a screen at the woman's midsection that blocks their view of the actual incision. When the baby is removed, either the screen is lowered, or the baby is lifted over it for them to see. Restate your positive emotional, interpersonal reasons for wanting to be together.

➤ *You will be told* that it is state law that the father cannot be there. This is misinformation or a lie on the part of the hospital representative. Most state health agencies require only that persons in an operating room be wearing "proper attire."

➤ *You will be told* that the hospital's insurance forbids it. This is also false. Usually one large insurance company covers all of the hospitals in one area. There is almost never a clause which specifically forbids a father, or anyone else, from being in attendance at an operation. Students, interns, and residents are frequently watching, and insurance doesn't exclude them any more than it does the woman's mate.

➤ *You may be told* that having the baby's father watch will create a mental strain on the doctor. Restate that your doctor has already agreed to your being together and supports the reasons for your request.

➤ *You will be told* that a cesarean baby has a higher chance of having some trouble breathing at first, and if there are any complications that the father would impede resuscitation attempts. Explain that you are aware that being together depends entirely on things going ahead *without complications*. The baby's father knows this—and is prepared to leave the operating room without question if the doctor or anesthesiologist asks him to. Explain that you realize this is for your baby's good and will also insure that other couples after you can have the option of staying together.

➤ *Most hospitals* will consider allowing a father to be present only if the couple is married. If you are not married, you have to deal with this in whatever way makes you most comfortable, including lying by omission. You can call yourselves Mr. and Mrs. Abrams, or you can use your own names as you do now. If there is any question, say that the woman has retained her own name. The best solution is not to raise the issue at all. But at least you are forewarned that if you let them know you aren't married they may reject the entire proposal for you to be together for the cesarean.

CERTIFIED NURSE-MIDWIVES

CNMs are nurses who have had special training and specialize only in normal pregnancy. They are trained to give prenatal care and attend a normal labor with normal spontaneous delivery with little or no intervention. If any medical problems arise during the pregnancy or labor—a nurse-midwife's training equips her to determine anything that is not normal—then a doctor is called in.

National recognition of certified nurse-midwives has widened only in the last ten years, although the statistics over the past fifty years are impressive. The statistics show an improvement in the outcome of births wherever nurse-midwives have worked, compared to the health status of mothers in other parts of the country who received traditional obstetric care.

At this point the majority of CNMs are practicing in hospital clinics. There are few places where a private paying patient can receive care from a nurse-midwife; thus, many women who could afford another alternative are becoming clinic patients. The future of nurse-midwifery—where CNMs will practice and the mushrooming demand for them—will be determined by the present and future society at large.

➢ *There are schools nationwide* that offer a course in nurse-midwifery. The school training lasts nine to twelve months, but when she is ready to practice, a nurse-midwife will have had a *minimum* of six years' training and experience. She will have had four years in nursing school and one or more years of practical experience, then a year or more of CNM schooling.

If you want to find a midwife, contact the American College of Nurse Midwives, 1522 K Street NW, Suite 1120, Washington, DC 20005 (202-347-5445).

➢ *A nurse-midwife follows your pregnancy* from prenatal exams right through postpartum care, when she teaches infant care and breast-feeding, and does gynecological exams as well.

➢ *Nurse-midwives usually practice through hospital clinics*, so the *total cost for maternity care is lower* than if you were to go to the hospital with a private doctor. Some CNMs also work in doctors' offices, others attend home births, and there are a few maternity centers either run by or staffed by nurse-midwives.

➢ *Health insurance reimburses for nurse-midwifery care*. Many states have mandated that private insurance companies must directly reimburse certified nurse-midwives (CNMs).

The American College of Nurse-Midwives keeps a list of health insurance companies which provide direct payment to the certified nurse-midwife or reimburse the insured for obstetric services, including labor and delivery, rendered by a CNM.

➢ *Prenatal care from a CNM* may appeal to women who like the idea of a woman-to-woman relationship. There are not that many female OB-GYNs, so those mothers who would prefer receiving care from another woman are more likely to find a nurse-midwife than a female obstetrician. With a woman caregiver you might feel less inhibited, feeling that another woman can be more empathetic to your physical and emotional experience.

➢ *A nurse-midwife has more time* than a doctor does to answer your questions about pregnancy and childbirth. With a doctor you might worry about "bothering" him with "petty" questions because he seems rushed. An important part of a CNM's training is parent education: she stresses prepared childbirth and non-intervention in the normal birth process.

➢ *A CNM will be constantly in attendance* throughout your entire labor. Since she will have given you prenatal care, you will have already developed a confident relationship with her. The importance of this trusted, constant-support person (in addition to or instead of your mate) cannot be stressed enough. If you have a long labor you may not necessarily have the same CNM with you the whole time, but you will have met her colleagues during prenatal care, so they will all be familiar to you.

➢ *A nurse-midwife usually is flexible* about omitting certain routine hospital procedures during labor and about the positions you choose for labor and delivery. Her training stresses a laboring woman's self-determination in a hospital setting, with medical technology available only in case of need. A nurse-midwife is committed to nonintervention, although she is also well versed in medical technology. She will support as natural and personalized a birth experience as you wish—as long as everything remains *normal*. When necessary, she will consult with or call in a doctor.

CASES IN WHICH A DOCTOR TAKES OVER FOR A CNM

➢ *Prolonged second stage:* A woman is fully dilated and in good labor, but has pushed for two hours and is either unable to continue or the baby isn't descending, at which point a doctor will use forceps or do a cesarean.

➢ *A breech presentation:* If the CNM and consulting doctors deem it safe, a CNM can attend a vaginal delivery of a breech, but a doctor is ready and scrubbed in the delivery room to use forceps or do a cesarean if labor doesn't progress or there is fetal distress.

➢ *If the baby is too large* for your pelvis, a doctor takes over surgically.

➢ *In cases of a prolapsed cord,* a doctor intervenes and does surgery.

➢ *If you are carrying twins* a doctor will be present, if only because an extra pair of expert hands will be needed.

➢ *A pediatrician is called in* and will be in attendance for a breech, cesarean, or multiple birth, and when there are signs of fetal distress.

CLINICS/HOSPITALS

A clinic offers lower-priced maternity care than a private doctor, although you usually receive the same quality of care as private patients in the same hospital. A teaching hospital often has the best clinic.

The main problem with a clinic is that you may see a different doctor at each prenatal visit, so you won't have an opportunity to build a relationship with the person who is going to deliver your baby. In fact, you don't know ahead of time which of these doctors is going to attend the birth; whichever doctor is on duty when you go into labor is the one who will care for you. This makes for a different experience than if you had a private doctor with whom you had developed a relationship. You will not be offered many alternatives during labor and delivery. Nor will you have the backing of your own hand-picked doctor if what you want is not within the hospital's routine. You are somewhat at the mercy of this unfamiliar doctor's philosophy because he will have the final word—for instance, if any medications are used, the choice will be his.

There are two schools of thought about the net result of getting maternity care from a clinic. Some people say that it makes it hard to have control over your own labor because your input doesn't carry the weight it would if you were being attended by a private doctor. Other people point out that since there is no constant "father figure" to depend on, it forces a couple to depend more on themselves. Not having the security of one doctor may motivate a couple to learn more about the birth process and then be more self-reliant and interdependent.

OUTSIDE-HOSPITAL CLINICS

The outside-hospital clinic is usually a community-oriented facility that offers prenatal care. Many of these are feminist and take a somewhat political stand on health care. These clinics can be the manifestation of the statements made by leaders in the feminist movement that the time has come for women to have control over their own health care. These clinics can be seen as a challenge to the U.S. health care system, which they see as profit-oriented, hierarchical, and expensive.

Expectant women who choose to receive prenatal care from clinics like these are encouraged to learn as much as possible about their pregnancy. You will be encouraged to actively participate in your own prenatal care, often checking your own urine, weight, and blood pressure. The idea behind this is that women have to break away from the traditional attitudes in obstetric care which presume that a pregnant woman has to be "taken care of." Feminist clinics try to stress the normalcy of pregnancy and childbirth and a woman's own capability in these areas.

There is an organization which maintains an up-to-date listing of all the childbirth centers or clinics across the country. The best way to get a current listing for your area would be to write to: National Association of Childbearing Centers, RD 1, Box 1, Perkiomenville, Pennsylvania 18074.

DOCTOR'S OFFICE

Many doctors refer to their offices as birth centers when they use them for deliveries, although usually all they have is a suite of examining rooms. One or two of them may have been decorated with a homelike style, like an alternative birthing room in a hospital, described earlier in this chapter.

> ➤ *A doctor's office is an option worth considering* for those who are totally against a hospital birth yet not interested in birth at home. There are no routine procedures in an office birth, little or no intervention, no drugs, and the mother and baby can leave within hours of the birth. A doctor's office is certainly more informal than a hospital, but it does not have any of the medical safety advantages, either. At the same time, it isn't your own home, so you don't get the benefits of familiar, relaxed surroundings in which you feel as if you are in charge. Thus a *doctor's office is neither fish nor fowl,* but it serves a need in communities that have not yet responded to people's changing expectations of childbirth.

> ➤ *Doctor's offices exist* as locales for birth for one reason: the *convenience (and economic survival) of the doctor.* In most cities a doctor who is doing out-of-hospital deliveries cannot maintain an OB/GYN practice *and* travel any distance to people's homes to wait during long labors. By having a woman come to his office, a doctor can attend her labor without sacrificing his office patients. Also, there are usually only a very few doctors doing out-of-hospital deliveries and they gain popularity through word of mouth. Some of these doctors are delivering over fifty babies a month; it would be impossible for them to attend all those births unless they all come to him rather than the other way around.

> ➤ *The requirements for being accepted* for birth in a doctor's office are the same as those for an alternative birthing room in a hospital or for a home birth. See the chart of "Factors That Rule Out Home Birth," on page 336–337. If any doctor tells you that he will let you deliver in his office, even though you have one of the conditions on that list, *distrust the doctor.* Not only would he be endangering you and your baby, he's just downright stupid. Anyone who would attempt out-of-hospital births for "high-risk" pregnancies is eventually going to have fetal deaths or problems.

> ➤ *If you develop any high-risk indications* during your pregnancy, a responsible doctor doing office births will refer you to an obstetric subspecialist. Ask the doctor ahead of time under what conditions he would refer you elsewhere and to whom he sends referrals. Some doctors have egos that have grown so large that they like to think they can handle anything and every-

thing themselves. Beware of a doctor like that: once a doctor begins practicing medicine with his ego, he is not using good judgment.

➤ ***Even though a doctor may be going against the grain*** of the majority of his colleagues by offering an out-of-hospital birth alternative, his training and orientation are still medical. The next chapter offers more information and insights to doctors, but the relevant point here is that *most doctors coming out of medical school have never seen a natural childbirth.* Modern medicine is oriented toward *controlling* childbirth . . . "improving" on nature. This usually means intervening in the natural progress of labor and delivery. The exceptions are the doctor who is an "old-timer" and has been doing out-of-hospital births for a long time, or a doctor who is assisted by lay or nurse-midwives with extensive experience of their own.

➤ *A doctor should have full admitting privileges* at a hospital close to his office. As with home birth, you are better off if you have paved the way for emergency backup care in the unlikely event that it is necessary. This is even more true with a doctor's-office birth, since a doctor is more likely to seek medical assistance if your labor seems abnormal.

➤ ***The chance of infection*** in a doctor's office is open to debate. Some say that there is less chance of infection because fewer personnel are involved in the process than would be at a hospital, and there aren't sick, infected people in an office. They point out that a baby has immunity to his parents. Those who do worry about infection possibilities in a doctor's office say that the room isn't sterilized, there aren't sterile gowns, masks, or drapes on the woman, while there have been patients coming through the doctor's office for gynecological exams who *do* have infections. However, most of these doctors contend that their sterile gloves are sufficient protection.

PAIN AND CHILDBIRTH

There have been important discoveries of substances produced by the body which are changing previous beliefs about pain. These morphine-like substances are called "endorphins," and they have been found in the brain and other areas of the body. They seem to have a special role in pain perception.

Studies have shown that individual differences in pain sensitivity are related to individual differences in endorphin production. Research has shown that treatments such as acupuncture and electrical stimulation which can reduce pain are associated with endorphin production. Each person's endorphin-production system responds differently; as more research is done, it may be especially useful in childbirth.

Childbirth preparation varies in its effectiveness for each individual. It is known that a small percentage of women are insensitive to pain during labor and delivery, even in cases where a woman has had no childbirth preparation. It is also known that childbirth education reduces pain for many women. More must be learned about these morphine-like substances and what can be done to stimulate production of endorphins in laboring women.

Keeping this information in mind, expectant mothers and those supporting her in labor must make some allowance for her individual endorphin system. It is not unusual for a woman to take childbirth education classes, consider herself well prepared for labor and delivery, and yet have unexpected difficulties with pain control despite her determination and training. It just may be that certain people's endorphin-producing systems are less responsive.

➤ *"Pain is evil"* is an American belief. Culturally we regard pain and even discomfort as evils to be avoided at all costs. Just look at the aspirin commercials on television to see the intensity of our national warfare on pain, with instant medication the moment there is the slightest discomfort. Medically, the goal is to control and suppress pain. These social attitudes will have an influence on your experience of labor contractions unless you can at least temporarily revise your outlook—for example, "the pain I am experiencing is not evil; it is a natural, normal aspect of expelling a baby from the womb."

➤ *Your expectations may be unrealistic,* which will make it difficult for childbirth education to be effective. The training methods which advertise "painless childbirth" are guaranteeing their own failure. We have to get away from the myth that if you can just find the right way to breathe during labor, it's going to be pleasant and easy. Childbirth education is *not* a magic tool that makes it all okay. It is going to be hard. It is going to hurt. Classes simply make it easier and less painful. But if you are looking for a way to have "natural childbirth" and feel no discomfort, you are in for a rude shock. Being prepared for the pain and knowing ways to lessen it is a realistic outlook on birth.

➤ *Another theory* that is somewhat contradictory says that *if you are expecting to feel pain* you will find the contractions painful. The point is "negative prophecy": you will create what you expect. The cultural conditioning says that childbirth is painful, and therefore that is how you perceive the sensory input. However, if you liken labor and delivery to a grueling sports event, it can give you a new perspective. A marathon runner is in great pain during the final stretch. The runner's entire body is in pain, but he or she expected it and keeps on going. Personally and socially their pain is not considered "evil" . . . therefore, no one would think to give them an anesthetic to finish the race.

HOW MUCH WILL LABOR HURT?

How much pain you will have will be partially determined by whether you have childbirth training and how committed you are to it. There is no doubt that a *belief in the techniques* is part of what makes them effective.

> ➤ *Studies show* that anywhere from 3 to 14% of women naturally experience no pain at all during labor and delivery (without using breathing techniques, etc.). In childbirth education classes, 10 to 20% of women report having felt no pain.

> ➤ *People differ greatly* in their anatomy and physiology. This means that there are *individual differences in the number of pain messages* reaching the brain. This is what is referred to as a low or high threshold for pain.

> ➤ *Your menstrual history* is an indicator of pain during childbirth. Women with irregular periods with acute cramps at the onset tend to have significantly more childbirth pain. There is less pain in women who menstruate regularly with little or no disturbance of their daily activities.

> ➤ *Do not make the mistake* of thinking that if you take childbirth classes you are going to have to suffer, and that if you don't, there are drugs which let you be fully awake yet feel no pain. *Every women* (except those 3 to 14%) *will feel discomfort; the trained ones are simply better able to deal with it.* Even if you decide absolutely that you want an epidural during labor, for instance, you are not going to be allowed to have it until you are halfway dilated (read the section on medication, pages 398–404). Ordinarily an epidural is not administered until at least five centimeters dilation: sooner than that and the anesthetic can slow down or stop the labor altogether, necessitating the use of synthetic hormones to speed things up again. This means that you are going to have to get through the first half of first-stage labor no matter what. The painkilling drugs you can be given during that time are not going to remove the pain entirely—only dull your senses.

If you had taken classes, you would be able to consciously relax and do breathing techniques to ease your way through it. A woman who hasn't gone through any training often can feel as if labor is one continual never-ending contraction—which soon becomes terrifying and overwhelming. With education you know that there is going to be time to relax between contractions and how to prepare for the next one. You learn that the discomfort will stop periodically and you'll have a break.

If you are unsure about whether you want to take the classes, *talk to couples* who have used or are planning to take prepared childbirth courses. Talk to ones who have gone through labor without any drugs and talk to those who had an epidural anesthetic as soon as they could. Regardless of how much they liked their teacher or how their birth went, you are going to have a hard time finding any couple who won't recommend that you take advantage of what the classes have to offer.

➤ *Accepting analgesia or anesthesia* is not a violation of childbirth education. Some methods of teaching are more adamant about refusing medication: for instance, the Bradley method (which is described on page 263), which can lead you to feel guilt and a sense of failure if you do accept drugs. However, the training is really just a tool. For some women its main benefit is to lessen fear by giving them an understanding of what is happening; for other women the techniques make them able to wait longer before having drugs; for some women the techniques mean they will need less medication; for many women it makes possible a drug-free labor and delivery. The important thing is not to allow a childbirth teacher, your mate, or your next-door neighbor to set up the techniques as a *test of your strength of character*. Don't fall into that trap if someone baits it and do not set it for yourself. The more you rely on the technique, the less you will need drugs; the fewer drugs you take, the better off you and your baby will be. However, childbirth should not be torture. The psychological harm of extreme pain during labor is greater than the potential harm from drugs. It is better to have a baby slightly groggy from medication than to have a woman so devastated by the pain her baby's birth caused her that it has a negative influence on her mothering.

EDUCATED CHILDBIRTH

Also known as prepared childbirth, educated childbirth is a far better name than "natural childbirth." The latter phrase has come to mean "martyrdom despite suffering," and that is not the desired result from educated childbirth. The point is to *inform* you about what will be happening to your body during labor and delivery and to *train* you to minimize the discomfort. Every expectant woman and/or couple can benefit from these classes. It does not matter whether you intend (or wind up) having analgesia or anesthesia: these classes are not supposed to set up a test of your bravery and fortitude. The intention is for you to have as much information as possible so that you can understand—and therefore be less overwhelmed by—what your body is going to go through. You have nothing to lose and everything to gain by taking classes.

Pain results from intense stimuli—noise, heat, cold, light—that are strong enough to cause, or threaten to cause, tissue damage. The *mental state* of an individual may alter the significance of the incoming pain impulses so they are minimized or exaggerated. Childbirth education classes prepare you to *control your mental state for the management of painful stimuli*.

How Childbirth Techniques Work

The theoretical explanation of childbirth techniques sounds more complicated than it really is. Laboratory studies on human subjects have defined five major psychological strategies that are effective in reducing pain. All childbirth methods utilize some or all of the following:

SYSTEMATIC RELAXATION is based on the repeated tension/relaxation of muscle groups in the body. Childbirth classes train you so that relaxation becomes a built-in response. When your coach says, "Contraction begins," you will have practiced enough so that you can automatically release any tension in your body. After a while during practice sessions you can add distractions like the radio or television and will eventually be able to relax in situations with stress or confusion. In labor itself you must remember to check for tension not only during a contraction but *between* contractions in order to insure complete systematic relaxation.

The goal is to relax all the body muscles to produce a mental state of *minimal anxiety*. This increases your pain tolerance: you are less fearful of the pain stimulus, therefore your mind decreases its awareness of the painful sensation. Thus, you can endure the pain for longer.

COGNITIVE CONTROL means involving the mind in mental activities other than the awareness of the incoming pain sensation. There are two types:

DISSOCIATION is concentration on a *non*painful characteristic of the pain stimulus with distracting imagery. For instance, putting your hand in ice water causes pain. The pain is lessened if you imagine yourself on a hot desert island where the water is coolly refreshing. In childbirth training this is applied in teaching you *how* to think about the sensations. If you think of them as muscular contractions of the uterus—not as "labor pains"—it is effective in reducing your pain perception.

INTERFERENCE involves two forms of cognitive control: *distraction* and *attention focusing*. Distraction works only for *slow-onset pain* such as labor contractions, which usually build slowly to maximum levels. The breathing techniques you learn are a form of attention focusing: active, intentional, mental attentiveness.

COGNITIVE REHEARSAL means a clear explanation of what the upcoming experience will involve. You rehearse specific fear images and accommodate them so as to reduce your anxiety. By discussing what you are afraid of and getting a description of what you can realistically expect during birth, your anxiety is lessened and therefore your tolerance for pain is increased. In order for this to be effective, you need to get both objective and subjective information—a factual explanation as well as personal accounts of how the childbirth training works. It is vital that an instructor is careful to provide accurate, verifiable information on a broad range of possible childbirth experiences. A lack of verifiability of subjective information at the time of exposure to pain will cause you to lose confidence. In plain English, if what you have been told doesn't jibe with what you experience, you will distrust the entire training.

HAWTHORNE EFFECT is a finding in psychological research that "more and special attention to a subject increases results in reducing pain." This is scientific proof of what prepared-childbirth advocates (and people who oppose hospital birth because it is depersonalized) have been saying for years: give a laboring woman constant and loving support and she will not need, or will need fewer, drugs. The childbirth instructor— but especially a woman's mate—can contribute immeasurably to her success in controlling her discomfort. The other side of the Hawthorne effect is that *insufficient* attention by a woman's attending doctor may actually be the *cause* of unnecessary requests for drugs. It may be her unconscious attempt to get attention and reassurance.

SYSTEMATIC DESENSITIZATION is what a childbirth class does for you, combining the preceding four other strategies in preparing you to manage the pain. This strategy is mostly for high-anxiety cases—women who need more intense and individualized preparation in order to go into labor with less fear and a well-developed ability to relax at will.

An example of systematic desensitization is a technique used in some classes in which the coach pinches your leg very hard to simulate the pain of a contraction. By the end of the course many women find their pain threshold has become higher: they can tolerate harder squeezing for longer. Some women find that even with their coach's hardest pinching, there is no pain (although he should not pinch so hard as to bruise you).

> *Studies have shown* that childbirth classes *shorten the length of labor*. The psychosomatic techniques applied in the training have a calming effect that allows labor to progress unimpeded by muscle and mental tension. One study showed a 14-hour duration of labor for the group of women who had taken classes, compared with an average labor of 18½ hours for the control group, who had no training.
> *One of the most useful things you learn* in classes is to *take labor one step at a time*. You deal with each contraction as it happens and are taught not to worry about the preceding contraction or about what is coming afterward. There is a misconception many people have about labor, sometimes not corrected even in classes: it is not true that labor gets worse as it goes on and that the contractions get stronger and stronger. Some

women don't take childbirth classes because they have this mis-conception and they figure, "It's going to get unbearable at some point and I'm not going to be able to stand it, so why bother with all the breathing?" Other women who have taken classes may lose heart part of the way through because they figure, "If it's this bad now, I'm not going to be able to handle it when it gets worse."

Labor contractions have an ebb and flow, like waves on a beach. You can have a very strong contraction which will do a lot of dilating and then it may be followed by several light con-tractions which consolidate the work of the strong one. As you will learn in the chapter on "Labor and Delivery," the uterine contractions are stretching and pulling your cervix open. A strong contraction accomplishes a lot of stretching, but it doesn't mean that every contraction after that is going to be progres-sively harder. In fact, if you can stay relaxed and your cervix is fairly cooperative, as labor progresses, the contractions can do more dilating with less pain as your cervix becomes more elastic. It is true that near the end of first-stage labor, when your cervix is close to full dilation, the contractions can last much longer and can have several "peaks" rather than just one. This interlude (known as "transition") is often the most difficult part of labor for a woman, but it is usually a great deal shorter than the early part of labor. Therefore, if you can remember to deal with each contraction as a separate event (rather than as "Oh, no, how many more after this?") your childbirth training will give you the greatest success in managing your labor and delivery.

➤ *Childbirth classes* were available in only 10% of the nation's 7,000 hospitals twenty-five years ago, but now it would be hard to find a hospital that doesn't offer them. Classes may be less expensive through a hospital than with a private teacher. How-ever, there are two problems with hospital classes: they may be larger than a private class, and teachers of such classes may have less freedom because they are beholden to the institution for which they work. Hospital classes may offer partial infor-mation or may give subtle support to hospital procedures. Ex-pectant parents may not know they might have other options (although if they've read this book they'll know!). Childbirth classes should teach about not only the birth process and how to manage labor contractions, but also how to cope with (and if necessary fight against) the hospital.

➤ *To find classes in your area,* ask your doctor or midwife for a recommendation. Ask any couples you know who have had prepared childbirth how they liked their instructor. You can write to the International Childbirth Education Association (P.O. Box 5852, Milwaukee, Wisconsin 53220) or write to ASPO (the American Society for Psychoprophylaxis in Obstetrics, which is the official namc of the Lamaze method) (1523 L Street N.W.,

Washington, DC 20005). You can also try calling the local chapter of the American Red Cross or the YWCA for suggestions.

➤ *All classes are essentially the same:* the exact breathing method they teach does not really matter. People from "rival" methods (Lamaze, Bradley, Dick-Read, etc.) would like you to think there is a difference to debunk other methods in favor of their own. Nowadays most classes have taken the best parts of all the methods and rolled them into one. The Lamaze method is the most well known and widespread—yet originally it did not include the husband as coach. That idea was initiated by Dr. Robert Bradley (whose method is also called Husband-Coached Childbirth). There are slight differences in the type of breathing they teach, but that is not central: it is your intense concentration on breathing patterns which reduces your experience of pain. The other important thing you learn is the ability to relax your body at will; it is the key to pain reduction. All classes are aimed at avoiding the vicious cycle of fear/tension/pain: the more afraid you are the more tense you become and the more you experience pain. The main difference between Bradley and Lamaze is that Bradley teachers tend to be quite adamant about their students having drug-free births. Bradley teachers are re-certified each year and sign a policy to strive for at least a 90 percent unmedicated rate. This is fine for expectant couples who have no doubts about having a drugless birth. It can be an extra incentive for those who are eager to deliver without any drugs. It can, however, be felt as pressure by couples who may have anxiety about "disappointing" their instructor, or may feel like failures themselves if they wind up wanting or needing medication.

➤ *A class can be a substitute for your extended family,* which you may not have nearby.

➤ *An important added benefit* of classes is that they are a support system for a couple. The camaraderie with other expectant couples is something you may not have during your pregnancy if your peers are postponing or deciding against childbearing. It is a great help to be able to share feelings and experiences with other people who are in the same situation. Discussing common problems and knowing that the things you feel are normal can help relieve tension and anxiety.

➤ *The class dynamic* depends on the individuals in your group. First you have to trust yourself, then you have to trust your coach, then the teacher, and finally the class. If the class dynamic is good, with shared participation and support, the personal bonds you make in these classes can be strong and the friendships can continue after your babies are born.

➤ *Classes usually start in your seventh month* and meet once weekly for anywhere from six to ten weeks. If you have not delivered by the time the class has finished many instructors will arrange for you to have "refresher" sessions to keep up your

practicing until the baby is born. Most classes meet in the evening and last two to three hours. The cost is usually around
$125, although it may be more or less depending on the part of
the country you live in. A good class size is eight to ten couples.
Any larger than that and you aren't going to get enough personalized attention or the kind of group interaction which can
give you so much support. Some teachers get a bit greedy and
take fifteen or more couples at a time: it really isn't fair to any
of them. The only time to consider a large class is if the teacher
lectures to all of you, then for the practical application of the
techniques splits the group up and meets with you in a smaller
section.

➤ *Choosing a class* is mostly a matter of finding a *teacher* you
feel good about. Trust in the instructor is essential in order for
the method to work for you. Most teachers will give you a class
outline, their credentials, and let you sit in on one of their classes
before signing up.

How to Choose a Childbirth Class

➤ *Find out whether films* are shown, and whether the teacher
has free discussion, formal lectures, or a combination of the two.

➤ *Is the teacher enthusiastic?* Does she have a sense of humor? This can be nice because it reduces tension and puts things
in perspective. A superserious and determined teacher can be
intimidating and make the classes a chore rather than fun and
interesting. A good way to judge this is whether the couples
seem relaxed yet enthusiastic.

➤ *If nonmedication is very important* to you, then you might
ask the teacher approximately what percentage of her pupils go
"drugless." At the least, make sure that the teaching in her class
is not aimed at "breathing until you're ready for your epidural."
That kind of class is a farce for any couple who is interested in
natural childbirth with commitment to prepared techniques. Instead it is just lip service, with the *assumption* of anesthetic
completely undermining any possible success with the training.

➤ *Ask whether "conditioned response"* is the basis of the
techniques that are taught. In Lamaze-type training the emphasis is on definite, repeated instructions by the coach to which
you will eventually have an automatic relaxation response.

The Man's Involvement in a Childbirth Class

➤ *The inclusion of the partner* is one of the important benefits
of childbirth classes.

➤ *It gives you a unique opportunity as a couple* to work as a team toward a common goal. The technique requires that you have total trust in each other. It elicits an intense nonverbal communication between you in which the coach is attuned to respond to your facial and body signals. When a couple is working well with childbirth techniques, they block out everything else that is going on and focus completely on each other. Some observers have noted that seeing a couple like this is almost like watching them "make love," they become so private and intense.

➤ *Most men feel somewhat reluctant* about starting the classes. Don't let that upset or stop you. All couples feel nervous at the first class, but as the man begins to see what his role is going to be during labor, he usually relaxes and becomes more confident.

➤ *Just how central a role your mate plays* during labor itself depends entirely on his personality, his attitudes toward childbirth, and how well you have been able to work as a team in practice sessions.

➤ *Some men are energetic* and determined to learn as much as they can about labor and delivery. This kind of man is probably eager to be fully involved in the birth, and it is important to him that he be your primary and sole support person during labor.

➤ *Some men remain baffled* and overwhelmed by the prospect of labor despite childbirth training (as do some women). A man like this will probably feel uptight and inadequate if he feels he has to be fully responsible for supporting you through the birth. Women who have mates like this often find that if there is someone additional to depend on, their mate can relax and enjoy the experience more and they still benefit from his emotional support. Their doctor, midwife, or an obstetric nurse experienced in prepared childbirth can all be useful for information and reassurance during labor.

➤ *Having your childbirth teacher as an additional coach* can either give you a wonderful feeling of security and support or it may be an extra burden. You may feel you have to do the technique perfectly and live up to your teacher's high standards. This really depends on how gung-ho your teacher is and your relationship with her.

Keep Practicing the Exercises

➤ *Practice is absolutely essential.* The techniques cannot work unless you practice them so that they become second nature.

➤ *Do not skip practicing*—or going to class—because your coach is not available. You are the one having the baby. You are the one who needs the conditioning. Practice by yourself. There are going to be times during labor when your coach may leave the room and you'll have to handle a contraction alone. Practice now; don't use his absence as an excuse to be lazy.

➤ *If your coach is unable to practice* with you routinely—because he has to be away during that time, for instance—tape-record his voice giving you instructions during a practice session. This will help condition your reflexes specifically to his voice.

➤ *Do not let anything interrupt* a practice contraction. Let the phone ring, the pot boil, or people ask you questions. There will be interruptions in labor, too, and this is good practice for your concentration. If you want, you can even *add* distractions once you've got the technique—turn on the radio or TV—and develop your concentration.

➤ *Practice your breathing* with a Braxton-Hicks contraction. Try it with a headache or to control the pain of bumping your shin. Test how well the techniques work and whether your use of them is improving.

➤ *If you do not have a coach,* prepared childbirth techniques can be done alone. Some mates flatly refuse to get involved. Trying to convert a man who feels this way may be a hopeless battle that causes a problem rather than solves one. If a man can't be gently swayed, you may be better off without him because you'd be worried about how *he* was feeling during labor and delivery instead of the other way around. You may not have anyone else in your life that you want to ask to be your coach. Don't worry; much of a coach's tasks are busywork anyway. The main importance of a coach is for emotional support—and to call out contractions and time them. To do it alone you have to have a strong will and motivation. You will be forced to depend more on yourself, knowing there's no one to lean on. It may be a rewarding experience.

➤ *Your anxiety level is high during pregnancy,* particularly as your due date nears. This may not be something you are consciously aware of, but it is certainly there. The effect of this anxiety level on your childbirth training is that you only hear about one-third of what you are taught and retain perhaps one-eighth of it. Try to remember that *you are not absorbing information normally* and that if you don't make a special effort to make things sink in, they may go in one ear and out the other. Ask the same question(s) of your teacher as often as you want to. Read and reread anything you want to be able to know during labor and delivery. It is common for an intelligent, seemingly calm woman who has had classes to ask questions during labor that sound as if she just awakened from a nine-month sleep and knows nothing about childbirth! There's nothing wrong with this except that you may not want to leave it to chance that there will be someone around at the time who can refresh your memory with accurate, reliable information.

FAMILY-CENTERED MATERNITY CARE

Offered by the more progressive hospitals nationwide, it means just what it says: that the hospital respects the importance of the family unit during labor and delivery and after the baby is born. Such hospitals usually have nurses in labor and delivery who are familiar with prepared childbirth techniques and can help you with them. However, the problem with the phrase "Family-Centered Maternity Care" is that *any* hospital can advertise it. Some institutions are using it as a catchphrase to attract patients, but the administration and staff are not genuinely committed— either in theory or practice—to what *should* be included or excluded from hospital routines and policies.

In order to determine just how family-centered a hospital is, you are going to have to take a tour and ask questions. Chapter 10, "Choosing a Doctor and a Hospital," describes the various family-centered options, including optional routine procedures on admittance, breast-feeding on the delivery table, Leboyer delivery, nonseparation of mother and baby after birth, rooming-in, early discharge, etc. If you decide that you want any or all of these options available to you, you will choose a hospital accordingly. Chapter 10 also discusses how to *change* a hospital so that it meets your needs.

THE FETAL HEART MONITOR (FHM)

This machine is hailed by some as the greatest advance in the history of maternity care. Others attack it as inaccurate, dehumanizing, and the cause of physical harm. In order to make a fully informed, balanced decision for yourself about fetal monitoring, it is necessary to learn how it works and then to look at it from three perspectives: theoretical, medical, and legal. Only then will you be able to formulate an opinion . . . as you will see, this is easier said than done. There is no absolute right or wrong about monitoring, but the issue *is* complicated by controversy about when it should be used, how it is used, and what medical action should be taken on the basis of the results.

How the Fetal Heart Monitor Works

➤ ***The monitor is a boxlike machine*** that looks like a large receiver for a stereo system. It is usually on a wheeled table that is approximately the height of your hospital bed.

➤ ***Two wide plastic straps*** (connected by wires to the FHM) are placed around your abdomen. The nurse will probably squeeze some electroconductor jelly onto your skin to improve transmission of signals. The upper strap has a pressure gauge to record your uterine contractions. The lower strap holds an ultrasonic transducer to pick up the fetal heart rate. The straps must be fairly snug to get readings, but if they are too tight for comfort, tell the nurse.

➤ *You must lie quite still* because the monitor produces indiscriminate *tracings* (called "artifacts") from your movements, the baby's movements, and other vibrations—the artifacts interfere with an accurate tracing of the fetal heart rate. These tracings come out of the machine on a narrow strip of paper and are two parallel squiggly lines with big dips in them indicating contractions. There is a microphone that picks up the baby's heartbeat, although the volume can be turned off in case you don't want to hear the steady, fast beat-beat-beating. A small light on the machine also flashes with each heartbeat and a digital number flashes (sometimes on a separate TV screen) a reading every second—153, 139, 146—which is a computation of the baby's heartbeats per minute.

➤ *An internal monitor* is more accurate and more artifact-free (and allows you to move around more freely in bed without disturbing the tracings). The internal monitor can ascertain variables in the fetal heart rate which are impossible to detect with the external monitor. The lower strap is replaced by an internal monitor. The internal monitor is either a clip or screw electrode—a small metal ending on a long wire. Your cervix must be dilated at least one to two centimeters in order for the electrode to be inserted, which can be painful for some women. The metal end is passed up inside you and clipped onto your baby's scalp or inserted just under the skin. There are as yet no studies determining whether this increases the risk of infection to the baby. The issue is rarely even raised as to whether this electrode causes the baby pain. Some hospitals use an internal monitor whenever a woman's membranes have already broken. Other hospitals use it only when fetal distress has been detected with external monitoring (in such a case the membranes would be artificially ruptured if necessary). A second catheter is sometimes inserted that measures the intensity of your contractions with more accuracy than the external monitor—and replaces the upper strap.

➤ *The purpose of an FHM* is to supply information about how your baby is responding to the stress of labor. With each uterine contraction the baby's blood supply is temporarily cut off. It seems a bit dramatic to make the comparison that it is like strangling the baby each time, but the baby does receive his oxygen via the blood and that flow is cut off each time you have a labor contraction. Some babies can withstand labor less well than others—depending on their size, the strength of the contractions, the length of labor, and other considerations. The FHM measures each of your uterine contractions and the baby's heart rate simultaneously. It is normal for his heart rate to drop with each contraction; it is also normal for the baby's heart rate to come right back up to where it was before the contraction. If the fetal heart rate is slow in returning to normal it is known as "late deceleration": if the monitor continues to indicate this is the baby's response to your contractions it is called fetal distress. A safe fetal heart rate is considered to be between 120 and 160 beats per minute. Distress is indicated when the rate goes above 160 or below about 110. This introduces an area of controversy about the FHM—in this section I am only *describing* how the monitor works. Pages 270 to 275 discuss the pros and cons of the fetal monitor.

FHM and Inaccuracies

The monitor's only dependable ability at this point is in telling you that everything is okay. The monitor's prediction of a normal outcome is more accurate than any other technique. When the FHM tracing is normal, you can be certain that everything is, in fact, normal. The problem is that the incidence of "false abnormal" tracings is high.

➤ **Monitoring patterns** may sometimes be indecipherable because of artifacts or a malfunctioning machine.
➤ **The external monitor** can give an inaccurate recording of data.
➤ **Even with the more accurate,** sensitive internal monitor, the data is subject to varying interpretations. The interpretation of distress patterns is not uniform: all tracings are subject to a wide difference in the way they are evaluated by doctors. Even the champions of the monitor agree that a refinement is necessary in the diagnosis of these patterns.
➤ **The maternal heart rate** may be counted by mistake or the fetal heart rate half—or double—counted.
➤ **There is a tendency to "overdiagnose"** when there is fetal distress. Some experts believe that an accurate interpretation of an abnormal tracing cannot be made on the basis of fetal monitoring alone: it is necessary to also do fetal scalp sampling (page 270).

What Happens if There's Fetal Distress?

➤ **If there is a distress pattern** the staff first tries conservative measures to restore a normal pattern.
➤ **They reposition you,** usually turning you on your side. A problem with monitoring is that you have to lie on your back, which invites *supine hypotension*. This means that the weight of the baby and your position press on the main vein returning blood to your heart: this can cause a drop in maternal blood pressure and ominous fetal heart rate patterns.

➤ *The staff will increase your blood pressure,* giving you intravenous fluids if you aren't already hooked up to an IV, and administering oxygen with a face mask.

➤ *The attendants will reduce or cancel any oxytocin* you are receiving (a synthetic hormone that increases your contractions), or will give you medication to inhibit contractions.

➤ *Fetal scalp sampling* is performed to determine whether the fetal distress suggested by the FHM is accurate. True fetal distress is almost always caused by a reduced flow of oxygen-rich blood to the fetus. When the oxygen supply is depleted, the pH of the baby's blood is lowered. The pH is a measure of the acidity or alkalinity of the blood; too low a pH level means that the baby is in jeopardy and must be delivered immediately, perhaps by cesarean. A low pH in the fetus is usually from a reduced blood supply, but it may also be the result of maternal disease like diabetic acidosis.

Scalp sampling is done by inserting a cone-shaped speculum into the vagina, which is moved up against the baby's presenting part (which is usually the head) and a tiny prick is made. A drop or two of blood is taken and examined for its concentration of oxygen, carbon dioxide, and its pH. The results of these findings help a doctor determine what course of action to take. Although the fetal heart monitor can be inaccurate, when used in conjunction with fetal scalp sampling the monitor becomes a much more reliable tool.

➤ *The rule of thumb* is that if an ominous fetal heart rate pattern in a previously healthy fetus cannot be restored to normal within half an hour, a cesarean section is performed.

➤ *The newest internal monitor* are hoped to be so accurate that fetal blood analysis will not be as frequently needed to verify the baby's condition.

Medical Arguments in Favor of Monitoring

➤ *The mother's condition does not necessarily determine the baby's condition.* You may be in perfect health, have had a trouble-free pregnancy, and therefore be considered "low risk." However, various studies show that the problems that develop during labor and delivery are not confined to women designated "high risk" (who gave prior indications that there might be complications). High-risk patients account for only one-half of the bad outcomes (newborns with problems). One study which eliminated all high-risk women, by every possible definition of high-risk factors, showed that one-third of all low-risk patients become high-risk during labor. Another study showed that 50% of newborns with problems resulted from low-risk pregnancies.

The argument has been made—and rightly so—that many

of the routine practices in the hospital can cause physical problems. A woman's emotional reaction to these routines—even to being in the hospital—can also cause complications. However, the larger issue rests on the fundamental position that *labor itself is what generates the problems*. Although the vast majority of births will be normal there is no way of knowing which babies will have trouble coping with the stress of labor and delivery. Thus, if you accept the premise that the mother and baby are independent of each other—that information you have about the mother's condition does not guarantee the baby's condition—then you accept the need to monitor. At the very least you accept that the designation "low risk" is limited in its usefulness as a prediction of how a baby will withstand labor.

➤ *The greatest benefit of the monitor is the confident prediction of a nondistressed fetus* regardless of its mother's condition. If properly administered and read, the monitor removes the guesswork about whether a baby is all right. The pitfalls in its prediction of an *abnormal* fetal condition have already been mentioned. Advocates of the monitor agree that the machine is in its infancy as a diagnostic tool and may be error-prone because the methods of its use and the terminology have not been universally agreed upon and authoritative texts are not available.

➤ *If your number-one priority in childbirth is the kind of safety* the monitor offers (i.e., the certainty of knowing everything is all right) then you will want the monitor. However, you have to decide whether you are willing to pay the personal price for the technology. Monitoring will necessarily inhibit other aspects of the birth experience that have their own importance; you have to be willing to forfeit those. You don't get something for nothing. There are many instances in modern American life where human personal qualities and experience are bartered for what machines have to offer.

At times our technology has outstripped our ability to know when, where, and how to use it. It may be true that the "right" way to use the fetal heart monitor has not yet been discovered. But if this sense of absolute certainty is your foremost concern (there is no way of knowing which baby has the cord tangled around his neck), then you may opt for a machine that can at least assure you that *your baby does not have a problem*. The warning must be added once again that you should not depend totally on the FHM: *normalcy* is the only absolutely reliable information it can give you.

➤ *A doctor cannot make these decisions for you.* If you are considered a low-risk patient, then you have to weigh the benefits and disadvantages of the monitor. There is no way of knowing ahead of time who the small number of women will be whose babies will become distressed during labor. Whether *all* women should be routinely monitored to determine if they are in the normal majority is a decision that should not be made by doctors and hospitals. If you are going to have a machine monitor your labor, you must know what you are gaining and what you may be giving up—each individual has to decide that for herself.

Arguments Against the Fetal Monitor

> *Inaccuracy in diagnosing distress* has already been mentioned. The rebuttal to this is that as it is improved, the monitor will become more reliable in predicting problems as well as normalcy.

> *The monitors must be monitored.* Just like the question of whether a falling tree makes a sound if no one sees it, a monitor is useless unless it is being watched. The machine varies from useless to dangerous unless it is being watched by someone who knows the subtleties of what to look for in yards and yards of tracings. This close surveillance which is required is not always available. When there *is* someone reading the tracing—whether it is a nurse or doctor—he or she may not be properly trained in interpreting the information. The good thing that can be said about the need to monitor monitors is that this increased surveillance may be helping to lower perinatal mortality, irrespective of the machine. There has been a lower death rate for infants at the large teaching hospitals that use monitors routinely on all women. This reduced rate can also be attributed to factors associated with monitoring: closer surveillance, enhanced alertness and education of the staff, changes in routines and procedures, etc.

> *All the attention is paid to the machine, not the woman.* The staff and even your coach can become absorbed in watching the strip that is continuously advancing from the machine. It is not uncommon for a doctor or nurse to walk into a labor room and the first thing they look at is the machine. They may not even make eye contact with you as they say, "How are you doing?" They pick up the long chart of paper that the machine has produced. It's almost as if they're asking the machine how things are going. The piece of paper has become the laboring woman. Even *you* may come to think of the machine as the controlling influence on your labor.

It is said in praise of the monitor that it can *alert you to an upcoming contraction.* It *is* true that you or your coach can see that a contraction is beginning by watching the needle making a tracing on the graph. But it is somewhat illogical to compliment the machine: after all, it is your body, and if you were focused on your uterus (instead of a monitor tracing) you could *feel* a contraction beginning! Very often the coach and staff will watch a contraction from start to finish on the tracing and exclaim afterward, "Boy, that was a big one." It becomes absurd; *they* are telling *you* about the contraction. Similarly you may have a hard time breathing your way through a particularly tough contraction and complain afterward how difficult it was. Your coach or the nurse may make light of it, saying, "No, that wasn't much of a contraction." They were watching the monitor tracing and it didn't look like much *there*. Nonetheless, a contraction doesn't have to look huge on a tracing to do a lot of dilation, which may cause you discomfort. If there weren't a monitor to "disprove" your subjective reaction, you might get some sympathetic support.

If you feel the monitor is getting all the attention, tell people. There is no use in having a coach and a well-trained obstetric nurse or a carefully chosen doctor or nurse-midwife if you aren't getting the attention and support from them that you want. Even the best-intentioned attendants can unwittingly fall into the trap of focusing on the monitor. There are serious pitfalls in it for you if the emphasis is on a machine.

➤ *The machine may take up so much room* or be positioned in such a way that the labor room is cramped and the monitor separates a woman and her coach. If this happens, simply tell the staff and move the bed, monitor, or your coach! If the room and machine are arranged so that there is no place for your coach to sit, take it upon yourselves to rearrange things for your comfort and convenience.

➤ *The monitor invites supine hypotension* (page 269) because a woman must lie flat on her back while it is in place. It is undeniable that lying on your back for long periods cuts off the vena cava (the vein that returns blood to your heart) and thereby shuts off the baby's oxygen supply.

There are *alternative ways* of using the monitor that guard against this hypotension occurring. However, you cannot count on your doctor or the staff to suggest them. *You* can suggest them to your doctor ahead of time and then do what you have agreed upon once you are in labor.

1. *Lie on your side.* The monitor tracing may not be quite as good when you lie on your side, and it takes more skill to interpret the results, but it does eliminate the problem of supine hypotension. You might want to shift to your side periodically.

2. *The external monitor can be removed* and you can walk around or go to the bathroom. The monitor can then be attached periodically to assure that all is going well. One way is to monitor only fifteen minutes out of every hour. In between you can take any position you want to, in bed or out. Physically and psychologically it is good for you to walk around during labor. Walking stimulates contractions, allows gravity to help the baby descend, and gives you a feeling of being normal, not a bedridden invalid. Another solution is to

monitor once every two hours: leave the monitor on for twenty minutes, and if you get a good tracing, then you don't need another for an hour and forty minutes. Discuss these options with your doctor ahead of time because even the strongest advocates of the monitor believe that these are viable alternatives.

➤ *A Doppler* can be used, some critics say, instead of a fetal heart monitor. Unfortunately this is *not true*. These hand-held instruments amplify the sound of the fetal heartbeat, which tells you only that the heart is beating and how fast. The Doppler *cannot* tell you how well the baby recovers after a contraction, which is the whole point of the FHM. It is said that human auscultation (listening to the baby's heart rate with the human ear) is a viable substitute for the monitor. Even if you had enough staff so that someone could stay glued to a woman's abdomen for hours and hours, however, it is *not possible to detect* the kind of late deceleration that indicates fetal distress and can result in problems for the newborn.

➤ *The fetal heart monitor has caused a rise in the cesarean rate.* It is true that there are babies with abnormal FHR patterns who are delivered by cesarean without appearing to have had any signs of problems of birth, for the FHM is not fully reliable at this point in its diagnosis of abnormality. Furthermore, the monitor's accuracy is only as good as the people reading its tracings. For example, a monitor can show a variable deceleration, which to an inadequately trained eye may look like a late deceleration but is *not* the same and does not indicate distress.

➤ *However, at Yale,* which was the birthplace of the FHM, after a period of increased C-sections when staff and physicians were still learning the intricacies of the monitor, their cesarean section rate leveled off to what it was in premonitor days: 10 percent. The goal for all doctors is to do cesareans on the women who do need them, and avoid C-sections for those who do not, particularly those high-risk patients whose babies register as normal on the monitor.

➤ *A drop in the FHR pattern may cause a woman or her mate to panic.* A coach may see something that doesn't look right to him on the tracing. He may get upset and perhaps interfere with your breathing techniques. To avoid this potential problem, ask to be shown a monitor tracing ahead of time—either on your hospital tour or in early labor—so that you know which drops are normal (i.e., variable deceleration) and which are late deceleration.

There have also been cases of an internal monitor dislodging from the baby's scalp. This means the fetal heart rate light on the monitor stops blinking and the beat-beat-beating sound stops. You might think your baby has died inside you, although it is only the electrode that has detached. This can be a terrifying and traumatic experience; it can disrupt your relaxation and concentration during labor, and it may be a long time before you recover from it. The only solution if this happens is to supplement the alarming information given by the monitor with what can be learned by the human ear. Ask a nurse or the doctor to listen to the baby through your abdomen to assure you that the baby is still alive.

➤ ***What do you do on the day the monitor is broken?*** A FHM is only a machine, and like any machine, it is far from perfect. They malfunction or stop working altogether. We are in the process of turning out an entire generation of doctors and nurses who *know how to assess labor only with a monitor.* They are lost without it. Medicine is fast becoming dominated by machines: that is where all the attention is focused and all decisions are based on machine data. Women have babies; machines don't. Women are going to continue to have babies whether or not the machines are ready for them on any given day! The staff of every hospital maternity unit needs training and practice in relying on their own personal experience and intelligence to assess a woman in labor, rather than on what a tracing on a piece of paper tells them.

➤ ***Official medical policy on FHMs has changed*** dramatically: in 1988 the American College of Obstetricians and Gynecologists (ACOG) overturned its long-standing policy favoring the use of electronic fetal monitors. The ACOG then stated that electronic fetal monitoring would no longer be part of the standard of care for maternity patients. But even when monitoring was "required" only for high-risk patients, it was commonly used on all women in labor.

The ACOG based its decision on the results of research which showed monitors didn't have any benefit over a nurse listening to the fetal heartbeat every fifteen minutes in the first stage of labor, and every five minutes in the second stage. One problem: where would you find enough nurses to listen that often to the belly of every laboring woman throughout her entire labor?

The bottom line is that there will probably be no difference in how often electronic monitors are used, despite the data which shows that using FHMs does not produce healthier babies. Obstetricians point to a combination of legal and economic pressures which make it almost impossible to stop using them. Because of the serious nursing shortage nationwide, hospitals could never hire enough nurses to take the place of the monitors.

The Legal Side of Monitoring

➤ ***"Established practice."*** Once a medical technique has become standard practice, a doctor can be judged on whether he has followed that standard or not. When a number of doctors state that a technique is necessary, it becomes so. Monitoring has become established practice. This means that if there is a bad outcome in childbirth and monitoring was available but not used, a doctor can be held responsible for the problem that resulted.

➤ *It could be grounds for a malpractice lawsuit not to monitor* once it has become a standard procedure. Theoretically, any doctor who disregards standard procedure is liable for the decision. It wouldn't even matter if a couple were to sign a release form ahead of time. For example, it would be malpractice for a cardiologist not to use an electrocardiograph—a machine which tells whether or not a patient has a heart problem. Even though it can be argued that childbirth is not a sickness or abnormality and therefore should not be treated as one, birth is becoming a high-risk, technologized field.

➤ *In the case of a lawsuit a fetal-monitor tracing can be used as evidence* by a doctor that a patient received thorough attention. The tracing on the strip chart (almost regardless of what is on it) becomes the doctor's defense in the event there is legal trouble later. In a day and age when people *are* litigious and *do* sue doctors, it is understandable that a physician would want every protection possible. A lot depends on the kind of relationship formed by a doctor and an expectant couple: one would imagine that if the relationship was good, then a lawsuit would never result. Not all patient-doctor relationships are optimal—and even those that are take unpredictable twists and turns.

FRIENDS ATTENDING YOUR CHILD'S BIRTH

This is a choice that either appeals to you or seems distasteful. In home births there are often friends present, both to help with practical matters and to share in the experience. In maternity center births and alternative birthing rooms in hospitals there is usually the option of having guests.

➤ *Your reaction* to having friends attend may be that birth is a private matter, and anyway, "who would even *want* to come?" However, in a hospital there can be a dozen people who see you during labor and delivery—it is hardly a private event. If you think of it this way you may feel differently about the possibility of *choosing* who is with you. As for "who would want to come," there are numerous people who would jump at the chance to see a baby born—it is a fascinating and awesome experience which is denied to most people. However, people with *unresolved feelings* toward births are not going to make good guests.

➤ *Emotional support* is most important during childbirth and being surrounded by friends can give you that feeling.

➤ **Guests are there to focus energy toward the birth.** Although people playing musical instruments or socializing with each other is fine, their activity should always be subject to how it affects you. If you get the feeling that there's a "party" going and you're left out of it (lying there doing hard work!) it can be counterproductive to your labor. Be sure to discuss this ahead of time with anyone you invite. Consider your friends' personalities. If you think they might be so caught up in themselves that they cannot take a back seat to the main event, then they may not be an asset to the birth.

➤ **Guests should not arrive too early in labor.** If people start coming before you are well-established in labor it may make you feel tense, which will slow your labor. See pages 396 for more on how your emotions can affect your contractions.

➤ **Curiosity-seekers** do not make good guests. They are voyeurs rather than participants—both physically and in an emotional sense.

➤ **If there are going to be children present,** be firm that there must be one adult per child to supervise and entertain them (see pages 286–289 on siblings attending for more on children at births).

➤ **Self-invited guests** may be tricky to uninvite if they are close friends. If you do not want them there for some reason, it may be awkward to tell them you do not want them there. You can ease out of it by telling a "white lie" and saying that your doctor or midwife has been very firm about how many people can be present and you already have invited as many as you can.

HOME BIRTH

Chapter 11 is devoted entirely to home birth, and includes a discussion of your various options with home birth: without any attendants except your mate; with a lay midwife; with a certified nurse-midwife; or with a doctor (who usually has midwives to "labor-sit" for him.)

INDUCED BIRTH

This is a choice in childbirth, but it can be a dangerous one. Elective induction is used in 15% of births: a woman and her doctor decide when to have her baby and then they start labor with synthetic hormones. There is only a small number of births that should be induced for medical reasons. Two common reasons for beginning labor artificially are *not* valid:

➤ **For a mother's convenience**, so she can arrange care for any other children, so she can be rested, etc.

> ➤ *For the doctor's convenience*, to fit in with his office schedule, or so he can be rested and alert, or so he can choose when the hospital is most heavily staffed.

Synthetic oxytocin is the hormone that stimulates contractions is used when you are admitted to a hospital but labor hasn't truly started. They will keep you in the hospital and administer *Pitocin*, the most commonly used oxytocin, or they may artificially rupture your membranes. This kind of medical interference with natural processes is not technically called "elective induction," although that is what it is. The reason behind inducing a woman in this situation is that she's tired out from being up all night with early labor contractions, that she's nervous and anxious to have her baby, etc. If that is the case, go home and go to sleep! Or stay in the hospital, if there's room, and sleep there. Most hospitals, doctors, and emergency rooms will either send you home or find you a place to pace or sleep if they think you're not ready to be admitted.

Do not allow anyone to tamper with the natural forces regulating your labor unless there are medical reasons (outlined later in this section). The use of Pitocin or artificial rupture of membranes with *no evidence of cervical change* after hospital admission (i.e., you aren't dilating naturally) must be considered elective induction with all its risks.

Many women would have stopped contracting naturally and at a future time delivered a mature fetus without the health problems of a baby whose birth was induced before it was ready for life on the outside.

Artificial Membrane Rupture

Some doctors do this routinely near your due date without your consent. It is known as an "amniotomy." Other doctors may "strip" the membranes: during an internal exam (in the office or in the hospital) a doctor can use his/her fingers to separate the amnion (bag of waters) from the uterine wall. One possible hazard is that you could have an undetected placenta previa: the placenta is nearer to the cervix than the baby is. Stripping the membranes could strip the *placenta* instead of the amnion away from the uterus, causing a critical hemorrhage. However, there can be an appropriate situation in which stripping the membranes is not dangerous and can have a beneficial effect.

The amniotic fluid is nature's protection for the baby, especially during contractions. Nature usually keeps the bag of waters intact until the last phase of labor. Most often the membranes rupture with the onset of second-stage labor, when you are fully dilated and the baby is nearing the end of her journey into the world.

Intact membranes are an excellent dilator. They maintain equal pressure on the cervix according to the laws of hydrodynamics. If force is applied to an enclosed liquid, the force will be transmitted equally everywhere throughout the liquid. An intact bag of waters makes a better dilator of the cervix than the contour of the baby's head and protects the head at the same time.

However, there are times when intact membranes can hold the baby's head up *off* the cervix and can slow down the labor. At such times an amniotomy is beneficial.

Artificial rupture can start labor but it often also *accelerates labor*, shortening it by thirty to forty minutes. This is not worth the risk of possible damage to the baby's head and other complications. When used to speed up labor, some of the possible ill effects are temporary deformation in your baby's head and even permanent damage. Although it is known that 95% of membranes will rupture in very late labor if left to themselves, there is a common obstetric practice of artificially rupturing membranes midway through first-stage labor, or at four to five centimeters dilation. *There is no good reason to do this except impatience.* Some doctors and even women seem to have lost touch with the concept of normalcy—they have no faith in the body's ability to do the best job in a normal birth. Birth is a normal bodily function and a woman's body is built for it. In a low-risk, normal situation, "hands off" is the best policy (and this goes for any kind of obstetric intervention). The birth attendant—doctor, midwife, or nurse—is there to watch as a lifeguard, not to interfere.

Rupturing the membranes can cause the umbilical cord to be compressed during contractions. This affects the baby's oxygen supply.

Ways to Use Pitocin (A Synthetic Oxytocin)

> *Injection* of Pitocin is less controllable than the other methods— it is hard to predict how a woman's uterus will respond and there is no way to reduce the amount in your system once you've been given the shot.
> *The hormone can be put into intravenous solution* and the flow into the IV can be adjusted. This is called a "pit drip." There is a measure of error in this method because the hormone is diluted in a large bottle of fluid, so the doctor doesn't know exactly how much you are getting.
> *IVAC or IMED infusion pump* is a small box mounted on the IV pole. The glucose solution contains the Pitocin, which flows through the IVAC box, regulating the amount you receive. This eliminates the hazards of a regular "pit drip."

Another Way to Start Labor

> *Prostaglandin is a synthetic hormone commonly used to stimulate labor.* It is applied to the cervix in a gel which is directly absorbed into the cervix and softens it. Prostaglandin stimulates the production of your own natural prostaglandin,

which readies your body to give birth. When softened, the cervix will be less resistant and will open more easily and naturally.

One of the problems with using pitocin has been that while it can create uterine contractions, they do not necessarily dilate the cervix. This means that some induced births have ended as cesareans because the contractions were not effective. However, if prostaglandins are used first when you are induced, it can help the oxytocin-induced contractions open your cervix.

Problems with Induction

➢ *More intense contractions*. It can make it *harder for a woman to stay in control* and use her breathing techniques. The result may be that she wants analgesia—or *more* of it. There is almost always an increased need for painkillers with induction (which stay in the baby's system longer than they do in yours).

➢ *Effect on the newborn:* There is a slightly higher risk of jaundice when labor is induced. One side effect of jaundice is that the baby spends more time sleeping and less time alert, which will interfere with "bonding" (see pages 391–393). A groggy baby will interact less with you and create a cycle, influencing the way you respond to her and she reacts to you.

➢ *Overdose of oxytocic substance*. The fetal heart monitor (FHM) has taken most of the danger out of induction, because you can get direct information from the FHM about the baby's condition. But problems do still occur when using oxytocic drugs to stimulate labors:

1) *The drug can overstimulate the uterus* and make the contractions so long and intense that not enough oxygen gets through to the baby.
2) *The drug can cause the placenta to separate* from the uterine wall before the baby is born, disrupting his oxygen supply. Unless a vaginal delivery is possible immediately, this will necessitate a cesarean section.

➢ *Your due date can be miscalculated.* The baby may be born *prematurely*. RDS, respiratory distress syndrome, also known as hyaline membrane disease, is a severe disorder of the lungs found in newborns, especially those who are premature (less than 28 weeks). Prematurity and RDS can be a problem in elective repeat cesareans and in inductions. RDS claims the lives of 20,000 newborns each year; many of those deaths could be prevented with fewer and more judiciously induced labors.

It is now believed that when a baby's brain reaches a certain state of maturity, it releases a substance that begins a chain of reactions leading to delivery. This is the reason that the *spontaneous onset of labor should be awaited whenever possible*.

➢ *Maturity studies should be done first*. Respiratory distress syndrome is preventable. If an induction is necessary, delivery can be postponed if the infant's lungs are not mature enough. The tests can be of lung maturity or measuring the baby's head by ultrasound. It is a good idea to have both studies done for greatest accuracy.

Medical Reasons for Induction

There are medical reasons to induce labor in approximately 3% of births. Basically, an acceptable reason is for the *safety of the mother and baby*.

➢ *A mature baby is overdue*. If through testing of the amniotic fluid, it is determined that *a mature baby is at least three weeks overdue*, then it is wiser to deliver than to wait any longer (see "Post-Term (Postmature) Pregnancy," pages 456–457). However, many doctors induce routinely after 42 weeks. The problem can be that your due date has been calculated from the last period and not conception, leaving a two-week margin of error. There are many healthy eight-pound babies born two weeks after their "due" date.

➢ *A medical problem with the mother*. With diabetes or toxemia, it is often mandatory to induce labor. Other medical problems might be severe Rh sensitization or a previous history of severe hemorrhage.

Premature Rupture of Membranes (PROM)

If the membranes have ruptured spontaneously and labor doesn't begin within a reasonable amount of time, it is standard procedure to induce labor. Studies show that if a woman has not *delivered* her baby (not just gone into labor) within 12 to 24 hours after her membranes have ruptured, there is an increased risk of amnionitis (infection of the amniotic sac). However, some birth attendants (both medical and lay midwives) point out that the decreased infection rate with a delivery within 24 hours was coupled with a policy of avoiding vaginal exams during that time. That may have contributed to the decline in the infection rate. Some doctors allow a woman to stay at home after ruptured membranes because the environment there has less bacteria than the hospital. Lay midwives may allow a woman to wait 48 to 72 hours after the ruptured membranes.

➢ *If dilation begins and then stops* some doctors advise induction. For example, it is possible to be dilated three centimeters for a week or two without labor beginning. However, with a dilated cervix, labor may progress quickly once it begins and you may be in the car on the way to the hospital when you're in transition (which may not be the ideal place to go through the toughest part of labor!). However, you have to compare that to the possible dangers of induction.

➤ *If an epidural anesthetic (or other drug) stops your labor cold*—if it knocks out the contractions altogether—pitocin may be necessary to get things going again.

➤ *If your uterus is atonic*—contractions are weak and ineffective in accomplishing any dilation—artificial stimulation by pitocin may be necessary.

LAY MIDWIVES

(Described in Chapter 11, "Home Birth.")

LEBOYER DELIVERY

Developed by a French doctor, Leboyer delivery has been misunderstood by some followers. It is not intended to be a blueprint of exactly how to manage a delivery: Leboyer's work is best applied if it is seen as an attempt to *sensitize people to understand that the newborn sees, hears, and feels*. The main concern is the baby's experience of labor and delivery.

The Psychology Behind Leboyer's Techniques

Leboyer was influenced by a group of psychiatrists who share the belief that later problems in life stem from birth trauma. They view the birth trauma as the "primal separation," which profoundly influences our later life.

Leboyer wants to reduce birth trauma. He says that we carry throughout life the imprint of our birth. He says that a baby is taken from the uterus and bombarded with thundering sounds, the cold openness of the delivery room, and the first breath of burning air. (Personally I find his book *Birth Without Violence* a bit fanatical and overblown. I think his methods are marvelous, but his rhetoric off-putting.)

Leboyer agrees with the previously mentioned psychiatrists that birth is a prototypic psychological experience of separation and loss. He believes that the process of birth involves deep pain, hurt, and fatigue for the baby. There are basic defense mechanisms which aid the newborn by blocking out these negative feelings—and it is these defenses which allow a child to become neurotic or preneurotic. The goal, therefore, is to reduce the trauma. Whether or not you agree with Leboyer's reasoning, you can still be interested in the net result of gentler, more loving birth.

Leboyer's Recommendations for Birth Procedures

➤ *Dim, indirect lighting.* This is more comfortable for the newborn's sensitive eyes. There is no doubt that a newborn will keep her eyes tightly shut beneath a bright light and open them and look around if there is reduced light. This can have an important effect in bonding, where eye-to-eye contact is so important.

➤ *A delivery-room temperature is adjusted to the comfort of the baby* rather than the delivery-room personnel. It can be quite chilly in a delivery room; the main reason for this is to reduce chances of infection since bacteria grow where it is warm. The other reason is so the staff can stay cool. One solution is to have portable radiant heaters under which the baby can be placed. The heater can also be positioned over the delivery table so you can hold the baby and have the heat source over you.

➤ *Immediate postnatal positioning of the newborn on the mother's abdomen.* Leboyer also suggests massaging the baby while she is on your stomach. This accomplishes skin-to-skin contact and lessens the shock of being in the open air because the baby can hear your heart and feel you. It can also hasten third-stage labor, the expulsion of the placenta.

➤ *A minimum of noise and talk throughout.* Leboyer is concerned that a newborn is shocked by noise outside the uterus, where all sounds have been muffled through the amniotic fluid. However, a newborn's ears are probably still filled with fluid at birth so the sound is naturally softened anyway.

➤ *A minimum of hard, jerky movements.* Leboyer is concerned about the somewhat rough way that babies are usually handled at birth and the trauma this must cause after the envelopment of the uterus. It is true that delivery-room personnel can be brusque in handing the baby to each other and rubbing her off; a Leboyer delivery focuses everyone's attention on the baby, thereby causing them to be more conscious about their treatment of her.

➤ *A delay in severing the umbilical cord until pulsation has ceased.* In many hospitals they routinely give an injection of oxytocin to hasten the delivery of the placenta. If you are going to wait for the cord to stop pulsating and delay cutting it, make sure you aren't given that shot of oxytocin at the time of birth because it can cause hemorrhaging. Also, be aware that cutting the cord is a medical procedure and is the doctor's "territory." Discuss it with him, but recognize that this is an area in which he may get defensive about being "dictated to." (See page 388 for a full discussion of late cord clamping.)

➤ *Placing the newborn in a tub of warm water* with gentle, firm support is perhaps the best-known aspect of Leboyer's recommendations. His reasoning is that birth trauma is lessened if a baby is returned to the weightless, wet environment he just came from. Some doctors and hospitals encourage the baby's father to handle the bath. Some offer practice classes before birth; in any case, a nurse or the doctor will assist your mate because a newborn is slippery. It is a wonderful way for paternal-infant bonding to begin, and if you are interested you should clear the way ahead of time. It is important that the hospital staff is alerted so that they can have a plastic tub and warmed sterile water ready at delivery time.

Objections to Leboyer Techniques

➤ *A baby has a poor ability to maintain body temperature.* One of the main concerns with any newborn is for her temperature to stabilize. A bath introduces *"cold stress"*—the water on her skin makes her feel cold when you remove her from the bath, just as it does to you after you step out of the shower and before you dry off. However, since the baby's temperature regulator is not very efficient, even drying her off quickly may not warm her. One solution: have a radiant heater placed over the tub of water and wrap the baby in warmed towels and blankets when you take her out.

➤ *A baby needs the shock of being born into air* in order to stimulate her lungs to breathe for the first time. Some experts say that placing her back in a warm liquid environment may not stimulate her enough to insure that she continues breathing. However, even with a bath there are still many stimuli unfamiliar to the baby's system that stimulate her to breathe on her own.

➤ *There is no "proof" for Leboyer's claims: this is absolutely true*. Leboyer's suggestions for childbirth sound kind and loving, but he makes unproven statements about the ways in which his techniques will improve children. He has nothing to back up his claims except his personal beliefs.

➤ *If your doctor disagrees with Leboyer's ideas*, ask if he'd arrange for *some* of Leboyer's recommendations. He might agree not to use the bright overhead spotlight; he might agree to hand you the baby gently and immediately, etc. Again, what counts about a Leboyer delivery is to focus the awareness of all attendants on the newborn's sensitivity to sights, sounds, and smells.

➤ *A Leboyer delivery may be redundant in a home birth* because it was originally intended to humanize hospital birth. The important benefit of Leboyer techniques in the hospital is that it allows a couple to identify themselves as wanting this kind of experience. It jolts caregivers out of their routines and makes them more aware of what they are doing to the baby and the way they're doing it. There is no problem about this kind of sensitivity at home. In fact, applying Leboyer techniques at home might *decrease* intimacy rather than increase it. Spontaneity would be sacrificed while you were trying to carry out procedures that were designed for a different birth setting. Having a Leboyer bath at home is like carrying the proverbial coals to Newcastle.

➤ *The bath may interfere with bonding.* Some women find that if they hold the baby immediately after birth and begin breast-feeding on the delivery table that it seems artificial and disruptive to hand the baby over for a bath. Try to be flexible and see how you feel at the time and *do not feel tied* to any of these techniques. Spontaneity—a natural, instinctive response—is more important than anything. If you feel like holding on to the baby, whether she is sucking or not, then do that. Of course your mate may be eager to give the bath, so you'll have your first negotiation over the baby!

MATERNITY CENTERS

Maternity centers are prevalent in many parts of the world, but there are pitifully few in America. A maternity center is a facility designed to meet the needs of low-risk women during a normal birth. (See page 336) for the chart of "Factors That Rule Out Home Birth" to determine whether you are eligible). If there are any complications during labor or delivery, in most cases you will be transferred to a nearby hospital. A maternity center is usually staffed by certified nurse and/or lay midwives with a doctor on call, with whom they consult if anything is abnormal. Affiliation with a doctor also enables them to prescribe medication during prenatal care or birth, and to admit a laboring woman into a hospital, if necessary.

Maternity centers emphasize the normalcy of birth. They require that a woman has had childbirth classes; they rarely have any analgesia available for labor, although they may have oxytocins and other drugs in case of complications with delivery. Some maternity centers have cooking facilities and room enough so that a couple can spend the night after birth.

It's unlikely that more maternity centers will develop. The ones that do exist are an anachronism in a day and age when maternity care in the United States is moving toward centralization. The medical establishment is trying to phase out the maternity departments of smaller hospitals, which traditionally have been the more flexible and humanistic for the very reason that they *are* small. The trend is to have all births take place at the largest, most technologically equipped institutions. This not only limits your choices in where the birth takes place, but it imposes high-risk obstetric management on all births, including normal, low-risk ones. The large, fully equipped hospital may be medically necessary for some women or it may be the choice for others who will feel more protected knowing the technology is present. However, each woman should have the right to decide where her baby will be born. There is uncertainty about risks *in* the hospital as well as outside of it. A maternity center offers a middle-of-the-road compromise.

SIBLINGS ATTENDING BIRTH

This practice is often part of a birth at home. However, parents choosing an alternative birthing room, a doctor's office, or a maternity center may also have that choice. In deciding whether your other child(ren) will be able to cope with and benefit from seeing their sister or brother born, there are several factors to consider.

- *Ask the child whether he or she wants to be there.* Explain a little of what it will be like. If the child does not want to participate or observe, respect that. Pressure on a child can be harmful.
- *Many people believe that ages one to five are too young to attend*. Some psychologists say that birth and death are trying experiences for any age, requiring maturity to handle them appropriately.
- *A child's negative fantasies cannot be predicted.* A child conceptualizes events differently than an adult does and if the child perceives the birth in a frightening way there is *no way to alter that negative fantasy.*

➤ A CHILD MAY IMAGINE THAT HIS MOTHER IS GOING TO DIE or be horribly changed. This is especially true if the labor is long and difficult and you make noises of discomfort and physical exertion.

➤ IN A CHILD'S LIMITED EXPERIENCE, a strained expression means anger or pain; blood means injury. The child may therefore have a frightening impression of what is happening to you—even if it is explained.

➤ A CHILD MAY BE FRIGHTENED seeing you in such a vulnerable state. Children perceive their parents as somewhat omnipotent. Although they must gradually develop refined opinions, it may be a shock to a child to see you in the physical and emotional vulnerability of birth.

- *What does your child know about sexuality?* The child's age will have some bearing on this, but a child's sexual knowledge and development should be considered.
- *What is a child's cognitive development?* This is related to the issue of negative fantasies and how a child perceives a situation. A younger child may have a harder time understanding explanations of what is happening and reassurances that you will be fine.
- *Birth is bloody*. How will the child handle that? (On page 287 there are suggestions on preparing a child.)
- *Sibling rivalry may be lessened* if a child watches his baby brother or sister born. Some people who have included a sibling in childbirth found that it enhanced family closeness and attachment. There was little sibling rivalry because the older child saw

the birth happen rather than being introduced to a wrapped bundle several days later.

It has been suggested that there is a critical attachment period for siblings and the newborn comparable to the maternal–infant bonding period right after birth. Only recently has the bond between the father and the newborn been considered; we can assume that the paternal–infant bond is similar to the feelings a sibling might have if allowed to get involved immediately with the new member of the family. This bond can result in permanently enduring and beneficial effects on the sibling relationship.

— *Small children are probably more influenced* by the reactions of adults around them than by the birth itself. A small child's sense of the world and expectations of it are not fully formed. If adults are happy with what is happening, the child probably will be. Of course, a child would be distressed if his mother were to scream or cry. This is a rare occurrence, but it could cause the child to fear for her safety.
— *Practice your breathing and pushing exercises when your child is around.* Simulate sounds of grunting, groaning, and moaning before birth. Tell the child what hard work labor is and how hot and sweaty and tired it can make you. If the child *does* get anxious during delivery, it may be better to encourage him to stay so there will be evidence of a happy outcome to all your hard work. This way the child can see that reality did not bear out the anxiety.

Suggestions for Siblings Attending Birth

➤ *Tell the child* as soon as possible that a baby brother or sister is going to be born.
➤ *Educate and expose* the child to everything you can about the birth process. If you can relate the discussions to what happened when the child was born, it may make it easier to grasp and relate to.
➤ *Take the child to at least one prenatal visit*. Let your child can meet your doctor or midwife and listen to the fetal heartbeat.
➤ *Show the child diagrams, drawings, photos,* and, if possible, a color movie or videotape about childbirth. Just as with adults, if a child is prepared and knows what to expect, the experience will be enhanced. It is important that at the child's level of understanding he learns about the physical process of labor and birth, including what uterine contractions are, dilation of the cervix, the stages of labor, etc. There are certain topics that should be discussed ahead of time with any child.

Topics to Talk About

— There will be *blood and amniotic fluid* on the mother and baby. The child must be reassured that it's okay, that it's normal, that it happened when he was born, too.

— The *sounds of work and/or pain* made by the mother can be frightening to a child. It is advisable to demonstrate to children the sounds that are common during labor and delivery.

— The fact that *labor is hard work* and an intense experience is something that should be thoroughly discussed ahead of time. This is an area that can be especially difficult for children: just when they feel they need their mother, she is unavailable to them. They have to understand that it is important that they let their mother work during contractions and not disturb her during them.

— *The mother's pain* during labor and the facial contortions that may accompany it should be talked about ahead of time. You must explain to the child that this pain is okay, that it's not like when you fall down and get cut. The pain of labor is good—the mother's body is doing the work it was made to do. However, stretching inside and opening to let the baby out can hurt.

— Discuss the *appearance of the newborn*, with special attention to the umbilical cord and placenta. The child should realize that the cord will be cut, which will not be painful to the mother or the baby. Explain that the baby may cry loudly in the beginning, which doesn't mean there's anything wrong; it's a sign of a strong baby. Describe, or show pictures beforehand, of the placenta, explaining what its function was for the baby in the womb.

— *Episiotomy (or tear) repair* should be discussed as a possibility. However, some of the people who favor siblings at birth feel that this may be too disturbing to watch. The decision should be up to individual parents, of course. You should see color photos or, better yet, moving pictures of an episiotomy before you subject a child to watching it. You might also ask yourself what can be gained by a child being present, and what the harm might be.

If the child has *never or rarely seen his mother naked*, or the mother is uncomfortable about being naked in front of the child, that must be sorted out before the birth. Perhaps taking a bath together, if they've never done that, is a natural and easy way to feel comfortable.

> ➤ **There should be an adult provided especially** for the child—or for each child if there is more than one attending the birth. It should be the sole responsibility of that person to see to the child's needs. Obviously it should be someone who can answer questions and give emotional support, who is comfortable with the child and vice versa. If the child needs entertaining, needs to go for a walk, needs to eat, and so on, make sure that the support person you pick will be willing to do all that.

Be sure you ask yourself an important question: Who does the child usually turn to if he or she needs someone? If it is always to the mother, *will the child be satisfied with a substitute?* If you don't answer this question honestly—or discuss it with the child if he's old enough—then you may be asking for trouble.

➤ *You might give the child a specific task during labor* to include him more actively in the experience. Depending on the child's age, you may want to give him the job of supplying ice chips or cool washcloths, for example.

➤ *Allow the child to come and go at will,* both in the birth room and in the house. Some children may be disinterested or may get bored with waiting. There's no use trying to encourage them to be more attentive, some just don't get very involved.

➤ *Wake up a sleeping child to see the birth* only if there is a familiar person to be with him. It can be disorienting to be awakened in the middle of the night and be confronted with the intensity of childbirth.

➤ *Reassure the child after the birth* that everything is all right. Both parents should do this, but the child may need particular reassurance from the mother.

ALTERNATIVES TO HAVING A SIBLING PRESENT

➤ *Include the child* as much as possible before birth. Bring the child with you to prenatal exams and share any information you have about pregnancy that a child can understand.

➤ *If you are having a birth at home,* you can *send the child to a neighbor's house* for the labor and delivery and have the child return immediately after birth.

➤ *Introduce the sibling to the new baby as soon as possible;* while you are breast-feeding is a good time. Just bringing a baby home with no preparation can create hostility. It can be compared to a man bringing home a beautiful woman and just announcing that she is going to be a "co-wife."

UNDERWATER BIRTH

Underwater birth may be something you'll hear about, therefore it is included as a "choice in childbirth." Fortunately, it is being done only by "fringe elements."

The justification for underwater birth is that it allows the baby to go from one liquid environment to another, thereby lessening birth trauma. There is no mammal on earth that goes into the water to deliver its young, other than whales . . . but then they live in the water, of course.

The fact about birth is that the baby is *supposed* to make the critical adjustment from intrauterine existence to the outside world. The baby's survival depends upon his making the many adjustments that are required for life outside the womb. The moment the placenta separates, the baby is on his own and his lungs must supply oxygen. If the baby is born underwater, there is no way to tell when the placenta has separated; the baby may take water into his lungs rather than air. The baby will drown. This has happened to some of the people practicing this fad in birthing.

The first few minutes of a baby's life are critical in assessing how he is adjusting to the extrauterine environment. If the baby is underwater, there is no way to monitor his responses, and therefore no way of helping a baby that may be having difficulty. Why anybody would be willing to take this life-threatening risk is hard to fathom.

❧ ❧

CHAPTER TEN

Choosing a Doctor and a Hospital

CHOOSING A DOCTOR

There is some debate about whether your choice of doctor or hospital should come first, but choosing a doctor seems to be the first and more essential task.

How to Find a Doctor

➤ **Ask women you know** who have had a baby recently whether they would recommend their doctor. However, it is not enough to simply accept a vague endorsement like "Dr. Stevens was really nice." Be aware that most women may not have had the benefit of the information you have gotten from this book and they may not know what options they could have had. If a woman you know recommends her obstetrician, ask her specific questions about areas that are important to you: "How much time did he give you in prenatal visits and how did he answer your questions?" "Was he with you during your entire labor in the hospital?" "Was she genuinely supportive of prepared-childbirth techniques, or did she suggest drugs at the first sign of your discomfort?"

Perhaps in addition to asking women, you could ask their husbands how they liked the doctor. Find out if they found the doctor straightforward, open-minded, and interested in the needs of the baby's father.

➤ **Write to the ICEA** (International Childbirth Education Association), P.O. Box 20852, Milwaukee, Wisconsin 53220. They

291

can send you a list of CEA member groups and individuals in your area who are supportive of Lamaze and other childbirth techniques. This is a particularly good way to find a doctor if you're moving to a new town.

➣ *The La Leche League* and other childbirth groups can make recommendations of doctors that their members have been pleased with. Although these recommendations will be coming from people you don't personally know, the doctors they endorse are probably progressive and responsive to nontraditional methods and attitudes toward birth.

➣ *Female doctors in obstetrics* used to be rare, but now half of the new doctors coming out of medical school to specialize in obstetrics and gynecology are women. However, just because a doctor is female does not necessarily mean that she will be more sympathetic or supportive. If you go out of your way to find a female doctor because you assume her attitude will be very different from a male physician's, you may be disappointed.

Medicine has been predominantly a male field: women who have entered that arena have had to deal with chauvinism and pressure. Some women obstetricians say that in order to finally gain acceptance by their male colleagues they had to become "more male than the men, like being hazed for a fraternity." This is not to say that many of the female doctors around are not excellent physicians—and they *may* be very understanding and warm as well. However, just because they are women does not give you any guarantee of this. If you are intent on receiving care from a woman, you might want to consider a hospital clinic that has certified nurse-midwives or an obstetrician who employs one.

Ask a Doctor Questions

➣ *Asking questions* is the best way of choosing a doctor. In order to have the best possible birth experience you have to make your needs clear to the doctor from the beginning. Then you have to be able to determine whether s/he is able or willing to meet those needs. This means that you first have to inform yourself and *decide* what your needs are before you even approach a doctor.

➣ *Time is limited*, so you should choose questions that reflect the aspects of birth that are most important to you. You don't want to bombard a prospective doctor with too many questions.

➣ *The way that you ask* questions is of utmost importance: it can influence the doctor's response. If you are too aggressive, it can make a doctor feel threatened or angry. Saying, "I demand . . ." is not a very good way to introduce a subject. A doctor has spent a great deal of time and effort reaching his level of accomplishment: if a patient announces "I demand . . ." she is diminishing the importance of the doctor's expertise. A less threatening way to begin a sentence is "How do you feel about . . . ?'' or ''What do you think about . . . ?'' This allows you to bring up an issue while acknowledging the doctor's intelligence and training.

Do not use a strong style of questioning. You'll only be harming yourself and your chances of getting what you want. Many of the controversial issues about birth require negotiation and cooperation between doctor and patient—if you assume a greater-than-thou (or even, depending on the doctor, an equal-to-you) attitude, it can put off a doctor. Keep in mind your final objective: to assure yourself the kind of birth you want. If getting that requires some self-control, or even role-playing on your part, it may be worth the sacrifice.

➤ *A doctor should answer your questions without rushing you*. Find out from the receptionist when you call for an appointment how many patients are scheduled per hour: appointments fifteen to twenty minutes apart is generally good. Then you can see for yourself how crowded the waiting room is— keep in mind that your doctor may share the practice with several other OB/GYNs, so a crowded waiting room doesn't necessarily mean you will be rushed. However, it can mean that the doctor is overbooked, rushed, or may be coming to the office straight from a delivery. A wait of up to an hour is not uncommon.

If you are compatible with a doctor, then you may have to make this sacrifice of your time; bring a book or something else to occupy you so that you aren't climbing the walls by the time you are called in. The realities of an OB/GYN practice usually mean a fairly long wait, but the essential point is whether *once you are with your doctor* she or he answers your questions without giving you the feeling that you are an annoyance.

➤ *Try to get direct, specific answers* to your questions. Some doctors may be unaccustomed to being questioned and feel they are being put on the spot. They may qualify their replies with statements such as, ''Depending on the circumstances . . .'' In this case, it is to your benefit to pin the doctor down to a more concrete answer. Tell him that his vagueness makes you anxious. Ask him under what conditions could the father *not* be in the delivery room, for instance, or would the Leboyer technique be abandoned. Although doctors cannot give you absolute promises (because labor is so unpredictable), you can get an idea of how the doctor's mind works by the way he answers.

➤ *Trust has to go both ways*. While it is important for you to find out as much as possible about the way a doctor thinks, it is equally important for him to believe that you respect and trust him. This is why you have to sit down *at the beginning* of your relationship with a doctor and clarify things. If a woman second-guesses a doctor constantly, throughout the pregnancy, then she needs another doctor. Of course, there will be questions which crop up about information you learn along the way, but it's best to settle important basics at the beginning. No doctor can work effectively if she or he is going to get the third degree every time you walk in.

➤ *Some doctors are going to react badly* no matter how you phrase your questions. Some MDs have grown so accustomed to having complete control that they consider any question an impertinent attack on their capabilities. Here's an example of how nasty a doctor can become if he or she feels threatened. A woman was trying to decide whether to stay with her longtime OB/GYN when she got pregnant. Until she asked these questions, he had been a charming, nurturant man. She asked the question, "Can I keep the baby with me for half an hour after it's born if everything's okay?" "What do you want to do that for?" he snapped back at her. She was stunned, but continued apologetically, "To get to know each other—for bonding." "Bonding, shmonding," he said in disgust. "You want to keep the kid between your legs for twenty-one years? You've got to cut the cord sometime." The woman said nothing, but she found another doctor immediately. This is just a warning that you may see a very different side of your doctor when you ask questions.

Making the Most of Your Relationship with Your Doctor

➤ Try to limit your calls to the doctor by first checking the index of this book to look for reassurance and answers.

➤ For issues that aren't urgent, make a note to remind yourself of the question for your next office visit. Keep a little notebook where you jot down your concerns so that you won't worry about forgetting it in the meantime, or arrive at your appointment and have it all fly out of your head.

➤ When there's something you really want to talk to the doctor about, you should feel free to make that phone call—but be aware of how limited his/her time may be. Before calling have your thoughts collected, perhaps with a few notes to yourself, so that you can be specific about any symptoms you're having.

➤ Some people feel so anxious at the doctor's office that they don't clearly hear or remember the information or instructions they're given. If this might be true of you, bring some paper and a pen with you so that you'll have a clear record of advice and facts, both for yourself later and for your partner if he isn't able to be with you at those appointments.

➤ Don't overreact when you hear or read something about pregnancy or birth that's news to you or contradicts what your doctor has told you. Share whatever you've read, or report on what you saw on TV or heard elsewhere, and give the professional a chance to respond. Certainly don't wave it at your doctor as a challenge: that's like waving a red flag in front of a bull. Instead of making your doctor your adversary, allow him or her to be your partner in health care, asking his/her opinion about the topic.

➢ Don't be afraid to speak up if anything is bothering you in your doctor's delivery of health care. If you're uncomfortable with how your physician speaks to you, treats you in the office, or you think she or he might have made a mistake or forgotten something, speak your mind. Doing so calmly, objectively, and with an open mind will encourage your doctor to respond in kind.

SOME QUESTIONS TO ASK ON THE PHONE

There are several revealing questions you can ask on the telephone before meeting a doctor. This gives you a chance to feel him or her out and perhaps save you both time if you discover you aren't on the same wavelength. Please don't misunderstand: the intention of these questions is not to trick or trap a doctor. It is simply a way of discovering whether you share the same ideas about pregnancy and birth. After that you can make an appointment for a preliminary visit.

➢ *"What percentage of your patients do you refer to childbirth education?"* A doctor may not know the exact percentage, so if he hesitates you might add, "One half? One quarter? None?" A doctor's reply will let you know his or her views about prepared childbirth. A doctor whose patients usually take classes is going to be more accustomed to expectant couples who want to be together, who ask questions and perhaps resist certain routine procedures in the hospital, and who generally want to be involved in the process. A doctor who isn't accustomed to this kind of patient is going to be more resistant to your requests for a personalized birth experience.

➢ *"Would you consider eliminating some routine procedures in the hospital?"* A doctor's answer to this lets you know where she or he stands in relationship to the hospital. A doctor may ask you to explain which procedures you're referring to—either because a patient has not made this request before *or* because he wants to get an idea of where you are "coming from." In the next section about choosing a hospital you can decide which of the routines (if any) you would want eliminated and why. Once you are specific with the doctor—for instance, if you would like an enema to be at your option—you can judge how flexible he is. Do not assume a doctor is *in*flexible, however, simply because she or he questions *you* after you bring up the issue. A doctor has just as much right—and need—as you do to discover if you're on the same wavelength. If you can give a doctor a valid reason for wanting a change from routine, he may be much more willing than if you become defensive.

A doctor who is open-minded about eliminating some routines is not intimidated by the institution of the hospital. A willingness to bypass routines suggests a belief that your desires are as important as some rules made for the efficiency of the system. For that reason, this question can tell you a great deal about the physician.

➤ *"Do you support breast-feeding on the delivery table and nonseparation for about forty-five minutes after birth?"* A doctor who is enthusiastic about this shows an awareness about maternal–infant bonding and its importance. A doctor might add the stipulation that he or she would allow this first bonding if there are no complications with the baby. (With any such request, there is the underlying presumption that it can happen only if there are no complications with the mother or the baby.)

A positive reply to this question can also show a doctor's awareness of the importance of keeping the family close after birth so that both parents can bond with each other and the baby. To give you an idea of how vital I personally believe the reaction to this question is, I made my initial choice of medical advisor for this book based on that. I said to Dr. Karen Blanchard: "Would you think it was irresponsible if this book suggested to parents of a healthy baby that they refuse to allow a delivery room nurse to take their baby away to the nursery?" "I think it would be irresponsible *not* to suggest that" came her immediate reply.

Some Questions You Might Ask in the Office

➤ *"What time will you get to the hospital?"* A very busy doctor cannot afford to arrive at the hospital when you do and stay there throughout your labor—he or she has a heavy schedule of office visits and perhaps other women who may be delivering around the same time you do. There are doctors, however, who want to be with a woman throughout her entire labor. If you feel that the physical presence of your doctor will make a huge difference in your feeling more secure and supported, you should say so. Even if the doctor does *not* usually sit with a woman throughout her whole labor, he might be willing to try to accommodate you.

A doctor may check in on you in early labor to be sure you are in true labor and then go back to the office. If the office is near the hospital, the obstetrician may tell the nursing staff to call when you are "complete and on the perineum" (meaning that your cervix is completely dilated and the baby's head is bulging on your perineum). Some women have felt abandoned and disappointed by doctors who arrive just in time to "catch the baby." Other women, depending on their relationship with their mate and the doctor, don't mind this at all.

You should discuss the issue of when the doctor arrives with your partner or coach and decide for yourselves how important the doctor's early arrival and/or constant presence will be for you. For some it can be comforting and reassuring just to have the doctor there; other women may feel a certain pressure in having the doctor hovering around. It depends on your attitude toward labor: how confident you feel about any childbirth training you'll have, what your relationship is to the doctor, how independent you and your mate or coach have become, how supportive the hospital appears to be, and so on.

➤ *"What kind of analgesia or anesthesia do you prefer?"* A doctor who says that it depends on what is happening with your labor is giving a fair answer—maybe none will be required. This will tell you that the doctor is familiar with natural, non-medicated childbirth and does not automatically assume that drugs will be used. You could then add, "If needed, which ones do you commonly use?" A doctor may be somewhat limited in his or her reply because of what is offered by the affiliated hospital. However, it is safe to say that a doctor who says he does "routine spinals" (saddle blocks) is not going to leave a lot of room for nature to take its course! In the chart "Medications During Labor" (on pages 402–404) you can see the pros and cons of "spinals" for yourself. (You should be wary of a doctor who routinely uses an anesthetic that can be administered only at the very end of labor, when you need it least, and that can give you a headache for months after delivery.

➤ *"What percentage of your patients are induced?"* For medical reasons this should only be 10% at the very most (the section on induction in Chapter 9 explains this). A doctor who has a 20% induction rate is a doctor who is unaware of or ignores the dangers of induction. She or he is also a doctor who is aggressive about interfering with the natural progress of labor. Depending on what sort of answer you get, you might want to ask the doctor how many patients' labors are *started* with synthetic hormones and what percentage are *stimulated* by them in early labor. A doctor may not know exactly what percentage of patients receive synthetic hormones at any time during labor, but the answer will tell you whether or not he or she favors the use of it. Doctors who are more conservative about medical intervention in labor will let you know that; those who see no harm in it will reflect that in their reply.

➤ *"When do you use forceps?"* The answer to this question may also tell you something about the extent to which a doctor intervenes in the natural labor process. The standard, conservative answer would be, "When a woman has been pushing adequately for two hours and the baby is not coming down." A doctor might qualify that answer by adding that, depending on how high up the baby is "stuck," he or she might elect to do a cesarean instead of a high forceps (a common practice nowadays because the outcome is better for babies). You could also ask, "Do you use vacuum extractors and when?" Although fairly popular in Europe, vacuum extractors have not caught on much in America, and, perhaps because of lack of practice, in the United States there is a high number of cerebral hematomas associated with the use of extractors. By asking, you can find out when and how the doctor favors helping the baby descend. Some women have strong feelings against forceps deliveries (because of bruising the baby), so by asking this question you can find out whether a doctor uses forceps routinely or is more conservative.

➤ *"Do you have any recommendations about diet or drugs?"* A doctor should, optimally, volunteer information about nutrition and medications during pregnancy, but we don't live in an optimal world. Doctors are busy; doctors aren't routinely taught nutrition in medical school; even worse, some doctors hang on to outdated ideas on the subject. Therefore, raise the subject, but don't get your hopes up too high. However, there are several replies that you should know the significance of. If a doctor says she likes to restrict weight gain to under 20 pounds, *beware*. There was at one time a belief that toxemia of pregnancy was caused by weight gain; it is now known that is not true. It is also know that a *minimum* gain of 20 to 24 pounds will result in a healthier baby. Doctors who try to limit weight gain to below that amount may also prescribe diuretics (water pills) and restrict salt in your diet. These practices are unhealthy for you and the baby and are discussed in more depth in the nutrition section of Chapter 4. If for some reason you wish to stay with a doctor who holds these ideas, you had better be prepared to deal with the fallout from disregarding improper nutritional advice. If a doctor simply says, "Eat a well-balanced diet" and gives you no specifics, it means that he or she does not know the specifics. There is no particular harm in this as long as you *inform yourself* and eat accordingly.

Considerations When Choosing a Doctor

➤ *A doctor should be supportive of your mate.* The most important support you should get is for your partner to take childbirth education classes with you and for you to be together in labor and delivery. Your mate should come with you to a prenatal visit at least once, even if you do not plan to have prepared childbirth. The baby's father should have a chance to meet the doctor and ask some questions of his own. One way to get a sense of whether a doctor is supportive of fathers is to say on the phone that your mate wants to come to the first appointment; you may be able to tell just from the doctor's (or receptionist's) attitude whether the office is accustomed to the participation of fathers-to-be.

➤ *If a doctor has a group practice*, ask to see the other doctors in rotation at subsequent prenatal visits. Some doctors already have their practice set up that way, but if not, you should say you'd like to meet the others. However, just because doctors share a practice does not mean that they share views about every aspect of pregnancy and birth. You can discover that although your doctor is a firm supporter of prepared childbirth, another doctor in the practice seems to give it only grudging lip service. You can also discover that while your doctor's bedside manner is comfortable for you, you feel ill at ease with his partner. If you have this problem, try to decide what is bothering you, whether you can talk about it and clear it up, or whether you can overcome the feeling.

Realistically, there is a fairly good chance that you will not be attended by your primary doctor if you don't go into labor during the hours that she or he is on duty. The only way most obstetricians can keep their offices running fairly smoothly—and get some sleep once in a while!—is to work with another doctor or doctors. If you have a long-standing relationship with a doctor, he might be willing to make an exception and promise you, within reason, that he will attend your birth. But do not fail to meet his colleagues even if you get such an assurance. For example, your doctor may have been up with another delivery for twenty hours when you go into labor and therefore wouldn't be able to attend your delivery.

Importance of the Doctor's Attitude

➤ *A doctor's attitude to your pregnancy will affect your attitude*. Even once you've chosen a doctor you like, you need to be aware of how subtle aspects of his or her style can affect your attitude about pregnancy. If she says, "I've examined your blood and urine and everything's fine," and says nothing about the *feelings* of pregnancy, the underlying message is, "Be a good girl and go home; I don't want to hear about your feelings." Yet you may be aware of emotional changes and want to discuss them. However, you may feel your emotions are petty and unimportant if your doctor doesn't encourage you to talk about them. A doctor who treats you as an intelligent, rational adult is supporting you during a time of personal growth.

By encouraging you to participate in childbearing decisions, a doctor helps you to build confidence in your own abilities. That feeling of self-reliance is important during pregnancy, and even more vital for motherhood and all the decisions you will be facing.

Your attitude toward your pregnancy—as a time of growth—will affect your attitude toward your child from birth. If a doctor discusses your expectations about parenthood, he is approving and setting into motion your exploration in this new world you are entering. If your feelings are denied during pregnancy and birth, it can influence your parenting, perhaps pushing you toward being a less sensitive or flexible parent.

➤ *Is a younger or older doctor better?* An advantage of older doctors is that they may be more attuned to natural childbirth because there was not as much technology when they began to deliver babies: they may have more patience and trust in natural processes. A doctor graduating from medical school in the last five to ten years *probably has never seen a "natural" birth*. (Anything less than a cesarean delivery is considered "natural" these days!) Some doctors are trained to view birth as a medical emergency, and intervening—with machines, drugs, and procedures—is normal for them. This is not to say that there aren't doctors who are aware of this problem and compensate for it in their practice. Some doctors do trust nature to take its course and have patience before intervening.

➤ *Flexibility on both your part and the doctor's* is essential. Right from the start it is vital for you to make your needs clear to your doctor if you want to have the best possible experience. At the same time, you have to leave room for any of the unforeseen developments that can arise in pregnancy and birth. There is no sense in having a doctor if you don't trust and listen to him or her. Remember that no doctor can honestly give you guarantees about labor procedures. You can discuss what you'd like in a "best case scenario," but until labor is in progress no absolute decisions can be made. If you try to demand absolute promises ahead of time, it can make a doctor feel boxed in. Your inflexibility can make a doctor feel helpless or powerless and she or he may become hostile. If your prejudices tie her hands (for example, if you refuse medication suggested by the doctor during labor), it leaves a doctor no room to exercise her best judgment.

➤ *A doctor has his or her own point of view*, which is based on medical tradition, training, and personal experience. This does not mean that you may not be able to change his or her point of view. Give *feedback* to your doctor: pass on what you've read and heard. Express how you feel about his or her style of doing things. A doctor will think that what he is doing is what people want unless you say otherwise. Be sensitive to the fact that some doctors may have trouble learning from patients, but they can overcome this tendency if you approach them with an unthreatening attitude. If you take the position that you are in this together and you want to share what you've learned, many doctors will make an effort to meet you halfway.

➤ *The doctor as God* is a social attitude that hinders doctors as much as it does their patients. Some pregnant women have been partially responsible for putting an obstetrician up on a pedestal and leaving all decisions up to him or her. In addition, our society treats doctors as deities. It may massage a doctor's ego to get better treatment in a restaurant, but in the long run it is an awesome burden for doctors that they be all-knowing and all-capable. Pregnant women can gain pride and strength as they exercise their intelligence and free will in birth choices: the doctors benefit, also. As prospective parents take more responsibility, it reduces the pressure on doctors. When a couple is involved in the decision-making process, it can reduce the tendency toward malpractice suits. Most of us are raised to believe that doctors are omniscient and omnipotent. The people who say they have *no* faith in doctors are simply rebelling against that social belief. Somewhere in between is the truth—that doctors are people like everybody else. They have training and experience, but the human body (particularly that of a woman in labor) is full of mystery and doctors cannot have all the answers.

➤ *How should you address a doctor?* Whether or not to call a doctor by his or her *first name* is tied up with the problem of social reverence. Would you call your lawyer "Mr.——"? If your doctor addresses you by your first name, you have the option to do the same. If she calls you "Mrs." (or "Ms." or "Miss"), you can suggest being less formal and call each other by your first names. It may only be words, but they carry a great deal of weight—it helps to equalize and demythologize the doctor/patient relationship if you call a doctor by name rather than by title. It may take a bit of getting used to for both of you, but you may find it eliminates some of the role-playing that unconsciously goes along with her calling you "Sally" and your calling her "Dr. Abrams."

LEAVING A DOCTOR

➤ *Don't stay with a doctor if you feel uncomfortable*. First try to identify what it is you don't feel right about. Then decide whether you can talk to the doctor and resolve the issue. Often just by pointing something out, you can clear the air and get on a better footing. You also have to determine whether your discomfort is a feeling you can overcome without confronting the doctor.

➤ *If you decide not to choose a doctor*—or if you decide to leave a doctor you have been seeing—you owe it to yourself, to the doctor, and to his present and future patients to explain why you aren't staying. Some women may feel comfortable talking to a doctor about this in person or on the phone: you may prefer to write a letter. Unless you take the time to explain why you aren't staying with a doctor, he will not know it is because you were dissatisfied with attitudes or procedures. In order for improvements to come about in the future, each pregnant woman has to make as much effort as each obstetrician. A doctor can only respond to consumer demands if he knows what they are.

If you have seen a doctor several times, then you must write a letter in order to retrieve part of any lump sum payment you've made, or to release yourself from any future obligation. For example, here's a letter to a doctor whose ideas on natural childbirth don't agree with yours:

Sample Letter to a Doctor You're Leaving

Dear Dr. X:

This is to inform you that I will no longer require your services for prenatal care and delivery.

My desire is to have as natural a childbirth as possible. I want to avoid medication and other intervention in the natural process of birth. I also feel very strongly about maternal–infant bonding—breast-feeding on the delivery table and nonseparation from my baby at birth. I did not feel that you (and your colleagues) share my beliefs sufficiently for my pregnancy and birth to be the kind of experience I want.

I do not underestimate the medical aspects of birth or you expertise in that area. The problem is really an ideological one of commitment to safeguarding the personal side of birth with childbirth classes, a Leboyer delivery, and nonseparation of parents and child after birth.

Thank you for the care you have already given me. Please send me a bill for the _____ visits I have made to your office. Would you please send my medical records to my new obstetrician Dr. _____.

Sincerely yours,

The Cost of an Obstetrician

➤ ***Payment of your obstetrician's bill*** is often required in full by the seventh month or six weeks prior to delivery. It may seem like an unusual financial arrangement to be paying fully in advance, for services *to be rendered* in the future, but that is how many doctors run their offices. There are some doctors, however, who send a bill after the baby is born. Of course, much of this, too, may depend on the policy of your health insurer.

➤ ***Preliminary interviews are free*** with some doctors, or they may charge a nominal fee. This can be a reflection of a doctor's awareness that it is best for both of you to discover ahead of time whether you are going to be compatible.

➤ ***Do not pay until absolutely necessary***. This gives you the freedom to change to another doctor if you develop problems with your doctor or her associate(s). It also gives you time to learn about ideological differences between you which may not be noticeable immediately.

➤ *Paying in installments* may spare you a lump sum at the end of your pregnancy, but it also reduces your freedom to leave. If you have been paying portions of the total bill during the early months of your pregnancy, it can make you feel wedded to a doctor without feeling free to change your mind.

➤ *Ask what the fee includes*. Will there be extra charges if there are complications in delivery? Are the prenatal lab fees for blood and urine included? Will the doctor see you more than the routine number of visits if necessary as part of the fee?

Retrieving Prepayment

➤ *If you want to change doctors* and have already paid the full amount for prenatal care and delivery, send a letter asking for "an immediate refund for the 'future services' paid for but no longer desired." State that you wish to pay only for the office visits you have already had up to that time. There is a time problem here: you have given $1,000 (let's say) to a doctor and you need that money back right away in order to give it to the doctor you have chosen as a replacement. You may have only a few weeks in which to do that.

Ways to Get a Refund from a Doctor

➤ *Follow up your letter* with a phone call to the bookkeeper at your doctor's office. Ask when you can expect a check. If he or she doesn't know anything about it, explain your situation and say you will call back the following day. Call every day until you get a result.

If you are told you cannot get your money back—or you do not feel assured that an honest effort is being made to get a check to you quickly—inform the doctor's office that their lack of co-operation forces you to write to the County or State Medical Association. This may improve their cooperation.

➤ *Write a letter to the Medical Ethics Committee* of your County or State Medical Association. Simply state that you have decided not to have Dr. X deliver your baby, but that you have paid in full, in advance, for those future services and they are not refunding your payments (excluding prenatal visits you have already had). Explain that you must have the money back right away to pay Dr. Y, whom you have now chosen as your obstetrician. Follow this letter up with a phone call and ask what action has been taken. (If the medical association's intervention is too slow, you can try the more direct method below!)

➤ *Picket the doctor's office*. If all else fails, this may work. Doctors are not accustomed to being picketed; it is not good for their image. All you need is two or three friends (pregnant ones are preferable) and a few signs that say "Dr. X Unfair to Pregnant Women," or "Dr. X Stole My Money."

If the street where you are picketing is not visible from the doctor's office, have someone call his or her office to inform them that their office is being picketed. You will probably be invited into the doctor's office within five minutes and things will be straightened out! These may sound like hilarious, strong-arm tactics to you, but if you were to get trapped in situation like this you would want a solution. Courts of law are expensive and can take years—which won't help you with only a few months to spare.

WHY DOCTOR VISITS ARE IMPORTANT

Visits to the doctor are vitally important. A pregnant woman is not sick, but regular checks to spot potential problems are essential. It may seem boring or unnecessary to you, but many of the complications of pregnancy and birth give advance warning. Regular doctor visits make it possible to identify problems before they get more serious, or make preparations for a potentially complicated delivery. Routine prenatal visits are scheduled once monthly until 28 weeks, twice monthly until 34 to 36 weeks, then weekly until delivery. The exam consists of checking your weight, blood pressure, and fundal height.

Blood Pressure

Blood pressure is checked to make sure that you are not hypersensitive (suffering from high blood pressure) and to learn what "normal" is for you so that your blood pressure during labor can be evaluated. A woman who is 130/80 to 140/90 during pregnancy can have a slightly higher blood pressure during the late stage of active labor or during pushing without any significance. But a woman who was 100/60 in prenatal exams may be having a problem in labor at the same 130/80 to 140/90 rate. Your pressure is a baseline learned during prenatal care.

The *rule of thumb* is that a 20-point rise in the systolic (top) number or in the diastolic (bottom) number is significant. It is the "resting" pressure. Your system is under maximum pressure when your heart is working hardest, which is the systolic (or "pumping") measurement. Thus, when the diastolic is as high, it may be a sign of problems. For example, a 110/65 to 120/90 might indicate problems.

CAUTION: A blood pressure of 140/90 is high for a pregnant woman, especially if this is your first baby. At the very least, you should question your doctor about it. If he is nonchalant, you should have another doctor (or clinic) do a second blood pressure exam on you. Some doctors feel that if a pregnant woman's blood pressure goes to 140/90, she should be put in the hospital for observation and bed rest.

Fundal Height

Fundal height is the distance in centimeters from your pubic bone to the fundus, which is the upper, rounded end of your uterus. The measurement of fundal height is taken externally with a tape measure and can tell the growth of both the uterus and the fetus in relation to the gestation age. The fundal height approximately equals the number of weeks of your pregnancy. So, at 24 weeks the top of your womb will measure about 24 centimeters from your pubic bone.

Normal, full growth is 38 to 40 centimeters, although some petite women will never reach that because their five-or six-pound babies won't force the uterus up that far. A large or unengaged fetus can measure as much as 40 to 43 centimeters at full term.

Extreme Measurements of Fundal Height

‣ *No fundal growth* means you are in nonpregnant state (in which case another pregnancy test should be done), or you've had a missed abortion (miscarriage). In the latter case, an examination by the doctor is very important because there can be complications.
‣ *Slow fundal growth* has a variety of reasons. There can be an error in the due date. You may have a baby who is small for its gestation age. Or the fetus may be in a transverse lie position, meaning that you get wider, but your uterus does not grow upward.
   There can be "placental deficiency"—the placenta is not nourishing the fetus properly. Some doctors will induce labor before 40 weeks in this case, because as this condition worsens the baby can die in utero.
‣ *Rapid fundal growth* can indicate multiple fetuses, a large baby, a miscalculation on your due date, uterine tumors, or hydramnios (excess amniotic fluid).

The Results of Any Prenatal Tests

Ask to see your chart. It is your right. It informs you more fully so that you are better equipped to participate in making decisions about your pregnancy and labor. Ask the doctor to explain anything you do not understand or are concerned about. It is your body and your baby: if you don't know your blood pressure during pregnancy, then you won't know the significance of your pressure during labor. If you know and understand these processes, you will better understand what your body is doing during labor.

Coordinate Your Obstetrician and Internist General Practitioner

Any medication that your doctor prescribes for any illness or allergy you may have should be double-checked with your obstetrician, even though your GP or internist knows you are pregnant. Similarly, any medication which your obstetrician prescribes for pregnancy-related drugs should be checked with your caregiver. It is a measure of safety well worth the trouble. Why not have the benefit of two expert opinions rather than one?

Some Thoughts About Doctors

A doctor graduates from medical school equipped with technical skills and knowledge relating almost exclusively to complex medical problems—to treating patients who are seriously ill. Yet pregnancy and birth and not a sickness: they are a normal, healthy biological process. In only a very small number of cases does anything go wrong. This can make an obstetrician feel useless having gone through many years of effort and expense to prepare for complications which rarely occur. It is no wonder that obstetricians so frequently intervene in the natural process of birth: that is what they are trained to do.

People complain that doctors view labor as a purely physical process. It is true that doctors often behave as if they do not understand that birth is an intensely emotional event in a couple's life. Perhaps we are asking too much. Some doctors view birth solely as a bodily process in which many things can go wrong and they are there to correct them. Perhaps we should accept the fact that doctors develop a particular viewpoint during medical training (outside of a few rare obstetricians). Their viewpoint comes from seeing dire emergencies: women hemorrhaging, babies in distress, blood, death, deformities. In large training medical centers they see a good deal of that: it leaves its mark.

Doctors see a lot of births. Many times women without childbirth education may yell and scream during labor, as much from their fear about the unknown forces taking over their bodies as from pain. It is understandable that a doctor may see his or her role as a white knight, who will rescue the woman from this ordeal of childbearing.

Patients put unrealistic demands on doctors, who are expected to have all the answers, know everything, and be totally responsible. As women start taking more responsibility for their own bodies, it's going to be easier on everyone, but in the meantime doctors are still expected to know all and do all. Giving up traditional procedures in obstetrics may be frightening to doctors because it leaves them hanging—the medical procedure is taken away as a protection and there is nothing to replace it.

Doctors did not design the dangers in being alive . . . they want to minimize them. This is one reason they fall back on traditional medical thinking. No two labors are alike. The physical and emotional intensity of labor and delivery is awesome. It is *still* not understood what triggers labor; often machines and medications cannot control it. Yet doctors are nevertheless expected to know what is going on, to be in charge, to be responsible for the outcome of a perfect baby.

We should keep in mind that doctors may also feel frustration, pressure, guilt, depression, and strain. Being a doctor is a complex and difficult task, perhaps even harder than some doctors recognize. Do not be angry with a doctor who may be rigid—be compassionate toward a person who has been channeled into playing God by other men and women.

Doctors are not bad people, although some of them may be. Nor are they great people, although some of them may be. Mostly, doctors are decent people under a lot of pressure trying to do the best job they can.

The one danger is a doctor who practices medicine with his or her ego. There are doctors who have gotten so caught up in the role and people's expectations that they actually come to believe that they *do* have all the answers. Beware of any doctor, in or out of the hospital, who does not separate ego and medicine. An example would be any doctor who will not listen to any point of view that differs from his or her own, or who refuses to consider any unfamiliar procedure.

A major facet of American medicine is its ever-growing technology. New machines and tests are seen as progress. Thus, a doctor who uses the newest equipment and procedures may believe he or she is offering you the best (newest, most advanced) care available. Doctors are also acutely aware of malpractice suits. By using the latest technique a doctor can "prove" that she gave the best possible care. In a society that worships technology, that makes sense.

The soaring price of malpractice insurance is driving a lot of obstetricians out of their field in what may become a health care crisis. Obstetricians are facing more lawsuits, and higher losses from lawsuits, because there is an inherent risk of "bad outcomes" in the course of delivering babies. Mother Nature doesn't guarantee that every baby will be 100% perfect: She cares only that the species as a whole is perpetuated. Yet we demand a guarantee of a perfect baby every time from our obstetricians, and sue them when anything goes awry. Many doctors can no longer afford the skyrocketing cost of malpractice insurance, or perhaps they can't tolerate a medical–legal atmosphere in which they have to look over their shoulders and make decisions based *not* on the health and welfare of the baby and the new family but on what could happen later in a courtroom.

The facts are sobering: more than 25% of American OB/GYNs have given up obstetrics. Half of rural Nevada's family physicians no longer deliver babies. Doctors in Brunswick, Georgia, stopped accepting pregnant lawyers, law clerks, or lawyers' wives as patients. By 1985 there were already seventeen counties in Alabama with no obstetrical care.

CHOOSING A HOSPITAL

The only way to find out what a hospital can offer you is to go there and *ask questions*. There is a questionnaire you can take with you to help you make your decision. (See "Questionnaire for Hospitals" pages 330–332.)

➤ *Take a tour of the hospital*, with your mate if possible. If there is no scheduled maternity tour, then ask for a personal tour. If a hospital will not allow you to see their facilities and ask questions, *be suspicious*: they are likely to be equally rigid in their maternity care.

➤ *Find out the location of the night entrance* to the hospital. Many hospitals lock their front doors at 10 P.M. and many women go into labor at night. Trying to search for the night entry during labor can be upsetting. Be sure your mate knows exactly where the night entrance is if he doesn't go on the tour with you.

Different Types of Hospitals

➤ *Catholic hospitals* can be quite restrictive in certain policies, but they account for 30% of hospital beds in the United States. There are certain procedures which are banned in Catholic hospitals: for instance, if you want to save time and money and have a tubal ligation right after delivery, *do not go to a Catholic hospital*. They will not permit contraceptive procedures. Ask what their rules are beforehand.

➤ *A teaching hospital has the best medical facilities*. Residents are always on duty, so if you were to run into complications and your doctor was not there, you would be attended by a doctor until yours could arrive. Doctors see more births and more complicated births, which may be transferred there from lesser-equipped hospitals. If a cesarean became necessary, it could be done in a matter of minutes in a teaching hospital, where they have facilities and staff at the ready, unlike smaller hospitals.

One drawback to a teaching hospital is that there is resident/intern traffic walking through your labor room. The trade-off is that you get better facilities and equipment in case anything goes wrong with you or the baby.

➤ *A smaller, community hospital* can be more flexible. A large medical center has more red tape than a local hospital, which has a smaller staff and fewer patients.

If there are certain procedures you wish or don't wish during labor and delivery, you can go to the hospital administrator's office in a community hospital and discuss it ahead of time. It is like the difference between going to the corner store and talking directly with the owner or going to a huge shopping complex.

However, while you may be able to arrange for a more individualized childbirth at a smaller hospital, you will probably be forfeiting the costly equipment and newer facilities of a teaching hospital.

➤ *Family-centered maternity care* is offered by some of the more progressive hospitals, both large medical centers and community hospitals. Family-centered care usually involves the optional elimination of certain routine procedures and the optional addition of other procedures, but this varies from hospital to hospital. Just because a hospital says that it has family-centered care *does not guarantee you anything*. You may have to use the questionnaire (on page 330) to find out just how committed a hospital really is to the concept behind the words.

Above all, family-centered care has to do with a philosophy about childbirth: individualized care aimed at nurturing the family unit during labor, delivery, and postpartum. A hospital that has adopted this kind of maternity care is showing its respect for the importance—both personal and for the society at large—of childbirth.

There are certain choices that are associated with family-centered care, including eliminating routine procedures, Leboyer delivery, breast-feeding on the delivery table, nonseparation of parents and baby during labor, delivery, and recovery, rooming-in, early discharge, etc. These are described in the following section, but few hospitals offer all of them. You have to find out what is available at the hospital you've chosen, and then see if you can arrange for further options if you wish them. If you are not able to make arrangements you're comfortable with, you may have to go to a more flexible hospital.

HOSPITAL CHOICES

Anesthesia Policy

A hospital's handling of anesthesia depends on whether there is an obstetric anesthesiologist on duty full time. Some hospitals that do keep an anesthesiologist on the premises *will charge you whether you use the service or not*. Some hospitals give a laboring woman an anesthesia release form to sign when she's in transition, the toughest part of labor.

(This can be when her resolve to give birth without medication is at a low point.)

Find out whether there is a anesthesiologist "on call" and how long it would take him or her to reach the hospital and administer anesthetic if you needed or wanted it. Perhaps you might prefer waiting twenty minutes for him or her to arrive so that you don't have to sign a form obliging you to pay whether or not you use those services.

Breast-Feeding and the Hospital

Breast-feeding can be overtly or subtly supported or discouraged by hospital policy and attitudes.

> ➤ *Ask whether babies are encouraged to nurse immediately* after birth on the delivery table. The reason this is desirable is because it reinforces the baby's natural sucking instinct while giving her the colostrum (which precedes the milk and is full of antibodies) in your breasts. Also, the baby's suckling releases hormones into your system that help contract your uterus and stimulate your milk supply.
>
>   Some doctors prefer nursing in the recovery room instead of on the delivery table; it may be more relaxed because there is less going on around you to interfere. This is just as beneficial.
>
> ➤ *Find out whether breast-feeding is supported by the hospital* by asking whether they distribute breast-feeding literature to new mothers and, if so, from what source: the La Leche League (which actively supports nursing), a formula company, or other sources.
>
> ➤ *Ask whether a test feeding* of glucose and water is given routinely in the nursery. Giving a rubber nipple to a newborn you want to breast-feed can sabotage your efforts. A baby won't suck properly at your breast if she has been satisfied by the sugar water that was so much easier to suck from a rubber nipple. A baby who does not suck energetically won't stimulate your milk supply to come in, which in turn will not stimulate the baby to suck. Your confidence can be undermined and with it your new relationship with the baby.
>
>   If you do not wish your baby to have these supplementary bottles (which can wind up replacing your breast rather than supplementing it), then discuss this ahead of delivery with your pediatrician and have him or her note on your chart: "*No artificial nipples*" or "*No supplementary bottles*." Some doctors believe that such a feeding cleans out mucus from the baby's system, although breast milk has the same effect.
>
> ➤ *Ask whether babies are allowed to breast-feed on demand*. This means that your baby is brought in to you (if she isn't rooming-in) when she cries, rather than on an every-four-

hours schedule imposed by the hospital. It is extremely hard to establish successful breast-feeding if a baby is not allowed to nurse on demand when she is hungry. When your baby is hungry, she will nurse with the enthusiasm necessary to stimulate your milk supply to come in.

If a baby awakens in the central nursery (assuming rooming-in is not available, or you have not chosen it) she may be given a bottle of glucose and water or formula to quiet her. When the baby is brought in to you on the hospital's four-hour schedule, she will be full and sleepy and won't suck properly. Breast-feeding babies get hungry sooner than formula-fed babies because breast milk digests more easily and quickly. The four-hour feeding schedule was instituted for the convenience and smooth running of the nursery staff; if you want to breast-feed, that schedule can frustrate you and your baby.

➤ **Do not assume** that just because a hospital *does* have on-demand feeding that every person on the staff understands or is supportive of breast-feeding. When you read the section on breast-feeding in Chapter 15, you will see that a large part of successful breast-feeding has to do with your emotions. If you do not get early encouragement and advice, your milk supply may not come in quickly.

Ask for help. If you don't get it from the nurse(s) assigned to you, then ask for the nurse supervisor and tell her you need help: breast-feeding is something you have to learn—it isn't instinctive. Many hospitals and birthing center have breast feeding advisors on staff. If you feel discouraged or as if you want to give up, don't. The beginning is always the hardest. Anyone who says, "Your baby doesn't seem to want to breast-feed," or, "Your baby isn't gaining much weight," can undermine your efforts. If you can't get support in the hospital, call up your pediatrician, if you've found one who is supportive of breast-feeding. Or call up the La Leche League in the phone book; they will have a member talk to you or even visit you in the hospital to show you the ropes.

Early Discharge

This means that you can be released from the hospital within 6 to 24 hours after your baby is born. This option is most attractive to couples who prefer spending the first postpartum days at home. Perhaps they have come to the hospital primarily for the medical care available "just in case."

YOU CAN CONSIDER EARLY DISCHARGE IF . . .

— *If you had childbirth education* and went through labor and delivery without any medication (except a local for the episiotomy, if there was one). The main worry about early discharge is that you can have postpartum bleeding if your uterus does not continue to contract—drugs used during birth would increase the chances of hemorrhage.

— *If the labor, delivery, and a two-hour postpartum* period were all normal for mother and baby.

— *If you get infant-care training* (for a first baby). Otherwise the shock and your sense of helplessness with a newborn can be overwhelming. Seriously consider taking American Red Cross (or other) baby-care classes before delivery. You also might want to have a trained baby nurse or relative/friend at home who is experienced with newborns.

— *If you know that you can force yourself to take it very easy* at home. Some new mothers try and do everything right away, which can be exhausting and even dangerous. Some women regret not having stayed in the hospital where everything was done for them. *Wait to see how you feel* once the baby is born: you may feel terrific and eager to get out of the sterile environment of the hospital and back to your own surroundings, or you may be exhausted and not want to move.

— *If the hospital has some arrangement for postpartum care.* Some hospitals send a specially trained nurse to your home on the first day postpartum and then once or twice after that; others have a 24-hour hotline you can call for questions or problems. Early discharge works best if there is some ongoing contact with professionals who can assist you and the baby if necessary.

REASONS FOR EARLY DISCHARGE

— *You save a great deal* of money because you do not have the three-to five-day hospital stay, which can be up to $300 per day. (You could hire a registered infant nurse to come to the house for a few days and *still* save money!)

— *In a hospital you have no privacy* because there are people constantly coming in and out of your room. If you don't have a private room, you have to contend with a roommate and her baby and family at a time when you probably won't want that intrusion.

— *A hospital is a place of sickness* and there will be patients around who are not well. You may be treated as a sick person: your temperature will be taken, your ''bathroom performance'' questioned, and so on. Being in a setting where people are not well can have a negative effect on you.

— *Most hospitals don't provide rooming-in*, so you will be separated from your baby at the time when you most need each other. When a baby is kept in a central nursery and brought out for brief visits every four hours, it can make you feel as if the baby "belongs" to the nursery staff and they are "allowing" you to see him. Many women report that they only begin to think of their baby as their own once they are out of the hospital. Also, as mentioned earlier, separation from your baby can make breast-feeding difficult.

— *Most hospitals don't provide facilities for the baby's father*, siblings, or close relatives to bond with the baby, whereas at home they have natural access to him.

— *Breast-feeding may be enhanced* by being together at home in relaxed, familiar surroundings. One study showed that women who chose early discharge developed their milk supply in 36 to 72 hours. Mothers who breast-feed, but stay in the hospital, usually have milk within 72 to 120 hours. This difference may be in part because demand-feeding is unavailable in most hospitals.

Father Participation in Childbirth

➤ *A father's presence is fairly widely accepted* nowadays, but some hospitals attach certain conditions. The first thing to ask is whether a father is allowed to be with his wife in the labor room, then ask whether he is allowed in the delivery room at birth. Ask under what conditions a father must leave his wife. Although there is no medical justification for it, some hospitals require a man to leave if regional anesthesia (like an epidural) is used (others ask only that he leave while the anesthesia is first administered).

There are hospitals with double labor rooms which allow a partner to stay only if there is no one sharing the labor room. If you find out that there are rules like this about staying together, discuss it *ahead of time* with your doctor. Find out whether she or he can intervene and arrange for some sort of exception so that you can be sure to stay together. If that doesn't work, have your partner contact the hospital administrator and explain how important it is for you both to stay together. Ask whether this can be guaranteed unless there is a medical emergency which would make it necessary for your mate to leave.

➤ *Once you are in labor* and the father is told to leave, *ask for a definite reason* for his exclusion from the labor room. Say that the doctor promised you could be together (assuming that the doctor is not there to protect your agreement). Do not just meekly have the father leave: don't back down unless the staff assures you that it is an emergency situation. Try to stay calm and reasonable, but do not have the father leave unless it is clearly in the best interest of the mother and baby.

➤ *Several recent court cases* have upheld the right of local hospital administrators and doctors to make the final decision about whether fathers will be allowed in the delivery room at individual hospitals. *All lawsuits by fathers demanding entry have been unsuccessful so far*—so if you were considering that challenge to the system before birth, forget it!

➤ *"Do it anyway"* is pretty radical advice, but it may be the only choice you have as a last resort. Legally the hospital *could* call the sheriff on the grounds that you are trespassing, but it's highly unlikely that the hospital will do that as a baby is being born; it's more trouble than it's worth to them. Besides, it is illegal—considered a tort—for anyone to seize you. The hospital will probably decide it's a one-time problem and they'll let you stay in the delivery room. They may be nasty, say you're crazy, and even threaten you, but if you're willing to go through that, you can probably get what you want in a hospital (which is cheaper and quicker than suing, with a better chance of satisfaction!).

➤ *Some hospitals require that the father take the hospital's own prenatal classes*. Ask whether this is true at the hospital you are considering.

➤ *Some hospitals require that a couple be married* in order for them to stay together during labor and delivery. If you are not married, call and find out hospital policy. If they do have that rule, when the time comes and anyone asks, there is always the option of saying you are married. Being together for the birth of your child is the most important thing.

There is no reason, however, not to use your own names since more and more married couples do that. If anyone questions why you have different names, say that the woman uses her own name. If they say, "Oh, you've kept your maiden name?" you can say, "Yes, and my husband decided to keep his maiden name also."

➤ *Be sure the father goes with you on a tour* of the hospital beforehand so that he knows where to change into hospital clothes for the delivery room. There can be a rush to the delivery room: if there isn't anyone free at that moment to show a man where to change, he may wind up missing the birth.

➤ *Ask whether fathers have unlimited visitation* hours or at least can be with the mother and baby at times in addition to visiting hours. Find out whether fathers may hold their babies. (Yes, there are actually hospitals that do not allow fathers to touch their own babies!)

➤ *Find out whether the father is allowed into the recovery room*. Most hospitals do *not* allow the father in, but it can be lonely for you if you feel wonderful and are separated from both your baby and your mate at a time when you most want to be with them. It can be even more unpleasant if you are alone feeling great and lying next to a medicated woman or one who is emotionally negative.

Fetal Monitors

Monitoring is discussed at length on pages 270–275. You should find out whether fetal monitors are used in the hospital you are considering and whether they are mandatory or optional. You can then discuss the pros and cons with your doctor.

Food and Drink Policy

Whether you can eat or drink during labor often depends on what your doctor has noted on your chart. Most hospitals allow a woman to have *nothing by mouth* once she is admitted in labor. This is to guard against vomiting in case general anesthesia is used. Some hospitals allow a woman to have ice chips during labor; others will allow her to suck on candy. (However, it's not a good idea to eat candy during labor: sugar stimulates stomach acids, which can be more dangerous than a stomach full of food.) You might ask whether you would be allowed to have spoonfuls of honey for energy, but as with all these options, you should discuss them ahead of time with your doctor.

Advocates of home birth believe it's unhealthy for the baby and mother to deprive her of food and drink over many hours. They say this adds to the "pathologic environment" of the hospital. In countries other than America, light food and drink are permitted during labor; even in the United States they tell you to stay at home during very early labor because you can have liquids and other nourishment there which will be denied you as soon as you enter the hospital.

Some hospitals will not allow a man to eat in the labor room. Some couples feel it is inconvenient and also disruptive for him to have to leave. Often it is nice for the man to have a break and go to the cafeteria or elsewhere for a snack, but that should be his choice, not the hospital's.

Labor Rooms

➤ **Labor rooms are an important part** of your childbirth because you'll probably be in one for many hours. The most important question is whether the rooms are single or double. If you have taken childbirth training and are not offered a private labor room, then ask to be paired up with a woman who has also had classes. It is hard enough to maintain your concentration, relaxation, and control during labor; if you have an unprepared woman in the next bed, it may be difficult for you to be successful. She will probably be frightened, ignorant of what is happening to her body, and in pain—it can be upsetting to listen to a woman who hasn't had the benefit of classes to prepare her.

If it is not possible for you to be alone with another prepared mother and your roommate is voicing a lot of pain and fear, then do your best to tune her out. Bring a radio or cassette machine and play music. Ask for soft foam earplugs or cotton for your ears. This is not a joke—if you do not have a suitable atmosphere it is very difficult to concentrate, relax, and breathe. Ask if there's anywhere you can be moved to—find out if another room has opened up since you were admitted (which happens just as soon as another woman is ready to give birth and is moved to the delivery room). *But don't ask to have the other woman moved* . . . she's got enough problems as it is.

➤ **Ask whether you will be confined to bed** in the labor room. Some hospitals require a woman to stay in the bed. Lying still, (especially if you have also been given some sort of tranquilizer) can slow your labor and circulation to the uterus, create muscle weakness and less effective contractions. On the other hand, walking during labor can stimulate your contractions, help your pelvis open, and take advantage of gravity to bring the baby down. If you are in a hospital with a stay-in-bed policy, at least get up to go to the bathroom frequently. (You can also walk around and let your partner deal with anyone who "orders" you back to bed!)

Leboyer Delivery

Leboyer delivery can be done in any hospital, but it is easier if the staff is familiar with the technique. Of course, first you have to discuss and agree on it with your obstetrician. If you are told that a hospital does do Leboyer deliveries, ask whether this also includes facilities for the Leboyer bath (see page 283 for more information about this).

All that is needed for the bath is (1) a plastic baby tub, (2) warm sterile water, and (3) a radiant heater. If a hospital has never done Leboyer deliveries but your doctor agrees to it, you can bring a plastic baby bathtub. Arrange ahead of time for the hospital to have bottled sterile water ready, or bring three or four bottles yourself. These can be put unopened in hot tap water to warm them and poured into the bath after the baby is born.

Since the main concern about the Leboyer bath is the possibility of the baby getting chilled, it is important to have a heating element over the bath. However, no special equipment is required. In every delivery room there is a radiant heater over the wiping/warming tray that the baby is put in after birth. Either that heater can be moved away from the tray and positioned over the baby tub, or the bathtub can be placed inside the warming tray.

This means that you can have a Leboyer delivery even if the hospital is not familiar with the procedures, as long as your doctor is in favor and will encourage the staff's assistance.

Photographs and Tape Recording

Both photographing and recording are forbidden in many large medical centers. The hospitals' main worry is that photographs could be used later in a malpractice suit. Hospitals that do allow photographing and recording may require you to sign a photography release form when you preregister; sometimes hospitals won't allow flash equipment to be used. If there is no rule against photos, you still must have the consent of the hospital and your doctor.

Many people have found, however, that although the hospital may have a policy forbidding picture-taking, their doctor is not against it: so they simply take pictures quietly. One way to do it without a flash is to use the fastest 35mm film and push the ASA to 1000. Be sure to tell the lab that you have done this—there may be an extra charge for developing the film.

Prenatal Education Classes

Some hospitals offer classes, either free of charge, or there is a fee but it is lower than for outside classes. The problem with in-house childbirth training is that the teacher is an employee of the hospital and therefore cannot comfortably criticize hospital policies. However, as long as you get the training in breathing, relaxation, and working as a team, it really isn't important whether the teacher challenges the hospital's policies or not: you can do that yourself, if need be!

If the hospital does have classes, ask whether they also include exercise sessions, an extra benefit you don't get in most private classes.

The most important question is what percentage of the women who deliver at the hospital have had childbirth preparation. This will give you a good idea of whether the staff is familiar with and supportive of the techniques: nurses can help coach with your breathing if necessary, or can just boost your morale at low points. There is a world of difference between that and a hospital where little is known about prepared childbirth and the staff interrupts you during contractions, refers to them as "labor pains," and offers medication, all of which can sabotage your training.

Preregistration

It can save you a lot of time and aggravation to be already registered when you arrive in labor. Preregistration allows you to fill out all the many required forms ahead of time so that you can go right in when you're in labor. Be sure to also find out how much money is required on admittance and discharge so that you can come prepared. If you can keep your hospital suitcase in a safe place at home, you could put the money or money order in an envelope so you don't forget it in the rush to the hospital.

If a hospital does not offer preregistration don't worry: you are not required to fill out all the forms when you arrive. It is not legally necessary to have the paperwork done before a birth takes place. You will have to sign a few things, but if you don't want to be separated from your mate and you're having some difficulty coping with contractions, *go directly to the labor room*. Your mate can complete the forms for you.

Rooming-In

➤ *Find out whether the hospital offers the choice* of rooming-in and then ask whether it is an all-or-nothing option. This one of the fundamental features of family-centered maternity care which provides for your baby to stay in your room with you. Some hospitals provide only 24-hour rooming-in, meaning that the baby is always in your room and you don't have the choice of sending her back to the central nursery at night. This system is most convenient for the staff; the logistics are more complicated if they have to bring a baby back and forth.

Some cynics suggest that a hospital may offer only full-time rooming-in as a way of discouraging mothers from choosing it because it is easier for the staff to keep all the babies in the central nursery, bringing them all out at routine four-hour intervals. This seems an unfair accusation, although rooming-in does require nurses to keep track of which babies are with which mothers, as well as going to their rooms to give them help.

➤ *Some hospitals offer the choice of having the baby with you during the day* but sending him back to the nursery at night. This can give you more rest, especially if you are tired out from a long labor. Of course, then there will be the shock of reality when you go home a day or two later and there is no central nursery at night!

➤ *A few hospitals have an innovative circular layout* with the central nursery in the middle and the mothers' rooms encircling it like pieces of a pie. There are "drawers"—the same plastic bassinets used in most hospitals to hold the baby. You can push the drawer in to return your baby to the central nursery if you want to sleep or go out of your room. You can get your baby back whenever you want him by pulling out the "drawer." This way you can choose how much the baby will be with you and the nurses can keep an eye on him when you want to rest or walk around.

➤ *An important advantage of rooming-in* is that you can learn your baby's needs and begin adjusting to her habits. The average American woman doesn't have previous experience;

you probably won't even know what a newborn's normal color, breathing, and bowel movements are like. With rooming-in you get exposure to your new baby before you take her home. It also gives you a chance to discover the realities of newborn care while you are still in the hospital and can ask for advice from the staff. Many women's ideas of what is good mothering come from magazines and television ads—rooming-in gives them a chance to test out what it's *really* like, so they don't go home and panic or make themselves miserable trying to be "Super-mom."

➤ *Rooming-in does not mean that you're totally on your own*, helpless and isolated in your hospital room with a crying newborn baby! Nursing care and teaching go with rooming-in. This is even better if there are unlimited visiting hours for the baby's father, because he can also benefit from baby-care demonstrations. This can help you and your partner feel more confident about caring for and sharing the baby once you're home.

➤ *If you don't choose rooming-in*, or if the hospital doesn't offer it, the father may not be allowed time with his baby. Needless to say, this is not helpful to his bonding with the infant! If rooming-in is the only way you can be assured that the father and baby can spend time together, that is one more advantage to consider.

➤ *The baby's adjustment to life outside the womb* is helped by rooming-in. Studies show that a rooming-in baby more readily organizes cycles of sleeping, waking, and crying by being cared for by one person in the first ten days of life. These babies cried much less and established a day-night rhythm more quickly than those in a traditional nursery with multiple caregivers and rigid feeding schedules. Thus, the baby you take home after rooming-in may be different than he would be if you had left him in the central nursery. There's also a chance that you will probably be more adjusted to the baby's cycles and the baby will already be settling into patterns of sleeping and waking that will make it easier to fit the newborn into your life at home.

Routine Hospital Procedures

There are procedures which most hospitals perform on all women who are in labor. There is nothing wrong with these procedures except that they are carried out *routinely* without any regard for individual circumstances or preferences. Hospitals are large institutions and function most efficiently when there are rules and tasks that are performed across the board. However, this disregards what may be your personal wishes in some areas.

The more subtle harm of routine procedures is that they can make a woman in labor feel as if the hospital is in charge of her body: it may undermine her feeling of strength and capability. A hospital and its staff are authoritarian by nature, which is magnified by automatically imposing routine procedures. The question to ask the hospital is whether any of the procedures can be eliminated if your doctor agrees to it and notes it on your chart ahead of time.

➤ ***Enemas*** used to be given routinely to women in early labor so that the lower bowel is emptied to give the baby as much room as possible. Another reason is so that during the pushing stage you will feel free to push. The fear (embarrassment) of pushing out fecal matter may make some women tense, and therefore they push with inhibition. Also, if fecal matter is pushed out with the baby, it can contaminate the sterile area into which he is born. These are legitimate reasons for an enema.

However, there is a natural "cleaning-out" process in many women's bodies prior to labor or in early stages of labor. In fact, one sign that labor has begun is that you may have several bowel movements or diarrhea. Also, an enema may be unnecessary because you may not have eaten much before labor began and may have had a bowel movement fairly recently. In those cases you might want to skip the enema. You should discuss this possibility with your doctor ahead of time so that he can note on your chart that the enema can be eliminated at your discretion.

An enema can bring on stronger contractions. It can also cause you considerable discomfort and anxiety, rushing to the toilet and then having to sit there while you are coping with intensified contractions. In addition, your mate or other labor coach will probably have been asked to leave, so you have to deal with this alone. If you choose to have an enema, or are given no choice, at least be prepared for this temporary difficulty.

Another word of caution: the nurse may administer the enema, see you to the toilet, and then leave, telling you to stay there for fifteen minutes. You do *not* have to stay there exactly fifteen minutes nor do you have to wait for the nurse to return— nurses get busy in other rooms and may not be able to get back right away. Many women feel they must "do as they are told" and get trapped on the toilet much longer than necessary! Once you feel your bowel has emptied, you can go back to bed or to a chair—the worse that can happen is that you feel the need to go back to the toilet or else you mess up the bed a little. It's better to have to clean up the bed than it is for you to feel alone and uncomfortable and have your prepared childbirth techniques disrupted.

➤ ***IV is the abbreviation used for "intravenous solution,"*** a bottle of liquid which is fed into your system through tubing which is inserted into a vein, often in the back of your hand. An IV of glucose and water is routinely hooked up to women in labor. The general thinking is that it supplies your body with energy and fluids when food and liquid by mouth are prohibited. Also, synthetic oxytocin such as Pitocin can be administered through the IV solution (although it can be an inaccurate method—see the section on "Induced Birth," pages 277–282).

If you object to an IV, it's likely you'll be told there's a critical reason that an IV has to be inserted: "just in case" you hemorrhage, or "just in case" they have to do an emergency cesarean. This raises the issue of "just in case" obstetrical science, which advocates the use of "preventive" measures—but an IV doesn't prevent anything. Interfering with the natural process of childbirth can create problems which then demand more interference.

This is not to say that an IV is *never* necessary. It is of great benefit in a situation in which a woman has had a long hard labor and could become dehydrated. But that can be determined at the time and an IV can then be inserted. The same would be true if Pitocin were necessary and the hospital did not have an infusion pump to administer it: putting it in the IV solution would be the next best way to stimulate contractions.

Some people believe that having an IV hooked up contributes to making you feel like a sick patient instead of a well person going through the normal bodily process of giving birth. It is often difficult for the nurse or doctor to insert the IV needle and catheter, so they may have to "stick" you more than once. This process can be painful; it is also disruptive . . . it can interfere with your relaxation and concentration if you are using prepared childbirth techniques. The IV limits your movement—it immobilizes your hand, or you may feel it does, and going to the bathroom, which you should do every couple of hours during labor, involves the IV hookup and tubing having to follow you into the bathroom. Veins can be aggravated for weeks afterward.

Some doctors feel strongly about having the IV hooked up. It makes them feel more secure to have that safeguard against the slight possibility of an emergency. As discussed in the earlier section of this chapter ("Some Thoughts About Doctors"), they have seen many frightening situations in maternity care. If your doctor won't eliminate an IV she or he may be willing to wait until delivery to insert it, giving you hours beforehand without it.

On the other hand, you might feel safer having an IV right from the beginning of labor. The point of this section is simply to let you know the reasoning that is behind having an IV inserted.

➤ *Shaving your pubic hair* is still done in some hospitals. It is not necessary. The reason given for it is that pubic hair harbors bacteria, although there has never been any proof that removing it reduces the incidence of infection. In fact, just the opposite was proven in one study, where *infection increased* with shaving. Your pubic area is washed down with antiseptic or iodine solution before the baby's head is delivered, anyway, so the chance of infection is eliminated by that.

The practical reason for the shave is to facilitate the episiotomy repair for the doctor. If an episiotomy is done, there is the alternative of pushing the hair aside or clipping it with scissors.

One option is to ask your doctor to note on your chart that you want only a "mini-prep," which means that rather than your entire pubic area being shaved, only the lips of your vagina will be. The other possibility is to arrange with your doctor ahead of time that you will trim the hair around the lips of your vagina beforehand.

➤ *Straps and stirrups* are part of the routine procedures in a delivery room. Some hospitals still require your hands to be strapped down to keep them clear of the sterile field where the baby is going to be born. This is a throwback to the days when women were so heavily drugged that they were not in control of themselves. Having your hands strapped down is undignified and degrading. If someone tries to strap your hands, do not allow them to: say that you respect the necessity of keeping your hands under the sterile sheets.

Stirrups are used on most delivery tables. They are not just the foot stirrups you've seen in the doctor's office: they are usually a metal and/or plastic molded form into which your entire leg is strapped. But when your feet are elevated and your legs stretched apart, it puts tension on the vaginal membranes during delivery and increases the chance of tearing and injury to your tissues. Also, if you lie flat with your feet high in the air, that position defies gravity instead of allowing it to help the descent and exit of the baby.

One option is to have the stirrups adjusted lower. You can agree on this with your doctor, but if he or she is not there, you are entitled to a reasonable voice in the matter: tell the attendants you are uncomfortable and cannot push effectively unless the stirrups are lowered.

➤ *Transfer for delivery* is done in most hospitals because it is more convenient for the doctor to deliver the baby with your feet in stirrups, at the edge of a hard surface, and with a stool for him to sit on. Right when the baby's head is crowning (is showing at the lips of your vagina) you are wheeled (often in a hurry) to the delivery room. You are then made to shift from the labor bed onto the narrower delivery table, which has stirrups. This transfer is awkward and disrupts the natural process of birth. Just as the baby's head is ready to be born, you are whisked down the hallways, often instructed to pant so that you don't push the baby out any farther, and then you have to get onto a different surface for the delivery.

Talk to your doctor and the hospital about the possibility of laboring and delivering in the same bed. If they'll agree to that, then ask if you can stay in the labor room to deliver if everything is normal. It will be more peaceful for you and won't put you through that last-minute rush and move. One reason hospitals may not agree to it is that you save a good deal of money if you don't use the delivery room—for which they charge a hefty fee.

The drawbacks of staying in the labor room are that you don't have the mirror overhead with which to watch the birth and you cannot give the baby a Leboyer bath in the labor room. It must also be mentioned that in the rare situation where something goes wrong (the baby cannot exit, or it has difficulty breathing, or you begin to bleed) you won't have the delivery-room facilities right at hand. You will have to be rushed into the delivery room at that point.

Separation of Mother and Baby

This is considered by many experts to be the most harmful routine procedure in a hospital. *Avoiding* this separation is often the primary reason why some couples decide against a hospital birth. Even those hospitals that have family-centered maternity care—which in theory is supposed to keep a family together—still separate mothers and their babies for hours after birth.

Taking a newborn away violates a mother's and baby's emotional and physical needs. Maternal–infant bonding begins with the "sensitive period" for the 30 to 45 minutes immediately after birth. However, it does not stop there. Birth *creates* a mother and a father and redefines them as a family with their new baby. The family is a unit, and its unity should not be broken at this crucial juncture in their lives (unless medically necessary).

In most hospitals a baby is taken at birth to the stabilization nursery for anywhere from 2 to 24 hours after birth. The medical reasoning is that a baby's body temperature has to stabilize, but delivery rooms are chilly and a small baby's system is not yet efficient at maintaining his temperature, so it can take quite a while for him to reach a temperature of 98.6° F. Opponents of routine separation point out that the best "baby warmer" is a mother's arms. A baby can be wrapped up and held close to his mother's body, and he will warm up *at least as well* as he would in a plastic bassinet!

The other reason given by the hospital for removing the baby is that a newborn needs constant observation. It is unrealistic, however, to think that in a busy hospital a baby is actually being watched constantly. His needs for holding and feeding are certainly not being met. The stabilization nursery staff is busy cleaning, weighing, and swaddling other newborns, so if you keep your baby in your arms while you spend the required postpartum hour(s) in the recovery area, the nurse checking on you could observe the baby as well.

Birth is rough for a baby and she has to make many physical adjustments to her new environment. Your baby needs the emotional assurance that all is well and she can depend on you. The first infantile needs are prompt satisfaction of hunger and the urge to nuzzle and suck. A baby needs the feeling of warmth and support from a nurturing mother and peaceful, undisturbed rest in between feedings. Look at a stabilization nursery and see the babies less than an hour old, looking around and trying to suck on their hands or the blanket, and you'll see that they belong with their mothers.

Nursing influences a child's later feelings about herself and other people. Are cries for help met? Are others to be counted upon? A baby needs to learn that crying results in being fed. This is a baby's first experience of trust and communication. When separated from her mother in the nursery, she is kept from forming this close relationship based on love and need. Hunger is a terrifying experience for a new baby: not only is it painful, but the child has no way of knowing that the pain will stop. In the nursery a baby may cry herself to sleep and then be too tired to nurse well when feeding time arrives. This can discourage you, too, and create a cycle of rejection and disappointment.

This section on the separation of babies and mothers may not seem objective, but I feel a moral responsibility to encourage new mothers to protect themselves and their babies from the sometimes unfeeling routines of the hospital. The issue here is about normal, healthy babies. Certainly a baby with any kind of problem must be cared for in the stabilization or intensive care nursery, and obviously a heavily medicated mother will not be sufficiently awake and aware to keep her baby with her. However, since the overwhelming majority of mothers and babies have no complications, there's no reason to separate babies from their mothers for many hours following birth.

Sibling Visiting

Another aspect of maintaining family unity during childbirth is the baby's older brother(s) or sister(s). Older children can feel frightened, angry, and rejected by your sudden absence from home, even if you explained it ahead of time. The first thing to find out is whether children are allowed to visit you in the hospital. Some maternity floors have visiting rooms for this purpose, and it gives your other child(ren) a chance to be reassured that you are fine and still love them.

Ask whether the hospital allows siblings to see the baby. A very few hospitals that permit viewing also allow the children to touch their newborn brother or sister. Some contact is better than none at all. It is hard for children to accept a new baby, who will be taking such a lot of their mother's attention. If you bring a new baby home without an introduction beforehand, it can increase the older child's jealousy and feeling of displacement. As noted earlier, it can be compared to how you might feel if your mate were to disappear for several days and then come home with his arms wrapped around another woman, stating that she was to become "co-wife."

HOW TO COPE WITH THE HOSPITAL

Although you should know what you do and don't want from a hospital birth experience, *you have to be realistic in your expectations*. Administrative and physical needs are going to be priorities. Emotional needs and individual requests and personalities impede efficiency. This is not to say that you should not make every reasonable effort to get what you want and refuse what you don't want, but don't set yourself up for confrontations and disappointment. For example, don't *expect* support and aid with breast-feeding—it will be wonderful if the hospital staff is able to help you, but in many cases assistance is not available. If you seek advice elsewhere, you can avoid being discouraged by an unsuccessful start to breast-feeding.

Hospitals Can Be Intimidating

Once you enter a hospital it is easy to feel overpowered by the authoritarian atmosphere, as if it's your first day of school. It is natural to feel "they" are in control and that you have to follow orders. Some personnel are bound to be particularly intimidating—don't let anyone push you around or make you do anything you don't want.

Keep in mind that *everybody in a hospital is following rules*. There is a chain of command that affects everyone. What often happens is that when people are ordered around from above, they try to exert control over other people "below" them. Nurses' aides and orderlies are at the bottom of the ladder and have to take orders from everyone else on the staff. Nurses are controlled both by hospital regulations and by any doctor, including interns and residents (who often know less than an experienced obstetric nurse). You may notice some doctors treat nurses with a callous arrogance, showing little respect for a nurse's opinion or expertise. Nurse supervisors have to enforce hospital policies, criticize their nurses as well as defend them, *and* answer to any doctor. Don't be surprised that hospital personnel can be bossy; they work in a system structured on authority.

The very atmosphere of a hospital can create anxiety—and its side effects—for you. As discussed earlier, your emotional state has a considerable effect on the physical progress of labor. If you are aware of the possible negative influence of the hospital atmosphere, you can attempt to minimize it.

> ➤ *A wheelchair will be used to transport you* from the hospital entrance or the admitting office to the labor area. If you are in hard labor you may welcome a wheelchair, but if you are able to walk comfortably, a wheelchair can make you feel like an invalid. It can undermine your feeling that you are well, not sick, and coping well with your labor. If you'd prefer not to be wheeled to the labor room, state your preference.

➤ **Personal effects are usually removed** when you get to the labor room, which can seem depersonalizing. It may seem like a petty issue, but taking away your personal belongings can undermine your sense of being in charge. The implication of putting on a hospital gown is that you are in their control. The army, prisons, and other institutions exert control by removing personal belongings and imposing institutional apparel. Make your own decision about how you want to handle this in the hospital—just understanding it may make it unnecessary to challenge it.

➤ **Confinement to bed** can make you feel powerless, particularly if the bedrails are raised. This can make the narrow bed seem like a crib. It can make you feel as if you're a sick child. Again, this is subtle intimidation, but it may affect you subconsciously unless you recognize it. You cannot help but be affected by being confined to a labor bed, hemmed in by metal rails on either side, with nurses and doctors (Mommy and Daddy figures) asking, "How are we doing?"

It can be important during labor for a woman to feel she is capable, self-sufficient, and has a say in what takes place. If the bedrails bother you, for instance, then ask to have them lowered. They are intended to keep medicated mothers from falling out of bed, but some hospitals raise them routinely even during unmedicated labors.

➤ **Questions, examinations, lights, equipment, needles** can all create anxiety. A hospital and its procedures make most people edgy and nervous—in addition, you have labor to cope with, and you may be anxious about how well you're going to be able to do that.

➤ **If you or your mate are frightened by hospitals**—if you have always felt queasy about seeing people in the hospital, for instance—then make a point of visiting the hospital several times before labor. The more chance you have to walk around in a hospital, the more accustomed you will become. If either of you knows beforehand that you dread hospitals, it is well worth the trouble of making a few trips there. To make it more fun you can find out what the hours are for viewing the babies in the nursery and make that your destination: you can look at all the newborns and decide which one yours is going to look like!

I personally know that this system of getting used to the hospital works. My mother was hospitalized several times before she died and I could never go into a hospital (then or afterward) without getting a migraine headache. To research this book I had no choice but to spend many hours in many hospitals. After the first few times the headaches disappeared; after that I was still uncomfortable for a while, afraid of seeing sick people on stretchers in the halls. Before long I could march into a hospital and feel right at home. Many people share my ex-phobia about hospitals; these feelings can interfere with both the personal and physical aspects of birth if you don't deal with them ahead of time.

➤ **Act at the time** if you aren't happy with a staff member or some procedure. Don't cave in to intimidation—you are only going to have this baby once. If you can't face it, have your mate go to bat for you. Confrontations are never pleasant, least of all when you have the work of labor to cope with, but if you don't stick up for what you want, you will have yourselves partially to blame for a less-than-optimum birth experience.

Avoiding "Routine Procedures"

Routine procedures can be avoided in a number of ways. It is important to find out hospital policies ahead of time so that you know what you are going to have to deal with. You should be aware that in side-stepping routines *you take on the responsibility for anything that goes wrong* as a result. Of course, one of the purposes of having a say in what happens during your labor is so that you can be more involved and responsible.

You've read the section on routine procedures in this chapter, so you know there really isn't much that can go wrong by avoiding certain routines in a normal labor and delivery (on the contrary, the routines themselves can cause physical and emotional problems). Also, just because you decide against a routine doesn't mean you can't change your mind. If you want to skip an enema you can always have it later in labor, or if you have decided against having an IV inserted in early labor your doctor can ask to hook one up at any point if he or she feels it is necessary.

➤ **Get a note from your obstetrician** stating that certain routines can be eliminated: this is a good way to protect your wishes. Some doctors will not sign anything, however. The only assurance you may be able to get is an understanding and agreement ahead of time. If there is any argument by the hospital, you, your partner, or the nurse can call your doctor to get permission.

➤ **Get a note from your pediatrician** stating that certain routines should not be used on your baby. This is especially helpful in a hospital that does not have family-centered maternity care. If there is a note attached to your chart that says, "Baby rooming-in. No supplementary bottles," it will protect your desire to breast-feed, for example. When the order comes from a doctor— rather than just being your individual request—it carries more weight with hospital staff, who are used to certain routines.

➤ **Admission forms can be a protection against routines**. There are forms you must sign when you preregister or when you are admitted in labor. Before you sign the form, write in: *All* *procedures subject to my complete understanding of need*. This makes it clear right up front that you question routine procedures in principle.

Getting What You Want in a Hospital Birth

➤ *Dealing effectively with the staff* will get you what you want with a minimum of hassle. Try tactful stubbornness in the face of opposition. Let the staff know you are knowledgeable, calm, and confident. In some cases it is probably best for the baby's father to speak up, but judge for yourselves.

➤ *Labor room nurses need information* about your labor prior to admittance. If you come well prepared it simplifies their job and can gain you their respect. You will probably be asked when your contractions began, how strong and frequent they have been, whether there's been any discharge of bloody show, if or when your membranes ruptured, whether you've felt nauseated, when you last ate, and any allergies you have to medications.

➤ *Tell any attendants that you've taken childbirth preparation classes*, whether they ask or not. Be sure to tell every new staff member with whom you come into contact. You might also add that you'd appreciate being kept informed of your progress during labor so that you can cope with it most effectively and cooperate with the staff. If hospital personnel know you will be using prepared childbirth techniques and want to be involved in the labor and delivery, they will deal with you differently than they would an untrained mother.

➤ *Refuse to answer anything during a contraction*. Some staff members may forget or not understand that you cannot be interrupted when you are in the middle of a contraction. Explain afterward about the need to answer any questions *between* contractions, or have your partner do so.

Diplomatic Ways to Communicate with Hospital Staff

— "We know this isn't routine, but we have our doctor's permission and he said you'd all be helpful if . . ."
— "You probably didn't mean to upset us but . . ."
— "We know you're trying to help and we appreciate that, *but* . . ."
— "We know you're very rushed and we appreciate the help you're giving us, *but* . . ."

➤ *Ask to speak to the director of nursing or the obstetrical supervisor* if you have a problem you cannot resolve comfortably with the staff. Don't let a staff member aggravate you so much that you or your mate get into a heated argument. If you cannot come to a reasonable understanding, then go above the person you are dealing with—not as a threat but to get your needs met. Getting upset is going to interfere with your labor. A supervisor is usually interested in helping make sure that customers are satisfied and will help smooth things over.

➤ **Write a letter as soon as possible after the birth** if you were unable to get satisfaction in some aspect of your hospital stay. It may be more effective coming from the baby's father—we are still a male-dominated society and a letter from a man, especially on business stationery, carries more weight. If your problem was with a nurse, address the letter to the nursing supervisor or the hospital administrator; call the hospital and find out their names. If your problem concerns a doctor, intern, or resident, address it to the chief of obstetrics.

Whichever official you write to, send copies of your letter to the other two and note at the bottom, for example, cc: Dr. William Brown and Mrs. Judy McDevitt, so that the person who receives your letter knows that the other officials in the hospital are now also aware of the problem. Be specific about dates, room number, names of people involved, and *exactly* what displeased you. By writing a letter you are not just finding an outlet for your disappointment and anger but, even more important, you are helping pave the way for future couples to get what they desire in a birth experience.

➤ **Write a letter as soon as you have time** if you were *pleased* with the individual care you received. It is just as important to support positive childbirth practices in the hospitals as it is to change policies and attitudes that get in the way of a good childbirth experience. Every person who praises a flexible, humanitarian hospital helps insure the survival of these qualities which are so important to making birth in the hospital a positive experience.

QUESTIONNAIRE FOR HOSPITALS

Anesthesia
1. Do you have an anesthetist on duty full-time?
2. If so, do you charge whether I use the anesthetist or not?
3. Do your anesthetists mostly use general or local anesthesia?

Breast-Feeding
1. Is breast-feeding encouraged here?
2. Do you encourage or allow breast-feeding on the delivery table?
3. Do you allow babies to be breast-fed on demand?
4. Do you give mothers breast-feeding literature? If so, from what source?
5. Do you routinely give a test feeding of glucose and water in the nursery? If so, can it be eliminated if my pediatrician requests it?

Early discharge
1. Do you offer early discharge?
2. If so, do you offer infant-care classes—or require them—ahead of delivery?
3. Do you have follow-up visits made by nurses or other professionals?
4. Do you have a way I can contact the hospital, postpartum, if I have questions or problems at home?

Father participation
1. Are fathers allowed in the labor room? Are there any exceptions (shared labor room, for example)?
2. Are they allowed in the delivery room? If so, under what circumstances are they asked to leave?
3. May a friend or relative substitute if the father cannot come? If so, must that person have taken the childbirth training with me?
4. Are fathers allowed to stay with wives in the recovery area?
5. Are there unlimited visiting privileges for the father? If not, can he be with me at times in addition to the regular visiting hours?
6. Are fathers allowed to hold their babies?

QUESTIONNAIRE FOR HOSPITALS (*cont.*)

Facilities

1. Do you have an alternative birthing room? If so, under what circumstances would I not be permitted to use it or be transferred to a regular labor room?
2. Do you allow women to labor and deliver in the same bed, either in the labor room or in the delivery room (so that there isn't the awkward transfer of beds when the baby's head is crowning)?
3. Are labor rooms double or single? If I can't have a private labor room, can you assure me that I'll be placed with a woman who has also had childbirth preparation classes? Am I permitted to walk around during labor?
4. Are fetal monitors used? If so, are they mandatory? Can an exception be made if my doctor were to agree to it?
5. Do you sponsor prenatal classes for parents? If so, do they include exercise sessions? Is there a fee charged?
6. What is your policy on food and drink during labor? Are ice chips provided? Is there any rule against fathers eating in the labor rooms? If so, do you have a cafeteria in the hospital?
7. Do you do many Leboyer deliveries? If so, do you provide a bathtub, sterile water, and a radiant heater? If not, to whom do I speak about bringing or arranging for these?
8. Do you have preregistration facilities? If not, would it at least be possible for me to fill out most of the forms and bring them with me when I arrive in labor? How much do you require as a cash deposit on admittance? Does the hospital bill insurers directly?
9. Do you allow cameras and/or tape recorders? Would you allow me to use them if I were to sign a release form of some kind?

The newborn

1. Are babies and mothers allowed to be together from birth?
   — If not, what is your separation policy? Are all babies automatically taken to the stabilization nursery?
   — If so, what is the *least* amount of time my baby would have to stay there, assuming it is normal and healthy?
2. What is the average length of a baby's stay in stabilization: the first two hours after birth? the first 12 hours? the first 24 hours?

QUESTIONNAIRE FOR HOSPITALS (*cont.*)

3. If my pediatrician agrees, would I be allowed to keep my baby with me in the recovery area?
4. If not, would the baby's father be allowed to stay with the baby in the stabilization nursery?
5. Do you have rooming-in?
   — If so, is it available to all mothers or only those with private rooms?
   — Must a mother commit herself to full-time rooming-in or is it flexible (so that she can have the baby or return it to the nursery as she wishes)?
   — Are babies all returned to the central nursery at night?
   — Do you have nurses available for questions and help in the room?
6. Does the hospital offer infant-care classes to new mothers? If so, are fathers encouraged to attend?

Routine procedures
1. Do you administer enemas, IVs and/or public shaves routinely?
2. If so, could any procedures be eliminated if my doctor agrees?
3. Are women's wrists ever strapped during labor or delivery? Are there cases in which they are routinely strapped down?
4. Are stirrups optional during delivery, and if so, is that my doctor's decision or hospital policy?
5. Do you routinely transfer from labor room and bed to delivery room and table?
   If so, with my doctor's agreement could I labor and deliver in the same bed?
   — Could I labor and deliver in the labor room in that case?

Sibling visitation
1. Are children allowed to visit their mothers?
2. If so, are they allowed in her room or is there a visiting room?
3. Are children allowed to see the newborn?
4. Are children allowed to touch the newborn?

CHAPTER ELEVEN

Home Birth

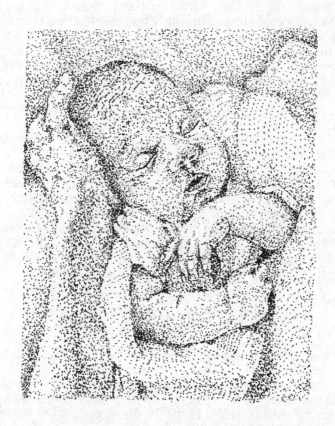

Some people in the medical profession believe that home birth is a fad and will go away. Medical caregivers often view home-birthers as ignorant rebels who have to be either punished or enlightened. In states such as California where home birth flourishes, just the opposite has been found: many of those choosing birth at home are middle- to upper-middle-class, well-educated couples. They are dissatisfied with the hospital system of birth and are not willing to make compromises; many of them would choose home birth even if hospitals were to suddenly make sweeping changes.

There is a basic philosophical position behind the choice for giving birth at home. Home birth reflects not just attitudes about birth but about life as a whole: to simplify one's life and to get back to real human values in a technologized society. Home birth is in most cases a matter of conviction, not of poverty, ignorance, or rebellion. Supporters of home birth view childbirth as a normal physiological process rather than an illness requiring hospitalization and aggressive medical intervention. Home birth is believed to be a necessary way of life for some people, just as hospital birth is believed to be a necessity of life for others.

The out-of-hospital birth advocates began to surface at the same time in the same communities in which aggressive obstetric care began to be applied to all women in childbirth in hospitals. The trend toward home birth was a reaction to the trend within the hospital to treat every birth as a potential high-risk situation. In a technological society there are constant trade-offs between technical advances and human values: people who choose home birth are not willing to pay the price tag of birth in a hospital, where they feel the personal aspect of birth has been compromised.

Home-birthers believe they are doing the best thing for their children and themselves. These are parents who judge the risks of the hospital to be greater than the risk of giving birth outside it. They are concerned about the routine administration in the hospital of often unnecessary treatments which themselves have not been proven risk-free. Some members of the medical community claim that those who choose home birth are endangering the lives of their children; these professionals are angry and frightened by the home birth movement, which threatens the core of their belief system. Most people choosing home birth do so in the belief that for them it is as safe or safer than a hospital.

SAFETY OF HOME BIRTH

The main question usually raised about home birth is whether it is safe. Those who choose home birth do not ignore the fact that things can go wrong, but they are also aware that *life* is fraught with danger (the odds are greater of harm coming to you and/or your child in a car than in giving birth outside a hospital). Those opposed to home birth ask why "flirt with danger" rather than take advantage of a hospital, which has machines and expertise *in case* unlikely complications arise?

For people who are considering or have chosen home birth, giving birth is not an event to be measured in terms of statistics or to be decided on the basis of other people's lists of possible problems. Birth is a personal and interpersonal experience—one of life's great events—and it belongs at home where this aspect is foremost. Home-birthers understand that there are no guarantees in life and that in birth there is no such thing as "absolute safety"—many people who give birth in a hospital go on the misguided *assumption* that the medical setting assures them absolute safety, which no one can provide. Those who have babies at home must know what to do and where to go if problems should arise; they also have to be able to accept that in nature there is a measure of unpredictability and cruelty.

There are two main factors to be considered in the safety of birth at home. One is that candidates must be carefully screened and receive excellent prenatal care. The other factor is the availability of emergency backup personnel and equipment. If these two elements are carefully taken into account, then home birth is relatively safe.

A study comparing the outcomes of a group of home births vs. hospital births in California matched two sizable groups of women so that those giving birth were as similar as possible except in the location of their babies' births. The result of this study was that the home birth outcomes were better than the California state average, with fewer complications than might have been expected. The conclusion of the study was that home birth is a safe alternative for women who have been medically screened as healthy. There was no increase in risk at home: in fact, due to an absence of medication in the home births there were higher Apgar scores.

In order to have the greatest margin of safety, those attending home births as well as those choosing to have them should employ very careful screening of candidates.

Emergency Precautions

You may want to take emergency precautions and plan ahead in case of an emergency to increase the safety of home birth. It's fine to maintain a positive attitude toward birth as a normal process of the female body, but you must also consider the "what if . . ." when you are planning a home birth.

➤ *Tape the emergency medical service's telephone number* on your phone. Find out ahead of time if there's someone in particular you should ask for in case of complications in childbirth.

➤ *Find the closest hospital* with emergency facilities or, preferably, with obstetric facilities. Find out whether it is necessary to have a doctor who has admitting privileges there in order to be cared for. It is sad but true that hospitals may reject a woman in labor who has chosen home birth. Most hospitals are ideologically opposed to home birth: in some states they may turn you away if complications arise. They may not want the responsibility of a situation that has already become serious. Feeling moral indignation at a hospital (which is presumably there

FACTORS THAT RULE OUT HOME BIRTH

* **Abnormal Presentation** . . . a baby in a breech, transverse, or other abnormal position might require last-minute obstetric procedures not possible at home.

* **Active Herpes Simplex Virus** . . . can be transmitted to your baby if you have lesions at the time of delivery. If you have a history of herpes, have a doctor examine you right up until your due date. If there are lesions, your baby should be delivered by cesarean section.

* **Bleeding** . . . with or without pain before labor can indicate placenta previa. In this case the placenta is covering the cervix, in front of the baby (who must be delivered by cesarean).

* **Cephalopelvic Disproportion** . . . if it is suspected that the baby's head is too large to fit through your pelvis, a sonogram can confirm whether this disproportion does exist. If cephalopelvic disproportion is not detected prelabor, labor will not progress after a certain point and you will have to be transferred to a hospital.

* **Complications in Previous Pregnancies** . . . includes anything on this list as well as previous cesarean or history of small-for-date babies (who have a higher risk or respiratory distress, low blood sugar levels, greater heat loss, and cerebral edema); complications have a tendency to recur in subsequent pregnancies.

* **Diabetes** . . . involves high risks for the baby and is a dangerous situation even in the hospital.

* **Grand Multiparity** . . . there is a higher incident of uterine inertia in women who have had six or more previous pregnancies.

* **Hydramnios** . . . too much amniotic fluid.

* **Hypertension** . . . also known as high blood pressure, is one of the unpredictable complications of birth. Some women develop hypertension during labor with no previous history of the problem. It gives no warning signals until you go into convulsions. *At least* have prenatal exams every week near your due date and abandon plans for home birth if your blood pressure rises.

FACTORS THAT RULE OUT HOME BIRTH (*cont.*)

* **Malnutrition** . . . involves risks to the mother in labor and may mean a small-for-date or otherwise compromised infant.
* **Maternal Anemia** . . . is determined by blood tests. It can result in low birth weight and prematurity; it also predisposes you to postpartum hemorrhage.
* **Multiple Pregnancy** . . . increases the possibility of: (1) small-for-date babies who require special care; (2) abnormal presentation of both babies or the second baby; (3) separation of the placenta before the second baby is born.
* **Postmaturity** . . . is best determined by a 24-hour urine test which indicates whether there is placental dysfunction (the fetus is no longer being properly nourished); determining postmaturity by dates (42–44 weeks gestation) can be incorrect because there may have been an error in calculation of dates.
* **Preeclampsia or Eclampsia** . . . can be detected in your prenatal exams.
* **Prematurity** . . . is any baby that goes into labor at less than 36 weeks gestation: he may be low birth weight or have other problems.
* **Primipara over 35** . . . if this is your first baby and you're over 35, more complications are possible. This factor is something you can discuss with a doctor sympathetic to home birth.
* **Rh Blood Incompatibility** . . . is a problem *only* if a blood test shows a rise in titer (maternal antibody production) before delivery. Otherwise, an umbilical-cord blood sample is sent to a lab, and if positive you must get a rhogram injection within 72 hours of the baby's birth.
* **Those who are not ideologically committed to home birth** . . . will depend heavily on the attendant(s) instead of themselves and may not be able to handle the physical or emotional demands of home birth. The wrong reasons for choosing home birth are religious (to avoid drugs, transfusions), financial (too poor to afford the hospital, not poor enough for government assistance programs), peer pressure (your friends have all had home births or your mate feels more strongly about it than you), or you just don't like doctors or hospitals.

for the good of society) won't do you any good if you're in need of medical care during childbirth. So line up a hospital that will accept you just in case.

➤ *Take a run-through of the hospital beforehand* so you know your way around if necessary. It also can't do any harm to preregister, just in case—this way if you do need the hospital's facilities there will be less hassle. Pack a bag with some night clothes, other necessities, and baby clothes in case you do have to be hospitalized. This may seem overly cautious, but it will smooth the way in the unlikely event that you have to leave home.

➤ *Make sure that your car is in good condition.* This is more than a precaution; it is a necessity. As your due date is nearing, be sure that you always have a full or close-to-full tank of gas. Sometime *during* your labor your partner, or someone he chooses, should start up the car just to be sure it's ready to go. If you have complications in your labor, the last thing you need is the anxiety of a car that isn't working. A station wagon or van is preferable because there is room for you to lie down in the back.

➤ *Do not be more than 30 minutes from a hospital.* If your house is too isolated, then choose a friend or relative's home that is nearer to a hospital where you can give birth.

➤ *Try to make a relationship* with a family practitioner or an obstetrician beforehand. You might even consider getting your prenatal care from a doctor so that you know each other. If you have no experienced birth attendant, or if you have a lay midwife, you must know ahead of time who will take over in an emergency.

It may be hard to find a doctor who is sympathetic to home delivery. Doctors spend years of their lives and a great deal of money on medical training—by choosing to give birth at home you are questioning the value of that background. By asking a doctor to give backup care, you are asking him or her to reject the hospital, which the doctor believes to be the right way and place to have a baby. A doctor's reaction to home birth may be fear, outrage, and indignation—you are threatening the foundation of obstetrical training. You should also keep in mind the pressure that can be put on doctors by hospitals. Some institutions indicate that any doctor who participates in a home birth risks having his or her admitting privileges at the hospital revoked.

It may not be wise to have a doctor as your primary *attendant* at home birth. A doctor is medically oriented, trained to intervene, and does not necessarily have the training for home delivery. Hospital deliveries are very different because labor is affected by drugs and other routine interventions. Many doctors with extensive hospital experience don't know what to expect at home. For example, they may never have seen a natural-length wait in the third stage of labor: they might expect the placenta to come out right away as it does in the hospital where synthetic hormones are routinely administered to speed things along. Therefore, a doctor might pull on the umbilical cord in third stage, a dangerous practice which could cause hemorrhaging.

Generally, a midwife (either certified nurse- or lay) is a better choice for a home birth attendant for the reasons above. If a couple feels strongly about having a doctor attend their home birth, they may wish to question whether they may not be 100% committed to home birth and may be choosing a doctor as a psychological crutch. There are two reasons why it might be advisable to have a doctor at home. In many states delivering a child is considered the "practice of medicine" and only licensed physicians are legally permitted to attend births. The other reason is that a doctor has hospital admitting privileges in case complications arise.

➤ *If you are not going to have a medically trained attendant at the birth* contact your local Visiting Nurses Association, which will probably be listed in your phone book, and find out if they have a nurse who specializes in maternity care. Find out whether she will make a postpartum visit *as soon as possible* after the baby is born. The nurse can examine your perineum to see if there are any tears and whether any stitches are needed. She can also check the baby. Even if you have insurance, you will probably need to pay for any VNA services to a home birth yourself.

➤ *Contact a pediatrician* ahead of time, particularly if there is not going to be a medical attendant at your birth and/or no visiting nurse is available. Find a pediatrician who is not opposed to home birth, because some may refuse to see babies who have been born at home. Then get the baby to the pediatrician (or to a clinic) for newborn checkup. Even though the baby may seem fine, *confirm that*—do not neglect an early checkup just because everything seems fine. There are some birth defects, such as cleft palate, which need medical attention.

➤ *Stay very quiet* for the first few hours postpartum. No matter how good you feel, you must stay still and rest quietly for the hours after birth. This is the time when hemorrhaging can occur. Make sure that your uterus is hard and that someone will massage it with a gentle downward pressure (within the limits of your comfort) so that it stays firm.

THE LEGAL ASPECT OF BIRTH AT HOME

The legal aspect of choosing to give birth at home is something you should know, especially so that you will not be intimidated by people who may be misinformed. *No state requires that childbirth take place in a hospital or forbids home birth*. There are laws about birth attendants, however, which vary from state to state. A doctor is legally free to attend a birth anywhere; the laws pertaining to certified nurse-midwives give the current, but frequently changing, regulations about lay midwifery. Standards vary widely among the states: in many states the responsibility for regulation is with state health or licensing agencies which determine the qualifications and training required.

Your legal obligation to your child does not begin until he is born. If at that time he is in need of medical assistance and you do not make every effort to summon that assistance or get the baby to medical care, and the baby dies—that is considered manslaughter. It is *highly unlikely* that such charges would be brought against you, just as it is highly unlikely that parents would not go to a hospital or doctor if their baby were in trouble. When efforts have been made to summon appropriate medical care, no charge of manslaughter has ever been brought.

There Is No Criminal Liability for Stillbirth

> **Nonprofessionals involved** in home birth have no legal liability unless there is death or permanent disability. In that case, the two possible consequences are a civil suit (money damages being sought) or a criminal suit (somebody wants to fine you or put you in jail). The "somebody" in these cases would presumably be the local authorities: although it is highly unlikely that any action would be taken, nevertheless, legal grounds do exist. It is conceivable that there could be enough fear and resentment toward home birth (i.e., toward people who are challenging the status quo of the medical establishment) to generate at least talk of such proceedings. Therefore, it's important that you know your legal rights beforehand.

> **If the mother dies** there is no legal liability as long as the mother knew what she was doing. It is her right to assume the risk of home birth. No one in the United States has to go to a hospital for anything, including childbirth.

PSYCHOLOGICAL ASPECTS OF HOME BIRTH

In a home birth the responsibility for labor and delivery and the outcome of the baby rest entirely with the expectant couple. The positive aspect of this is that it gives you a sense of power and control over the situation, a feeling that you are running your own life. This responsibility also means that if anything goes wrong there is no one else to blame— you can't pin the fault on other people or factors that are out of your control.

You will probably encounter some social pressure against your decision to give birth at home. In most cases it is in your best interest not to get dragged into emotional discussions—no purpose is served by them. If it is important to you that particular people *understand* your decision for home birth, then make the effort to explain it to them, but do not set out to persuade them you are "right" or to get their sanction: it will frustrate you and them and perhaps strain your relationship. If you find that it's important to get validation from other people, then you should talk again with your partner about your decision for home birth until you are sure it is what *you* want.

Giving birth outside of a hospital is not the norm in America. You have to prepare yourself for a lack of support for your decision. A value judgment will be directed against you for choosing home birth if anything goes wrong (even if it's something that could not have been prevented in a hospital). Our society does not hold it against you if your child is damaged or her intelligence is stunted by too many drugs or other procedures in the hospital. However, if a baby is born at home with a birthmark or a clubfoot or cleft palate, you will be held to blame. Even though you *objectively* know that this is senseless reasoning, *subjectively* it can be upsetting. Recognizing these potential psychological problems ahead of time and discussing them with your mate is the best way to protect yourself.

Fear

Fear is the worst enemy you can have in home birth. It can prolong your labor and even impede it to the extent that you have to transfer to the hospital. The way to avoid this kind of fear is for a couple to be truly committed to birth at home. Even the man must feel at ease, or he will transmit his doubts and fears to the woman. *Communicate* your fears and fantasies when you are discussing home birth. Talking about them may resolve some fears; other fears can be eliminated or lessened by making all the "just in case" arrangements listed in the preceding section.

➤ ***Our social conditioning*** says that home birth is dangerous and painful. People who choose to give birth at home are affected by this belief and they have to *un*learn it. Taking excellent care of yourself during pregnancy, having regular prenatal examinations, choosing a qualified birth attendant, and making careful preparations for any eventuality help to inform and prepare you. It is vital to acknowledge that we are all deeply conditioned by social attitudes. If you believe that birth is dangerous and painful, you will contribute to making it so. People who want to give birth at home have to make a conscious choice to experience it differently . . . which is to say, as a *positive* event.

➤ ***Pain in labor*** may be related to fear. A woman who is frightened and tense is going to create the fear/tension/pain cycle that childbirth training attempts to avoid. If you are giving birth at home and the pain becomes unbearable and you cannot cope, it is advisable to go to the hospital. The pain may be the result of extreme fear that you were not conscious of before birth. At the hospital they can give you an artificial relaxant. You may not have been as committed to home birth as you'd thought; just being in the hospital may relax you.

Intense pain may also mean there is something wrong physically, so going to the hospital may be a wise choice.

➤ *A prolonged and difficult* labor may be the result of fear and tension on your part. Home birth attendants find they can sometimes relax a woman by repeating over and over, "Let your baby come down, let your baby come out, let your baby get born." The need for physical contact is also a factor, and being held or stroked by your mate and other attendants has also brought successful results where labor was impeded. There is always the possibility that labor is prolonged because of physical impediments to the baby's descent and these must always be taken into consideration.

➤ *See a home birth* or a film of one before deciding on home birth. This will give you and your partner a sense of what to expect even though every birth is different. The more information you have, the greater sense of control you will have over your own birth experience.

Dealing with Unexpected Hospitalization

Going to the hospital is a possibility that all home-birth couples must consider. Practical and emotional preparation will make it less traumatic.

➤ *Emotionally the first step* is for you and your mate to *express your sorrow and disappointment* that you could not complete the birth at home. You should avoid feeling guilty.

➤ *A woman feels let down by her own body*. Part of your self-esteem comes from depending on your own body, and when it fails you, it can lead to feelings of anger, reduced self-worth, and disappointment in yourself. This *can* lead to depression if you don't clearly understand it. Eventually you can accept the fact that bodies do sometimes let us down. Where home birth is concerned there is a great deal of emphasis on a woman's self-reliance and freedom from dependence on the medical establishment. It will help you to accept the reality that nature is unpredictable and that bodies do not function like well-oiled machines. If you don't make allowance for this going in, then you will feel like a failure if you have to be hospitalized.

➤ *The primary concern* of loving parents is *the baby's well-being*. A laboring woman may have to give up the satisfaction of the natural process of birth and go to the hospital. In doing this she is putting the baby's welfare before her own needs, which can make her feel good as a woman and a mother.

REASONS FOR CHOOSING HOME BIRTH

➤ To be in a relaxed, familiar environment.
➤ To choose who will be present at the birth and make it a positive personal event.
➤ To choose supportive birth attendants who will stay with you throughout the labor and delivery.
➤ To be free to move around during labor and have the food and drink you want.
➤ To wear what you want as well as to keep on jewelry, eye-glasses, or other personal effects (often removed in the hospital).
➤ To be free to use your own bathroom as often as needed without waiting to be taken or having to use a bedpan.
➤ To labor and deliver in the same room and same bed in whatever position you find comfortable.
➤ To have family members together during the birth and after-ward, which may lessen the jealousy of siblings, whose bonding to the baby may be enhanced if they have participated in or witnessed the birth.
➤ To be free to reach down and touch the baby before he is fully born and assist in the rest of the birth if desired and/or to allow the father to be the first person to touch the baby.
➤ To be able to breast-feed immediately and on demand.
➤ To feel as if your baby belongs to you rather than feeling she belongs to a hospital staff, who bestow her upon you at certain times, or to have to ask permission for you or your mate to hold her.
➤ To be able to follow your own natural rhythms and those of your baby after birth so that you can rest, get up, nurse, and eat when you want and have visitors, including children, whenever you want.
➤ To not be awakened to have your temperature taken or to be offered pills to sleep, for pain, or to dry up your milk.
➤ To promote paternal bonding so that a man is an integral part of the entire experience, on his own territory, without feeling he is imposing.
➤ So that a man doesn't have to view his baby through a pane of glass or be considered the bearer of bad germs and have to scrub and change clothes or put on a gown before touching his own baby.
➤ To avoid the hospital's overbearing environment, which can un-dermine a woman's self-confidence.
➤ At home a woman is encouraged to get in touch with her own

body and she is listened to when she describes what is going on—good or bad—with her body in labor. The hospital interferes with most women's abilities to tune in to their bodies during birth, and/or no one listens to them.

➤ To avoid excessive routine intervention in a natural event (fetal monitors, IVs, pubic shave, enema, synthetic oxytocin).

➤ To avoid routine episiotomies with a birth attendant knowledgeable in the methods which minimize the need for episiotomies and the possibility of tears.

➤ To avoid aggressive obstetric intervention, such as routine cesarean section of breech babies, routine induction after 24 hours of ruptured membranes, and routine induction of labor at 42 weeks gestation.

➤ To avoid the feeling of being pressured to "perform" according to preconceived medical notions of what "normal" labor is, and to be made to feel inadequate or to have technical intervention if your individual labor does not fit the standard description.

➤ To avoid the temptation of drugs during labor, particularly during transition, when you may be tired and frustrated and your resolve may be lowered.

SUPPLIES NEEDED FOR HOME BIRTH

➤ *A very firm bed is necessary*; this can be achieved by putting a board under the mattress. Otherwise, your hips may make a depression, making it harder for the baby to get out. Also, a puddle of amniotic fluid may form under your hips which the baby will emerge into, with the danger that she will breathe in some of the fluid. Some elevation under your hips may be necessary anyway (pillows, for instance). If you are not able to stiffen the bed sufficiently, then you should lie on your side with your knees drawn up for delivery so that your genital area will be up and out of the soft mattress. A water bed is comfortable for first-stage labor but is not recommended for birth because of this lack of firm support.

➤ *A plastic sheet should go over the mattress*. You can use an old shower curtain or a plastic tablecloth—anything that will be large enough to protect the mattress.

➤ *Old linens can be tucked in over the plastic sheet* and then can be discarded after birth or soaked in cold-water detergent to get them clean later.

➤ *Wash the sheets* and any towels you'll use for delivery in hot water using chlorine bleach. Tumble-dry in a clothes dryer at the hottest possible temperature. As soon as the dryer stops, fold the sheets and towels *while they are still hot* and put them in new, unused plastic bags. Seal them completely with tape and store in a closet until labor begins.

➢ *The most convenient way to arrange the bed* (once labor has begun) is to make the bed as you normally would with fresh sheets. Then put on the plastic sheet. Get out the sealed old linens and put them on over the plastic. This way the old sheets and the plastic can be stripped off the bed after birth, leaving a freshly made bed for you and the baby.

➢ *Newspapers should be collected for several weeks* before your due date. Newsprint is considered clean and even inhibits the growth of germs. The newspapers can be used for extra protection instead of or in addition to the plastic sheet on the mattress. They can also be used to make a pathway to the bathroom from the bed to catch any drippings. And if you don't object, they can even be used under you as bed pads.

➢ *Disposable bed pads* (Chux or Johnson & Johnson) will be necessary for absorption under your buttocks. They resemble large disposable diapers and during labor will absorb amniotic fluid and then can be discarded.

➢ *A Fleet enema should be used* if there is any chance that you have hard feces in the lower intestine. Most women go into labor having had several bowel movements or diarrhea, which is nature's cleansing process, but sometimes women are constipated. In this case an enema makes labor easier; the baby has more room if there is no fecal matter in your lower bowel.

STRICT HYGIENE IS VITAL

— *A small bottle of rubbing alcohol* is used to soak and sterilize any instruments that the attendants need. The alcohol can also be used afterward on the stump of the umbilical cord.

— *A saucepan or Dutch oven* is needed to boil instruments, although you can check first with your birth attendant(s), who may bring presterilized equipment with them.

— *The mother should wash her hands* past her wrists in the same way, especially if she thinks she might want to reach down and touch the baby before he is fully born. In addition, at the beginning of labor you should wash your pubic region, including your pubic hair and the inside of your thighs, with the same careful sudsing and rinsing.

Before the birth do it again. Your thighs should be washed 12 inches down on either side. This time when you wash your pubic area you should finish with the antiseptic soap or solution on a fresh sterile cloth or gauze pad, making one clean motion from the top of your vagina downward. Repeat with a second *fresh* sterile cloth in the same way.

— *Everyone should "scrub up" carefully.* Birth attendants should scrub their hands and arms up to the elbow with either an antiseptic solution or surgical soap and plenty of water. *Use repeated sudsings and rinsings for at least four minutes.* Make sure that fingernails are short.

➤ *The hygiene of attendants* is incredibly important. Everyone at the birth should wear freshly laundered clothes. Anything coming into contact with your vagina needs to be kept scrupulously clean. No one with any infected sore on their hands or a sore throat should attend you.

— *A bottle of antiseptic solution*, either pHisoDerm, pHisoHex, Betadine, or Zephiran Chloride (which must be carefully diluted according to directions on it), is needed for washing up. A broad-spectrum antiseptic surgical soap can be used instead. Washing up should be done by the mother and birth attendant(s) at the beginning of labor and *again* during the pushing stage of labor, when many hours will undoubtedly have passed.

➤ *Antiseptic solution is also a good lubricant* for perineal massage because it is antibacterial.

➤ *Antiseptic solution is necessary if the attendant is going to do vaginal exams* to determine how far dilated you are. However, *as a precaution against infection, vaginal exams should not be done at home*. (An alternative way to determine full dilation is to try a few pushes when you have the bearing-down urge. If it hurts, it means your cervix is not quite fully dilated but will be soon, perhaps when your breathing has a "catch" in it during contractions.)

— *Two large boxes of sterile 4" × 4" gauze pads* have a variety of uses.

➤ *As* **compresses** to support, relax, and soothe the perineum while the baby's head is crowning to prevent tearing or lacerations.

➤ *Instead of sterile pads you can prepare 10 or more washcloths or old towels or flannel cut to washcloth size, washed and stored, as described on page 344.*

— *A work area* can be a cleared tabletop or a dresser within easy reach of the bed for the attendant's supplies.
— *A place for attendant(s) to lie down* is something to plan for, because labor can go on for many hours.

EQUIPMENT FOR THE BIRTH

— *An infant ear syringe* is sometimes used to suction excess mucus from the newborn's nose and mouth.

➤ *Some home-birth attendants do not suction.* They believe that the mucus stimulates the baby to breathe. (This is not logical because even after suctioning a lot of mucus remains.)

➤ *If you do not suction then at least* hold the baby's head lower than her feet so that gravity helps the mucus to drain out.

➤ *The ear syringe should not be boiled*—rubber loses its retractability and sucking power when boiled. Wipe it off with alcohol before use.

— *One pair of infant shoelaces* to tie the umbilical cord. They should be boiled for five minutes anytime before labor begins and then soaked in alcohol until needed.

— *A large bowl* is needed to catch the placenta. If you line it with a plastic bag, it will make cleanup easier.

— *Receiving blankets* are needed to cover the baby and maintain her warmth. Even with skin-to-skin contact, a newborn's "thermostat" doesn't work efficiently yet. Towels can be used, but flannel blankets are softer. Launder them several times before labor so that they are comfortable to the touch and then seal in plastic bags to keep them sterile until they are needed to wrap up the baby.

— *Clothes and diapers* for the baby after the birth, and a fresh change of clothes for you.

— *Hospital-sized sanitary napkins and belt* are difficult to locate, but some drugstores carry them.

➤ *They are slightly more expensive than regular napkins but they are more absorbent.*

➤ *If they are unavailable, there are thick pads like Depends for incontinence that are more absorbent than regular sanitary napkins.*

➤ *Do not use Tampax* (although the way your vagina may feel after birth, you probably would not consider it anyway!).

— *It is mandatory* by law to protect your newborn baby's eyes with antibiotic ointment at birth.

— The issue of whether it is really necessary to guard against the blindness which gonorrhea may cause is discussed in Chapter 12.

— However, be advised that even late-pregnancy gonorrhea tests are not reliable. You may have been exposed and still test negative.

— The ointment can be delayed until after the initial bonding with you and your mate has taken place.

Scales are needed to know the baby's weight for the birth certificate and registration. If there are no baby scales available, someone can step on a bathroom scale alone and then step on holding the baby; the difference in the two weights is the baby's weight.

THE PLACENTA

— ***Most people dispose of the placenta*** in a plastic garbage bag.
— ***Some people plant it under a tree*** so that it symbolically nourishes the earth, and so they can watch the tree grow as their child does.
— ***Some women eat a small portion of the placenta raw***. Many animals do this in childbirth: any bleeding stops when the placenta comes in contact with the mucous membrane of the animal's mouth.

CHOOSING A LAY MIDWIFE

Most people choosing home birth will be attended by a lay midwife because they are the birth attendants most willing and available. The southeastern portion of the United States has the highest number of lay midwives (Alabama, Florida, Georgia, Kentucky, Mississippi, North and South Carolina, and Tennessee), but there are fewer of them all the time. The legality of lay midwives is different in each state, where legislatures rule on whether attending a birth is the "practice of medicine." The legislative trend has been to make it illegal even for a licensed certified nurse-midwife to attend home birth unless accompanied by a doctor.

An example of a unique home birth service is Maternity Center Associates in Bethesda, Maryland, which offers certified nurse-midwives with a doctor on call. In normal pregnancies and deliveries the primary care is given by the nurse-midwives; the doctor is notified when the woman goes into labor and is on call by telephone or in person. The definition of "normal" is the same as for any home birth or birthing room. If the pregnancy or labor is abnormal, the nurse-midwives and doctor jointly manage the birth in a hospital. A woman choosing this service must agree to a hospital transfer in case of complications.

Unfortunately there aren't any other organizations in the United States which offer trained medical attendance at home. But you can get information about what home birth services are available in your community by contacting childbirth instructors, the La Leche League, birth-control and feminist health clinics, Jehovah's Witnesses, and the Christian Science Church, which often have connections to home birth attendants because their religious doctrine shuns doctors and medication.

However, the laws have not stopped home birth or lay midwives, although many of them are cautious about how they work and with whom. The important thing to realize is that many lay midwives have had *no training*. In some areas where there are not enough attendants for home births, there are women who have been at one or two births who are calling themselves midwives. If you choose to have a woman like this at your birth, it is the same as having an *unattended* home birth—beware that this is what you are opting for if you don't ask for a midwife's qualifications.

Try to meet with several midwives with the following questions in mind. Ask around locally about each woman's reputation. Then choose one midwife after careful deliberation with your mate and notify the other(s) you met with that you won't be needing their assistance (which is common courtesy).

There is no formal training available for lay midwives, so one way to judge expertise is to find out whether a midwife has worked on an apprenticeship basis with a more experienced midwife and has been present at 50 to 100 births. (Of course, it is possible to attend many births without gaining practical knowledge of how to cope with certain problems or prevent difficulties from becoming dangerous.)

SOME QUESTIONS FOR MIDWIVES

What Is Her Training and How Many Babies Has She "Caught"?

➤ *If a midwife has caught fewer than 50 babies* or is doing fewer than two or three births a month, she probably qualifies more as a helpful and knowledgeable assistant than as a professional midwife. Her presence can still be valuable, but she may not have acquired some of the skills and techniques you might require. It is really a question of evaluating the risks and the degree of service you feel you need. About 90% of births are normal, so if all goes normally, you might not desire more than a friendly helper. However, often problems do not arise until you are already in labor and frequently there is no warning beforehand.

➤ *Training for dealing with infants in distress* is also very important. A midwife who knows the basic ways to resuscitate a baby in distress can make the difference between life and death or damage. There are textbooks in hospitals and the Red Cross offers courses to anyone in mouth-to-mouth and cardiopulmonary resuscitation; a midwife can get instruction from these sources.

➤ *A midwife who subscribes to professional newsletters* and journals in the childbirth and home-birth field and/or attends local or national conferences shows her interest in broadening her knowledge. A midwife can become more competent by staying in touch with other midwives and childbirth organizations and reading new publications.

"What Complications Has She Seen and Handled?"

It is a great advantage to have a midwife who has handled breech birth or other unusual presentations or complications. At the very least she should have the experience and knowledge to recognize danger signals during labor and delivery and know when she is out of her depth. A midwife is fulfilling her role if she is honest about her limitations, can identify problems, and can get you to appropriate care in time.

A midwife should discuss the possibilities of complications and give you detailed information about what is happening in pregnancy and during labor. A midwife should explain to you what she sees or is looking for: she has to be strong and intelligent enough to share her knowledge so that you understand the consequences.

You and your partner have the final decision and responsibility. You cannot choose wisely unless you have reliable information. A midwife who tells you nothing can go wrong at home, or that she can handle whatever does occur, is doing you a disservice. There are no guarantees in birth, especially home birth. You need a midwife who is as clear about that as you are.

"Does She Have Medical Backup?"

Ideally a midwife should have a working relationship with a physician so that if complications arise she can supply him with a written pregnancy and labor record. If you have to be admitted to a hospital during labor she may be able to continue supporting you through the birth (though this is rarely possible; most doctors are antagonistic to home birth and many lay midwives are antagonistic to doctors).

A midwife should be familiar with local hospitals and public health facilities and be able to transport you there in case of an emergency. She needs to know the procedures required to admit you for care. You should also inform yourself beforehand and take responsibility for these precautions even if a midwife is well prepared. By making a connection in the medical world you are also acknowledging that you might have need of it.

Pediatric backup is also very useful. It is probably best to find your own pediatrician who will agree to check the baby (see page 503, "Choosing a Pediatrician"). It can be helpful if the midwife has access to phone or office consultation with a pediatrician if it is needed. If not, she should know how to obtain care for a baby through public health facilities.

"Does She Do Prenatal Checkups?"

Good maternity care is based on thorough prenatal care, careful screening of high-risk mothers, and good nutrition. A midwife should either refer you to prenatal care facilities or be able to follow your pregnancy herself. She should check your urine for sugar and protein, your blood pressure, general heath and appearance, and follow the growth of the uterus and the position of the baby and placenta. As with any pre-natal care, you should be examined once a month until the seventh month, every two weeks until the ninth month, and then weekly until the baby is born. It is also helpful if she is knowledgeable about nutrition and breast-feeding. Beware of a midwife who does not help you arrange for this time and effort in your prenatal care.

At some point in early or mid-pregnancy you should have a lab screening done to determine the following:

➤ *what your blood type and factor are (A, B, or O, and Rh negative or positive);*

➤ *whether there are abnormalities or infection in your urine;*

➤ *whether there is evidence of syphilis in your blood;*

➤ *whether you are anemic (hemoglobin less than 10.0, hematocrit less than 33%).*

If you show problems in any of these areas you should be retested during the last two months of your pregnancy so that you can receive medical care for any severe problem. A midwife should require that you get this lab work done and should be able to interpret the lab findings and assist you in dealing with any problems.

"What Does She Carry in Her Birth Bag?"

A midwife's minimum equipment should include a thermometer, blood pressure unit, stethoscope, clamps and small scissors, sterile string or other means of tying off the cord, alcohol, antibacterial agent for cleaning and scrubbing up, and small bulb syringes to clean the mucus out of the baby's mouth and nose, if necessary. As of 1990, all also carry and use surgical gloves and masks as a precaution against AIDS.

➤ ***Does she have any drugs to stop bleeding?*** Although there is antidrug sentiment among home birth couples and attendants, it only takes one experience with postpartum bleeding for a mid-wife to carry oxytocins. These can usually stop bleeding by con-tracting the uterus (either Ergotrate tablets or Pitocin with disposable syringes). A midwife may not have access to these medicines because they are available by prescription only. She— or you—may be able to get some from a friendly physician be-fore your due date. It is worth the trouble to have these drugs on hand just in case.

➤ ***Does she use tetracycline or erythromycin ointment in the baby's eyes?*** This prevents damage or blindness to the baby's eyes from infection picked up from gonorrhea. This sexually transmitted disease can be unsuspected and without symptoms in your vagina.

Discuss antibiotic ointment with a midwife ahead of time and be sure that you are in agreement about using a preventive substance. In some states, public health facilities are required to supply the ointment; in others it can be obtained by taking the baby within three or four hours of birth to a hospital emergency room, laboratory, doctor's office, or a similar facility. A midwife can also get a supply from a friendly physician or over the counter from a pharmacy.

"Do You Feel Comfortable with Her?"

➤ *Does she charge a fee?* If she does and it seems fair to you, pay it. If you think she charges too much, then you may disagree with her about other things as well. If she doesn't charge a fee, you may not feel right taking her help for free. You can devise a monetary or barter exchange that seems fair. You need to feel comfortable about the issue of paying a midwife, or it can interfere with a good working relationship.

➤ *Do you feel confident, open, and trusting* with her? Listen to your own instincts about this regardless of how well trained or how highly recommended a midwife is. She might be great for someone else, but you may not feel comfortable with her. Discuss this with your mate and see if perhaps you can overcome your doubts; if not, try to talk to the midwife about what is bothering you. There are some lay midwives, for example, who "manage" a home birth with the same dominance and authoritarianism that is often found in hospital management of birth. That may be reassuring to you at home or, more likely, it may put you off. If you don't determine what is making you uncomfortable, it is bound to cause a problem sooner or later.

➤ *Is she dependable?* Does she make and keep appointments with you, for instance? Is her car in good running condition and does she live within a reasonable distance to you? It is important that you feel a midwife is organized and responsible so that you can depend on her.

COMPLICATIONS IN HOME BIRTH

Early Rupture of Membranes

This happens when the bag of water breaks and you don't go into labor. It can be an indication that the baby is in a bad position for delivery. The safest time for rupture is when the baby is well down in your pelvis, labor is advanced, and your cervix is fully dilated.

WHAT TO DO

— Remain in bed after your membranes rupture.
— If labor has not begun within 24 hours call a doctor; the infection rate rises dramatically after this 24-hour period, so the traditional decision is to deliver the baby before that time.
— Less conservative doctors may allow you to wait 48 or even 72 hours at home as long as you stay in bed to avoid infection.
— The most dangerous possibility with early rupture is that you can have a *prolapsed cord*—the umbilical cord comes down before the infant and can *mean death for the baby*. If your membranes rupture and a loop of umbilical cord washes out with the fluid and is protruding from your vagina, get into a knee-chest position (head down, behind in the air).
— Rush to the hospital or call the rescue squad. *The baby's oxygen supply is being cut off.* If the cord is still protruding in the knee-chest position, it should be gently supported (not compressed) with warm wet gauze pads or any damp clean cloth. Stay in this position on the way to the hospital—it reduces pressure on the cord.

Bleeding Prior to Birth

➤ Any bright red bleeding of a tablespoon or more is a sign to rush to the hospital. It can indicate a placenta previa (the placenta is covering the baby's exit) and can mean death for you and the baby.
➤ Bleeding is clearly different from the "bloody show," or the blood-tinged mucus plug that comes out before labor begins. Bleeding can be an indication that you have a placenta previa and an internal exam can cause a major, life-threatening hemorrhage.
➤ **WARNING:** Under no circumstances should you allow anyone outside the hospital (including a doctor) to do a vaginal or rectal exam on you if you have bleeding in the third trimester.

Bleeding After Birth

There are two possible sources for blood: from the *uterus* (darker blood that comes in gushes and starts a few minutes after the baby is born) or a *vaginal tear* (brighter red blood that starts right after the baby is born and is a continuous trickle). It is normal in birth for there to be bloodstained water (amniotic fluid) and perhaps some blood on the baby from vaginal tears.

If there's going to be bleeding it usually occurs with third-stage labor: the birth of the placenta, which pulls off from the uterine wall where it has been anchored. It is normal for there to be a gush of about one cup of blood (sometimes as much as two cups) following delivery of the placenta. Then the uterus contracts and the blood vessels close off.

Postpartum hemorrhage can be caused by:
- trying to hurry the placenta by pushing on the uterus and/or pulling on the umbilical cord;
- a long labor which leaves the uterus too tired to contract properly after birth;
- a full bladder during second and third stages of labor; or
- an unhealthy mother.

If there is more than two cups of blood, this is considered excessive bleeding: the other symptoms are paleness, faintness, slowed pulse, and other symptoms of shock.

WHAT TO DO

— Lie flat with your feet elevated, covered enough to avoid losing body heat, but not enough to add extra heat; you are better off cool than too warm.

— Drink plenty of liquids, preferably mild saltwater—one quart of water to one teaspoon salt—with one-half teaspoon of baking soda added. Rush to the hospital.

— Encourage the baby to nurse on the way there; this will release oxytocin, which helps the uterus contract.

— Do not panic. A massive hemorrhage following delivery is usually very brief and shuts off before a dangerous quantity of blood is lost. Fatal hemorrhages are usually slow, continuous bleeding that is not stopped.

— To control excessive bleeding if the placenta has not been delivered and the uterus is soft, massage the abdominal wall with gentle downward pressure until the uterus gets hard. Do not massage to the point of extreme pain (this can increase instead of decrease bleeding). Within the limits of comfort no damage can be done to a hard womb.

— If the placenta has been delivered and there is excessive bleeding, *compression of the womb* will stop it. An attendant should push down with the edge of one hand, in a fist, beneath your uterus on the abdominal wall just above the bone which marks the lower limit of the abdominal wall. Her other hand should be placed above your womb: she is now holding your womb externally between her hands. After gentle massage has caused it to harden, she can hold your uterus pressed very firmly between two hands for at least five minutes. If bleeding starts again when the pressure is released, she should resume holding it firmly.

— Do not stuff gauze or cotton packing into the vagina: this should be done only by a doctor.

Prolonged Labor

This is usually defined as:
- more than 20 hours of labor-breathing;
- transition that lasts longer than a couple of hours without full dilation occurring; or
- a second stage (pushing) that lasts longer than two hours with no sign of progress.

Most long labors are not a result of physical obstruction to the baby's birth but may have an emotional or nutritional cause. Prolonged labor is *not* damaging to the infant *as long as there is evidence of some progress, however slow*. A change in position, walking around, or stroking and other relaxing support from attendants may all speed things along. No progress may be a result of the baby's head being too large to fit through your pelvis, or the baby may be malpositioned. If either of these things is suspected you should transfer to the hospital.

Unusual Amniotic Fluid

Any deviation from the normally clear fluid indicates that the baby is in distress. If it is foul smelling, yellow, green, or brown, you should get to the hospital. The abnormal color and/or smell comes from meconium in the baby's bowel, which is passed by the baby when the anal sphincter relaxes during stress. Although such a baby can seem fine at birth, in some cases of "meconium staining" (as the discolored fluid is called), *there is no way of being sure of this at home*. You need to be near sophisticated infant resuscitation equipment in a hospital in case your baby needs help.

Fetal Heart Rate Drop

This indicates that the baby is not tolerating labor well. Normally the fetal heart rate (FHR) is 120 to 160 beats per minute. During a contraction it usually slows and then returns to normal after the contraction is completed.

An increase or decrease of 20 beats per minute may indicate that the baby is not receiving enough oxygen. A rate of under 110 per minute or over 160 per minute is a cause for alarm. Also, a change in the rhythm (a long first sound and a short second sound instead of the reverse, or an intermittent or irregular FHR) is a sign of distress.

Breech Presentation at Home

It is foolish to attempt birth at home if you know the baby is in this position. Some home birth advocates believe a breech birth is not dangerous, but their belief is based on ignorance of the serious danger.

In a a normal vertex (head-down) position, a baby's head is an effective dilator of the cervix. The baby's head is the widest part of his body and is equal in width to the shoulders, which it precedes through the cervix and birth canal, making room for them. A breech baby comes down buttocks first: the buttocks are not as wide as the head and shoulders and therefore are not as effective in dilating the cervix or in molding the birth canal. A common problem is that the baby simply does not descend far enough down in a breech presentation for vaginal delivery to be completed. The great danger is that in a fairly small baby *the buttocks can go through the cervix before it is fully dilated*. This means that even if the shoulders can also get through, the head cannot (being the widest part) and the baby is trapped, with the partially dilated cervix like a collar around his neck.

Just because you have heard that other people have successfully given birth to breech babies at home does not mean you should try it. There are women who smoke two packs of cigarettes a day and eat poorly and manage to have large, healthy babies—that doesn't make it safe for you to try the same thing. The odds are against you.

If you are unaware that your baby is in a breech position, or if he flips into it during labor, the first indication will be the appearance of buttocks or feet instead of the head.

WHAT TO DO

— *Get into a hands-and-knees position*. This adds the baby's weight to the pull of gravity.

— *No one should try to support the emerging baby*—allow his body to hang down freely so his own weight is pulling him down.

— *One attendant should stand by* to steady you from falling and another attendant should take responsibility for the baby.

— *When a breech is born to the point where the navel and cord can be seen*, this means the umbilical cord blood supply is shut off and with it the baby's oxygen supply from the mother.

— *The baby must be delivered to the point where his nose and mouth can get air within the next 8 to 10 minutes or he will suffocate*. Usually, the mother's bearing down accomplishes this.

— *Never try to help a breech until after the navel appears* and the mother has had two more contractions with strong bearing down.

— *Never pull on the legs or buttocks before the navel is born*. If birth from the navel to the baby's armpit takes more than two contractions, then gentle pulling on the legs is all right. The pulling should be in a general downward direction so that the baby's back is kept toward the mother's belly or side. Do not allow the baby to turn toward the mother's back.

— *The arms should be brought out before the head*. When the armpit appears, use one finger to push the baby's shoulder blade over toward his spine—this usually helps the arm to drop down. If this doesn't work, then slide two fingers up along the baby's arm and sweep the arm down across the baby's chest and out. It is usually easier to do this with the arm nearer to the mother's back because there's more room in that part of the birth canal.

— *When two arms are out, insert a finger in the baby's mouth* in order to flex his head so that his chin is bent down on his chest. The head cannot exit if the chin is raised because it can get caught.

— *When the head is flexed, strong pressure from above* on the mother's abdomen will often deliver the head.

— *Pulling from below may permanently injure the baby's spinal cord, the nerves of the arms, and his breathing apparatus*.

— *If you can't help the baby to deliver without using undue force*, then help him to breathe by creating and maintaining an air passage to his nose. Use two fingers or your whole hand to press back the wall of the vagina from the baby's face. In this position he is able to breathe and can live for an indefinite amount of time until a doctor can complete the delivery.

Hand-First Presentation (Transverse Lie)

This makes delivery mechanically impossible unless the baby is very tiny. You must get to the hospital if the baby is in this position.

In this position there is no sign of the baby's head because his body is wedged crosswise in the birth passage with one shoulder and hand pointing downward, his head shoved off to one side of the passage and his body to the other.

Cord Around the Baby's Neck

This is a common occurrence and happens in as many as 25% of births. The cord can usually be felt as soon as the head is delivered and can be slipped over the baby's head.

If the cord is too tight to slip over the baby's head, an attendant can cut it between two clamps; *however*, the infant must be *delivered quickly*. The umbilical cord is the baby's lifeline—if you cut it, the baby must be ready to breathe with his lungs.

Shoulder Dystocia

This means that the baby's shoulders can't be born without help, but it happens in less than one percent of births. In a normal birth there is a gap of two to three minutes after the birth of the head and the next contraction. With that next contraction, the baby's anterior shoulder slips under the pubic bone, the posterior shoulder is born (the one toward the mother's back), and then the rest of the body slips out. If the baby begins to breathe after the head is born, an indefinite amount of time can pass before the shoulders are born, giving you time to summon medical assistance.

However, if the baby does *not* breathe after his head is born, then the attendant should wait for only two contractions before helping the shoulders. Shoulder dystocia is a rare complication and is listed here only for thoroughness.

Do not be hasty. After the birth of the head, the mother must push through two contractions with verbal assistance. If the shoulders still have not been born, then for the next two contractions an attendant must put pressure on the uterus, pushing on the top (fundus) of the uterus.

If that doesn't work (and only if it does not), the attendant should insert a finger and hook it into the armpit that is toward the mother's back. Then she can pull it gently out in a spiral fashion, rotating the hooked shoulder toward the baby's own face.

The Baby Doesn't Breathe Properly

There may be fluid or mucus in his airways, or the baby is brain-damage (this is a major cause of improper breathing, although lack of breathing can also *cause* brain damage).

If a baby is crying, this is good—do not get sentimental and think it means the baby is upset. Let the baby cry until he's pink—this is the way the newborn's breathing and circulatory systems start working. If the baby is silent, you want to stimulate him to cry to take in oxygen.

WHAT TO DO

— First place the baby on his stomach over your thigh, lowering his head and chest.
— Suction out his mouth again as thoroughly as possible with a syringe.
— Cover him with a warm blanket and massage his back and flick the soles of his feet. Gentleness is very important in trying to stimulate breathing in a newborn.
— An occasional shallow gasp means the baby is taking shallow breaths, although they may be imperceptible to an observer.

— If the baby is still not breathing, tie and cut the cord if the blood has drained (it will have a light color).
— Wrap the baby warmly and turn him on his right side.
— Holding him securely in both hands rock the baby *slowly and gently* by tipping first his head down and then his feet.
— Shifting the weight of the internal organs is often sufficient to compress and release the lungs, facilitating breathing.
— Artificial respiration (mouth to mouth or rib compression) is not a good idea. The air capacity of a baby's lungs is only a mouthful of adult air, so it is easy to accidentally blow out a baby's lungs. He can also contract pneumonia from contamination. With rib compression you can apply too much force and damage the ribs and internal organs.
— A form of artificial respiration you can use:
  • Hold two hands under the baby, one under his shoulders and head, and the other under his hips.
  • Keep his head level.
  • Bring your hands together and gently raise them, turning them so that you gently bend the baby's body in the middle like a hinge to the point where the stomach is decidedly compressed.
  • Then straighten your hands so that the baby's body straightens out again.
  • This produces movement of air in and out of the lungs. The approximate rate should be 12 per minute, or once every 5 seconds.
— A pale, limp baby is in danger. A baby with no facial expression, no limb movements, and no resistance to outside efforts to move his arms and legs has little hope of survival. If gentle efforts do not succeed, he probably cannot be helped.
— Even if a baby is breathing, *check the breathing*. Normally a baby will breathe about 60 to 70 times a minute for the first couple of hours after birth and then slow down to 40 to 60 times per minute. A newborn's respirations are frequently irregular and easily altered by internal and external stimuli.
— The baby's breathing should be fairly regular and it shouldn't seem as if he has to work hard to breathe. If the baby has any of the symptoms from the following chart, she may be suffering from respiratory distress syndrome (RDS) *and should be taken to a doctor or hospital immediately to be checked.*

Examine the Umbilical Cord Stump

Be sure that no blood is oozing and that there are *three blood vessels in the cord*; if there are only two, you should have the baby checked by a pediatrician right away. Sometimes an abnormal number of cord vessels is associated with certain kinds of abnormalities.

SIGNS OF RESPIRATORY DISTRESS SYNDROME (RDS)

* Respiratory rate of more than 70 breaths per minute in the second or third postpartum hour.
* Chest retraction: the chest drops down (is sucked in) right under the rib cage or between the ribs while the baby is breathing.
* Grunting on exhalation.
* Gasping for breath.
* Flaring of nostrils while breathing.
* Cyanosis: a blue color, especially at the lips and ears (indicating that the baby is not getting enough oxygen).

Retained Placenta

This means that the placenta does not detach from the uterine wall or doesn't detach fully. Normally the third stage of labor lasts anywhere from 20 minutes to 2 hours. If there is bleeding and cramping and the placenta is not delivered, you have to go to the hospital right away to have it removed.

When the placenta is born, lay it flat and examine it. Any torn piece should fit together with another piece like a jigsaw puzzle. If there are any missing pieces, they may still be in the uterus.

Go to the hospital, because a retained placenta can lead to hemorrhaging.

Registering Home Births

Keeping a record of home births is important to demonstrate their safety. Many people giving birth at home do not file birth certificates. However, the law requires that deaths must be reported. Therefore the statistics showing the fetal death rate in home births are inaccurate, *but* neonatal mortality is computed by *comparing* the number of births with the number of deaths. Obviously this makes the infant mortality figure for home births look much worse than it is.

The medical community believes the neonatal mortality is greater at home than in the hospital because current statistics are grossly inaccurate. This inaccuracy gives the medical establishment ammunition to bring greater pressure against home birth. What is at stake here is maintaining the *choice* of home birth for those who want it. Those who are considering home birth deserve accurate information on which to base their decision. Home-birthers who do not register births are creating a false impression of lack of safety. Their nonreporting also gives a false impression that there are fewer home births than actually take place.

Adequate medical backup for home birth will not be available until the statistics show that a sufficient number of people are giving birth at home to justify the expenditure of public or private funds for emergency facilities if they become necessary.

One reason that couples do not register home births is because of the harassment they may encounter from health officials who are opposed to home birth. But children really need birth certificates. The long-term consequences for a child are worse than whatever discomfort her parents may have to withstand. A birth certificate is necessary for getting into school, getting a driver's license, a social security card (and therefore being able to prove citizenship to get a job), a passport, proving majority, voting, establishing citizenship, claiming inheritances, qualifying for old-age pensions, Social Security, and Medicaid. A couple should take the responsibility of reporting a birth not only for their child's sake, but also so a more accurate picture of home births will be available.

In order to register a birth, look in the telephone book under County Health Department, Department of Public Health, or Registrar (or Bureau) of Vital Statistics. It does not require a doctor's signature, only that of a witness to the birth. Anyone can register a birth if he or she was present; it can be the mother herself. Depending on the state, there is a time limit on registering anywhere from a few days to a year. After that time, late registration can be considered a misdemeanor—which may be a hassle (but is still worth the advantages to the child).

CHAPTER TWELVE

❧❧

Labor and Delivery

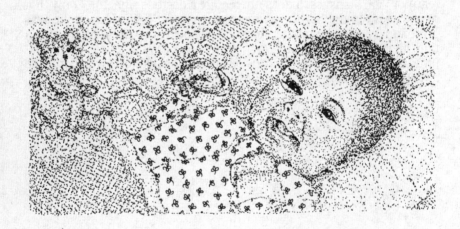

The labor that your body goes through, which ends in the birth of your child, is divided into well-defined stages.

1) Indications of prelabor (see below).
2) Perhaps a stage of false labor (when your uterus is contracting but not effectively opening up your cervix).
3) Early first-stage labor.
4) Late (or active) first-stage labor, which culminates in:
5) Transition, the hardest part of labor, when your cervix completes the process of dilating (opening to the fullest).

6) Second-stage labor: the time when you push your baby down the birth canal.
7) This stage ends with the birth itself.
8) Third-stage labor: the expulsion of the placenta, the organ that has nourished your baby in utero for nine months.

THE SIGNS OF PRELABOR

— *Lightening (also called engagement)* usually takes place two or three weeks before the onset of labor if this is your first baby. The baby's presenting part (in most cases, her head) settles down into your bony pelvis: it is "engaged" in the pelvis. If engagement takes place more than four weeks before your due date, it may mean that the baby will be early, although the head may also dislodge.

    The degree to which the baby has descended is measured in "stations." Before the baby's presenting part is engaged it is at a negative (−) station, meaning she is moving or floating freely. A baby may engage in your bony pelvis and then dislodge, which some babies do even during labor, so that she is floating again. In that case, the baby could return to a −1 or −2 station, meaning that the presenting part is that much above the ischial bones of the pelvis. Each station is approximately one centimeter. As the baby moves down through your bony pelvis, she is at plus (+) stations.

➤ *In a woman who has had a baby previously*, lightening may not occur until early in labor. Her abdominal muscles may not be as firm, especially after more than one baby. Therefore, the uterus tends to bulge *out* rather than being pushed down by those muscles.

➤ *You will know when engagement has taken place*. Your breathing may be easier because the baby has settled lower down. You may feel pressure behind your pubic bone and you may need to urinate more frequently because of the increased pressure on your bladder.

➤ *After engagement,* walking becomes more difficult because of the increased pressure on your hip joints.

— *Braxton-Hicks contractions* increase in strength and frequency.

➤ These are "practice" contractions, which are more common in first pregnancies. The uterus is getting ready for labor, flexing its muscles to prepare for the work of labor.

➤ You can use them to practice your childbirth training: test your release of tension, your breathing techniques, light massage of the hardened uterus, and get used to how a contraction feels at its peak and when it is falling off (although with Braxton-Hicks there is rarely any discomfort).

— *Increased vaginal mucus* is another sign of prelabor.

➤ Vaginal discharge may increase the day before active labor begins. Then the tiny mucus plug blocking the cervix breaks loose: it is called "pink show" or "bloody show" because it may be blood-tinged from the blood capillaries that had attached it to the cervix.

➤ Although "show" is usually a sign of early labor, it can occur as many as 12 days before active labor begins.

— *Weight loss of two to three pounds* often occurs three to four days before the onset of labor.

— *A spurt of energy*, which can be considered a "nesting instinct," affects some women and motivates them to rush around doing chores and the like. *Resist* this urge: you have to conserve this energy and save it for the hard work of labor to come.

— *Premenstrual feelings may precede labor*—the same sort of physical and emotional changes that often precede a period. You may also feel crampy with pressure in your rectum or the need to urinate frequently.

FALSE LABOR

False labor is also known as "prodromal phase" labor—the symptoms of labor without any noticeable changes accomplished in the cervix. Prodromal contractions are different from true labor contractions: the uterine muscles contract differently and they can be quite painful, sometimes more so than true labor contractions. It can be discouraging to be hurting yet told that it's a "fake": it can make you worry that if it's this bad and is "false labor," you'll never make it through true labor! Don't despair.

Although it can be embarrassing and discouraging to be examined and sent home, you are *better off going home*—you can relax, drink, and move around. Especially with a second baby it really shouldn't be called "false labor" anyway: it is prelabor, during which the cervix is softened so that it is ready to thin and dilate.

Some people say that if you have to ask yourself whether you're in real labor, then you probably are not—that you will know you are when the time comes. This is not always true: some women go through much of the first stage of labor without really knowing it. As your due date nears, you become understandably anxious and excited, and when contractions begin you have every reason to suspect you are in labor. Early labor is, in fact, ill-defined. It's hard to distinguish between "warm-up" contractions and true labor.

How to Know if It's False Labor

➤ *In false-labor, contractions won't occur on a regular 15-to 20-minute schedule*. However, this is not always true. For some women nonregularity of contractions is not a reliable measure; their contractions *never* become regular.

➤ *Contractions may subside* if you walk around, whereas true labor usually worsens when you get up. To test if you are having true contractions, change your activity: they will stop or decrease if they are false contractions, whereas the opposite will be true if it's the real thing.

➤ *One big difference in contractions* is that in true labor they get stronger and longer as the interval between them gets shorter. In warm-up labor, after maintaining a plateau of intensity, the intensity diminishes as time passes. However, contractions feel different to each woman and are different in each pregnancy. They can be like menstrual cramps, gas pains, or a mild backache—some women think that early contractions are indigestion.

➤ *Call your doctor, midwife, or childbirth educator*, because often they can tell from your voice during a contraction whether it's the real thing. True labor usually requires your full attention and you will stop your end of a conversation during a contraction.

➤ *A good rule of thumb* is that if you have to use your breathing techniques to stay comfortable during a contraction, you're probably in true labor.

➤ *Ask your doctor about having a glass of wine* which may sound like a contradiction to previous warnings. Wine can relax prodromal contractions and stop them, which is more help than harm at this point. Wine can help relax you if you are in TRUE labor, but will not stop the contractions.

➤ *A warm (but not too hot) bath* (if your membranes are still intact and have not yet ruptured) is also excellent. Your energy will be conserved and you can rest at home until the labor begins.

➤ *Get medical reassurance* if you want it. Go to the hospital and have them check you to see if your cervix is opening. If you are told it is not true labor, *do not be embarrassed*—this happens to many people. But *do* ask your doctor about going home rather than staying in the hospital, where you may be confined to bed without fluids by mouth and may get tense and tired. Unless you live very far from the hospital, go home and rest there.

WHEN TO GO TO THE HOSPITAL

— *If, during the space of an hour,* the contractions are one minute in duration and occur approximately fifteen minutes apart and don't go away when you move around, call. The doctor will probably tell you to come to the hospital (or your midwife will come to your home) when the contractions are five minutes apart.

— *Don't rush to the hospital.* The average first stage of labor lasts 8½ hours with the first baby. If you are unsure of the doctor's and/or hospital's attitude toward childbirth education techniques, wait as long as you can before going there. Another problem with going in early can be that you won't be allowed any liquids and, for example, you might not be allowed to use a hands-and-knees position to do pelvic rock for a backache. Of course, if you live far away from the hospital, or have a special fear about not getting there in time, then go as soon as you want to. Some hospitals may send you home if you arrive too early, but others may let you walk their halls.

— *A rule of thumb about when to leave for the hospital* with a first baby is when contractions are between 55 and 65 seconds long and the first level of breathing exercises is no longer adequate: this means your cervix is probably four to six centimeters dilated. This is a good time to go in because it's early enough to complete all procedures but doesn't leave you with too much time in early labor in the hospital.

➤ Your mate should know how to get to the hospital and how much time is needed for the trip. It is wise to have thought of an alternate route in case of heavy traffic, construction, or other impediments. Choose smooth roads when possible for a more comfortable journey.

➤ Be sure you know which hospital entrance to use during the day and whether it is necessary to use a different one at night.

➤ Although you may plan for your partner to drive you to the hospital, *you should know all this information*, too, in case he is not available and you have to call a taxi or ask a friend to take you.

— *The car trip to the hospital* will be more comfortable (if it's longer than 15 minutes) if you lie down on the backseat. If you want to sit in front, you may be more comfortable with a pillow behind your back, which allows your uterus more room to contract.

What to Bring to the Hospital

- **2 nightgowns** that open in front, if you're breast-feeding
- **robe and slippers** for walking around
- **2 nursing bras**, if you're breast-feeding
- **baby clothes:** diapers with pins and plastic pants if you're using cloth, nightgown or stretch suit, receiving blanket, and something warm if it's cold out (such as an infant "snuggle" suit)
- **sanitary pads and belt** if you don't want to pay the hospital charges for each one they issue you
- **washcloths** for your face during labor and to suck on if there are no ice chips. Some hospitals don't supply washcloths
- **radio or cassette player** for music during labor, to relax you, to drown out other noises
- **camera and/or tape recorder**, if you have gotten permission
- **heavy socks**, as it can be cold in the delivery room
- **watch or clock**
- **books, baby announcements,** for your hospital stay

FIRST STAGE OF LABOR

In the first stage of labor your cervix is effaced and dilated by the uterine contractions: "effacement" is the softening and thinning of the cervix, which is the lower, necklike part of the uterus. Effacement is measured in percentages; for example, your doctor or midwife may tell you that you are 30% effaced before you ever go into labor.

By the time that you are about three centimeters dilated, your cervix is usually 100% effaced. "Dilation" is the opening up of the cervix so that the baby can pass through it into the birth canal. Dilation is measured in centimeters; the cervix is completely open at 10 centimeters. Some attendants speak in terms of how many "fingers" you are dilated—in this case, one finger equals roughly one centimeter. When you cervix is fully dilated, the first stage of labor is complete. The diagram on page 381 shows the stages of dilation. The circles are the actual sizes to which your cervix opens.

The Signs of First Stage

The signs of first-stage labor are sometimes the same as the signs of false labor. The important difference is in the contractions and whether they increase or decrease if you change your activity and walk around.

➤ *Your membranes may rupture* at any time. Have a plastic sheet or a double mattress pad on your bed during the final weeks of pregnancy. You might want to wear a sanitary pad if you are out of the house a lot and are nervous about the possibility that your water will break. Most often the membranes of the amniotic sac do not rupture until late in first-stage labor, when the cervix is opened up.

It does not hurt when the membranes rupture: you will have a sensation of a warm flow of water. There may be a lot or a little fluid depending on the location and size of the break; usually once it ruptures there is continuous leaking with gushes during contractions until the baby's head is far down enough to act as a "stopper" in the neck of your uterus. When you are standing up, the baby usually pushes against the cervix like a cork, and when you lie down fluid may escape. You can lose as much as one quart of liquid, although amniotic fluid continues to be manufactured at a rate of about three-quarters of a cup per hour.

➤ *Pink show (also called bloody show)* may appear. This is the blood-tinged mucus plug that was blocking the cervix and breaks loose before labor or at the onset of labor.

➤ *An achy feeling in the pelvic floor*, similar to the feeling of sore muscles from exercising, is a sign that dilation is beginning.

➤ *Contractions feel different to every woman*, but early labor often feels like menstrual cramps with a mild backache. Some say that a contraction feels like a wave rising, breaking, and receding. There is a gradual tightening of the uterine muscles that increases in intensity until a peak is reached and then the tightening slowly relaxes. The longitudinal muscle fibers on top harden and the circular muscles below relax with each contraction. These lengthwise muscles of the uterus are involuntarily working to pull open the circular muscles around the cervix. In early labor it's slightly crampy, like a period, and sometimes the intermittent tightening in your lower abdomen is strong enough to awaken you at night.

The action of the uterine muscles is like the contractions of the intestinal tract—they are activated by the autonomic nervous system. You are not voluntarily controlling these muscles, but like the intestine, they are affected by your state of mind. Just as you may have experienced "butterflies" in your stomach or diarrhea from excitement, your state of mind during labor has a definite effect on the contractions. If you go into the hospital and are uptight or there are hassles with the staff, this can affect your contractions. Your hormonal balance gets set for "fight or flight," as with animals that react to *external* stimuli. A mother deer can be giving birth and if she hears a frightening sound, she gets up and her hormones halt labor; she goes back into labor when she has found a safe place again. Your uterus can respond to your emotions as well—it holds on to the baby or spits her out too fast. So it's important to create and protect a good atmosphere around yourself when you're in labor.

➤ *A common misconception about labor* is that contractions start out weak and get stronger and stronger, ending in birth. But there is an ebb and flow to contractions, like waves on a beach. There will be a strong contraction and then a weak one, each contraction doing the work that is necessary at that time. Each contraction consolidates the work accomplished by the preceding one, slowly stretching and pulling open the cervix.

➤ *The length of contractions* is timed from the *beginning* of one contraction to the *beginning* of the next one. In early labor contractions are 30 to 60 seconds long with 5 to 20 minutes between contractions. This is the stage of labor that lasts an average of 8½ hours for first babies. In the *active phase* of labor, which accomplishes dilation from 4 to 7 centimeters, the contractions are 45 to 75 seconds long and 2 to 4 minutes apart.

➤ *The length of labor* varies, but the average total length of labor is 12 to 14 hours for a first baby and an average of 7 hours in subsequent labors. The longest part of labor is the easiest part— in a first pregnancy it takes an average of 9 hours to get to 3 centimeters of dilation. Generally, the longer the labor, the lighter the contractions will be. Fast labors start with long, strong contractions and usually without much preliminary labor. The optimal length of time for labor is 11 to 15 hours: this is long enough for your tissues to stretch, long enough for the fetus not to be traumatized by a too-fast birth, but short enough so that maternal fatigue doesn't cause stress for the baby.

➤ *Late first-stage (or active phase) labor* is when the cervix is opening from 4 to 7 centimeters. After about 5 centimeters dilation your prepared breathing techniques usually become necessary to maintain comfort. For many women this is when they will go to the hospital. Dilation from 4 to 10 centimeters is usually more rapid in women who have had childbirth education. They are able to relax so that their contractions can have maximum effect in dilating the cervix.

➤ *Frequent position change* is important, especially in early labor. Try to walk around as much as possible. Moving around is discouraged in some hospitals, but again, you should check with your doctor or the hospital. Walking takes your mind off contractions and encourages more rapid engagement of the fetal head, meaning that it settles into your pelvis and helps to dilate the cervix. Walking is restful because it aids circulation, which is better for you and the baby. Walking can also increase the intensity of contractions—*which is good*. You want good, strong contractions. Your goal in labor is to get your cervix open and get that baby out. So if the contractions get harder when you walk, think of that as *positive*.

Backache

Backache during labor is experienced by most women, but it is severe for only a few. It feels as if your abdomen is tensing with an ache in the back. It occurs more often and more intensely if a baby is in a posterior vertex position during labor (her head is pressing on your spine), or is a breech presentation.

THREE REMEDIES FOR BACK LABOR

— **Counterpressure** is the most effective; you "counter" the pressure the baby's head is putting on your spine. You can make fists, put them under your back where the pressure is worst, and press down on your fists during a contraction. Tennis balls are recommended by many Lamaze teachers to be used in the same way. You can also stuff a pillow or two behind your lower back and press back into them. Both these techniques should be done in a sitting or semi-sitting position. You can also have your coach apply counterpressure with his hands if you lie on your side.

— **Position changes** can help. *The worst position for backache is flat on your back*: the baby's head presses hardest there. You can lie on the side toward which the baby is rotating (usually the left) or you can try tailor-sitting, knee-to-chest, forward-leaning, or a pelvic rock. Any position that gets the baby off your spine will relieve or reduce the pressure.

— **Application of heat**, either during or between contractions, helps some women.

Examinations During Labor

Vaginal examinations during labor are done periodically to check for cervical effacement and dilation. The attendant also checks for the position and station of the baby. These examinations are done vaginally or rectally by an attendant, who puts on a sterile rubber glove and inserts two fingers.

The "station" is how far down the baby's presenting part is in relation to the ischial spines (the two bony projections of the pelvis). A "minus station" means the baby is that far above the ischial bones; a "plus station" means that the presentation part is below. Each station is approximately one centimeter. At a +4 or +5 station, the baby's presenting part is out in the world.

➤ *Ask how you are progressing after each exam* if you are not told. Each time that an attendant begins to examine you, ask what she or he is doing, so that you are prepared. Some attendants use the term "fingers" to describe dilation, but it is a less accurate measure. If you are unclear, ask for your progress in terms of centimeters.

➤ *If contractions are getting longer and stronger* and you haven't been checked for quite a while, you can *ask for an examination*. It can boost your morale if you find your cervix has dilated more than you realized.

➤ *Examinations can be quite painful*, so you will need your relaxation and breathing techniques while you are being examined. Some attendants are more gentle then others: if you are being hurt, *say so*. The back-lying position is the most common for exams, but if it's particularly uncomfortable for you, ask if the exam can be done with you in a side-lying position.

➤ *In each contact with a new staff member* tell them that you have taken childbirth classes: they may not be accustomed to women with a positive attitude toward labor who want to be given information about their progress. *If a new staff member enters and begins to examine you without saying anything*, have your mate interrupt the attendant by saying, "Excuse me . . . I'm Simon Harrison and I don't think we've been introduced." (This is particularly effective with male interns!) The point of this is that it is *your* labor and your labor room: anyone coming into it should introduce himself or herself, explain any procedure he or she is going to perform, and then tell you the results.

➤ *Ignore any questions during a contraction*. Keep up your concentration and breathing. If your coach is there, he can explain that your concentration is essential during contractions, but that you will be glad to answer their questions between contractions—otherwise you can explain this when your contraction is over.

➤ *Your coach may be asked to leave* during examinations for no reason other than it is customary. Even though staff members who are strangers to you go in and out of your room and see your legs spread open, there is a residual "modesty" in some hospitals about a woman's mate being present for examinations. In fact, you may need your coach more than ever because the exams can stimulate stronger contractions. The coach has every right to stay and the woman should just say, "I need my coach here during contractions. It might not be routine, but we have Dr. Ray's permission, so I'd really appreciate it if you could let us stay together."

➤ *"Forced accouchement"* (also referred to as a "vaginal hysterectomy" or a "vaginal hys" for short) is what some doctors do during an internal exam in labor to speed things along. They force open your cervix with their fingers. One way to tell if a doctor is trying to do this is if a vaginal exam is especially painful. Some doctors' internal exams can be painful anyway, but if one exam feels more painful than previous ones ask the doctor to stop immediately.

Another clue that a doctor may have performed forced accouchement on you is if you go from 6 centimeters to complete dilation in a very short time (especially in a first labor). If the doctor then takes more than 15 minutes for the episiotomy repair and asks the nurse for a lot of sutures, it may mean he is repairing your cervix as well as the incision.

Advice to the Coach During Labor

In most cases a woman's husband or partner will be with her during labor, so the coach will be referred to as "he" in this section. However, *anyone* can be a coach—friend or relative, male or female—as long as you feel comfortable and they are committed to going through childbirth training with you. Since this section is intended for the coach, the "you" will refer to the coach, not the pregnant woman (as in the rest of the book), who is referred to here as "her."

Early Labor

➤ *During prelabor you should encourage her* to sleep or conserve her energy.

➤ *There is often a burst of energy*, a sort of "nesting instinct," before labor really begins. Often a woman needs someone to *tell* her to put her feet up. If there is some chore she insists is essential, *do it for her*, even if it doesn't seem important to you.

➤ *Suggest that she take a warm (but not too hot) bath* or a shower to relax if her membranes are intact. Once her water has broken, there is a chance of infection while bathing. Help her get in and out of the bath so that she doesn't slip.

➤ *Unless she feels nauseated, suggest she drink*. Natural fruit juice, which has fructose (natural fruit sugar), is good. Tea with honey has natural energy. Jell-O has gelatin, which is protein (although not readily assimilated by the body) and sugar, which gives energy (but is not as healthful as honey or fructose). You can make some "slush cubes" in an ice tray: frozen orange-juice concentrate mixed with honey and a little water.

Dairy products are a bad idea: they are hard to digest and remain in the digestive system for a long time. You want to give her fluids and quick energy, but you don't want to burden her digestive system, because her body is focused on the uterus. (Remember to eat something yourself—coaching is emotionally and physically strenuous.)

➤ *When contractions begin* you should time them. Note the interval between contractions and how long they last: they are timed from the beginning of one contraction to the beginning of the next. Make a note of the time when (if) she has any "bloody show" or her membranes rupture. This information will be useful for the doctor or midwife.

➤ **When you leave for the hospital**, bring your childbirth class certificate in case they require proof that you have completed the training. Bring this book with you if you feel more comfortable having the reminders with you. Bring a sandwich or other snack for yourself (don't choose tunafish or anything with a strong odor because a woman in labor can be hypersensitive to smells!).

➤ **When you arrive at the hospital** don't get hung up filling out forms if your partner is having a hard time with contractions. Just sign the essential documents and *go directly to the labor area*. You can fill out the forms later. The important thing is to get your wife comfortably settled so that the move to the hospital does not make her anxious or upset her control of labor.

➤ **The father's waiting room** is where some hospitals send a coach while a woman is being "prepped" (hospital gown, shave, enema, IV). Although your wife may say to the nurse that she wants you to stay with her, some hospitals may be strict about excluding you. If you do go to the father's waiting room, *do not wait there longer than 20 to 30 minutes*. They may forget to come and get you, and your partner may be waiting for you, increasing her anxiety. Identify yourself to a nurse and ask to join your mate—or if you know where her labor room is, just go there.

Reminders to the Coach

Coaching her through contractions is your primary task, along with the basic comfort and support of your presence.

➤ **Use positive words**—don't criticize her and don't point out negative things. Don't say: "You aren't relaxing properly." Use supportive phrasing, such as: "You seem to be having trouble with _____. Would you like to try _____?"

SOME COMFORTING WORDS

- "Good."
- "Go with it."
- "Easy, easy."
- "Let your *shoulders* [for example] go loose."
- "Breathe, breathe."
- "Steady, steady."
- "Hang in there."

➢ *Make sure each breath is complete* with the emphasis on the *exhalation*, not the inhalation. A breath that is completely blown out makes way for the next complete breath and the complete exchange of gases in her lungs.

➢ *Place your hand* on her abdomen so that you can feel when it begins to tighten and you can help her anticipate a contraction. A fetal monitor can also tell you when a contraction is beginning, if you ask a nurse to show you how to read the tracing coming out of the machine.

When her uterus starts to harden and rise up, tell her to take a deep, cleansing breath. By helping her anticipate what's coming, she won't be caught off guard and can stay on top of the contractions.

➢ *Encourage her to maintain each breathing level* for as long as possible. She should change from deep chest breathing only *when it is no longer working* to keep her comfortable. Each successive breathing technique is more tiring and more damaging and should be used only when it becomes necessary. You want to get maximum effectiveness out of each breathing technique and not "use up" the effectiveness of a higher level of breathing before it is needed.

➢ *Breathe with her when the going gets rough*, sort of like breathing "in stereo." To do this you have to establish *eye contact*, sometimes referred to as "catching eyes." Many people are not comfortable with prolonged eye contact, so this is something you should practice before labor. It can give a feeling of "oneness" between two people whose gazes are locked and are breathing in rhythm. Breathing this way can have a positive effect even if a stranger does it with a laboring woman, so it is that much more powerful if it comes from her mate.

If a woman is struggling with a difficult contraction and loses her perspective, she may feel as if she is "disintegrating," or losing her center. Say to her—and you may need to be firm if she has become agitated and distracted—"*Open your eyes and look at me—I'll breathe with you.*" Keep your face as close to hers as is comfortable and take deep, calm breaths along with her. If a woman will do this and trust you enough to maintain eye contact, you can get her through almost any kind of contraction just by the power of your being there and experiencing it with her.

➢ *Hyperventilation can occur* if she is not making a complete exchange of gases in her lungs during breathing. The signs of hyperventilation are dizziness, tingling, and numbness of the nose and extremities. Cup your hands over her nose and mouth while she is breathing to correct the problem (but do not cut off her airflow completely).

➢ *Shaking during labor* can be strange and overpowering to a woman. If a woman does not know that shaking is normal, it can be more upsetting than the contractions. Do not let yourself be thrown by this shaking, which can sometimes be strong. Soothe the woman, remind her that it is normal and that it will pass.

➤ *Touching*—or any kind of skin-to-skin contact—can help a woman so much. Touching and stroking are emphasized in home birth. There's a saying that a loving touch is worth at least 75 mg of Demerol to ease a woman's discomfort! Don't underestimate how soothing it is for a woman to be fondled during labor: wiping her face, massaging her back or abdomen, holding hands, etc.

➤ *Watch for signs of tension* during *and* between contractions. Her forehead, neck, shoulders, or feet will be the first places to show tension. Constantly be on the lookout for tensing in those areas—you can remind her to relax an area of tension before it builds up and interferes with her relaxation and breathing.

➤ *Remind her to keep her mouth loose between contractions*. There appears to be a connection between tension around the mouth and the pelvic area. If a woman keeps her mouth and jaw loose, it may influence the relaxation of her vagina and allow her cervix to dilate more easily.

➤ *Remind her to empty her bladder every hour*. A full bladder can cause pain during contractions. Standing up and walking may increase her contractions, so stay near her when she goes to the bathroom. You can coach her, even through a closed bathroom door if necessary. Try to start her to the bathroom at the end of a contraction so that she has the maximum amount of time before the next one.

➤ *Follow her moods*. Talk if she wants to, play cards (or any game you may have brought), or let her doze between contractions if she wishes. But alert her to upcoming contractions so that she isn't taken off guard.

➤ *Medication is an area in which you can be helpful*, although you cannot presume to tell her that she shouldn't have any. If she asks for drugs, ask the nurse what a particular drug is for, how long before it will take effect, and how it may change her behavior. Be sure your partner knows this information before she accepts the medication.

— *Try to get her to wait 15 minutes*, or, if possible, half an hour after the time she requests a drug. A great deal of dilation can take place in that time, particularly in the active phase of labor. You may be able to breathe with her through a rough time and help avoid unnecessary medication.

— *Medication is definitely indicated* when contractions continue, but effacement, dilation, and descent of the baby do not occur, *or* if the doctor will use forceps and needs the vagina to be totally relaxed.

Transition: The Hardest Part of Labor

- Try hard to get her to relax.
- Ask questions that need only a word, or shake or nod answer.
- Wipe her face with a cool cloth if she's warm.
- If she tells you to take your hands off her, do so, but *stay near the bed*. Her moods will swing and she may need to hold your hand a moment later.
- If she feels sick or wants to vomit, get a basin and encourage her. She'll feel better afterward.
- Express affection and praise—continue coaching her through contractions with simple, firm commands. She may be confused and may also be irritated by talking. *Remind her to take it one contraction at a time*.
- If her legs are trembling, put socks on her, cover her with blankets, and hold her legs firmly, stroking them.
- If she grunts or makes pushing movements during a contraction, notify the nurse or doctor immediately. These are signs that the "bearing-down reflex" is starting and her cervix may be fully dilated. However, before she can push she must be internally examined to be sure that none of her cervix is in the way. *Use "don't push" techniques until an attendant has examined her and says it is okay to push.*
- A woman may turn to a supportive female instead of you. Don't be offended or take it as a personal rejection or sign that you have "failed" her. A professional female who has years of experience may give her more confidence at some point during labor. Whatever gives her the most strength in labor is in your mutual best interests.

The Delivery

The delivery is imminent when the baby's head has crowned (is visible at the lips of her vagina). Your role changes as the birth begins. The teamwork now is between the woman and her doctor or midwife. You are more of an observer, although you can still be involved.

> ➤ *Change quickly* when you know that delivery is near, or better yet, try to change before this time. Some hospitals give you a sterile gown to put on over your street clothes; others require you to remove them and put on hospital pants and top. It is important that you do this before the transfer to the delivery room takes place—it is very hard for her to make that move and keep her attention on contractions if you aren't with her.

> ➤ *Remind her to relax her pelvic floor during pushing*. She should take two or three deep breaths and push her hardest at the peak of the contraction—it is less tiring and makes fullest

use of the force of the uterus. The pushes should be long, strong, and steady.

> ➤ *Remind her to look in the mirror at the baby emerging*   in all the hard work and excitement, she may forget. Don't forget to look yourself!

> ➤ *If asked to leave the delivery room, do so without question.* In a medical emergency they have to move quickly and you will be in the way. Go outside the delivery room, but *stay nearby*. The problem may be handled quickly and you can go back in.

LABOR POSITIONS

In most U.S. hospitals the supine position is used, lying flat on your back. However, there are some drawbacks to the supine position, so you might want to practice and try different positions (were back to you being the pregnant woman). The squatting and hands-and-knees positions are rarely allowed in most hospitals, but they may be more comfortable for you as well as beneficial to your labor. You can also try lying on your side. If you are laboring at home or in an alternative birth room in a hospital, you should try a beanbag chair placed on the bed—it is popular because it gives you support, but also molds to your shape.

Supine (On Your Back) Position

> ➤ *The supine (lithotomy) position* has so many drawbacks that you might want to try a sitting, semi-sitting, or side-lying position for at least part of your labor.

PROBLEMS WITH THE SUPINE POSITION

— The uterus compresses the aorta, a main artery supplying blood to the fetus. This causes a fall in your blood pressure, which can mean the baby doesn't get enough oxygen because her blood supply is reduced.

— The normal intensity of contractions is decreased.

— Voluntary efforts to push the baby out are inhibited because gravity is not working in your favor. This increases the need for forceps to assist delivery.

— It inhibits the spontaneous expulsion of the placenta for the above reason, increasing the need for cord traction (pulling on the cord), manual removal of the placenta, and related procedures that increase the possibility of hemorrhage.

— It increases the need for an episiotomy because it increases the tension on the pelvic floor and stretching of the perineal tissue.

Other Positions

➤ **The dorsal position** has many of the same drawbacks as the supine. In this position you lie on your back with the soles of your feet flat on the delivery table. Contraction intensity and effective pushing are not hindered as much as with lying flat on your back, and it is more comfortable because it gives you more freedom of movement. Also, your feet are not spread as far apart, so there is less tension on the perineal floor. This position permits your spine to curve so that you are working with gravity in pushing the baby out.

➤ **The side-lying (left lateral) position** takes the weight of your uterus off the main blood supply to the baby and also reduces tension on the perineum. During the pushing stage of labor, either you, your coach, or another attendant has to hold up your right leg during a contraction. If you are in the delivery room, your right leg can be placed in the stirrup usually used for the left leg in the supine position—this is less tiring and more comfortable for some women. The problem with the side-lying position is that it is difficult to see the birth in the overhead mirror because your upper (right) leg blocks your view. You can solve this by having someone adjust the angle of the mirror.

➤ **The semi-sitting position** is good for birth because the contractions are not hampered, the perineum is not stretched, and the force of gravity aids the descent of the baby. Your upper torso is propped at a 45-degree angle with your knees flexed and your feet flat on the table. Some labor beds and delivery tables can be adjusted to support your back in this position; otherwise, you can use pillows.

➤ **The hands-and-knees position** is good because it gets gravity to work for you, especially with a baby in a breech or posterior position. It also takes the weight of the uterus off your back just as in the pelvic rock exercise, so it is good if you are having painful back labor. This position can be dangerous for delivery, however: the baby emerges face up, horizontal to the floor, and just as his head is fully born, the afterwaters (the amniotic fluid that remains in the uterus) flood over his body and into his mouth and up his nose. It would be like lying on the edge of the surf and letting a wave break over you. The afterwaters can surge in any delivery position, but if you are sitting or squatting, the baby's face is toward the floor and therefore doesn't get the full force of the liquid.

➤ **A birthing chair may be available in some hospitals**. It is a chair specially designed for labor and delivery. Some women like the idea of sitting up for delivery, while some doctors dislike the difficulty in doing episiotomy repair. If there is a birthing chair available where you intend to give birth, try it. But give it up if you find it doesn't suit you. It is important to keep in mind that devices like the birthing chair tend to be something of a fad.

Labor is hard, slow work. No bed, chair, or particular piece of equipment is going to change that very much. Use whatever facilities are available to you wherever you give birth, but remember that in the end you are the one who makes it happen.

TRANSITION

This is the time in labor before you are fully dilated: it is the transition from the end of the first-stage labor to the beginning of second-stage labor, when you will be pushing out your baby. Transition is the hardest part of labor, but it is also the shortest. It occurs when you are 7 to 8 centimeters dilated and may last for only 10 to 30 contractions. The *average* length of transition with a first baby is 90 minutes, but it usually lasts only 30 to 60 minutes and maybe less.

➤ *The signs of transition* are important to look for because you will need extra encouragement during this stage. It means that soon you will be ready to push. Oxygen is being concentrated in the uterus rather than the brain, which means there is an increased need for coached breathing during contractions and to alert that a contraction is coming. There are many signs of transition and a woman may have only a few or many of them.
  — Discouragement ("I can't go on")
  — Shaking, shivering
  — Irritability ("Don't touch me")
  — Nausea (to the point of vomiting, which you should not resist because you'll feel better afterward)
  — Restlessness, excitement
  — Disorientation
  — Anxiety for your safety and the baby's
  — Dizziness
  — Prickly skin (especially on the fingers)
  — Sleepiness between contractions

Transition is the emotional booby trap of labor, the time when many women lose faith in their own abilities and turn to medication. They get the feeling that the contractions are just going to get worse and worse until it is unbearable and there's no one to reassure them.

For the Coach

➤ *A woman needs absolute support* to get through transition. Do not leave her alone. Encourage her—she is more dependent now on outside feedback.
➤ *Explain that her loss of faith is normal* and that she is in transition. Remind her that transition is short and temporary:

first-stage labor is almost over. Tell her how well she has done until now and that it's only a little longer.

➤ **It is essential to maintain concentration** because contractions come very close together and may have three or four peaks which makes them hard to manage. If she is worrying about the previous contraction, she may lose control. If she isn't ready for a contraction, she may panic and feel she cannot go on with her prepared techniques. Transition is the ultimate test of how well the woman and her coach work together.

➤ **Contractions are erratic in transition:** they can last anywhere from 50 to 120 seconds, with 3 or 4 peaks, and can be anywhere from 30 seconds to 3 minutes apart.

Most women have a continuous backache during transition, which makes relaxation more difficult. The remedy for this is to lie on your side and have your coach apply counterpressure to your lower back. This is what the tennis balls and paint rollers recommended by Lamaze instructors are meant for!

You can get up in a nearly sitting position with pillows behind the small of your back: bend your knees up with the next contraction and press the small of your back into the pillows. This releases some of the pressure of the baby off your spine. You can also try a hands-and-knees position during a contraction, arching your back to take pressure off your spine and breathing through the contraction in this position.

The psychological hazard of transition is that you may be afraid to move into another position thinking that it's bad where you are but it might get worse if you move. But you might be more comfortable sitting upright or changing positions during transition.

The end of transition is often marked by a catch in your labor breathing. It may be a hiccuping sound, as if your vocal cords have gotten in the way of your breathing. This means that the bearing-down reflex is beginning to be established and you will have the urge to push soon. From this time on you should be propped up (if you aren't already), so that gravity helps you move the baby down and out. Your coach must be alert to whether you begin to grunt or to push involuntarily so that he or she can *alert the staff that you are ready to push*. You may be able to tell them that you have the bearing-down urge, or it may come as a surprise to you. When you have the urge to push, transition is over and second-stage labor is about to begin.

SECOND-STAGE LABOR

The second stage of labor lasts from complete dilation of your cervix until the baby is born. This is the pushing stage of labor and it usually lasts one to three hours for a first baby and 30 minutes to an hour for women who have already had a child. It is routine procedure in most hospitals for forceps to be used if you have not been able to push the baby out after two hours of strong pushing.

<u>Pushing</u>

➤ *The urge to push,* also called the bearing-down reflex, is an instinctive urge caused by the pressure of the baby on the perineal floor and the rectum. Many women feel an overwhelming urge to bear down while others are not overcome by the feeling. Notify your coach when you feel this urge, *but do not push until you have had an internal exam* to determine that your cervix is fully dilated. Sometimes you can get the urge to push and a vaginal exam will reveal that you "still have a lip"—there is a little lip (small portion) of the cervix that still has to recede. If

DILATION OF THE CERVIX IN CENTIMETERS

This is a life-sized diagram of how much your cervix opens.

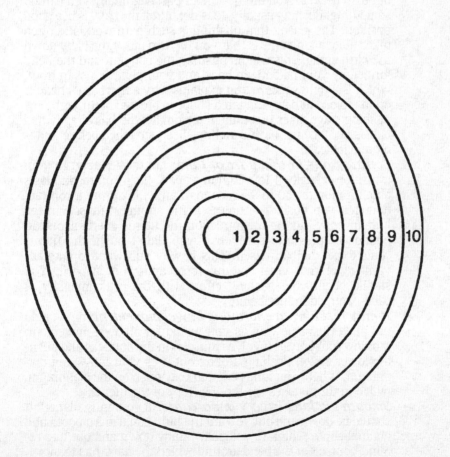

you were to push before a complete 10 centimeters of dilation, you could rip your cervix. If the urge to push is very strong, you may have to use a "pant" or "blow" breathing technique to avoid pushing until you're told it is safe.

➤ *Coach should put on greens (sterile covering) by* this time in labor. Usually the coach is sent to get changed when the baby is ready to be born and you are being moved to the delivery room. His absence at that point can be upsetting to you and may even mean that he will miss the actual birth depending on how long it takes him to get changed and how quickly the baby comes. By changing before now, he avoids a last-minute rush and can be with you during the sometimes disorienting transfer from labor to delivery room.

➤ *Pushing is the most strenuous work of labor* but also the most satisfying. Once it's okay to push it can be a great relief, not only because the discomfort of the first-stage labor is over but also because you are no longer passive: finally you can *do* something. Pushing usually does not hurt if the baby is in a good position. The reason that pushing is such hard work and often takes quite a long time is that you have to move the baby down the birth canal. This means pushing the baby around the bend formed by your tailbone in back and your pubic bones in front, which is a tight squeeze and explains why a newborn's head is often molded into an elongated shape in order to fit through. The pushing stage takes less time in a woman who has already had babies because her birth canal has been stretched before and is more pliable.

➤ *Contractions in this part of labor* are further apart than in transition, usually 4 to 5 minutes apart. Each contraction lasts about a minute (60 to 90 seconds), and it is *during* a contraction that you push. The uterus is the strongest muscle in the human body: during a contraction the uterus exerts about 50 pounds of pressure; so even if you didn't push, the uterus could expel the baby itself. This is why you want to take advantage of that great natural force and work *with* it. You should begin your pushing effort with the peak intensity of each contraction, not before.

➤ *It may feel like an enormous bowel movement*, but you do not push the same way as you would for a bowel movement. Moving your bowels involves muscles in the buttocks and pushing lower down. Pushing a baby out uses your lungs and diaphragm. When your lungs expand they push on the diaphragm, which in turn pushes the fundus (top) of the uterus.

➤ *Smooth pushing is very important*. All your muscular effort should be down and out, toward the birth canal in a smooth and gradual curve. Think to yourself, "Baby down and out," to remind yourself of the bend around which the baby has to move. If your pushing is not smooth and the baby comes out too quickly, you can get a vaginal tear even if you've had an epi-siotomy to make more room.

➤ **Relaxation of the pelvic floor and anal area** is very important during pushing. You may be unconsciously tensing your anus to keep fecal matter in—even if you've had an enema. The urge to push can feel as if you have to make an enormous bowel movement. Make a conscious effort to relax this part of your body when pushing or you won't get the maximum benefit of your efforts. If there *is* any fecal matter in your bowel, don't worry about it—birth attendants have seen all this before.

➤ **You may urinate during a push**. Don't be embarrassed by it; this happens to many women, especially if they've forgotten to empty their bladder in the late part of first-stage labor.

➤ **Two cleansing breaths before and after** a push are very helpful. You need more oxygen at this point and the cleansing breaths also help you to relax.

➤ **Don't relax too quickly at the end of** each contraction. Don't let your coach lower you too quickly from a semi-sitting position after pushing. The baby will retain more of her forward progress if you relax slowly and gently.

➤ **Positions for pushing are** the same as those listed for first-stage labor. The hospital usually encourages back-lying or semi-sitting, but if you have tried other positions at home ahead of time and would prefer kneeling, squatting, hands-and-knees, or side-lying, tell the attendant(s).

➤ **Pushing contractions are good for the baby**. The contractions squeeze the water and mucus from her breathing passages. They also massage the baby's skin, which has been fairly free of stimulation in the amniotic fluid and will soon be rubbed and held by people. Contractions also increase the baby's circulation.

➤ **After two hours of pushing** most doctors intervene. It usually takes 45 minutes to 2 hours of good pushing to get the baby's head to crown (to be visible at the lips of your vagina). At the end of 2 hours you may be too exhausted to continue, it is hard on the fetus to stay in the birth canal that long, and the baby may be hung up somewhere and need help getting out. In this case a forceps delivery is indicated.

The Birth Itself

The birth of the baby is imminent when she has crowned. If it is your first baby you will probably have done most of the pushing in the labor room, but if you have already had a baby you will most likely be moved to the delivery room before the baby crowns because a second (or third) baby will exit more quickly.

➤ **Giving birth in the labor room** is an option you should discuss with your doctor and check out hospital policy ahead of time. This choice is mentioned under questions to ask of the hospital. One benefit is that you are spared the rushed transfer to the delivery room which can be emotionally disruptive. Also you save money—the birth itself can cost half as much if you stay in the labor room. However, if there is any indication that your baby is having distress, or if you or your doctor feel anxious about giving birth in the labor room, it is preferable to make the move.

➤ *The transfer onto the delivery table* can be awkward but there will be attendants to help you: your labor bed is pushed alongside the delivery table at the same height and you have to shift sideways. This move is clumsy and the delivery table is narrow. This may make you lose your pushing rhythm for a few contractions afterward or may even slow down your contractions. Try to relax. It is best not to make the move during a contraction.

➤ *Face masks* will probably be worn by everyone in the delivery room except you, and you will all probably be wearing caps to cover your hair. It may give you a slightly creepy feeling that things are now depersonalized and seem serious with everyone masked. Your mate may look strange because you can see only his eyes, but smile at him: his eyes can smile back!

➤ *Arm straps* are used in some hospitals to keep your arms strapped down so that you don't touch the sterile area into which the baby is being born. This procedure comes from the days when women were so heavily drugged that they could not be counted on to control their own hands. You should discuss arm strapping with your doctor and the hospital *ahead of time*, but if you get into the delivery room and an attendant does try to strap your arms, tell him that you understand the need for a sterile field and that you will keep your hands away. Then be very careful not to touch any of the sterile area, including the drapes over your legs and your perineal area, which has been swabbed with antiseptic.

➤ *Stirrups are used in most delivery rooms*, but you can ask to have them adjusted lower so that your legs are more comfortable and there is less strain on your perineum (thus decreasing the chance of tears). Once your legs are put into the stirrups, which are actually molded supports for the entire leg, your vaginal area will be washed down with antiseptic solution and sterile drapes will be placed over your legs and abdomen.

➤ *The mirror above* and in front of the delivery table makes it possible for you to watch the baby emerging. Make sure it is adjusted at an angle that gives you the best view. Even if you think you or your mate may not want to watch, have the mirror tilted at a convenient angle—you may very well change your mind(s). Be sure to push with your eyes open . . . many women squeeze their eyes shut when they are pushing hard and they miss the sight of the emerging baby.

➤ *If your doctor or nurse-midwife has not arrived* and the baby is ready to be born, you may be told to "pant" or "blow" until they arrive. The urge to push, plus the baby's head crowning, can make it hard to pant for even 5 minutes. *Do not let anyone hold your legs together to delay the birth*: this can lead to brain damage. If your baby wants to be born and you cannot comfortably delay it, do not let anyone interfere. A nurse, intern, or resident can catch the baby—they have done this before when doctors were delayed or babies were more eager to be born than was expected.

➤ *The birth itself* begins with the first sign that the baby is coming: your anus and perineum begin to bulge, distended from within by the baby's head. With each contraction more and more of the head shows, receding back into the birth canal between contractions. Don't get discouraged: you push the baby down two steps and she slides back one step, but this is the normal pattern.

When the baby gets around the curve in the birth canal formed by your tailbone and pubic bone, the baby's head stays in sight. When the whole top of her head is visible it is called crowning, and the next contraction or two will bring the baby's head out into the world. The baby is born facing your backbone, but as soon as her head is out it turns toward one thigh or the other, depending on the position of her body, which is still inside. This puts the baby's shoulders in a position to be born easily with the next contraction or two.

➤ *A stinging, burning sensation* is normal as the baby stretches the outlet of the birth canal. This is your signal not to bear down with the contraction. When you feel the burning and stretching, stop pushing, lean back, and go completely limp. It is especially important to let go of the muscles of the perineal floor: tensing at this point can cause a perineal tear. This burning sensation is short-lived and is followed by a natural anesthetic effect caused by the baby's head. It is at this point that an episiotomy can be cut without injection for pain. Thus the birth itself is not painful but feels like a sliding sensation. Some women are actually surprised by the baby's first cry because they don't realize that she's actually been born.

➤ *A feeling of being split apart* is something a woman may feel as the baby is stretching the birth canal. It may feel that way, but it won't happen! If you get the feeling that you're being split open do not tense up—it will cause you discomfort and hinder the baby's exit.

The Episiotomy

An episiotomy is an incision made in the perineum, between your vagina and your anus. If an episiotomy is cut when the baby's head is stretching your perineum, there is a natural anesthetic and you won't feel it; if a doctor cuts an episiotomy before the baby gets that far out, then he or she will inject a local anesthetic.

In the United States almost every woman giving birth in a hospital gets an episiotomy. There are some women who are rebelling against the routinization of episiotomies: they say that women are treated like links of sausage on an assembly line, as if no woman is capable of giving birth without a tear.

DOCTORS' REASONS FOR EPISIOTOMIES FOR EVERYONE

- A clean, straight incision is easier to repair and heals better than a laceration or tear, which can happen if the baby's head doesn't have enough room to get out.
- There are fewer third-degree lacerations following an episiotomy.
- The episiotomy prevents fetal brain injury because it reduces the pressure of the fetal head on the pelvic floor.
- It shortens the second stage of labor, which in turn helps prevent damage to the pelvic floor.
- An episiotomy will help keep a woman from becoming "stretched out" for intercourse.

There is no clear proof, however, that an episiotomy prevents third-degree laceration, which is an incision or tearing of the tissue that extends into the anus. In fact, the data even shows that sometimes episiotomies tear further and can extend into the rectum.

In hospitals in the United States, episiotomies are performed nearly 99% of the time, whereas in birthing centers where nurse-midwives have primary responsibility, the rate runs between 15–25%. In hospitals in other countries, the rate is around 10%. Detractors of the "American way" claim that it is the positioning of a woman for delivery (in a supine position, in stirrups, and in a rush), and especially the lack of perineal massage, which *creates* the need for routine episiotomies. The technique of massaging the perineum with warm compresses and oil before and during labor is used by midwives worldwide to help gently stretch the perineum and decrease the laceration rate. Doctors in the United States are not taught perineal massage in medical school: they are trained to cut episiotomies. Therefore although there may be no scientific support for cutting an episiotomy on every woman in labor, it is done since that is what American doctors know how to do.

There's no proof that a woman's sex life will be adversely affected if she doesn't have an episiotomy. Under the influence of pregnancy hormones, your whole vagina softens and stretches. If you do the Kegel exercise during pregnancy and exercise those same perineal muscles after birth, they regain their tone quickly.

VALID REASONS FOR EPISIOTOMY

- The perineal tissue hasn't had enough time to stretch gradually, even with the help of massage.
- The baby's head is too large for the opening.
- The woman's pushing isn't in control: she isn't able to stop pushing when necessary and be smooth and gradual when she does push.
- A speedy delivery is necessary, i.e., there are signs of fetal distress.
- A laceration seems imminent: a tear is more difficult to repair than a cut.

The basic point about episiotomies is that they should be done *if and when* necessary. It is not really possible to know *until delivery* just how elastic and yielding an individual's perineal tissue will be. For this reason you should not decide ahead of time that you absolutely refuse an episiotomy: once you state your desire to avoid one, you have to be flexible and trust that your caregivers have your best interests in mind. However, you should know that the perineal muscles have an 8-to-1 stretch ratio, which means that your perineum has been designed to stretch considerably. Ideally, an episiotomy should be used on the small group of women who have unusually tight perineums.

You may want to trust your doctor's judgment about whether you need an episiotomy, but realistically you will probably get one: American doctors are taught to believe that every woman does need one.

There are two types of episiotomy incision: a "medial lateral," which goes off to the side at an angle from your vagina downward, and a "lateral," which goes straight down from your vagina toward your anus. The lateral heals better, whereas a medial lateral can cause permanent muscle scarring. If the repair on an episiotomy is not good, a woman can suffer spasm upon entrance during sex later on. The healing period for episiotomies is very uncomfortable: the wound can cause so much soreness that it is painful to sit down and the stitches usually cause annoying itching.

Cutting the Cord

➤ *Clamping/cutting the umbilical cord* is routinely done at 45 seconds to one minute after the baby is born. The cord is clamped in two places and is cut between the clamps. The cord pulsations cease after about four minutes. It is often a nice symbolic ritual for the baby's father to cut the cord: you should discuss this ahead of time with your doctor to see if she or he will agree to it, assuming all else is normal.

At birth there are two major changes which must take place in order for the baby to survive. First he must start to breathe, filling his lungs with air. Then his circulation must accordingly change from the fetal to the neonatal pattern. At birth, oxygen is reaching the baby via the umbilical cord while his lungs are taking over the breathing. The small vessel which links the blood flow while the baby is in utero seals itself off and the lungs take over fully.

There is controversy about the traditional practice of immediately clamping and cutting the cord right away versus the practice of "late cord clamping." Delayed cord clamping gives a large placental transfusion of blood to the baby and is advocated in a Leboyer delivery. About 25% of the placental blood volume is transferred to the infant in the first 15 seconds after birth. The remaining 75% is partially transferred by one minute and almost completely by three minutes. Those who favor late cord clamping state that the baby receives an additional 25% of his blood supply if the cord is clamped late. They claim that the red cell volume in these infants can increase by as much as 50%.

Even if claims about late cord clamping are correct, it is vital to point out that this additional blood transfer only takes place *if the infant is held below the uterus*, where gravity allows more blood flow. But if the infant is held above the uterus, it almost completely prevents this blood transfusion regardless of whether the cord is clamped or not. An essential part of the Leboyer delivery, for example, is to place the newborn immediately on his mother's stomach to be massaged. Obviously this means the baby is higher then the uterus and is not getting the additional blood transfer even with late clamping.

There are some ill effects on late-clamped infants that have been noted in scientific studies. The additional blood volume distends the circulatory systems of normal newborns, who are able to adjust to this circulatory overload. But late clamping does cause increased effort and duration in respiratory and circulatory adaption. There are no long-term problems recorded, but the baby has to compensate for the increased blood volume: a late-clamped baby will have a greater urinary output, for example. He will breathe faster during the first 2 to 6 hours and have some difficulty breathing. Both full-term and premature babies have a higher serum bilirubin count at 72 hours than babies whose cords are cut right away, and the incidence of jaundice is higher in late-clamped prematures. Late-clamped infants are red, more irritable, and cry more. There is a higher percentage of "quiet sleep states" and fewer "quiet awake states" after birth than with an early-clamped baby, who has more "quiet awake" periods. This means that a late-clamped baby spends less time awake during the day, leaving less time to bond with his mother during the early days.

THE NEW BABY

➤ *The newborn at birth* is wiped off immediately to prevent cold stress. The baby is wet with amniotic fluid, perhaps some blood, and with vernix, the white cheesy substance that protected its skin in utero. Wetness increases cold—the same way that adults feel cold coming out of a shower until they dry off.

➤ *Suctioning with a rubber bulb* is usually done when the baby's head is born, even before the body is fully out. The baby's mouth and nose are filled with mucus and amniotic fluid, and when they are cleared out the baby can breathe more easily. The baby is then suctioned again when he is wiped off. If you have a Leboyer delivery, the baby is covered and wiped off a little while lying on your stomach. After this skin-to-skin contact has been made, his nose and mouth are often suctioned out again.

Some home birth attendants say that suctioning a baby is a bad practice. They say that mucus in the nose and mouth is desirable because it irritates and forces the baby to cough and spit, reminding him to breathe, which a baby can forget to do at first. Most doctors do suction a newborn, however, claiming there is still a good deal of mucus and fluid in the baby's breathing passages even after suctioning. Removing some of the fluid helps the baby, who has to cope with learning a new skill: breathing.

➤ *Apgar rating* of the baby is done at one minute after birth and again at five minutes. This is a two-point test that rates five aspects of the newborn: heart rate, respiratory effort (or "cry"), muscle tone, reflex irritability, and color. Dr. Virginia Apgar developed this test when she was an anesthesiologist to judge how well and how quickly a baby adapts to his new environment and as an indicator of how well he will continue to adapt.

The five-minute score gives a more accurate prediction of a baby's survival and normalcy. A low score at five minutes is much more serious than a low score at one minute. However, the problem with the Apgar rating is that it is subjective, and therefore an unreliable evaluation. Each birth attendant might give a different score to the same baby.

➤ *Antibiotic ointment* is always applied to the baby's eyes, a treatment required within two hours of birth in most states. Tetracycline ointment or erythromycin ointment is used, with delays of up to one hour after birth before applying it and the cautionary reminder not to flush the baby's eyes after any of these agents are used.

The purpose of these agents is to guard against eye infection that can lead to blindness. This infection can be caused by a mother who has gonorrhea, which often shows no symptoms in a woman who has it and often cannot be detected even by repeated tests before birth. It is therefore virtually impossible to be sure that a mother does not have gonorrhea, and thus much safer to medicate all babies as a precaution.

The ointments may not be irritating, although most babies shut their eyes after these agents are applied. Since this interferes with maternal-infant and paternal-infant bonding because it eliminates eye-to-eye contact, it is a good idea to delay applying the medicine until the baby has had a chance to look around and perhaps nurse. Then the baby will be less likely to cry and the drug won't interfere with bonding.

➤ *Vitamin K is routinely given by* injection to newborns. The reason for this is that all babies are deficient in vitamin K because they have inadequate intestinal flora-bacteria. There are parents who object to this shot because they reason that if all babies are deficient in vitamin K then that is *normal* and should not be tampered with. Also, babies that breast-feed do have intestinal flora-bacteria. You should discuss this with your pediatrician before birth if you do not like the idea of the vitamin K shot.

➤ *A band will be put on your baby* with your name and the doctor's name. Banding a baby at birth has replaced the old system of footprinting infants, so that the baby you give birth to is the same baby you take home!

➤ *The Stabilization nursery* (or central nursery) is where most babies are sent very soon after birth. The issue of separating mothers and babies at birth is discussed on page 323. The stated reason for not leaving a baby with her parents after birth is that she will get cold: her temperature has to stabilize at 98.6°. Hospitals point out that the highest mortality rate for infants is in the first 24 hours of life, but that has nothing to do with a normal baby, who needs only to warm up.

Studies have shown that normal newborns who are dried, swaddled, and held by their mothers for up to an hour after delivery arrive in the nursery without significant cooling. The difference in temperature between these babies and those who were put in heated cribs was *less than half a degree* Fahrenheit.

There are strong reasons for keeping a mother and baby together after birth. If the hospital's routine procedure does not have a valid, provable reason, then it should be challenged, if you wish. Home birth advocates who are opposed to babies being taken away and put in heated containers have been saying for years that "a mother's arms are the best baby warmers." There is now scientific proof to support what they instinctively knew was right.

Discuss with your doctor the possibility of keeping your baby with you after birth if all is normal. If you cannot find any support for keeping the baby with you, there is an alternative: *Just don't give the baby up*!

First you must make sure that everything is normal and the baby is okay. Ask the doctor or nurse, "Is the baby okay? Is there anything wrong?'' It is natural for any new parent to ask this. If they say the baby is fine and they hand him to you after drying and swaddling him, don't let them take him away. Tell them that they can come and look at the baby anytime they want to—but that your baby belongs in your arms.

MATERNAL-INFANT BONDING

Maternal-infant bonding is the process of a mother and newborn getting to know each other and to bond. This bonding process with the mother is the wellspring for all of the infant's subsequent attachments and will affect the quality of future bonds to other individuals. The newborn sees, hears, and moves in rhythm to your voice in the first few minutes and hours of life. He will turn his head to the spoken word; mothers seem instinctively to use a high-pitched voice to a new baby. A newborn alerts and attends best to a high pitch, perhaps because his ears are stilled filled with amniotic fluid and he may not be able to hear a lower pitch. In turn, the infant's appearance evokes responses from you: eye-to-eye contact especially establishes the baby as a reality after all the months of waiting to meet him. Skin-to-skin contact is yet another way of establishing these channels of communication.

➤ **The "sensitive period"** is defined as the first hour of life: the infant is alert and quiet during this time and after that goes into a deep sleep for three to four hours. A baby in a "quiet alert" state is at his most responsive, and thus this crucial time right after birth is ideal for attachment. The 30 to 45 minutes immediately after birth are the most rewarding for skin-to-skin and eye-to-eye contact.

— *It is important to ask* that the application of antibiotic ointment to the baby's eyes be delayed until after this meeting has taken place.

— *You may not want to face the baby instantly*—you may want a few minutes to compose yourself after the baby is born. No one should insist that you take the baby right away. Your mate can hold him until you are ready.

— *Bonding should be a private session* with a minimum of interruptions. Affectional ties can be easily disturbed and may be permanently altered during the immediate postpartum period. Medical attendants may not be aware of this, so you should protect yourself: any questions or procedures that are not essential can wait until after you and the baby have gotten to know each other.

— *A heat panel* can be placed over you and the baby so that he doesn't get cold during this sensitive period. The radiant heater usually found over the newborn warming tray can be shifted next to the delivery table just as it can be placed above the bathtub in a Leboyer delivery.

➤ *A Leboyer delivery* can interfere with the bonding process because the baby is taken away from you to be given a bath. It is probably best to wait and see how you feel after the birth and decide *then* whether or not to give the baby the bath. If you and the baby are lying together touching and watching each other, then it doesn't make sense to take the baby away just because a Leboyer bath was planned. On the other hand, if your mate really wants to give the bath, it is equally fine to let that happen. Don't worry that the baby is in the "sensitive period" and his bonding with you can be so disturbed. *Do not get hung up on rigid ideas about what is "right," what you "should" do.* Know the facts and then be spontaneous—do what feels right to you *at the time*. If you try to go "by the book" with Leboyer, bonding, or any other technique, you'll be falling into a trap of rigidity.

➤ *Anesthetics and analgesics may depress the infant*, depending on how soon before birth you were given drugs. This is not true of an epidural. A newborn with drugs in his system from labor and/or delivery is going to have depressed responsiveness, which will influence the first mother/baby interchanges. If your birth was medicated, the baby can be somewhat groggy and you won't be getting the positive feedback that you would from an unmedicated baby.

➤ *Your interaction with the baby* is good for both of you. The more contact you have with your newborn—and the sooner you touch, hold, and fondle her—the less bleeding you will have, and the better and stronger you will feel. It appears possible that contact with the baby causes the release of maternal hormones which help your body return to normal. Studies have shown that a newborn adapts best when she is soothed, held, and given the opportunity to suck at will. Thus, a baby who is allowed to bond with her mother at birth may have a smoother time adjusting to life outside the womb.

➤ *Paternal–infant bonding* is as important as the mother's attachment to the baby, but in the rush to the delivery room and the procedures after birth, the father may be forgotten. However, eye-to-eye and skin-to-skin contact with the newborn has the same effect on the man and his baby as it does with the mother. But, unlike the mother, the father may not be biologically or culturally primed to be responsive to cues from the infant. For this reason, extended early contact between a father and his baby is particularly important.

➤ *The foundation for maternal–infant bonding* is laid during pregnancy. There are certain events that are important to the formation of your attachment to the baby, and if you skip any of the steps it can affect bonding.

During pregnancy these steps are:

1) confirming the pregnancy
2) accepting the pregnancy
3) fetal movement (the baby first asserts his presence)
4) accepting the fetus as an individual in utero: you begin to think of the baby as a separate person even before he is born

After birth the events that affect bonding are:

1) the birth itself
2) seeing the baby
3) touching the baby
4) giving care to the baby

Anxiety about your baby's health or survival in the first few days—even when the problems are resolved—may affect the way you feel about the baby afterward. For instance, sometimes women who are heavily drugged and do not see their babies at birth then believe something is wrong with the baby and no one is telling them. Even after they see the baby this feeling may linger, and it can affect the delicate bonding process. Be aware that if your baby has trouble breathing at birth, for example, which then passes, your continued anxiety can influence bonding.

THE THIRD STAGE OF LABOR

The third stage of labor is the expulsion of the placenta, which normally takes from a few minutes to an hour (30 minutes is about average). In hospitals, doctors often give Pitocin, a synthetic hormone, to increase your contractions in order to expel the placenta more quickly. This can be painful and cause cramping later on. Some doctors even pull on the umbilical cord to hurry the expulsion—this is a common cause of hemorrhage and can cause excessive bleeding in the hours after birth. It can also mean that a woman has to return to the hospital for a D&C (dilation and curettage) for suspected retention of a fragment of the placenta which may have remained in her uterus when the doctor pulled the placenta out.

What happens in third-stage labor is that at the site where the placenta was attached it detaches and pencil-thick blood vessels are torn across. Women usually do not bleed, however, because the uterus is constructed of crisscrossing muscle fibers with blood vessels in the spaces in between, like lacing the fingers of one hand between the fingers of the other. The blood vessels of the placental site are shut off when the walls of the vessels are squeezed together by the tightly contracted muscle bundles surrounding them on all sides. This is why it is essential that the uterus remain firmly contracted after the third stage of labor. This is usually done by kneading the uterus periodically for an hour after the placenta is expelled.

➤ *The average length of third-stage labor* at home, where there is no interference in the natural process, is 20 minutes. At the hospital the average time for third stage is five minutes, because doctors so frequently intervene.

➤ *A hormone shot as the baby is being born* is given in many hospitals to stimulate the uterus to contract and decrease the possibility of hemorrhage. Sometimes the uterus contracts so violently that the placenta is retained. In this case, the doctor has to remove the placenta by hand, reaching up into the uterus, detaching the placenta, and scooping it out.

➤ *Doctors are often impatient*—they are used to "improving" on nature and getting the placenta expelled in a few minutes, even though it is natural for a placenta to take 20 to 30 minutes to be born. If a doctor says that he has to perform a manual removal of the placenta after only 10 minutes without a medical reason (i.e., that you are bleeding), then ask him to wait. Manual removal can cause hemorrhage.

➤ *If the placenta doesn't detach spontaneously*, the doctor and nurse will push on your abdomen. This can be uncomfortable and you may need to use the breathing techniques you used during first-stage labor. There are cases of a *retained placenta* that have nothing to do with the hormone shot that can sometimes create this problem. In a case like this, a doctor should explain that your placenta is not detaching and that he or she has to retrieve it. This is obviously different than a doctor who rushes in to perform manual removal because of impatience.

➤ *The placenta is examined* to make sure it is complete and none of it was left behind. If any piece of placenta is left in your uterus, it can cause hemorrhage later on. You might want to see the placenta after the doctor has examined it so that you and your mate can see the amazing organ that nourished your baby inside for nine months.

➤ *Shaking after birth* can sometimes be quite strong. It is caused by a combination of the adrenaline released by your system, the sudden change in your circulation (the 25% of your blood volume which was directed to the placenta is suddenly routed back into your circulatory system), and the adjustments your body is making and the big stress it has just gone through. Don't be frightened by this shaking; ask for a blanket and try to relax.

➤ *Nursing on the delivery table* reinforces the baby's instinctive rooting and sucking reflexes while releasing hormones into your system that cause the uterus to contract. If you think you might want to nurse on the delivery table, discuss it before labor with your obstetrician and pediatrician.

　　Some pediatricians object to nursing on the delivery table because the newborn has too much mucus in her nose and mouth to nurse properly, which may then make the mother insecure about her ability to breast-feed. The objection is also made that a baby won't be warm enough (but remember the home birth belief that a swaddled baby in her mother's arms is in the "best baby warmer on the market"). Some doctors also believe that the hospital should give a test feeding of glucose and water to a baby before she ingests anything else to make sure that her digestive system works properly. You should discuss all this with your pediatrician ahead of time and make sure you are in agreement.

➤ *The recovery room* is where you are sent after delivery for one to three hours. The nurse there will check your pulse and blood pressure frequently and knead your uterus to make sure it remains firm. If you have arranged ahead of time to keep your baby with you in recovery (if all is normal) this can be a peaceful time together. If you cannot have the baby with you, you might to arrange ahead of time for your partner to stay with you. Otherwise the recovery room can be lonely and frustrating if you are elated about your baby's birth, feeling fine, but cut off from your baby and your mate.

➤ *Hunger may overtake you* after the baby is born. You probably will not have had anything to eat for many hours and—particularly if you're unmedicated—you'll most likely be ravenous. Try to get the hospital to bring you some food, although this is fairly difficult—they usually serve food only at designated mealtimes. Maybe you'll be able to persuade your mate to go out and bring you back a wonderful "birthday treat."

THE PSYCHOLOGICAL ASPECTS OF LABOR

The way you *feel* and *think* before you go into labor (and during it) influence how labor progresses physically. If you understand how your mind may be functioning—or how it may play tricks on you—there is a better chance that you will have a positive birth experience.

➤ *However you get through it, labor is an accomplishment*. This has to be said before anything else. You and your partner should practice saying this before, during, and after the birth!

➤ *Birth may be more difficult and painful if the mother is fearful.* The most anxious time usually comes before you go into labor. You fear the unknown and you fear that you will lose control. Sometimes these fears are the reason that a woman chooses to have labor induced—it gives her a feeling that she has control over *when* labor will happen, at least. But induced labor is dangerous and cannot reduce fear.

The more you know and understand every step of labor beforehand, the less possibility that you will be surprised—and so the less anxiety you will feel. Also, the less anxiety you have during birth and the immediate bonding period after birth, the better your first relationship with the baby will be. This is reason enough to take childbirth education classes.

Your attitude toward pain is a major factor once you are in labor. Do you have a high or low tolerance for pain? Does the idea of pain make you frightened? Don't get trapped in fixed ideas that don't relate to your experience and your personality. If you have unrealistic expectations of how you're "supposed" to handle labor, or if you let your mate or childbirth teacher intimidate you ahead of time about accepting medication, you're setting yourself up to fail. Try to learn as much as you can, practice your childbirth exercises, and keep an open mind—say to yourself and your mate that you're going to "wait and see" how you feel once you're in labor. This way you won't feel locked into any promises or high standards you feel you have to live up to (or, on the other hand, give up before even trying).

Everyone's anxiety level is high during the end of pregnancy and especially high right before and during labor. No matter how calm you feel, how prepared you are, how positive you feel about the birth, your anxiety level is high. You may forget breathing techniques; you may forget how to push; you may forget a lot of the information you learned during classes. This is normal. Ask for help. Do not expect perfection from yourself.

Studies have shown that stress, fear, or anxiety are known to increase levels of substances in the blood called *catecholamines*, which can interfere with natural hormones such as oxytocin that help labor progress. Maternal anxiety can cause increased catecholamine levels in the mother's circulation, which can adversely affect the progress of labor. Catecholamines can also decrease circulation to the placenta, thereby affecting the baby.

Another consequence of stress and/or anxiety during labor is the uterine muscle tension, which can turn simple contractions into painful cramps. Research indicates that women with higher levels of anxiety may be more likely to have complications in pregnancy, including dysfunctional uterine contractions: painful contractions that do not accomplish their function, which is to open the cervix.

The reason to point this out is not to alarm you, but to make you and those attending your labor aware of how important it is to conquer fear and anxiety so that it does not become physical interference to the natural process.

➤ ***Depend on those around you for support***. Turn to your partner and any attendants for advice, encouragement, and just plain friendship. If a woman feels neglected or misunderstood during labor or delivery, it can mar her experience. *Never be left alone when you're in labor*. Births at home tend to have shorter labors in part because of the constant support, encouragement, and reassurance from the people who are in attendance.

Protect yourself against anything that interferes with a positive emotional and physical experience of birth.

➤ *A feeling of autonomy* is an important aspect of birth for a woman. Just as you need people to depend on, you also need to feel you have some control over this intense and even overwhelming experience. Your feeling of strength and self-reliance comes in part from feeling that you *have a choice* about what happens to you and your baby during birth. This feeling of independence, a feeling that you are able to handle your own life, may be very important to you as a woman.

It is easy to feel overpowered by the authority of the hospital, its equipment and procedures, and its efficient, uniformed staff. The criblike bed, the parental figures, and the imposition of routine procedures can make you feel childlike and powerless.

Some women feel so overwhelmed by the authoritarian atmosphere in a hospital that they are afraid to "disobey." It's your body and your baby; even if your anxiety level *is* high, you still have the power to reason. Do what seems reasonable and right and don't fall into the trap of feeling you're back in grade school and have to do exactly what you're told.

When you're in labor it's not unusual to be hypersensitive to caregivers' reactions to you. If a nurse simply says, "Is this your first baby?" it can make you feel judged and incompetent, although it wasn't meant that way. This can be because you've set unrealistic standards for yourself, therefore you imagine that everyone else is judging your "performance." If you find yourself saying things during labor like: "I'm sorry," or "I'm doing terribly, aren't I?" you will know that you are in danger of wrapping yourself into an emotional pretzel. There is no "right" way to cope with labor; no one is keeping score. If you see that you're doing this to yourself, rip up your scorecard and relax.

➤ *A feeling of inadequacy* affects some women after birth, although they may not want to talk about it. The feeling of inadequacy can be strong for women who planned on having a birth at home and have to be transferred to the hospital: they have the problem of feeling they've failed because they wound up in the hospital, which they were determined to avoid.

One way to protect yourself against feeling inadequate is not to set up rigid expectations that will spell failure if you don't meet them. A small example would be if you were laboring in the hospital and you gripped the bedrail during a contraction. That may be what works best for you, but it contradicts what you were taught in childbirth education: that total relaxation is the "right" way to deal with a contraction. That's why you don't want to lock yourself into an inflexible belief system which dictates that you "fail" if you deviate at all.

➤ *Romantic notions about togetherness with your partner* during labor can be a disappointment. Don't either of you get your expectations high about staying in loving unison. You may withdraw from everyone—the force of the physical changes may consume all your energy. Or when the baby starts to descend, you may tune out everything but getting that baby out—and after that you may care only about holding him.

Avoid unrealistic fantasies about sharing every magical moment, about how this powerful experience will bring you closer than ever. Childbirth can be enhanced by being a shared experience, but that doesn't mean you have to be totally tuned in to each other every minute—just being there together is sharing it. Don't try to second-guess how it will be. There's enough pressure on you without adding the additional burden of expecting a spiritual experience of togetherness. You might *very* well have it anyway!

MEDICATION DURING LABOR AND DELIVERY

The American Academy of Pediatrics recommends the least possible medication during childbirth. It is best for your baby if you do not take any drugs during birth, but sometimes it is best for you to have medication.

➤ *All drugs except epidural anesthesia reach your baby*. There are many women who come into the hospital in labor and ask for epidural anesthesia right away, since they have been told it cannot harm their baby. Often the hospital staff offers a laboring woman a small dose of painkiller to "take the edge off the contractions"—more often than not that drug is Demerol. Demerol can drop maternal blood pressure, which reduces the blood supply (and therefore oxygen) to the infant. It is not known the degree of oxygen deprivation an unborn or newborn baby can tolerate, but if more women knew this, they might be slower to accept drugs.

➤ *The "walking epidural" is a new variation* on the idea of handling labor pain. Some doctors are calling it "epidural light," but the amazing thing about this new procedure is that it allows a woman to feel her contractions without pain and even to walk around during labor while anesthetized.

In the traditional procedure the doctor puts a catheter into the woman's epidural space—the area of the back lying between the vertebrae and the spinal cord—and pumps in anesthetics to numb the abdomen and legs. Some anesthetists have found that they can get by with much smaller doses of anesthetic if it is mixed with a narcotic. Generally narcotics are avoided because of their effect on the baby; however, it does not affect the baby when it's injected directly into the mother's spinal fluid.

The new procedure dulls the pain, but you still feel the pressure of your contractions so you know when to push. And whereas with traditional epidural you're too numb to even turn over, this version gives you control of your leg muscles. There is disagreement among doctors about whether a woman should be allowed to walk once this lighter epidural is injected, although no study has shown any problems associated with walking and some caregivers feel that walking speeds the delivery.

➤ *Patient-controlled epidural anesthesia (PCEA)* is another option now available at some medical centers. The epidural is set up as usual, but the woman can add more medication by pushing a button when she feels the pain returning. The button is attached to a pump which is programmed to prevent overdose.

Not all hospitals provide PCEA for childbirth, although it is frequently used for certain postoperative patients and those with cancer. The PCEA cuts down on the reaction time—usually you'd have to wait for a nurse, who then has to summon an anesthesiologist, who might have to reach the hospital or is already there but involved in another procedure. By giving the woman the ability to self-medicate, you relieve her anxiety about how much worse the pain is going to get and how long it will take relief to arrive. It has been found that patients actually use less pain reliever in long-term pain management, or for the intensity of postoperative pain, if they are in charge of their own pain management.

Is Medication Safe During Labor?

➤ *Consider the "price tag" of drugs* before you take any. There can be a domino effect in which one drug necessitates using another—often an epidural "knocks out" contractions and oxytocin has to be used. When your bearing-down reflex is lost through anesthesia, forceps are often necessary to get the baby out. If you have childbirth training, a minimal dose of some drugs can cause you to lose control of your techniques and therefore need more drugs to cope with the contractions.

➤ *You have a legal right to refuse all medication.* Some doctors have standing orders for routine medication for their patients in labor. Some nurses may make it sound as if you have to take what's ordered. Make sure your doctor is aware of your wishes about drugs and ask him to write that information on your chart.

➤ *Wait before accepting drugs.* A few encouraging words from your partner and some physical contact can get you past a tough time. Have an attendant examine your cervical dilation—if you know you're making progress that can be as good as drugs to sustain your strength. *Find out how far dilated you are* before taking any drug in labor: if taken early in labor, it may stop the contractions. And if you are almost fully dilated, then you have gotten through the worst of it and have only a little longer to go. If you accept medication you may regret it later, so be cautious. Try to wait 15 minutes to half an hour before taking medication: you may make a lot of progress in labor during that time, and you may find you can manage without chemical help.

➤ *Alertness is impaired* by any drug. Even a minimal amount of Demerol, for example (offered to "take the edge off contractions"), can affect your ability to work with contractions. A drug may make you fall asleep between contractions and you may be panicked if you wake up in the middle; you might temporarily forget how to breathe and will therefore experience more pain. The domino effect here is that you would then request more medication, further impairing your ability to cope with labor.

➤ *The baby's body takes longer to break down drugs* than yours does. Your kidneys and liver rid your body of medications in several hours, but the baby's organs are too immature to eliminate the drug from his system. This is true even of a healthy, full-term baby—it is harder for a premature baby or one that has any kind of complications. Medications can affect the baby at birth, often making him groggy and unmotivated to suck; it can take several days for the effects to wear off completely.

➤ *There are times when medications can be helpful during labor*. Be aware of the dangers, but leave an open mind for the possibility that you may want or need help. The foremost reason for accepting drugs is if you become so tense that you cannot relax. If tension mounts, it not only increases your perception of pain, but it can even slow down labor, which then causes fetal distress. In a case like this, drugs to reduce tension may be beneficial.

Some physicians believe long periods of pain can lead to chemical problems and hormonal imbalances, which can reduce blood flow to the uterus.

➤ *Advances in technology* allow a more subtle use of medication during labor. More is known now about how drugs interact with the fetus. For example, doctors are now using one-fourth the previous dosage of Demerol, the narcotic most commonly used for women in labor. Many physicians feel that the quantity of medicine used today does not cause problems in the normal, healthy fetus (and the dosage can be adjusted for a fetus showing distress).

Another important advance is the ability to deliver the epidural block on a continuous basis, either through a pump or by injection. In the past, the epidural was given in a single shot. With the newer continuous administration, the anesthetist can lighten the dosage and stop giving the drug as the mother is ready to push, then give it again as the baby emerges.

➤ *Your doctor may want you medicated*. You may find yourself having to withstand pressure from your doctor, who wants
to give you medication during labor. There are some doctors who
feel drugs are "more humane" and make it easier on a woman.
They assume that all women want medication since so many
women have in the past. These doctors want to relieve "unnecessary suffering": their intentions are good . . . but misguided.

No man can fully understand the experience a woman goes
through in labor, but obstetricians stand by and watch hundreds
of women give birth and they *imagine* what it feels like. Based
on these projections—and the fact that they've seen many unprepared women crying and screaming in labor from the vicious
cycle of fear/tension/pain—doctors want to protect women from
that. You can insure your chances of not needing medication by
taking childbirth classes. And you can protect yourself from an
overprotective doctor by explaining your desire to avoid drugs.

➤ *Try not to be too rigid about drugs*, however, because you
may want them or your doctor might advise them for medical
reasons. Some women just cannot tolerate the pain of labor. It
is better for you to have an epidural, for example, than to start
a relationship with a baby following a painful or traumatic labor
and birth (which can be bad for maternal–infant bonding be
cause you can feel as if the baby has assaulted your body, which
will affect your attachment to her).

Three Kinds of Labor Medications

There are three basic types of drugs used for labor. *Analgesia* is used
to relieve pain. These drugs inhibit the reception of pain stimuli and
therefore raise your threshold for pain. There are several kinds of analgesics—tranquilizers, barbiturates, narcotics, amnesics, and inhalation
analgesia—all of which are listed on pages 402–404. *Anesthesia* is used
in late first-stage labor and during expulsion of the baby to block sensation in an area of the body or to block consciousness. *Oxytocics* are
the third type of drug used during labor, which are synthetic hormones
given to stimulate contractions.

MEDICATION USED DURING LABOR

ANALGESICS (TO RELIEVE PAIN)

Tranquilizers
(Miltown, Vistaril,
Phenergan, Largon,
Sparine)

— Reduce anxiety
— Good for long labors if tension mounts
— May have little effect on fetus
— Excess can cause loss of control over contractions
— NOTE: Valium should not be given because of the length of time it remains in the newborn's body

Barbiturates
(Seconal, Nembutal)

— Sedates and produces sleep
— Effects on the newborn last up to a week after birth

Narcotics
(Demerol, Phentinyl,
Dolophine)

— Relieve pain, sedate, relieve anxiety
— Negative effect on the newborn's respiration

Amnesics
(scopolamine)

— Used in combination with pain-relieving drugs
— Hallucinogenic
— Drawbacks outweigh any advantages
— Causes violent, odd behavior

Inhalation
analgesia
(nitrous oxide,
Penthrane, Trilene)

— Inhaled during peak of contraction
— Self-administered
— Have to learn to time self-administration so maximum effect coincides with peak of contraction

OXYTOCICS
(TO INDUCE OR SPEED UP LABOR)

Pitocin

— The most commonly used oxytocic
— Often given through the IV. The doctor cannot easily control the dosage when administered this way.
— The alternate method is through your vein via infusion pump. With this method the doctor can increase or decrease the dosage instantly depending on how your body reacts.

MEDICATION USED DURING LABOR (*cont.*)

Ergotrate — Oxytocic given in pill form after delivery to contract your uterus
— If you are breast-feeding, the hormones that will contract the uterus are naturally excreted

ANESTHESIA

General anesthesia — Seldom used in normal births
— Inhaled to produce unconsciousness
— Forceps necessary
— Side effects include grogginess and amnesia

All other anesthesia is regional (local)

Caudal — Administered in your lower back after six centimeters' dilation
— You are turned on your side while a thin tube is inserted and taped in place
— Blocks sensation, but you can usually still move
— Removes the urge to bear down but trained women can still push
— Passes quickly to baby and can cause a drop in maternal blood pressure, which can affect baby's oxygen supply
— Forceps often required
— Risk of puncturing rectum or baby's head

Epidural — Administered after six centimeters' dilation in a procedure similar to caudal
— Does not cross placenta
— Thought to be the safest drug with minimal side effects
— You can feel pressure but not pain, yet you lose the urge to push
— 75% of epidural deliveries use forceps
— 25% of babies show dramatic slowdown in heart rate when given in early labor
— Epidural necessitates the following:
  • IV hydrating solution
  • Blood pressure taken every fifteen to thirty minutes
  • Fetal monitoring—to monitor baby's reaction and tolerance to it

MEDICATION USED DURING LABOR (*cont.*)

Spinal	— Injected into spinal fluid at eight centimeters or after full dilation (i.e., no relief of first-stage labor)
	— Necessary to lie flat on your back for four to eight hours after delivery
	— Used when mother is too tired to push
	— Does not cross placenta
	— Relaxes tense perineal area for forceps delivery
	— Slows labor as contractions weaken
	— Blood pressure drops, reducing oxygen to baby
	— Forceps often necessary
Saddle block	— Injected into spinal fluid lower than a spinal
	— Given close to delivery
	— Deadens area you would touch with a saddle
	— Less drug required than for a spinal
	— Drug does not cross placenta
	— Can lower mother's blood pressure
	— Can cause spinal headache, even if you lie on your back for twenty minutes afterward
Paracervical block	— Administered on side of cervix—active labor must be under way but still some cervix remaining
	— Stops pain from uterus and cervix
	— Good for cervix not dilating well
	— Lasts about one hour but crosses placenta in about three minutes
	— Fetal heart rate can slow; can be accidentally injected into fetus
Pudendal block	— Injected into pudendal nerve in vagina or into buttocks
	— Numbs vagina and perineum (area between vagina and anus)
	— Urge to push usually lost, but you can still push when told
	— Transfers to baby in fifteen minutes
Local infiltration for episiotomy	— Xylocaine or procaine injected into perineum
	— "Local" only in terms of where it's given
	— Reaches entire system instantly

CHAPTER THIRTEEN

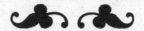

Complications in Pregnancy and Childbirth

TESTS FOR COMPLICATIONS

Ultrasound

Ultrasound (or sonography) can be used to detect many complications of pregnancy. It is a quartz crystal placed on a woman's abdomen; high-frequency sound waves (two million cycles per second) are beamed toward the fetus: the ultrasound machine produces a picture of the fetus in utero. Unlike X-rays, ultrasound can show soft tissue in detail and offers none of the hazards of X-rays.

This device is used to investigate development of the fetus: its exact placement, the size of its head, and the location of the placenta. It can identify disorders such as hydrocephalus (fluid on the brain), uterine tumors, and ectopic pregnancy (pregnancy in the fallopian tube rather than in the uterus). It can detect fetal life or death and measure the growth of the baby. Ultrasound is used before amniocentesis is done so that the doctor knows precisely where the baby and placenta are and won't touch them with the needle.

Ultrasound can be used to measure the biparietal diameter (BPD) of the fetal skull, a measurement that gives a general idea of the baby's age. A BPD of 9.0+ centimeters indicates that the baby is mature. However, fetal lung maturity is the most important consideration of whether a fetus is ready to be born. The BPD can confirm whether a baby is full-term when the lung maturity test (L/S ratio, see page 406) indicates otherwise.

If you have an ultrasound and are told that your placenta is low-lying, near the cervix, don't worry: this will change as your pregnancy progresses. The placenta moves around in your uterus just as the fetus does. The placenta seems to move upward during most pregnancies and by the third trimester the majority have moved into the upper part of the uterus. In only a small fraction of pregnancies does the placenta remain low in the uterus and cover or partially cover the cervix, potentially causing a problem. As delivery gets near your doctor will let you know where your placenta is: the odds are you won't have a problem.

Amniocentesis Late in Pregnancy

Amniocentesis is a test in which a painless needle is inserted in your abdomen to extract some of the amniotic fluid for microscopic examination. There is a small risk of complications of pain, bleeding, infection, and premature labor, *but* it is the most reliable test for determining postmaturity syndrome—whether a fetus is postterm and should be delivered.

> ➢ ***Discovering whether there is meconium*** in the amniotic fluid can be done best with amniocentesis, although it's also possible to determine it with an endoscope, a device inserted into the vagina and placed against the cervix to view the amniotic fluid.
> ➢ ***Fetal lung maturity*** is the most accurate indicator of how mature the baby is. The lecithin/sphingomyelin (L/S) ratio in the fluid determines lung maturity, which is reached when the L/S ratio reaches 2.0 or greater. The L/S ratio tells you whether the fetal lungs contain enough "surfactant" to allow oxygen to pass in and carbon dioxide to pass out.

Late in pregnancy this test may not be possible or can be hazardous for some women because the quantity of amniotic fluid decreases after 42 weeks.

Fetal Monitor Testing

There are three kinds of fetal monitor testing: the nonstress test, the oxytocin challenge test, and breast stimulation. In all three tests a monitor belt is put around your waist. This belt measures the fetal heart rate (FHR) as well as uterine activity. The results are shown on a video screen and also printed on paper.

In nonstress and stress testing the terms "negative" and "positive" indicate a reaction or lack of reaction by the baby, but the meaning is different in both cases. "Positive" in a nonstress test means a normal *acceleration* of the fetal heart in association with movement or some external stimulus; a lack of acceleration is "negative." In stress testing, "positive" means an abnormal *deceleration* of the FHR is response to uterine contractions; the test is "negative" if no deceleration pattern is observed.

➤ *Oxytocin challenge test (OCT)* is done to evaluate the baby's well-being and the function of the placenta. Some reasons for doing this test include: hypertension (high blood pressure), toxemia, falling estriol levels, suspected postmaturity, and suspected intrauterine growth retardation.

An OCT is done before labor begins, from 31 to 44 weeks gestation. It consists of stimulating the uterus to contract as it would in labor. It is usually done in the hospital as an outpatient: an IV is started and the mother is given a synthetic hormone similar to the one her own brain produces to produce uterine contractions. Abnormalities can be detected if there is deceleration, or slowing, of the baby's heart rate following each contraction.

If certain patterns are recorded on the test, it can show placental insufficiency and the likelihood that the fetus will not tolerate "real" labor well. Such patterns, which are called a "positive OCT," are an indication for immediate delivery, usually by cesarean. A negative stress test is one in which there are no worrisome changes in the FHR in response to the contractions during the test. A negative OCT is often repeated to make sure it was accurate the first time.

There are some disadvantages to this test: one is that the OCT requires the constant presence of trained hospital staff. It also may need to be repeated on several occasions. This can be costly and inconvenient.

➤ *The nonstress test* is a simpler exercise: the monitoring belt is attached and the mother makes a mark on the monitor's printout when she feels the baby move. If everything is normal, that mark will be accompanied by an acceleration of the baby's heart rate. This test was devised as an alternative to the OCT

➤ *Breast (or nipple) stimulation* is a combination of the previous two tests. The mother is asked to stimulate her nipples until they become erect and create uterine contractions. She is asked to mark the printout when she feels the baby's movements. The monitor will detect acceleration of the FHR with movement, which is normal. It also detects deceleration (or slowing) of the fetal heart rate after a contraction, which would be abnormal.

PROBLEMS WITH THE MOTHER

Miscarriage (Spontaneous Abortion)

Miscarriage is fairly common: it happens in about one of eight pregnancies and some studies show it may be as common as one in four as tests for pregnancies become more exacting. Your own chance of miscarrying depends on certain factors such as your age, how quickly you got pregnant, and whether you've miscarried before.

An early miscarriage may feel no worse physically than a heavy period. With a late-first-trimester miscarriage there can be bleeding and cramping on and off for days until your uterus has expelled everything. If you miscarry in the second trimester, it is a "mini-labor," with strong, regular contractions that dilate your cervix.

➤ *Go to bed and phone the doctor* if you have cramplike pains in your lower abdomen and/or bleeding (not necessarily heavy). It's possible that the pain and bleeding will stop and the pregnancy will continue. However, if the fetus is definitely aborting, the cramps and bleeding will worsen, with large blood clots in the flow.

➤ *Collect the fetus and afterbirth in a clean container*. This can be very hard on you, but it will yield information about why you miscarried. It may show a "blighted pregnancy," which is a random natural event. But if it shows genetic abnormalities, or suggests you have an illness or infection, the doctor may be able to help correct the problem. There are also treatments available if you had insufficient hormone levels or an "incompetent cervix" (see "Causes of Miscarriage," below).

➤ *The miscarriage is complete* when a large clot is expelled and the bleeding stops. You'll be physically fine in a few days. If bleeding persists, it means placental tissue remains in the uterus and a D&C (dilation and curettage) is necessary: the doctor must dilate your cervix to clean out the tissue remaining in your uterus.

➤ *The sight of blood*, especially a heavy flow of blood with clots, can be upsetting. If it is a second-trimester miscarriage, the woman is actually in labor and it can take several hours of strong uterine contractions to dilate the cervix sufficiently to expel the fetus.

Causes of Miscarriage

➤ *Blighted ovum* is the most common reason for a first-trimester miscarriage, which is when most miscarriages take place. The fertilized egg never develops into a normal fetus: the majority of miscarriages reveal a deformity that is usually a random mistake of nature.

➤ *DES daughters* (women who were exposed to DES in utero) often have malformations of the cervix and uterus that put them at higher risk for premature labor and habitual miscarriage. If your mother took DES while she was pregnant with you, your doctor will want to check you more frequently than usual during the first half of your pregnancy. Being a DES daughter is an important factor to mention to the person giving you prenatal care. For more information about DES daughters, see page 14.

➤ *Hormonal deficiency*. If the estrogen or progesterone levels diminish in your uterine lining, the attachment of the embryo is jeopardized. The risks to the fetus from hormone treatments must be considered if you are in danger of miscarrying.

➤ *Ordinary tap water* may contribute to miscarriages. Studies have shown women who drank bottled water had fewer pregnancy complications and miscarriages than those who drank tap water, even in neighborhoods where tap water was not polluted. You may want to consider drinking bottled spring or distilled water during your childbearing years.

➤ *Research has linked HLA* (human leukocyte antigens) to spontaneous abortions. Doctors have found that if the mother and father have similar types of HLAs, the pregnancy has a higher than normal chance of aborting, usually around the twelfth week of pregnancy. Both the mother and father should be tested to pinpoint the cause of repeated miscarriages, and the aborted fetus should be tested as well. This helps provide a diagnosis so the family can be advised about the next pregnancy, since physical and chromosomal abnormalities are common in these pregnancies.

➤ *Anatomical problems of the uterus*, such as a bicornuate uterus (divided inside with a central wall) or fibroid tumors can cause miscarriage.

➤ *Anatomical problems of the cervix* are relatively rare. The cause may be a congenital defect, most commonly in women who were exposed to DES in utero. An "incompetent cervix" may also have been caused by a previous pregnancy, too many dilations of the cervix for tests, previous miscarriages, or elective abortions. The result is that the cervix does not stay tightly closed and weakens with the increased weight of the fetus. A doctor can do a cervical circlage: she or he threads a ring of stitches around the cervix to keep it closed until labor, then takes out the stitches.

➤ *Incompatible blood type*: An Rh-negative-sensitized woman, or a woman who has an antagonistic blood type with the baby's father, may develop antibodies to the hostile blood type. This can cause fetal death and miscarriage.

➤ *T-mycoplasma virus* is a microscopic organism that infects a man or a woman without giving any symptoms. This virus may be a factor in habitual miscarriage (more than three), but antibiotics can easily eliminate it.

➤ *A late habitual aborter* is a woman who has had three or more miscarriages. The problem may be due to factors such as thyroid or another endocrine imbalance, or a major disease such as syphilis or renal-hypertensive disease. Some doctors find that dietary instructions plus thyroid treatment help some women; some doctors use hormones, others prescribe psychotherapy plus liberal amounts of vitamins B and C. There seems to be a strong psychological component in repetitive abortion: if a woman is reassured by a doctor's authoritative attitude, it can help eliminate this element of habitual abortion.

➤ *Second-trimester miscarriage*: an autopsy should be done to determine the cause and indicate any necessary treatment to prevent the problem from recurring.

➤ *Miscarriage is considered an obstetrical admission* (if it's necessary to go to the hospital). *This is very hard emotionally*. You are taken to the labor area to miscarry and the maternity ward to recover. Hospital staff and others don't know your situation and are bound to ask about your baby. Every effort should be made to isolate you from these insults to your feelings—if possible, request a room on another floor. Most important, your mate should have unlimited 24-hour visiting privileges—speak to your doctor about arranging this. Unlimited access to each other and privacy will help the grieving process.

Mourning a Miscarriage

➤ *The depth of grief* that a woman can feel for her lost infant may be downplayed by friends and relatives. They may think this will lessen the intensity of the parents' grief. However, health professionals are often aware that these couples should not have to suffer in silence, perhaps thinking something is wrong with them for mourning so deeply. Parents who lose a baby before, during, or soon after birth can have profound grief, which is not related to the length of a baby's life. Unresolved grief over a miscarriage can leave lasting emotional scars. Many women say they are still grieving over miscarriages that happened many years ago because they didn't have a chance to come to terms with it. Both parents can get very attached to their unborn baby. Other people never got to know the baby and therefore may not be able to appreciate the depth of your affection and subsequent grief.

➤ *Please refer to the section* on "Death of a Baby" (page 469) for more information and advice about how losing your baby can affect you and how to understand and deal with these emotions. "Resolve" has groups all over the country that offer counseling to parents who have lost infants. To find a group near you, ask your hospital, VNA, childbirth educator, local Family Health Association, or your doctor(s).

➤ *Naming a baby can be important*. Women who lost fetuses or babies many years ago have found that even giving the lost child a name now can help them put the grief behind them. It can also help to do something tangible, such as plant a tree. Do anything you can think of to help you deal with your sadness.

➤ *Having a funeral or memorial service* is suggested by some groups, which encourage parents to view miscarriage as the loss of a family member. The ritual involved in a small funeral can be an important part of a healthy grieving process, as well as encouraging the compassion and support of loved ones. A funeral for a lost fetus may seem strange to others, but it can be important as a way for some people to express their love for that child.

➤ *A man will react differently* than his wife to the loss of a baby. Men in our society are taught not to cry or otherwise show grief, but a women who is grief-stricken may mistakenly perceive her husband's lack of tears or signs of grief as an indication that he does not share her sadness. He may throw himself into his work or a sport after losing a child, which can be his way of handling grief. A man's ability to bounce back right away and apparently return to normal can be upsetting to his wife if she perceives him as uncaring. Exerting control over his life can be one way a man copes with feeling powerless and helpless: he may behave in an authoritarian way to mask what he's feeling underneath.

➤ *A woman's reaction to a miscarriage* can include all the obvious signs of grief, from crying to not eating to difficulties sleeping. There are also psychosomatic ways in which your body may symbolically grieve for the lost baby. A mother's arms may hurt at some point after the miscarriage, which can be a natural part of grieving—it may be your body's way of wanting to hold and cradle the baby you lost.

➤ *Hopes and dreams are lost* when you lose a baby. Your fantasies and plans for the baby and her future life are lost when you lose the planned-for child. Many parents become attached to their unborn babies early in the pregnancy, even giving the child a name from the beginning. The father may talk to his baby through the mother's abdomen, and the mother may sing or talk to the unborn infant, stroking the child through her belly.

The Experience of Grief

Four Phases of Mourning	Four Tasks of Mourning
1. Shock/Numbness 　　Lacks rationality 　　Healthy avoidance 　　Delusions/hallucinations	1. To Accept Reality of the 　Loss 　　Reunion impossible 　　Benefit of viewing dead 　　　body 　　Opposite—Denial
2. Searching/Yearning 　　Desire to get loved one 　　　back 　　Painful repetition of loss 　　Denial of permanence of 　　　loss 　　Anger and guilt	2. To Experience Pain of Grief 　　Need for assurance that 　　　pain is OK 　　Opposite—Not feeling
3. Disorganization/Despair 　　Life falling apart 　　No meaning/purpose 　　Helpless hopelessness 　　Fatigue, apathy, 　　　depression 　　Lack of self-esteem	3. To Adjust to Environment in 　Which the Deceased Is 　Missing 　　To make sense of loss 　　To modify one's 　　　assumptions 　　Opposite—Not adapting
4. Reorganization/Recovery 　　Putting life back together 　　Reinvestment in new 　　　activities/ 　　　relationships	4. To Withdraw Emotional 　Energy and Reinvest It in 　Other Relationships 　　Not loving deceased any 　　　less, but beginning to 　　　love others too 　　Opposite—Not loving

Once life has gone back to normal, there may be some painful reminders (anniversaries of the due date or the date of the loss) which may revive some grief symptoms for a time. Grief takes time and is different for everyone, but if any of these symptoms *persist*, you and your partner should investigate counseling alternatives.

➤ **The reactions of friends and relatives** are important after a miscarriage—they can help you recover or add unnecessarily to your sadness. Some psychologists believe that people who are mourning need to have their grief acknowledged by others, although it's natural to be uneasy talking about it. You may have to be the one to raise the subject and explain to those close to you that they can help you by listening. You may find comfort

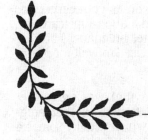

MANIFESTATIONS OF NORMAL GRIEF

Feelings	Physical Sensations	Behaviors
Sadness	Stomach	Sleep disturbances
Anger	hollowness	Appetite problems
Guilt	Throat tightness	Absentmindedness
Self-reproach	Chest tightness	Social withdrawal
Anxiety	Oversensitivity	Dreams of deceased
Loneliness	Depersonalization	Avoiding reminders
Fatigue	Breathlessness	of deceased
Helplessness	Muscle weakness	Sighing
Shock	Lack of energy	Restless
Yearning	Dry mouth	overactivity
Emancipation		Crying
Relief	**Cognitions**	Visiting places or
Numbness	Disbelief	carrying objects
	Confusion	that remind you
	Preoccupation	of deceased
	Sense of presence	Treasuring objects
	Hallucinations	that belonged to
		the deceased

and release in talking to a few close friends about the details of the pregnancy and miscarriage.

Friends may be sympathetic to your pain and want to help, but they may not know how. Some will say the wrong thing and hurt you unintentionally. You may think others don't care about your pain because they say nothing at all, when they're remaining silent only because they don't know what to say.

The easiest and most helpful thing for a friend to tell you is that she is sorry you miscarried. You may be hurt by the thoughtless clichés people utter, which are listed below. However, if you're prepared for these comments, they may have less negative impact. Don't resent well-meaning friends who leave you feeling even lonelier in your grief just because they've said the wrong thing.

Hurtful Clichés About Miscarriage

- *"It's normal, people miscarry all the time."* This doesn't make you feel any better: miscarriage is hardly a "normal" event for you.
- *"You'll get pregnant again in no time."* Whether you can or will conceive again has no bearing on the traumatic experience you've been through.
- *"There was probably something wrong with it anyway."* It is no comfort to be told your baby was probably defective. Doctors can tell you that half of all miscarried fetuses have genetic defects, but hearing it from friends is no consolation.
- *"It was God's will."* This is unintentionally cold, like telling you not to be sad over the death of a beloved grandparent "because he was old anyway."
- *"You have other child(ren), be grateful."* This comment is maddening because children you may be blessed with have nothing to do with the baby you have lost. Children are not interchangeable—it's frustrating to be told "to go home and love the son you already have" when your heart is breaking for the one you'll never know.

When to Get Pregnant Again

You can resume sexual relations again as soon as your cervix has closed (to prevent infection) usually 4 to 6 weeks after a miscarriage. Check with your doctor about attempting another pregnancy, but depending on the cause of your miscarriage it is advised to wait for one or two normal menstrual cycles.

- ➤ *If a defective germ plasm* (blighted ovum) was proven responsible for the miscarriage you can attempt another pregnancy immediately after the first period, which usually comes 4 weeks to the day after the abortion. The doctors who advise this reason that the miscarriage was just a natural random event and implied nothing wrong with you—and that psychologically it may be better to try again right away.
- ➤ *Some doctors* believe it is best to wait about three months before trying to conceive again. That allows you time to correct any known medical problems, go on an excellent diet, get plenty of rest and exercise—in general, build yourself up.
- ➤ *Doctors are more conservative* in cases where there was no known cause for the miscarriage; i.e., the fetus and the placenta were normal. They say that a six-month wait is best, hoping that whatever the cause was will correct itself in that period of time.

Ectopic Pregnancy

Ectopic pregnancy occurs when the egg is fertilized in the fallopian tube and, rather than passing into the uterus, remains in the tube. This is dangerous because if the pregnancy is allowed to continue, the tube will burst.

Call your doctor immediately if you suspect you are pregnant and have any of the following symptoms:
- Vaginal bleeding
- Pain in the lower abdomen (often on one side)
- Weakness and/or fainting

A pregnancy test and a physical examination can determine whether you have an ectopic pregnancy.

Treatment

Surgery must be performed for an ectopic pregnancy. Sometimes the fallopian tube can be rebuilt; other times it has to be removed on the side where the pregnancy occurred.

A woman treated for one ectopic pregnancy tends to be infertile. There is a 50% chance of not conceiving again. You *can* have a normal pregnancy the next time, but you have an increased risk (15% chance) of having another ectopic pregnancy.

Bursting the Tube

➤ ***The tube usually bursts between the eighth and twelfth weeks*** of the ectopic pregnancy. If it does, you get the symptoms mentioned above: vaginal bleeding, pain on side of the abdomen and weakness or fainting.

➤ ***That first sharp abdominal pain*** might mean a rupture. Go quickly to the doctor.

➤ ***You are bleeding internally*** when the tube bursts. It may be a sudden, acute bleeding, or more frequently, a slow trickling of blood into the abdominal cavity. You might feel an aching pain in your diaphragm or a sharp shoulder pain caused by blood flooding up to your diaphragm.

   If the bleeding is heavy, you might be in shock. The symptoms include: hot and cold flashes, nausea, dizziness, fainting.

➤ ***It's possible to confuse ectopic pregnancy with miscarriage***. Before or after a ruptured tube you might have a late period with mild menstrual-type bleeding or fragments. You—and the doctor—might misinterpret this as as an early miscarriage. If uterine lining is passed with the blood it should be examined microscopically. If there is no evidence of early fetal tissue, then an ectopic pregnancy should be suspected.

Fibroid Tumors

Fibroids are small, nonmalignant growths in the inner walls of the uterus. They usually occur in women over 35, who may have had them for many years before becoming pregnant. The majority of women with fibroids get pregnant and give birth without problems, but it is a condition that your doctor will want to keep an eye on throughout your pregnancy.

Once in a while a fibroid can cause an ectopic pregnancy, miscarriage, problems with the placenta, or complications during labor. If you have fibroids you should be aware of whether you have pain or pressure in the abdominal area, with or without fever. Don't be alarmed, but do call your doctor, who might want you to rest in bed for a few days until the pain passes. And don't worry about the birth itself: rest assured that if your doctor thinks your fibroids could hamper a safe vaginal delivery, she or he will suggest a cesarean.

High-Altitude Pregnancy

If you've been living at a high altitude for a while, your body is already used to breathing thinner air and it's unlikely for it to have any effect on your pregnancy. There's a very small risk of pregnancy complications, but you should be fine if you concentrate on getting good prenatal care, high quality nutrition, and are careful to avoid the known pregnancy risks.

However, if you're planning on moving from sea level to a higher altitude during pregnancy, it may be hard on you to adjust. If at all possible it's probably best to put off a move to a high altitude—or even a visit there—until after you've given birth.

> ➤ *Avoid smokers and smoky rooms* at a high altitude because they deprive the growing baby of oxygen and can stunt her growth no matter where the mother lives. At high altitudes smoke seems to have an even worse effect on the baby, so it's extra important to stay away from tobacco smoke when you're living up high.
> ➤ *Take it easy exercising* at a high altitude because strenuous exercise can cut down the oxygen reaching the baby. It's also harder on your body, so choose activities that put less strain on your breathing and always stop exercising before you reach a point where you're really tired.

Pregnancy with Long-Term Health Problems

If you have a chronic health condition and get pregnant, you'll probably be under the care of a specialized doctor who will follow your pregnancy along with your obstetrician. This section is not intended to replace the high level of medical surveillance that women at risk need during pregnancy. Think of this as brief notes about how some of those long-term health conditions can affect your pregnancy (and vice versa).

Eating Disorders: Anorexia or Bulimia

If you have been afflicted for years with an eating disorder, your body is at a disadvantage right from the beginning of your pregnancy because your nutritional reserves are low. (However, you may not have suffered as much as some women who have eating disorders, as anorexia and bulimia disrupt the menstrual cycle and most sufferers are never even able to get pregnant.)

A woman with an eating disorder can have as healthy a baby as any other woman, provided she has the mental strength to get control of the disorder. There are several things you need to do for yourself and your baby as soon as you decide to try to have a baby or discover that you are pregnant.

➤ *Stop the binge/purge habits* as soon as you learn you are carrying a baby.

➤ *Pregnancy is your chance to make up for the abuse* you have done to your body by taking special care of it now for your baby's sake.

➤ *You must tell your medical caregiver* of your eating disorder, even if you are so thin that it seems obvious. This problem is something you need to address out loud, for your sake as well as that of the person caring for you.

➤ *Get professional counseling from a therapist* who specializes in eating disorders. This is advisable for anyone who suffers from eating disorders, but is especially true for you now with the special needs of pregnancy. If there are any support groups in your area, this can be very helpful, too.

➤ *You must stop using laxatives or diuretics (water pills)*, which are commonly used by people with eating disorders. If you take them during pregnancy, they remove the nutrients and fluids from your body that the baby needs to grow properly. These medications can lead to abnormalities in the developing baby.

➤ *Weight gain during pregnancy* is obviously going to be a loaded issue for someone who has been anorectic or bulimic. Even women for whom weight is not a big issue can have trouble with their growing belly and the change in their body image. Read the section about weight gain starting on page 59 so you'll understand when and why your body begins to get bigger, how the weight is distributed, and how you'll regain your prepregnancy weight about six weeks after the baby is born.

➤ *You may have to be put in the hospital* if you can't get

control of the eating disorder. If you aren't able to stop vomiting, binge-eating, taking laxatives or diuretics, or you can't force yourself to eat frequent meals of proper foods, then you need to talk to your doctor about how to get this disease under control for the baby's sake. Hospitalization may be your baby's only hope of developing properly, if you decide that you do want to be pregnant and become a mother.

Lupus, Also Known as SLE (Systematic Lupus Erythematosus)

Lupus, or SLE, is an autoimmune disease in the rheumatoid arthritis family that primarily affects women between the ages of 15 and 65. There is a great deal not known about this disease, but it now appears that getting pregnant does not have a long-term effect on the disease. Some women who suffer from lupus find that their condition improves during pregnancy, while for others it worsens, and it can change from one pregnancy to the next. For most women there is a flare-up after the baby is born.

➤ *The best time to conceive* is when there is a quiet period in the disease.
➤ *If your kidney function is impaired by SLE*, it is recommended that your kidney function be stable for at least six months before you conceive.
➤ *The effect of lupus on pregnancy is not fully known*, and although the risk of miscarriage is slightly higher for women with lupus, you have an excellent chance of having a healthy baby.
➤ *Lupus and SLE are diseases that can be genetically passed on to the baby.*
➤ If your lupus requires daily doses of a NAISID and prednisone (a steroid), taking the lowest effective dose (with your doctor's orders, obviously) appears to reduce any risks to the pregnancy. Talk to your rheumatologist about taking steroids: some don't cross the placenta and even those that do are not considered a risk to the developing baby. Antimalarial drugs like Plagrenil should be discussed with your arthritis specialist if they have been ordered for you.

Diabetes in Pregnancy

There are an estimated 10 million diabetics in the United States, half of whom are unaware of their condition. Women are 50% more likely to become diabetics than are men. There is a great risk of complications in a diabetic woman's pregnancy: she is more prone to toxemia, infection, and congenital malformations in the baby. Even though all diabetic pregnancies are dealt with as "high risk," there are still many problems that even advanced obstetric science cannot resolve. The best results during pregnancy and delivery occur if you are under the joint care of an expert in diabetes and an obstetrician who specializes in high-risk pregnancy.

The *earlier* the onset of diabetes and the *longer* you've had the disease, the worse the prognosis for pregnancy. The risks are greater for insulin-dependent diabetics. Maintenance of a normal glucose concentration in the blood brings the best fetal and maternal results, but this may be extremely difficult and require frequent hospitalization. Even under constant care there is no certainty that your baby will be born alive and healthy.

RISKS TO THE BABY OF A DIABETIC MOTHER

➤ *The characteristics of the offspring of diabetic women* are: hypoglycemia, low serum calcium levels, elevated bilirubin level, large fetal organs (the heart and adrenals), and relatively small brain and thymus.

➤ *The risk of respiratory distress syndrome* (RDS) is five times greater in a diabetic pregnancy. RDS usually affects a baby whose lungs are not yet mature enough, which can be determined by the L/S ratio in the amniotic fluid. An L/S ratio of 2.0 is normally considered a measure of fetal lung maturity, but doesn't necessarily guarantee that a diabetic's baby will *not* have RDS. In a normal pregnancy a 2.0 L/S ratio is usually reached at 35 to 36 weeks gestation. In a diabetic pregnancy it is safest to wait, if possible, until at least 36 weeks and an L/S ratio of 2.5 or higher before delivery.

➤ *The fetus of a diabetic woman has a tendency to die*. The risk of death before labor is greatest in the last two or three weeks of the pregnancy. The optimal delivery time is 36 to 37 weeks: most doctors deliver a diabetic pregnancy by cesarean or induction from three to six weeks before the calculated due date. Insulin-dependent diabetics cannot go to term and are nearly always delivered prematurely.

Toxemia of Pregnancy

Toxemia is a complication of pregnancy which usually happens in the third trimester. It used to be blamed on gaining too much weight during pregnancy, but that is not true. *Poor nutrition* is thought to play an important—perhaps the most important—part in causing toxemia, but the full causes are not known. Toxemia is also called preeclampsia. If it reaches the severe stage, it is known as eclampsia: in this case, a doctor may decide to deliver the baby by cesarean to protect the baby from the additional stress of labor.

> ***The signs of preeclampsia*** include: swelling, vision disturbance (from cerebral edema, usually a sign of second-stage toxemia), high blood pressure, and protein in the urine. The signs of second-stage are abdominal pains, vision disturbance, severe headaches, and mental dullness. The last three result from cerebral edema, "water on the brain."

> ***Water pills (diuretics)*** are sometimes prescribed to treat toxemia, but they deal only with the symptoms, not the cause. They should not be used to "cover up" the swelling of toxemia, which is one of its danger signals. Along with the fluid they force out of your tissues, diuretics also cause the loss of essential nutrients and can deplete the amniotic fluid.

> ***Malnutrition***—insufficient protein, in particular—has been linked to toxemia in various studies. The best way to prevent toxemia is to eat a well-balanced diet with a focus on high-quality protein.

> ***The signs of the eclamptic (severe) stage*** of toxemia are convulsions and coma, but this stage is rarely reached if you are under medical care.

> ***A psychosomatic basis*** for toxemia is being studied. The effect of the mind on the body is being examined more fully in all aspects of health care, and there is an apparent link between high blood pressure and stress and anxiety. Toxemia may fall into this category, but more investigation needs to be done.

> ***Toxemia affects the baby*** because the placenta does not function as well, which may cause a small-for-date baby or fetal death. Since labor must be induced early in some cases of toxemia, prematurity is another danger to the baby. There is also a higher incidence of placenta abruptio along with toxemia.

Hypertension (High Blood Pressure)

Hypertension is one of the signs of toxemia, but it can also exist in a pregnant woman as a separate complication. There is usually some sign of high blood pressure in the last trimester of pregnancy, but some women having a first baby develop it during labor with no prior indication. This is one of the reasons that blood pressure is monitored in the hospital during labor—because if it does develop, it gives no warning until the woman goes into convulsions. It can cause temporary or permanent blindness if the blood pressure is not lowered.

Blood pressure is usually not monitored in most out-of-hospital birth settings, but it would be of little use anyway because there is no medication at home to correct the problem. In the hospital a "magnesium drip" is started (magnesium is added to an IV hydrating solution), which has an excellent ability to lower the blood pressure.

A blood pressure of 140/90 is universally recognized as hypertensive, especially in a first pregnancy. Some doctors will hospitalize you before labor for observation and bed rest with this pressure reading. But it is possible to be hypertensive with a lower reading than this. A doctor knows what your blood pressure has been during pregnancy and uses that as a baseline—you will be diagnosed as hypertensive if there is a 20-point rise during labor in either the systolic (top) number or the diastolic (bottom) number. For instance, if you are 130/80 during pregnancy, you can have a slightly higher pressure in the late stage of active labor without any concern. But if your baseline blood pressure was 100/60, you may be having a problem in labor at the 130/80 or 140/90 reading.

A diastolic rise is more significant because this is the "resting" pressure of your heart. Your system is under maximum pressure when your heart is working hardest, which is the systolic, or "pumping," measurement. Thus, when the diastolic number is high, it may be a sign of problems because theoretically this is when your heart is supposed to be resting. For example, a 110/60 rise might be normal in labor, whereas a 110/65 rise to 120/90 might indicate problems.

Herpes Simplex Virus II

"WHAT IS HERPES?"

Because herpes is a common venereal disease in the United States, it is not a rare complication of pregnancy, but it is a complication which must be monitored. Herpes consists of clusters of fluid-filled blisters on any part of the body, although usually around the genital area. If you have active lesions at the time of birth, there is a strong possibility that you will pass the disease to your baby, who may suffer damage to the nerves or eyes or may die.

"HOW CAN YOU GET IT AND HOW DO YOU KNOW?"

You can get herpes by having sexual contact with someone who has herpes (but may not have the symptoms). Three to 14 days after being exposed you would notice some symptoms yourself: sometimes there is a fever accompanied by a headache or just generally not feeling well. Urination can be very painful and there can be severe burning or inability to urinate. The blistery lesions usually open and group together, forming larger open sores which heal within a few weeks.

Once infected, a victim will probably have recurrent outbreaks, but the disease can be sexually transmitted to another person only during an active recurrence. Between times, the virus becomes inactive. There is a drug which can be used to control herpes called acyclovir (brand name Zovirax). However, it is not yet known whether it is safe to use this drug during pregnancy; studies are being conducted

"HOW CAN THIS DISEASE AFFECT MY BABY?"

Active vaginal or cervical lesions at the time of delivery can give the virus to your newborn: 50% of infants that pass through an infected birth canal will get herpes. This means they will suffer serious nerve or eye damage or may even die. *A woman who has had herpes* **at any time in her life** *must be examined for recurrent infection in the cervix and birth canal as she gets close to her delivery date.*

The fetus can be infected *before* birth if the membranes are ruptured for a prolonged time. If a woman has herpetic lesions in the genital area near her due date, it is essential for the baby's well-being that the baby be delivered by cesarean section, before the membranes ruptures, or if they do, within 4 hours. Most newborns will be protected by this precaution.

"IS THERE ANY WAY TO CONTROL HERPES?"

The best way to prevent recurrences of herpes is through good health habits. If you are an expectant mom with a history of herpes, take extra care to eat well regularly, get plenty of sleep, keep your body clean, and wear loose-fitting undergarments. Mental and physical stress are both important factors in whether herpes recurs: knowing this, do whatever you can to maintain a low-stress environment for yourself during your pregnancy.

Diet therapy is another way to control herpes outbreaks. Studies have shown that certain viruses like herpes, mononucleosis, and chicken pox are affected by the protein composition of their environment. Research has shown that one of the protein building blocks, an essential amino acid called *L-lysine*, inhibits the growth of the herpes virus. At the same time, researchers found that another amino acid, *arginine*, enhanced this viral growth. The research is not conclusive, but there is reason to believe that changing your diet can reduce the chance of infection and the recurrence of the virus, as well as help heal any lesions which are already present. See the chart on page 21.

Since this treatment doesn't involve the use of medication, it doesn't pose drug-related risks. If you have a history of herpes you should take care, especially in the last six weeks of your pregnancy, to avoid arginine-rich foods. You should also supplement your diet with an L-lysine supplement. It is available in health food stores and many drugstores. The usual recommended supplement is 1,500–3,000 mg a day, taken in three doses.

HIV Infection

The epidemic of AIDS in America has reached a point in recent years where the most rapid increase in cases of AIDS (acquired immunodeficiency syndrome) in our population is among women. As the incidence of HIV infection has increased among women of childbearing age, so has the number of infants who have become infected through mother-to-infant transmission. This perinatal transmission of HIV accounts for 90% of cumulative AIDS cases among children, while practically all new cases of HIV infections among children came from their HIV-positive mothers. As a result, HIV infection has become the leading cause of death for young children.

However, it has been discovered that the majority of these babies and their families can now be spared this suffering. *Just because a woman discovers she is HIV-positive does not necessarily mean that she has to pass this deadly disease to her unborn child.* The exciting news is that for the first time ever, it has been discovered that HIV infection can be prevented with a drug. An HIV-infected woman's baby may be spared if she is treated with AZT (zidovudine, also known as ZDV) during pregnancy and labor and if her newborn is treated from birth. In fully two-thirds of the pregnancies treated with AZT, the mother's HIV infection was not transmitted to her baby. AZT treatment was found to be highly effective while also causing no serious short-term side effects for the mothers or infants.

"WHAT CAN I DO TO PROTECT MY UNBORN BABY?"

The first step in protecting yourself and your unborn child is to be tested to determine whether you have become HIV-infected. Without realizing it, you may have been exposed to AIDS at some time, although you are not yourself in a high-risk group (injecting drug use or unprotected sexual contact with a high-risk sex partner). The frightening fact is that an increasing number of babies contracted AIDS in the womb from their mother, who acquired HIV infection through heterosexual contact with a partner she didn't know was high-risk or who was already infected. Optimally you would want to learn whether you are HIV-infected before becoming pregnant, but if you are already pregnant, then it is best to learn early in your pregnancy so you can get the best possible treatment for yourself and your baby.

"WHEN IS THE FETUS MOST AT RISK?"

HIV can be transmitted from an infected woman to her fetus during pregnancy, during labor and delivery, or to the newborn during the postpartum period through breast-feeding. HIV can be passed to the fetus as early as the eighth week of gestation. It is thought that at least half of the perinatal transmissions take place shortly before or during the birth process. Because of this, the baby of an HIV-infected mother is often delivered by cesarean section. Since breast-feeding can increase the rate of transmission by 10 to 20%, bottle-feeding is also recommended.

"HOW IS AZT GIVEN TO AN HIV-INFECTED WOMAN?"

The current use of AZT to prevent perinatal transmission is for the mother to start AZT orally between the 14th and 34th week of pregnancy and continue until she goes into labor. The drug is given intravenously during labor and delivery and orally to the infant for six weeks after birth. This AZT regimen caused only minimal side effects in the mothers and infants who were studied; the only adverse effect was mild anemia in the infants, which was resolved without therapy.

"WHAT IS DONE FOR THE BABY AFTER BIRTH?"

A baby who is exposed to HIV infection in the womb is at risk for a variety of illnesses and has to be closely monitored by healthcare professionals. Although AZT can save two-thirds of these babies, there are still many who will become infected with HIV from their mothers. Of these infants, approximately 10 to 20% will develop rapidly progressive disease and die by twenty-four months of age.

There is frequently the chance in children who have been perinatally exposed to HIV of becoming infected with PCP (pneumocystis carinii pneumonia): this disease usually occurs at three to six months of age and is often fatal. Because of this, it is recommended that babies of HIV-infected mothers should be identified as early as possible and preventive treatment be given promptly to all of them. The guidelines for these children are to put them on prophylactic therapy to fight against PCP at four to six weeks of age. HIV-infected infants usually continue treatment until they're twelve months old, at which point the pediatrician will evaluate how your child is doing. Babies infected perinatally should also be carefully followed for prompt diagnosis of other potentially treatable HIV-related conditions, like severe bacterial infections or tuberculosis.

Since HIV-exposed infants are more at risk for childhood illnesses pediatricians know that they also need to change the usual schedule of routine immunizations, as early as two months of age.

"WHAT ARE THE GENERAL RECOMMENDATIONS FOR HIV PREGNANCY?"

➤ **The hospital should be notified of your baby's status.** You need to ask your healthcare providers to notify the pediatric medical staff at the hospital where you are planning to give birth that your baby has been HIV-exposed during pregnancy. Your medical records are confidential, of course, but for your baby's sake the hospital caregivers should be prepared for any anticipated complications with the baby and be informed about the advisability of administering AZT (ZDV) after birth.

➤ **Discuss the advisability of a cesarean section with your doctor.** It is believed that avoiding vaginal delivery may lessen your baby's chances of becoming infected with HIV.

➤ **Know your rights as an HIV-infected mother.** It is against the law to discriminate against you in matters such as housing, employment, state programs and public accommodations, including physician's offices and hospitals. However, there are potential negative reactions to expectant women who are HIV infected. If you anticipate or experience problems in your personal relationships or your employment or you have psychological difficulties you may want to arrange for counseling.

➤ **Avoid breast-feeding.** To reduce the risk for HIV transmission to your baby it is advised that you should not expose her to your breast milk.

➤ **Arrange for HIV testing for any other children you may have.** Protect the health of any children born after you became HIV infected (or if you don't know when you became HIV positive, any child born after 1977) by having them tested. Children older than twelve years of age should be tested with their understanding and your informed consent. It is possible for a baby to be infected during pregnancy and not have any signs or symptoms for several years: just because a child does not have signs or symptoms of HIV infection does not necessarily mean he is not HIV infected.

➤ **Follow-up medical care of your child is essential.** Discuss with your pediatrician the need for the baby's infection status to be monitored; whether preventive therapy for PCP should be administered; if she's infected, her need for medical treatment; she should be watched for disorders in growth and development which often occur before twenty-four months of age; the need for altering the vaccination schedules for HIV-infected children and other children living in households with HIV-infected persons.

For more information, or for free, anonymous and/or confidential testing, you can contact the National AIDS Hotline at 1-800-342-AIDS.

Intrauterine Devices (IUD)

It is recommended that if you become pregnant with an IUD in place you have it removed as soon as possible. If you wish to continue the pregnancy, you should have the device removed immediately when the pregnancy is confirmed. Spontaneous abortion (miscarriage) is the main problem of continuing to keep an IUD in place once you are carrying a child. Another problem of continuing a pregnancy with an IUD still in place is the possibility of premature delivery.

Syphilis

A pregnant woman with infectious syphilis can miscarry at any time after the fourth month or have a stillborn. Early diagnosis and treatment of the mother will cure infection in the unborn baby. If the mother is treated with drugs before the eighteenth week, the disease will not cross the placenta and affect the baby. Most states require a syphilis test for pregnant women even though they may have had a premarital test which was negative.

One-quarter of syphilis-infected babies die before birth and nearly one-third more die after birth. Babies can be born with congenital syphilis. They can also have such abnormalities as saddle nose (lacking a bridge), blindness due to an opaque cornea, deafness due to syphilis of the auditory nerve, abnormal pegged teeth, and internal problems. These babies can also have three symptoms known as Hutchinson's triad: baldness, rashes, and lesions.

Complications During Labor

About 10% of women can be diagnosed as high-risk before labor and delivery so that they and their doctors are prepared for possible complications. However, the majority of all complications during labor, birth, and the immediate postpartum period occur in women with no indications during pregnancy. Some studies have shown that during labor itself one-third of all women who were designated "low-risk" become "high-risk."

The problems that arise vary in seriousness, but the medical community points to this one-third proportion as an argument for birth in the hospital; advocates of the fetal monitor cite these figures as a rationale for routine fetal monitoring of all women, since it isn't possible to know ahead of time who will develop complications.

However, those who favor out-of-hospital birth question what proportion of complications are a *direct result of aggressive obstetric procedures.* Some examples are inducing labor by starting it or speeding it up with synthetic hormones for the woman's or doctor's convenience; keeping the woman comfortable at the expense of jeopardizing the integrity of the fetal brain; artificially rupturing membranes to speed labor or insert an internal fetal monitor; and other procedures that may provide a learning experience for medical students, interns, and residents.

Labor Is Best Left to Nature Unless Nature Falters

There *are* times when nature falters and only medical intervention can correct the problem. However, there are several ways in which you can insure that labor will not falter and several things you can do if problems arise.

➤ *A peaceful emotional state* is essential for a successful labor. The peak time for delivery is from 3:00 to 4:00 A.M., and the onset of labor signs occurs more frequently during the nighttime hours. This is when you are most likely to be in a calm state of mind. If you realize the importance of your emotional condition, you and your mate can do everything possible to protect it.

➤ *Environmental disturbances* may affect the timing, strength, and efficiency of your contractions. Contractions often decrease or disappear temporarily in the move from your home to the hospital and from the labor room to the delivery room. Medical caregivers usually ignore the psychological component of labor complications, so you have to be aware of them and try to improve your emotional state so that it doesn't interfere with labor.

➤ *Anxiety may be related to the length of your labor.* Also, uterine dysfunction may be associated with concealed anxiety. If you are feeling frightened or worried during labor, *talk about it.* Share your feelings with your mate or coach; ask the doctor or nurse for information that may reassure you. If you simply try to "forget" the anxiety, it may assert itself by slowing down your labor or undetermining the efficiency of your contractions.

➤ *Reaching a plateau* in which dilation slows or stops is a common occurrence. This can be discouraging if you are having strong, regular contractions, but dilation is not progressing. Do not let this upset you. Take cheer—and don't take artificial relaxants or stimulants right away. When the plateau has passed, your dilation often progresses rapidly. Try to keep a positive outlook, stay calm, and try some of the suggestions below.

Helpful Suggestions for Labor Complications

➤ *Change positions often*—moving your position or walking around may cause the baby to move into a more favorable position. Moving may engage her head more firmly in your pelvis, which is a better wedge to dilate the cervix.

➤ *Check your release of tension*. You may be getting tense although you're unaware of it; this can slow your dilation. Use all your relaxation techniques. Have your mate give you a light massage. Concentrate on a feeling of floating in water.

➤ *Massage or pull on your nipples*—this can increase contractions that have stopped or slowed. By stimulating your nipples, you trigger the release of oxytocin into your system. This is the natural form of the hormone Pitocin, with which labor is often medically administered, but can have side effects which mandate other medical procedures as a result.

The Problems That Can Arise During Labor

➤ *Hypotonic contractions* are weak, infrequent, and do not produce normal labor progress. They can occur any time in labor but are more frequent in advanced stages. Oxytocic stimulation usually works.

➤ *Hypertonic contractions* are severe but with little or no progress. They may occur in early labor, in which case you can be sedated to rest before resuming a more normal labor, or you can be given an oxytocic to regulate the contractions.

➤ *Incoordinate uterine activity* resembles hypertonic labor in that the contractions are difficult to predict or control and bring little progress. A change of position is the most helpful treatment, along with a mild sedative (or meditation instead!) and analgesia if the pain is severe.

➤ *Prolonged latent phase* (0 to 4 centimeters dilation) is considered anything longer than 20 hours for a first baby or 13½ hours for subsequent pregnancies. This complication may be the result of excessive analgesia, a breech presentation, a large baby and small pelvis, or if your membranes rupture when the cervix is still unripe and has not yet effaced (thinned out). A mild sedative can help you rest, or oxytocin can be used to stimulate the efficiency of the contractions.

➤ *Prolonged active phase* (above 4 centimeters dilation) is usually caused by a malposition of the baby—either his head doesn't descend into the pelvis, he is a breech, or his head is too big to fit through your cervix. Patience and close supervision are often the best means to deal with the problem.

➤ *Secondary arrest* is when the progress of labor stops altogether in the active stages. This may be from too much medication or because the baby's head is too big for you. Oxytocin can be used to stimulate contractions or a C-section can be performed if the problem is a pelvis that isn't large enough for the baby to pass through.

➤ *Precipitate labor* starts out with very strong, frequent contractions with rapid dilation—more than 5 centimeters per hour for a first baby or complete dilation within an hour in later pregnancies. Labor can last a few contractions to a few hours, but things are happening so fast that it will be hard for you to stay in control. Do not let anyone hold your legs together: it can cause brain damage in the baby. Do not push with contractions: the uterus does not need any help—keeping the baby from coming out *too fast* is desirable. If it happens when you're in the hospital, the doctor may try to slow labor down because a gentle birth is easier on you and the baby, who needs the hours of contractions to stimulate its skin and lungs; she can also suffer oxygen deprivation from the hard, frequent contractions. The reasons for precipitate labor are now known, but there is a tendency for it to recur—so be prepared for the next time you get pregnant!

➤ *Soft tissue dystocia* is a rare occurrence that may follow previous treatment or an operation on your cervix, or there may be no discoverable cause. The cervix dilates at an abnormally slow rate despite strong contractions, a normal pelvis, and an average-size baby in a satisfactory position. It may prolong labor many hours and the very last stages of dilation may have to be completed by some operative means. Sometimes a doctor or nurse can massage your cervix during contractions to help it open up. The treatment is patience—on your part and that of the doctor.

Resistant vaginal tissues may prolong second-stage labor (pushing). It is especially common for women over 35 who are having their first baby. Strenuous athletics, especially riding, can thicken vaginal muscles, which can produce soft-tissue dystocia. An episiotomy can overcome this problem.

SOME SIGNS OF ABNORMAL LABOR

* *Continuous and severe lower abdominal pain,* often accompanied by uterine tenderness.
* *Discontinuance of good strong contractions* during first-stage labor.
* *Excessive vaginal bleeding*—some reasons could be a cervical laceration, placenta abruptio, or delivery before full cervical dilation.
* *Abnormality in fetal heart rate,* in which case you should be moved onto your left side to take pressure off the major blood vessels on the right.
* *Abnormally slow dilation* of the cervix, which is a subjective judgment made by attendants based somewhat on your pain tolerance and the strength of the contractions.
* *Abnormal presentation or prolapse* of the cord, placenta, or an extremity of the baby.
* *Adverse change* in the condition of the mother (fever, high blood pressure) or the baby (fetal heart rate, meconium staining).

Cesarean Birth

One out of every ten women reading this book is going to have her baby by cesarean section—depending on the particular area of the country and the hospital involved, it may be as many as two out of every ten pregnant women. This may mean you. Many women don't know they are going to have a cesarean until partway through labor. Cesareans are not something that "happen to other people"—*every* pregnant woman should know about cesareans. *Please* read this section and inform yourself ahead of time.

Understanding what procedures will take place and why (the preparation, the catheter, the operation itself) will make it less frightening and less emotionally wrenching if you have to "be sectioned"; a cesarean section is often referred to as a "C-section" or a "section," and the verb "to be sectioned" has grown out of that. Many childbirth classes and books don't discuss cesareans, but preparation for the possibility makes it much smoother. You and your partner should know enough about the whys and wherefores of cesareans to be able to participate with your doctor in the decision to have a cesarean. You should talk to your doctor *ahead of time* about what options are available if you have to be sectioned. Don't accept a doctor's reply of "Why worry about that now? Everything's going to be fine." Most of the time a doctor doesn't know any better than you do whether you'll need a cesarean until you're in labor. There are several options available to you and you should negotiate them beforehand with the doctor. It may be possible to have your partner in the operating room with you; you should also have the choice to be awake and have regional anesthesia or to be unconscious under a general anesthetic. Sometimes medical factors determine this, but often it's decided by a doctor's or hospital's habits.

The Increase in the Cesarean Rate

The high cesarean rate sounds ominous until you look at the reasons for it. Cesareans now account for 15 to 20% of all births in the United States—the number has doubled over the last decade. Some people "blame" the increased cesarean rate on fetal monitors, but this increase came before widespread monitoring. There are a number of reasons for the increase.

> ➤ *The operation is now safer*. Although a cesarean is major surgery, and therefore carries with it the risks of any surgery, the operation has evolved to the point where it is a relatively safe procedure. This means that a doctor can decide in favor of a cesarean when its risks are low compared to the alternative—which may be a high-forceps delivery, a baby in a breech position, or signs of fetal distress. A cesarean has become so safe that it can be considered more risk-free than many complications of vaginal labor and delivery.

➤ *Women are waiting until their late thirties and early forties* to have their first baby. They are approaching the age where the risks of a deformed child increase and when there can be complications in labor. These women often want only one or two children and they are demanding that nothing be wrong with the baby—they have waited a long time and don't have many childbearing years ahead of them. Thus, if things are not going smoothly, a cesarean will be performed rather than riding it out and "taking chances."

➤ *Ultrasound and electronic fetal monitors can predict* which babies might be compromised by the rigors of labor, indicating a cesarean rather than attempting a vaginal delivery. Monitoring also detects which babies do not tolerate labor well once it has begun. The stillbirth rate has been cut in half at many hospitals since fetal monitors were introduced there.

It is also true that cesareans can be performed before they are really necessary by doctors who are newly introduced to monitoring and do not read the monitor properly. *A fetal monitor is only as good as the person reading the tracing*: reading the monitor properly is a skill that has to be developed. Often the cesarean rate will rise at a hospital when fetal monitors are first introduced and the rate will drop back down once the personnel have become more practiced in deciphering the information correctly.

➤ *Defensive medicine causes many cesareans*. Doctors are afraid of malpractice suits. They are afraid of the dangerous effect on the baby of prolonged labor, in which there can be oxygen deprivation. They are afraid of being sued for failing to do everything possible to deliver a perfect baby. It is the attitude and actions of prospective parents that have backed doctors into a corner so that the only way they can deliver what people demand is to do a cesarean and eliminate the risks of the unknown. Nature is whimsical and wasteful—yet many Americans are not willing to accept that. They expect a doctor to present them with a "perfect" baby, and they often feel justified in blaming him/her for *any* problems. Doing a C-section gives a doctor more control over the outcome and therefore a greater chance of meeting the parents' expectations.

One study showed a higher cesarean rate for women who had taken childbirth classes. Doctors have a greater fear of malpractice litigation from educated, affluent, sophisticated, middle-class parents. The resulting irony is that those women who care the most about having a normal, natural birth may be more likely to have their baby by cesarean.

➤ *The higher cesarean rate* at some institutions may be high because they are just getting accustomed to the monitor, but there are other related reasons. Until now the monitor has been reserved for high-risk pregnancies. And although there is now routine monitoring of all women in relatively few well-endowed institutions, in most hospitals the $6,000-per-machine cost (not counting maintenance, etc.) means that the monitor is still reserved for high risk. *But the high-risk group has grown.*

WHY ARE THERE MORE HIGH-RISK MOTHERS

* **There are couples with genetic or fertility problems** who might have adopted in the past, for instance. Because of improved prenatal testing and fertility cures, they are now able to get pregnant but remain at risk.
* **New tests that determine fetal maturity** can indicate when an insufficient placenta begins to jeopardize the fetus. This alerts doctors to a potentially complicated labor and delivery, so they elect to do a cesarean instead.
* **There is a relatively higher proportion of first-time mothers** because parents are electing to have only one or two children, and there are relatively more older first-time mothers because women are waiting longer to conceive. Both these groups are at higher risk.
* **There are also more legal reasons** for doing a cesarean, which are discussed in the following section.

Indications for a Cesarean

There are two categories of reasons for performing a cesarean. The *absolute indications* are those in which there is no question or doubt as to whether a C-section is required. The absolute indications listed here can sometimes even be emergency cesareans, in which immediate delivery is necessary to save the baby's and/or the mother's life. They involve the subjective opinion of your doctor, perhaps in consultation with another physician, or with you and your mate. The decision depends on your body, the baby's condition, your desires, and your doctor's beliefs, based on his experience. *Relative indications* can be divided into two categories: determining factors that are known before labor begins, and those that are evaluated once you are already in labor.

Because some experts believe that a little labor is good even when a cesarean has been decided upon, your doctor may wait until you go into labor and then allow you to labor for a while before doing the cesarean. Cesarean babies sometimes have respiratory problems, and labor contractions help stimulate the lungs, compressing them to remove some of the fluid and to prepare them for breathing. Therefore, if you have a relative indication, you might want to discuss this possibility with your obstetrician ahead of time.

DIRECTORY OF REASONS FOR CESAREANS

Absolute Indications

— *Placenta previa* means that the placenta is preceding the baby; vaginal delivery is either physically impossible or you can hemorrhage. In the United States, six out of every ten women with placenta previa are given a cesarean. A *total placenta previa* means that the placenta is completely covering your cervix, blocking the baby's exit. A *partial placenta previa* is sometimes not an absolute indication for a C-section, depending on how much of the placenta is covering the cervix. If the doctor can feel only a silver of placenta, he may allow you to deliver vaginally, usually in the operating room so that a cesarean can be performed instantly if it becomes necessary.

— *Placenta abruptio* means partial or complete detachment of the placenta from the uterine wall before the baby is born. It normally detaches after the baby is delivered. There is grave risk to the mother from hemorrhaging, and to the baby, whose oxygen supply is cut off.

— *Prolapsed cord* means that the umbilical cord slips down in front of the baby's presenting part. Vaginal delivery would compress the cord in the birth canal, endangering the baby's life because her oxygen supply would be cut off.

Relative Indications Before Labor

— *Rh incompatability*: Depends on whether your antibody titer is high or rises before your due date. With a vaginal delivery there would be a greater chance of your blood's mixing with the baby's.

— *Malpresentation of the baby*: If the baby is in a breech position (buttocks first) or transverse lie (sideways in the uterus), the risks may outweigh the benefits of vaginal delivery.

— *Previous cesarean*: Depends on what the reason was for the previous C-section and what kind of incision was made (see detailed discussion later in this section).

— *Postmaturity:* If determined by tests that the baby is at least two weeks past the due date, and placental function is diminishing, then a cesarean may be better than the risk of waiting for spontaneous labor or the potential hazards of induction, which can place added stress on an undernourished, postmature baby.

DIRECTORY OF REASONS FOR CESAREANS (*cont.*)

— *Maternal disease*: In some cases of *diabetes, renal disease*, and *toxemia* the mother's health may be further endangered by the stresses of labor. In the case of *herpes simplex virus II*, if the mother has active vaginal lesions at the time of delivery, this viral infection can be fatal to a baby going through the infected birth canal.

Relative Indications During Labor
— *Cephalopelvic disproportion*: If prelabor tests suggests CPD are proven correct when baby does not descend.
— *Primipara over 40:* A woman having her first baby past age of 40 may lack the elasticity in her pelvis to give birth vaginally.
— *Fetal distress:* Continues after changes in position and other corrective measures designed to improve oxygen supply to the fetus.
— *Ruptured membranes:* Without the commencement of labor, or prolonged labor after the membranes break. The infection rate rises if a woman has not given birth within 24 hours of the time her membranes rupture.

The Operation Itself

If you are going to have an elective cesarean (one you have decided upon beforehand), there is the decision as to when it should be done. The main concern is not to take the baby out before it is mature enough because premature babies are at risk for many complications after birth. There are a number of tests to determine fetal maturity, all of which are described earlier in this chapter. At about 20 weeks gestation, ultrasound scans are done to determine the baby's general size and the fetal biparietal diameter, which correlates, although imprecisely, to gestational age. Amniocentesis can be done to determine the L/S ratio—the amount of lecithin/sphingomyelin increases as the baby's lungs become more mature. Unfortunately, the more reliable amniocentesis is not done as frequently as ultrasound, because the latter does not have any risks. Thus, there is almost always the chance that a cesarean may be premature.

Two Kinds of Cesareans

➤ A *classical* incision is vertical, a longitudinal cut made on top of the uterus. It is the quickest way to cut a cesarean and therefore may be done if speed is essential, or if you have a placenta previa located so it might be cut, or if the baby is especially large or in a transverse-lie position. The uterus is quite thin at the top and a classical incision is more difficult to repair and more likely to rupture in future pregnancies.

➤ A *transverse* incision is also called "a bikini cut" because it is done right below your pubic hairline, allowing you to wear a bikini afterward without the scar showing. It is done if the doctor has more time. The horizontal incision is made at the bottom of the uterus and is easy to repair and unlikely to rupture in the future. A third incision, a low-flap vertical, incorporates the other two cuts. It is made in the lower portion of the uterus, but the incision is made up and down, so that it can be enlarged if necessary.

Although a cesarean is a relatively safe operation, it still carries the risks of any major abdominal surgery. You are left with a scar on your uterus that can rupture before or during labor or delivery in a subsequent pregnancy, although this is highly unlikely. The uterus has an almost infinite capacity to stretch and is able to hold up to 15 to 18 pounds—the fetus plus the other "products of conception."

Preparation for a C-Section

Most C-sections are scheduled for early morning so that the doctor can then go to his office and see patients. Knowing ahead of time exactly what will be done to you makes a cesarean easier—just as childbirth education makes vaginal delivery less frightening. Be sure to *ask* about any procedures that are done to you—the more you know the less scary it will seem.

➤ **You will check into the hospital** about two hours prior to the operation or the preceding night. If you feel jittery, nervous, and afraid, that's normal! Samples of your blood and urine will be taken and your abdomen will be "prepped": a nurse will shave your stomach from about your belly button down through the upper portion of your pubic hair. You can request not to have your entire labia shaved because there is no need to shave *all* your pubic hair. Also, the routine enema is unnecessary unless you are constipated, so you can ask to forgo an enema.

➤ **A sedative before the operation** may be given by injection. It is your right to refuse this medicine. This is something you can discuss with the anesthesiologist, who will probably discuss what she or he will be doing during the operation. This drug will reach the baby and may make him groggy, as drugs used in vaginal labor and delivery often do. It can have the same effect on you, too.

➤ *The anesthesiologist is an important part* of a cesarean—you should discuss with your obstetrician whether you have a choice of anesthesiologist or whether you simply have to use whoever is on duty at the time (which is usually the case). The man or woman administering the anesthesia is the only person during the operation who will be relating directly to you (unless you're fortunate enough to be able to have your partner with you). Your doctor and the other staff will be too busy with their tasks. If an anesthesiologist is friendly and supportive of your feelings of fear and excitement, it can have a calming and cheering effect on you. The anesthesiologist is the person who has the final decision on what kind of anesthesia you get and will probably use whatever she or he feels most comfortable administering.

➤ *A catheter* will be inserted into your bladder. This is usually done in the operating room. It is a rubber tube placed up your urethra and into your bladder so that urine is drained out of your body during the operation. The catheter is left in afterward, depending on how you are feeling after the cesarean and how soon you're ready to get up and walk. It doesn't usually hurt, but it feels strange when they take it out.

How the Operation Is Done

➤ *A cesarean takes 45 minutes to one hour* to perform. Right before it begins, you will be given oxygen by mask to insure that the baby has plenty. The mask may smell medicinal, but you are getting pure oxygen. If you had a previous C-section, the first step is to cut around the old scar so that the normal skin edges can be brought together at the end. After the initial incision the abdominal muscle fibers are separated and then the peritoneum (the lining of the abdominal cavity) is opened, exposing the uterus. If you are having a "classical" C-section, a small incision is made in the lower midportion and is enlarged upward and downward to about 6 inches in length. In the low type of incision first your bladder has to be detached from the front of the uterus and then is pushed down in the pelvis beneath the pubic bone. A 6-inch longitudinal incision is made in the lowermost portion of the uterus, which was previously overlain by the bladder.

➤ *At this point the membranes usually rupture*. The doctor then gets the infant's head out of the incision, extracts the body, and clamps the umbilical cord. From the beginning of the skin incision to delivery is the shortest part of the operation: 5 to 6 minutes. The repair of the uterine and abdominal walls takes the most time. The placenta is manually removed and an oxytocic drug (usually Pitocin) is given intramuscularly or intravenously to encourage your uterus to contract. These contractions may be painful, so if you know breathing techniques you may want to use them. Your uterus is not massaged, as it would be in a vaginal delivery, because it might bleed.

➤ *If stitches are used* they will probably be of nonabsorbable silk and have to be removed between the fifth and seventh postoperative days. Some doctors use metal clips to close the skin, which can be removed in a week or less. There are 12 to 14 external clips or stitches.

➤ *An epidural is the anesthesia most often used* for a cesarean (see page 403). After the baby's birth the mother is often given a drug called Duramorf, which is administered via the epidural catheter. This is a morphine drug which stays in a woman's body about 24 hours, during which time it will eliminate or greatly reduce any postoperative pain. Many women do not need any other pain medication in recovering from the cesarean. Duramorf has a few mild side effects, such as itching and dizziness. The drug also has an uncommon but dangerous complication of respiratory depression: a woman has to be monitored carefully to be sure she's breathing normally during the 24-hour period after the drug is administered.

➤ *General anesthetic after the birth* is still used by some anesthesiologists, who may put a new mother lightly to sleep after the baby is born. You might want to discuss ahead of time the possibility of *not* being knocked out, since this can make you groggy or even sick at a time when you might want to be with your partner and/or baby.

➤ *When the anesthetic begins wearing off* in the recovery room, you will become aware of the pain from the incision. The return of sensation is more abrupt after general anesthesia. You will probably be given an injection of pain medication, and this—especially after general anesthesia—may make you nauseated to the point of vomiting. Retching is most uncomfortable after abdominal surgery, so if you are prone to nausea, you should ask your doctor before delivery about receiving an antiemetic drug. This is sometimes given routinely along with pain medication to prevent nausea.

The Emotional Aspects of a Cesarean

A simple thing like the choices of words used about cesareans can be negative. Some women feel it is dehumanizing to be spoken of as "a section" or having been "sectioned"—they say that grapefruits are sectioned but women give birth! Another example is when it's said that someone had a cesarean rather than a normal birth—this implies that a woman who had a C-section is abnormal, which can translate as "bad." The words you use can have a subtle influence on the way you feel about a cesarean; it helps to be aware of this.

To avoid potentially negative feelings about a cesarean, it is important to keep your perspective. The most important thing is that a baby is being born. If this idea can be kept foremost (without losing sight of the fact that a C-section is also major surgery with its risks), it allows you to focus on the joy of birth rather than the anxiety about the operation or the disappointment at not being able to have a vaginal delivery.

> *Anxiety* often dominates a woman's feeling about a C-section. If the cesarean is planned, you may be apprehensive for the entire time beforehand. If it is unexpected, often following a long and arduous labor or a frightening alarm for the baby's well-being during labor, it can be emotionally shattering. In the second case your choices and participation are often eliminated, so it can also make you feel helpless.

> *Braxton-Hicks contractions* before your due date and other normal uterine twinges during a pregnancy can be frightening if you know you are going to have a cesarean—you can fear that your uterus will rupture. Talk to your doctor to get reassurance if you do have these fears.

> *Another worry can be the expense* and separation from your other children during the traditional 5-day stay for a cesarean. Find out whether your insurance covers a cesarean: many that don't cover vaginal delivery do pay for a C-section. Try to have your other child(ren) visit you in the hospital once you are up and moving around.

> *Get a second opinion* about whether you need a cesarean, if your doctor tells you it's necessary ahead of time. That way you and your mate can satisfy yourselves that the decision is justified; it eliminates the possible doubts later that the cesarean could have been avoided.

> *Maintaining control* is a factor in making a women feel positive about her birth experience. If you are self-sufficient and feel like an autonomous, active participant rather than a passive object of care, it can enhance your feelings about yourself and the birth. It is a great disadvantage to cesarean women—especially those given a general anesthetic—not to have the opportunity to participate in the experience in that way. Make an attempt to involve yourself as much as you can in the decision about the operation and the postoperative procedures to overcome this feeling of helplessness. Your mate may also feel this way, so encourage him to be as involved as possible.

➤ *Negative feelings afterward* are fairly common. A woman's self-esteem often suffers. You may feel like a failure at mothering if you have trouble moving around and doing chores right from the start. You may also feel that your body didn't work "right," and in addition you have a scar as a constant reminder. Some women feel mutilated and no longer whole. If you feel this way you can take heart that the scar will be less evident as time goes on and may eventually disappear altogether.

➤ *Your partner may feel inadequate* and like a failure after an unexpected C-section. He may interpret his banishment to the waiting room as a punishment for not having helped enough— although the feeling is usually not a conscious one. If a man feels he was inadequate during labor ("If only I had been more supportive, labor could have gone on normally"), these feelings may be carried over into the early fathering role. A man who subconsciously feels he failed his partner and his baby may continue these feelings as a new parent.

➤ *Discuss the reasons for the cesarean* with the doctor beforehand and also afterward if you still have any questions. Get any information you want and talk about your feelings as well as plans for future pregnancies. Often these issues are left up in the air. Repressed feelings and a lack of understanding can cause fears, frustration, uncertainties, and anxiety.

➤ *Allow yourself to feel and express* negative feelings after a cesarean. You may feel jealous or resentful toward other women who talk enthusiastically about their nonmedicated birth and the ease of mothering. You may feel angry at the baby for having caused the cesarean; then you may feel guilty and blame yourself for "letting the baby down" because a cesarean was necessary. These feelings may be irrational, but you have to confront them. There may be a "C-sec" group you can call in your area and talk to a member or join a discussion group. If you don't get these feelings out of the way, they may haunt you or interfere with your relationship with the baby.

Some New Twists on the Traditional Cesarean Experience

There are some options you and your partner might want to consider. These can help counteract some of the possible negative aspects of a cesarean and enhance the experience for yourselves and your baby.

➤ *Allowing the baby's father into the operating room* has gained popularity. Birth is a time for togetherness, and this is especially true of a cesarean. You need each other at a time of stress for mutual support. Your mate may feel helpless, unneeded, and worried. You may feel lonely and scared. At the same time you may want to share the excitement and joy of seeing your baby's first minutes of life. For more information about how to make this option possible, see pages 249–251. "Prevailing practice" is what is considered in a hospital's decision to permit a couple to stay together. This means that if other hospitals have already allowed husbands to stay with wives, the path will be opened for the more cautious hospitals to try it. If they will not allow your mate in the delivery room, they may allow him to join you in the recovery area—ask about this. If it is a general recovery room—with various postoperative patients and not just women recovering from childbirth—it is less likely they'll allow your partner and/or baby to keep you company.

➤ *Lowering the screen* when the baby is born allows you to see the baby being born. This eliminates the problem that some women have in making a connection between the baby they have been carrying inside and the one that is placed in their arms, usually many hours later. The baby can also be examined near your head rather than the routine of examining her over in the warming tray or in the nursery. This gives you a chance to see the baby and assure yourself she is all right.

➤ *Holding the baby*, if only for a few minutes, can make a big difference. If the baby is not having respiratory distress (cesarean babies sometimes have trouble breathing right away), then ask if you can hold her for a little while. This is not routine in cesareans, but can make you feel closer to the baby, particularly if the hospital policy is to take her away for many hours. Unless the child needs immediate medical attention at birth there is no reason why the father cannot cuddle her, too. It is an important opportunity for paternal–infant bonding.

➤ *Breast-feeding on the delivery table* or in the recovery room is possible if the baby is fine and you've discussed it with your obstetrician and pediatrician, preferably beforehand. Breast-feeding often has a special meaning for cesarean mothers who may feel "At least my body can do *something* right!" The sooner a baby sucks, the better the chances of successful breast-feeding, because the sucking reflex is reinforced at birth. A cesarean mother who experiences difficulty breast-feeding, perhaps because of an immediate and prolonged separation after birth, may have feelings of *two* failures.

Don't forget that any medications you take for pain relief after a cesarean pass into your breast milk. To whatever extent you can, try to avoid drugs, because they can affect the baby. To lessen your reliance on medication you should rest as much as possible. Overexerting yourself makes your incision hurt more. Use hot-water bottles or a cold pack on the incision, change positions, and get comfortable by using pillows.

➤ *Postdelivery observation of the baby* usually means separating you and the baby: you may want to do everything you can to minimize it. Bonding immediately at birth is particularly meaningful for cesarean mothers and babies. Usually, the prerequisite for releasing you from the recovery area is that the anesthetic has worn off—this means you will be feeling pain, which will inhibit your first encounter with the baby if you cannot bond in the delivery room.

Some hospitals require that a cesarean baby go routinely to the intensive-care nursery (ICN) or the central nursery for a minimum number of hours or days, regardless of her condition. But a healthy baby is healthy no matter how she was born and many experts now believe that some alternative to this separation is necessary. Although the routine is to send the baby to the ICN or CN for a long observation, there is no reason the baby and mother cannot be watched together postpartum. If it isn't possible to keep a healthy baby with you, *make every possible attempt to have the baby released from the ICN to the central nursery or to your room* as soon as possible. Just having your baby in the ICN can make you feel she is ill or there is something wrong, which in most cases is *not* so.

If that doesn't work, you and your partner should visit the baby and *insist upon touching her*. As soon as you feel able to, you should arrange for the baby to room with you. The possible trauma and separation of a cesarean birth are something you have to work to overcome.

Vaginal Birth After Cesarean (VBAC)

In 1980 the National Institutes of Health released a report recommending vaginal birth after cesarean (VBAC) when appropriate. In an effort to reduce the rising number of cesarean births, the American College of Obstetricians and Gynecologists (ACOG) adopted new guidelines in 1988 to encourage attempts at vaginal births by women who had previously had cesareans. Repeat cesareans represent 25% of the recent increase in cesarean births. Data shows that 50–80% of women have successful vaginal births after a low-flap transverse incision (bikini cut).

➤ "*Once a C-section, always a C-section used to be the belief,*" but research has shown that a woman who's had a cesarean before doesn't necessarily have any higher risk in vaginal delivery. The ACOG changed its long-standing policy and declared that VBAC is perfectly safe for mother and fetus, even if the mother has had two or three cesareans, unless there is a medical indication for a repeat cesarean.

➤ *The basic rule of thumb* now is that the only reason for a repeat cesareans should be for a repeat of the *reason that the first cesarean was performed*. In other words, you won't need another cesarean if the first C-section was for reasons of the baby: he was breech or transverse, it was a multiple birth, or distress showed on the fetal monitor (unless of course the same conditions apply with the next birth). Nor will you need another cesarean if your first C-section was for placenta previa or abruptio, toxemia, or infection, and you have no history of surgery on your uterus other than the first cesarean.

ACOG GUIDELINES FOR VBAC

- There should be only one fetus, with an estimated weight of less than 4,000 gr.
- The previous cesarean should have been transverse: VBAC is not safe with a previous classical incision, but vertical incisions are rare, occurring in only 1% of cesareans.
- If your previous baby's head was too large for your pelvis, you can attempt labor this time if ultrasound shows that your pelvis is adequate for the head of the new baby. Studies show that subsequent trials of labor are successful for up to 70% of women who were originally given a C-section because of "failure to progress in labor." Remember that absolute cephalopelvic disproportion (the baby's head not fitting through your pelvis) is rare.
- There should be continuous electronic monitoring of fetal heart rate and uterine activity throughout labor.
- Staff and facilities should be able to perform an immediate cesarean if it becomes necessary.
- Blood of your type should be in the hospital blood bank and 24-hour blood-banking capabilities should be available. When you arrive for the delivery, your blood should be typed and screened for irregular antibodies.

ARE YOU CANDIDATE FOR VBAC?

➤ *The kind of incision on your previous C-section* is one determinant of whether you are a candidate for VBAC. If it was a bikini cut, then it's possible to try a vaginal delivery. A high "classical" incision (rarely used anymore except for emergency cesareans) would allow your uterus to rupture too easily. The incision on your skin may not parallel the internal incision on your uterus, so your doctor has to know how the previous surgery was done. If he or she wasn't the one to do it, your previous medical records are necessary.

➤ *Whether you're a candidate for VBAC* depends on whether you meet certain criteria. While every doctor and hospital will have individual guidelines for making that decision, the chart below outlines most criteria used to determine who can be considered for a vaginal delivery.

WHO IS A CANDIDATE FOR VBAC?

— Previous low transverse incision (bikini cut)
— Normal pregnancy
— Delivery within 12 to 24 hours after rupture of the membranes
— Willingness to avoid pain medications or use minimal amounts so that you have full feeling in case of pain due to rupture
— Avoidance of Pitocin to induce or augment labor; Pitocin (or other forms of oxytocin) to be used only in conjunction with an internal fetal monitor
— Understanding that general anesthetic may be used if a serious problem develops requiring an immediate cesarean

➤ *Previous abnormal labor* (which often results in a cesarean) should not disqualify you for VBAC. It doesn't mean you shouldn't try a vaginal delivery the next time around. The conditions causing the problem in labor do not necessarily repeat themselves. In fact, some physicians feel that there is less chance of uterine rupture when the previous C-section was performed because of abnormal labor. This is because the uterus had a good chance to stretch during the previous labor, permitting the incision to be placed lower, where it is least likely to rupture.

Cesarean birth is being performed for abnormal labor far more often than in the past. Cephalopelvic disproportion (CPD), prolonged labor, "failure to progress," arrested labor, uterine inertia, and prolonged second stage account for about one-third of the increase in the cesarean birth rate. Doctors don't wait as long as they did in the past before resorting to a C-section. This is because cesarean birth used to be viewed as a risk to be avoided, whereas today the thinking is that a cesarean is safer for the fetus than a complicated forceps delivery. Also, the medical-legal climate has doctors practicing "defensive medicine" for fear of being sued if the baby is compromised.

RISKS AND BENEFITS TO VBAC

➢ ***There are multiple benefits*** to VBAC. You eliminate operative and postoperative complications and postpartum pain, and have a shorter hospital stay (depending on your insurance situation this can reduce your financial costs). Infection rates in mothers after cesarean birth range from 10 to 65% and are much lower after vaginal delivery. Also, labor can be beneficial to the baby, readying her lungs for life outside the womb. After cesarean birth, the infant is usually taken to the nursery for observation, severely limiting the time parents can have with their newborn at that special moment.

    Finally, it can be psychologically important for you to have a vaginal birth. You may have really wanted natural childbirth before, and you may have felt like a failure after your cesarean. Also, your sense of control and participation in the birth are enhanced by attempting a vaginal delivery.

➢ ***The risk of VBAC is uterine rupture***, but this rarely happens. What "uterine rupture" actually refers to is any separation in the wall of the uterus. The most common ruptures are incomplete, which cause separations of the previous scar in the uterus. However, rupture is highly unlikely: the statistical risk of rupture is less than 1% for a woman who had a lower segment incision (bikini cut) and is undergoing a trial of labor.

    Massive uterine rupture, which is life-threatening, is extremely rare. The possibility of excessive strain on the uterus is feared only for those women who have weakened uteruses from many pregnancies and deliveries or who receive too much oxytocin during labor. Because of the potential risk of uterine rupture with the administration of oxytocin, some physicians choose not to use it to induce or augment labor in VBAC. However, several studies have shown that using oxytocin for women undergoing a trial of labor after a prior low transverse cesarean delivery carries no greater risk than using it to augment labor for women who haven't had previous cesareans.

➢ ***Finding a supportive doctor*** can be the most important element of VBAC. The best way to find one is by word of mouth: ask friends, ask childbirth educators, ask the OB/GYN department of your local hospital, contact local childbirth organizations, or find out if there are going to be childbirth workshops or conferences in your area.

➢ ***Accepting the realities of VBAC*** is important to the experience you will have. You're setting yourself up for disappointment if you expect a vaginal birth to make up for what may have been an unsatisfactory birth experience the first time. You might want to make a list of the things you liked and didn't like about your previous cesarean delivery and discuss how you want things to be different this time. If you and your mate can discuss these feelings and requests with your doctor, it gives you a chance to clarify what your priorities really are. If the physician has concerns about any of the items, listen and take this into account. You may have to be more realistic in the kind of birth experience you can expect with VBAC, and/or you and your doctor may be able to compromise so that you're both comfortable.

➤ **Making the decision is difficult**, and whatever you decide, you'll probably have moments of ambivalent feelings, wondering whether you've made the right choice. The important thing is to consider the option of VBAC. You may decide after talking to even the most open-minded and supportive doctor that you want a repeat cesarean anyway. You may want the convenience of a scheduled birth to arrange child care and time off from work or other responsibilities. You may feel that a vaginal birth is too frightening a prospect for you, or that you have specific medical problems that make it an unacceptable risk for you. What it comes right down to is this: trust your instincts. The most valid factor in making a decision is to think it through with your partner and respect your own feelings about what is best for you and your baby.

➤ **What if you have another cesarean?** If your vaginal birth doesn't work out, will you be devastated and hurt? Or will you be disappointed but glad you made an attempt at labor? Most couples are able to accept a disappointing outcome of VBAC if they are well-informed and prepared before labor and have established a good line of communication with their physician. Be sure that your doctor understands that you and your mate want to be active participants in the management of the VBAC and that you want to be kept informed about the options available as your birth situation unfolds.

If a couple participates in the decision-making process throughout VBAC, it can be a positive experience even if it results in another cesarean. A woman's feelings of failure—that she "could" or "should" have done more—can come from the feeling that the labor was out of her control and she had no say in what was being done to her and her baby. Even if the outcome is disappointing, by being involved you'll know you did the best thing for your baby and yourself under the circumstances.

THE FIRST DAYS AFTER CESAREAN

➤ **The IV is kept in after surgery** depending on your condition usually for 24 to 48 hours. The intravenous solution keeps down postoperative fever, which is especially important if you're nursing.
➤ **The catheter that emptied your bladder** during the surgery will be removed within 24 hours, but you may find it hard to

urinate afterward. It is important to drink plenty of fluids. This keeps you from becoming dehydrated, encourages urination, and may shorten the length of time you have to stay on IV fluids. The catheter may increase your chances of getting a urinary tract infection and/or urethral irritation. If you develop any of the symptoms of such problems, notify your doctor.

➤ *Bowel movements may be difficult* following your operation. The operation itself, plus your postoperative limited diet and activity, may contribute to sluggish bowels or constipation. Straining in an effort to have a bowel movement is nearly impossible after you've had an abdominal incision. It is important to do everything possible to get your bowels moving and keep your stool soft. The first few postoperative days you'll be put on a liquid or very soft diet. Drink plenty of fluids, eat roughage and whole-grain cereals and bread as soon as you're able. Get on your feet and move around. Your doctor may prescribe a stool softener, which is a capsule that you swallow, to ease your first bowel movement.

➤ *Gas and gas pains* are a sign that your intestines are beginning to function again, which will probably be about the third day after the operation. Although you may be upset by these sharp pains, your doctor will view them as a good sign that your body is recovering from the surgery. The fact that gas is being moved down the intestinal tract is a good sign there's no infection causing intestinal difficulties.

Getting up and moving around is the best prevention and cure for gas. Rolling from side to side in your bed and changing positions will also help your body get rid of the gas. Sleeping on your stomach may help, although getting into that position may be uncomfortable.

Try placing the baby on your upper abdomen when you give her a bottle, or put her on a pillow on your stomach if you are breast-feeding. In both cases the baby's weight will tend to push the gas down and bring you relief.

There are certain foods and drinks you should avoid until at least 10 days after the cesarean. Carbonated drinks and bubbly water can make gas pains worse. Some women find that apple juice, which is frequently given to postoperative patients in the hospital, can cause gas. The worst offenders for causing intestinal gas are leafy green vegetables and beans of any kind. Avoid these until your body is functioning normally or you may feel like you're going to explode!

➤ *Pain in your shoulder(s)* may occur due to blood and air that collects under your diaphragm and irritates, pressing on the nerves that go to your shoulders. This shouldn't last very long.

➤ *Medication can be tailored to* breast-feeding—some drugs will not harm the baby as much and are suited for nursing (see Chapter 12). The small amount of colostrum in your breasts the first few days won't contain enough medication to pass on to the baby. However, when the painkillers wear off the pain may seem worse: try to take as little medication as you can. Some doctors routinely prescribe tranquilizers in addition to pain medication. It is better not to have your perceptions and emotions blunted after birth. Be sure to ask what drugs you are being given and why.

➤ *Walk around as soon as you can.* This will get your body systems like digestion and elimination working and start you on the road to feeling well. Walking may be quite painful at first: try taking short walks with tiny steps. Your lower abdomen will probably feel bruised and tender, as if you've been beaten up. Try to stand upright, although your instinct will probably be to hunch over like an old lady because the incision will feel like it's pulling. Don't worry: the stitches will not come out.

➤ *A belly binder is a large bandage* used by some hospitals to support your stomach after the operation. It may be uncomfortable, in which case you should ask to have it removed.

➤ *Abdominal discomfort will lessen* within 7 to 10 days. On the third day after surgery the intestinal tract begins to function normally again, and sharp gas pains may occur when you sneeze, cough, laugh, or hiccup. The involuntary movement of your abdominal muscles may hurt. Hold your hands pressed against the incision or press a pillow against it when you laugh or cough.

➤ *Lochia is the same as after a vaginal delivery*—it is a menstrual-like flow of the uterine lining that lasts for a week or two after delivery. If you are given a sanitary napkin with a belt, the metal clasp may irritate your incision. You should try beltless napkins that attach to your underpants or pin the napkin to your underpants with safety pins.

➤ *Look at your incision before leaving the hospital* in case you have any concerns. Have your partner look at it, too. The scar can be itchy, numb, it may pull or may ooze a little—all this is common and not a cause for alarm. If the stitches are nonabsorbable, they will be removed about a week after surgery. The procedure is uncomfortable, but there is no reason to fear that it will be very painful.

The incision bandage is usually removed a day or two postpartum. The incision can hurt a bit more afterwards because it has no support. Your clothes can rub your stitches or clamps, if you don't have the absorbable kind of stitches.

➤ *The breathing exercise to clear your lungs* should start as soon as possible after the operation. Place a pillow over the incision: breathe deeply in, exhale, breathe deeply in and hold for 5 to 10 counts, then exhale and breathe in and out normally.

➤ *Modified rooming-in might be the best solution if* you are feeling less than terrific and need to rest. A woman who has had a cesarean may have a hard time focusing on the newborn's needs instead of her own real and pressing needs. You should ask for lessons in infant care from the nurses and get accustomed to the baby as soon as you can.

➢ **Nursing may be uncomfortable at first**—putting a pillow over your abdomen may be a solution. Remind the staff that you are breast-feeding and don't want the baby to be given bottles of glucose water or formula. Your baby may be sleepy from the effects of general anesthesia if that's how you were medicated for the delivery. The baby may have been placed in the intensive care nursery for observation, since cesarean babies have more respiratory problems—both these factors may interfere with initiating successful breast-feeding. You may have to be more patient than a woman who had a vaginal delivery. Also, don't forget that all medications enter your breast milk; see the chart on page 564. If you're taking pain medication, realize that it reaches the baby and may affect nursing.

➢ **Emotions in the first days can be depressed**—you may feel tearful, cheated, or like a failure. Feelings are not right or wrong—they just *are*. Try writing your feelings down. Your mate may feel he was thrust out of the picture by the cesarean and may feel cheated himself. You two must *talk to each other* in order to overcome the feelings and recognize that you aren't alone—you're going through it all together.

MAKING THE ADJUSTMENT AT HOME IS ESSENTIAL

➢ **Help at home is essential.** Unless your partner is already a house-husband he cannot handle the household alone. A well-meaning man may try to stay home and handle everything, but he will exhaust himself and you'll probably feel obliged to get up and help him. That is the last thing you should do. You'll recover more quickly and fully if you take it extremely easy. Yet taking care of you postoperatively and taking care of a new baby and a house is a *big job*. If you have parents or in-laws who are willing and able to help out, that's great—if not, hiring someone for the first week or two would make a great gift from the new grandparents if you can't afford it.

Do not be a stoic—it will needlessly prolong your convalescence. Hired help might be less taxing emotionally than friends or relatives, because if you are paying someone, you won't feel it's an imposition or that you have to help them.

➢ **Avoid stair-climbing for the first week or two** if at all possible. Your abdominal muscles are healing; climbing stairs puts a strain on them that may cause you pain afterward, tire you out, and otherwise hamper your recovery.

➢ **Avoid lifting until about fifteen days** after surgery, when the incision heals and becomes strong. This even means lifting the baby in the first postpartum days. Have someone hand the baby to you.

➤ *Medication for the first week at home* will probably be the same kind you used during the end of your hospital stay, if you were taking painkillers then. Beware of codeine-based drugs, which are constipating.

➤ *Wear a lightweight girdle* (a stretchy and inexpensive Lycra-Spandex type) if you get the unpleasant sensation that your belly is about to fall out. The girdle will give you support until your stomach muscles tighten up again.

➤ *Try never to be left alone, at least for the first week*. It is important to have someone around at all times, if only to lift the baby and hand him to you. You shouldn't lift anything after abdominal surgery. Guests are going to tire you out a lot the first week, but you can ask *certain* friends and relatives to come be with you—then you won't feel helpless or that you have to get up and do things you aren't ready for.

➤ *Siblings may be suffering* from a feeling of jealousy and abandonment since you've been away a week or so. One good way to overcome those feelings without tiring yourself is to let the older child come into bed with you and read, draw, or cuddle.

➤ *The feeling of failure* can be overwhelming for some time after you get home. Some women feel incomplete as a result of having had a cesarean and some become obsessed with the feeling of failure. You can have periods of nonstop crying and serious depression. If this happens, seek professional help—these feelings can be detrimental to your newly forming relationship with the baby.

SEX AFTER CESAREAN

➤ *The obstetrician usually gives the okay* for you to resume sex after your six-week postsurgery checkup. However, your mate may still be fearful of hurting you. Let him talk to the doctor to get reassurance.

➤ *Your vagina probably won't lubricate* as quickly as in pre-birth days no matter how much foreplay you have. K-Y lubricating jelly can solve this problem until your hormones are back to their previous levels.

➤ *Sex is something you probably won't be in the mood for* right away. The sheer physical exhaustion and hormonal changes after birth may cause the lack of interest. Some women say it took 6 to 9 months for their previous level of sexual interest to return (see Chapter 8 on sex).

➤ *The man-on-top position may be uncomfortable*. Experiment with other positions for lovemaking that don't put a strain on the incision, which can still be tender.

➤ **You may be feeling unattractive**, which would make you shy away from sex. Your new scar and bulging stomach may make you feel unsexy. Start exercises to get back in shape as soon as you can both for your health and self-image.

Premature Labor and Delivery

Premature labor is calculated on the baby's birth weight rather than the duration of pregnancy because the latter is so difficult to determine with exactitude. When a newborn weighs less than 5½ pounds (2,500 grams), it is considered to be a premature infant. Ordinarily a 5½-pound baby is about four weeks from its expected delivery date and at that weight is at greater risk. There is a critical difference in the final two or three weeks of gestation for fetal development, particularly of the lungs.

Some causes of prematurity are multiple birth, toxemia, placenta previa, premature separation of the placenta, or maternal illness with severe infection, such as pneumonia or untreated syphilis. But in most cases there is no obvious reason: in an apparently normal pregnancy, labor begins or the membranes rupture between 20 and 36 weeks.

When labor starts, there is nothing that will definitely stop it, but doctors can make an attempt with medication. An intravenous alcohol solution given by a continuous-drip technique over several hours may inhibit labor by blocking the release of oxytocin. The alcohol acts on the pituitary gland by preventing the discharge of the chemical hormone that stimulates uterine contractions. In some instances when the alcohol is stopped it has shut off the trigger mechanism that initiated labor. The side effects of IV alcohol drip can include a headache and nausea. Alcohol can also have an effect when taken by mouth—a glass of wine or a mixed drink can stop the contractions of prodromal labor (see page 364).

Several other drugs to stop premature labor have had varying degrees of success. However, bed rest may accomplish as much as any drug. If the membranes ruptured prematurely but contractions do not begin, a woman may be put flat in bed in the hospital (perhaps on antibiotics to guard against the infection that can develop with ruptured membranes). The hope is that labor will not begin for the crucial final weeks of pregnancy.

➤ **Get to the nearest large medical center** if you do go into labor prematurely. If your labor begins six weeks early, a community hospital is most likely going to be inadequate to meet your premature baby's needs. Have your partner (or the police) rush you to the nearest perinatal center where there are specialists and facilities intended for the care of premature infants. Premies' first hours are crucial, and if they are born in a hospital with a neonatal intensive care unit, they generally do better.

Hospital Equipment for Premies

CPAP (continuous positive airway pressure). A tube is inserted into the baby's windpipe, or a pressurized hood is fitted around his head, so that a continuous supply of low-pressure air is directed to the sacs of the immature lungs, preventing their collapse.

BILIRUBIN lights detoxify the jaundice that often affects premies.

SKIN SENSORS monitor oxygen and other blood gases.

BLOOD ANALYSIS is done with several drops pricked from the newborn's heel or from a plastic tube inserted into the umbilicus and left there (which eliminates the need to keep pricking the baby). Blood sugar, blood acidity, and blood gases are measured and analyzed for any changes.

AN ELECTRONIC THERMOMETER is taped to the baby's skin to insure that his temperature remains constant.

AN INFUSION PUMP is a tiny tube inserted into the umbilical cord to deliver intravenous fluids at a preset rate to the baby's bloodstream.

A NASOGASTRIC FEEDING TUBE is inserted into the baby's nose, and breast milk or formula is fed through it if the baby is not strong enough to suck.

ALARMS SOUND if breathing or other life signs become too fast or slow. Neonatal intensive care specialists are in constant attendance to correct any such problems.

➤ *The survival rate of premies* depends on how early they are born. A premie is technically any baby born more than three weeks early. The most troubled babies are those born at the current limit of viability: about 24 weeks (6 months) old. At this point, a baby's lungs have developed to the point where he can breathe with the help of a machine called a ventilator. Before 23 or 24 weeks the lungs are so rudimentary that the infants have virtually no chance of survival. Infants have been known to survive at a weight of about 500 grams or one pound; infants weighing less than two pounds currently have about a 70% chance of survival. Larger babies do better: 90% of infants weighing from two to three pounds survive. Sex and race are important factors. Statistically, black girls seem to do the best, while white boys are the least likely to survive.

➤ *Lung failure used to be* a major reason that premature babies died. A substance known as surfactant provides surface tension in the air sacs of the lungs. Natural surfactant does not develop until 35 weeks into the pregnancy, so it has not developed in many premies: without it, the tiny air sacs collapse and stick together with every breath, causing respiratory distress.

The newborn's tiny lungs have to be expanded and contracted mechanically by a ventilator. With the increased use of this ventilator, more babies are surviving. However, there are side effects. Some infants' fragile lungs are damaged by the ventilator and they develop chronic lung disease. Others become ventilator dependent. Researchers are working on methods of injecting natural or artificial surfactant into the babies' lungs at birth to aid pulmonary functioning.

GROWTH PATTERNS OF PREMIES

24 WEEKS
Height: 13 inches
Weight: 1¼ pounds
Lungs have developed just enough for mechanical ventilation. All babies have a dark red appearance because skin pigmentation has not begun. Skin is unable to help regulate body temperature or ward off infection. Eyes are often fused shut, earlobes are just skin flaps. Baby has a 5 to 20% chance of survival outside the womb.

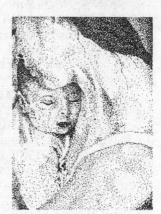

29 WEEKS
Height: 14½ inches
Weight: 2½ pounds
Lungs have developed enough to increase chance of survival outside womb to 90 to 95%. Baby takes a more rounded, plump appearance because fat layer is developing. Pigmentation is present. Eyes partly open. Baby can follow objects with his eyes and has longer periods of alertness. Some babies begin to suck.

35 WEEKS
Height: 18½ inches
Weight: 5½ pounds
Baby sees almost as well as a full-term baby and shows a preference for a human face. Testicles in the male have descended. Baby can coordinate sucking, breathing, and swallowing to allow nipple feeding. Skin is smooth because there is a substantial fat layer. Muscle tone is developed.

40 WEEKS
Height: 20 inches
Weight: 7 pounds
Baby is plump and fully developed. Baby has received iron, calcium, vitamins and immunities against infection from her mother.

The Psychological Aspects of Premature Delivery

A premature delivery robs you and your mate of the final weeks of physical and psychological preparation for the new baby. Aside from the physical risks to a premie, there is also a tremendous psychological impact on the parents. In order to understand and cope with those feelings it is necessary to know what they are.

BASIC PSYCHOLOGICAL STEPS

— *The mother prepares herself for the possible loss* of an infant whose life is in jeopardy.
— *She must face and acknowledge her failure* to deliver a normal, full-term baby.
— *She must then reorient her perspective* from preparing herself for a potential loss to viewing the situation with hope and anticipation.
— *She must learn the premie's special needs* and growth patterns, which will eventually become normal.

ANXIETY

— *Fear is probably the primary emotion* you will feel. Most premature babies do survive, but pessimistic remarks by medical caretakers can deeply affect you. If you prepare yourself for losing the baby, it can interfere with your bonding process with the infant. You might repress the natural bonding to the baby because you fear she will die. This can cause *years* of anxiety; you may remain unconvinced for a long time that all is well with your child.
— *Involve your partner in the situation* as much as possible. Including him in assessments of your baby's condition will lessen his anxiety and give you support at the same time.
— *Try to understand that if the doctor says*, "Your baby may not live," he or she may not recognize the irreversible psychological damage to you. Doctors are accustomed to dealing with life-and-death situations and discussing them in a somewhat casual way. A doctor may not recognize that new parents are unable to hear certain comments without jumping to unwarranted conclusions. For example, some doctors might mention the general possibility of brain damage or eye problems with premies. However, it is not possible to tell what the outcome for *your* baby will be at such an early age, and you might be upset unnecessarily by such discussions.

A doctor should certainly not withhold information or lie to parents, but should tell them negative information only where it can be accurately predicted (such as with Down's syndrome). If your doctor is having such theoretical conversations with you, ask the actual odds of such an outcome for your baby. You may find that the risk is actually quite small.

— *Rebel against rigid visiting hours*. The visiting hours for fathers are often shortened with a premie, but this is the time

when *you need your mate the most*. Do whatever you have to in order to have as much time together as possible—whether it means getting special permission from the hospital administration or just ignoring the rigid visiting hours.
— ***Consider moving to a different part*** of the hospital, or at least getting a private room, so that you are not subjected to the routine care of full-term babies. It is hard enough to deal with the complex emotions of a premature delivery without having other mothers and babies right under your nose. You will probably have an empty feeling: your uterus is empty, but you have no baby to hold in your room. It can only hurt more to be around full-term babies and their mothers.

GUILT

Guilt can be a strong feeling: a premature delivery can make you feel like a failure and be a blow to your self-esteem. You may perceive it as a comment on your "inferiority" and feel guilty that it is your "fault." These feelings are irrational, but they are common feelings nevertheless. Unless you face these feelings, they can affect your relationship with the child. This underlying feeling of your own "badness" translates to your being an "unfit mother," with the net result of distancing you from the child.

It is important to *verbalize* these feelings. Talk to your partner. Talk with sympathetic doctors, midwives, or nurses. Group sessions with other parents of premies can be helpful. Wrestle with the guilt you are feeling because of the prematurity: withdrawing makes it even harder to adjust.

THE SHOCK OF SEEING A PREMIE

You should have a chair nearby the first time you see your baby in the neonatal intensive care nursery in case you feel faint. It helps to see pictures of premies ahead of time and get a verbal description of the equipment that will be attached to your baby. This will lessen the discrepancy—and therefore the shock—between what you dreamed of (a chubby "Gerber" baby) and what you will see.

A premie bears little resemblance to a full-term newborn. Earlobes are often just skin flaps at the sides of their heads and their eyes maybe fused shut. Skin is a dusty red color no matter what race the baby is: normal pigmentation comes about a month later. The premies can't control their body temperature; their skin is like gelatin, not a good barrier to infection or water loss. Very premature babies are so delicate that their brittle bones can break easily: the amount of calcium a full-term baby naturally gets from her mother cannot be reproduced in the intensive care nursery. The chart "Growth Patterns of Premies" on page 452 can give you some idea of what you might expect your premature infant to look like.

You may feel frightened and repulsed by the sight of your baby. Those feelings toward your own child may make you feel guilty unless you know they are normal reactions. The baby will most likely be scrawny and naked with tubes coming out of her nose and/or umbilical cord, wires attached to her chest, labored breathing, ominous-looking equipment like a plastic hood around her head, flashing and beeping machines, and perhaps bandages over her eyes. She will hardly resemble the cuddly pink infant you had fantasized snuggling in your arms! The sight of all this equipment may not only turn you off but will probably also increase the anxiety you've already been feeling. Ask the nurse assigned to your baby to explain all the contraptions. It will help you feel less intimidated while appreciating the good they are doing for your baby.

PROBLEMS FEELING CLOSE TO THE BABY

— *Your relationship to the baby will be influenced by your "coping attitude."* It is better to be worried, to ask questions, or to *grapple* with your feelings than to repress them. Your coping behavior can be measured by the presence of four elements: high anxiety, seeking information, maternal feelings (even before seeing or holding the baby), and support from your mate. If you are experiencing these feelings, it is a good sign of effective coping.

— *Feeling that the baby belongs to the hospital*, that the staff and machines control the baby, is common. Premie mothers and fathers often don't think of the baby as "theirs" until they get her home, *but that is too long to delay your bonding*. There is a tendency, especially in the medically overwhelming setting of the intensive care nursery, to feel inferior to the nurses. You may feel "bad" or "inadequate"; nurses should encourage your participation in diapering and other tasks.

— *Involvement will overcome these feelings*. Get confidence and lessons from the nurses in holding, feeding, and diapering your baby. Participate where possible and make a special effort to establish eye-to-eye contact with the baby—this gives you reinforcing feedback and is fundamental to maternal-infant bonding.

— *Breast-feeding is excellent* because it gives you a chance to make a tangible contribution. If the baby is not yet strong enough to suck, you can express breast milk with a pump and with the help of a nurse, and it can be fed to the baby through the nasogastric tube. When the baby gets stronger you can actually breast-feed. Breast milk can reduce infections and other complications, which is particularly important for a premie. (See page 543 of the breast-feeding section for important information about the special qualities of breast milk for premature babies.)

— *The longer a woman delays in becoming attached* to a premie, the harder it will be. It is *very serious* if a woman does not visit the nursery or ask about her baby. Delay in naming the baby and referring to him as "it" can also indicate a critical problem.

— ***Maternal-infant bonding is vital for premies*** and their mothers. Studies have shown that simply by touching and stroking a premie, a mother can improve the infant's breathing, physical development, weight gain, and relaxation. Hospitals that recognize this benefit allow a mother to hold her baby while he is being fed through a nasogastric tube. If you hold the baby during feeding, he relaxes and digests more easily. You should bottle-feed the baby only if a doctor or nurse has successfully bottle-fed the child several times already—it can be devastating to your self-esteem about mothering if it does not go smoothly.

The premie's development is improved by close contact with you. He does better if the mother feeds and cares for him through the incubator. If a baby is touched, rocked, and fondled daily, he develops better and more quickly—and since there is a personnel shortage in any hospital, you should get into the intensive care nursery as much as possible.

A premie has only short periods of wakefulness, so it can be discouraging for you. If the baby is usually asleep, you will need encouragement from the staff and your partner.

Postterm (Postmature) Pregnancy

A pregnancy prolonged past the week 42 is considered postterm. In many cases the due date has been miscalculated. One reason for error in calculating postmaturity is that ovulation took place several weeks later than the usual fourteenth day of the cycle—impregnation therefore did not take place until 40 or 50 days after the onset of the last period. The other reason is that there has been an error in menstrual dates.

In some cases, however, a pregnancy actually does go beyond the usual 40 weeks. After 280 days in utero a baby gains little weight. In fact, he may lose weight: a typical postmature baby is thin, scrawny, and old looking, with loose, baggy skin, long nails, an abundance of scalp hair, and a very alert look. He will gain back the weight after birth.

There are several tests which can be done (amniocentesis, ultrasound, OCT, ect.) to determine whether a baby is postmature. If these tests are not normal—if an OCT is positive or meconium is present in the amniotic fluid—delivery should be immediate. The reason to determine whether a baby is postterm (and if so, to deliver him immediately) is because there is a risk of fetal distress for postterm babies during labor. One solution might be to allow such a fetus to go into labor, then use fetal monitoring with particular care to watch for distress.

Your estriol level is another indicator of whether the baby is postmature. Estriol is a hormone created by the baby's system and the placenta, which convert it from certain substances excreted by your body. The amount of estriol in your urine can be measured, giving an indication of the condition of the baby and the placenta. If the estriol level is low, or not increasing as it normally does, this indicates that the baby needs to be delivered.

Cervical ripening by self-stimulation of nipples can be done at term. Some doctors recommend it for low-risk patients, as it may shorten labor and prevent the complications of postmaturity. The woman is instructed to stimulate her nipples until they are erect for one hour, three times a day for two days. **WARNING:** THIS SHOULD ONLY BE ATTEMPTED UNDER A DOCTOR'S INSTRUCTIONS.

Prostaglandin gels are used to stimulate prostaglandin production, which helps to thin the cervix in preparation for induction of labor.

Breech Presentation

In over 96% of births the baby is in a cephalic (fetal head leading) presentation; in 3% of cases the baby is in breech position (buttocks lead). In less than 1% of pregnancies, a baby is in some other unusual position. There are several types of breech presentations: *complete* (the baby is cross-legged in the bottom of the uterus): *frank* (his legs are straight up with his feet near his face); *footling* (a rare position in which one foot or both come down first); and *knee* (an even more rare occurrence with the knee presenting).

Other positions can cause complications. *Posterior vertex* (the baby faces your abdomen on his way down the birth canal; normally he would face your tailbone) can cause painful back labor. If the baby does not turn before he is born, the doctor may have to rotate his head with forceps. There are also two very rare versions of the cephalic position: *face* or *brow* presentation. The fetus's head, instead of being flexed down chin on chest, is extended so that he delivers with his face presenting rather than the top of his head. His features may appear swollen with contusions, as if he's been in a fight, but this will disappear within 48 hours. The final unusual position is *transverse lie*: the baby is lying sideways in your uterus, and (unless he can be manipulated into a cephalic position) he will have to be delivered by cesarean.

Causes of Breech Presentation

- A small or premature baby
- A large baby who may not have enough room to settle head-down into your pelvis
- Excess amniotic fluid, which allows the baby to float around instead of engaging in your pelvis
- Multiple pregnancy
- Placenta previa

- Contracted pelvis
- Uterine tumors
- A hydrocephalic baby with water on the brain, making the head oversize

The Dangers of a Breech Presentation

Because there are risks in a breech presentation, the current medical practice is to deliver all breeches by cesarean section. There are *some* situations in which *some* doctors will attempt a vaginal delivery (see below), but generally the dangers outweigh the benefits of a normal delivery.

> ➤ *Labor can be longer or simply not progress* because the buttocks are not as good a wedge to dilate your cervix as the head would be. The birth canal cannot be as effectively molded open. Also, when the head exits last it has no time to be molded in the birth canal and may not be able to descend all the way out.
> ➤ *The after-coming head is usually larger* than any other part of the baby that has come down first. Therefore, especially with premies or small babies, the cervix does not need to dilate fully because the body is small enough to get through. But the cervix may not have opened enough to allow the head to pass through, *or* the cervix may close around the baby's neck after the shoulders have slipped through.
> ➤ *Prolapse of the cord* occurs in 5% of breech births. This is ten times the normal frequency of this dangerous complication in which the umbilical cord comes down before anything else. With prolapse the cord can be compressed, cutting off the baby's blood supply. It necessitates an immediate cesarean section.
> ➤ *The cord can be compressed* in its passage through the pelvis, cutting off the baby's oxygen supply.
> ➤ *Fractures, dislocations, and nerve damage* are all more common in vaginal breech deliveries because of the complications in getting out.

Vaginal Delivery with a Breech Presentation

If you are aware of the potential complications in a breech delivered "from below," yet a vaginal delivery matters a great deal to you, seek out a doctor who will try it. (This does not mean seeking out a doctor who will deliver a breech vaginally because she or he does not respect the potential dangers, or who has not had experience but needs your business.) It is essential that you find a doctor who will do every possible examination ahead of time and knows what to do in the possible event that labor does not progress normally.

You should also be aware that you may be disappointed if you want a vaginal delivery because you want a "natural, normal birth." A vaginal delivery of a breech calls for high-risk management. If you meet the requirements for a vaginal delivery, you will have to be closely watched on a fetal monitor. The prevailing attitude will be "poised for emergency." You might even be required to go through labor and delivery in the cesarean section room with an anesthesiologist in attendance so that surgery can be done immediately if it becomes necessary. There are very real potential dangers and the atmosphere may be tense.

In a breech delivered vaginally the baby's buttocks and genitals are often swollen and discolored. They can be black-and-blue because they came down first and were battered against your cervix and the walls of the birth canal. This clears up quickly and causes no permanent damage.

Vaginal delivery of a term breech can be an acceptable choice for delivery when the following conditions are present: (1) anticipated fetal weight of less than 8 pounds, (2) normal pelvic dimensions and architecture, (3) frank breech presentation without a hyperextended head, and (4) delivery to be conducted by a physician experienced in vaginal breech delivery.

> ➤ *Before you can attempt a vaginal delivery,* the doctor will want to know whether your pelvic structure will allow the baby's head through. What they want to learn beforehand is whether there is cephalopelvic disproportion—whether, given the baby's size and position, and given the shape and size of your pelvis, there may not be room for the baby's head to fit through. Ultrasound can be used to get a measurement of the baby's head size (her "biparietal diameter"). The problem with a breech is that this disproportion may not be discovered until after the baby is born. If you have what is known medically as an "inadequate pelvis" (a rather insulting term for it!) or if the baby's head is not well flexed (with the chin up rather than resting down on her chest), a vaginal delivery would not be safe.
> ➤ *The baby's weight should not be less than 5 pounds or more than 8 pounds*. A baby over 8 pounds is likely to have a large head that may not be able to descend, while a small baby's body could slip through a partially dilated cervix, which may then close around her neck. One reason that routine C-sectioning is done on breeches is that it isn't possible to accurately predict a baby's weight ahead of time.
> ➤ *Once you are in labor if there is any fetal distress* or labor does not progress well the doctor will undoubtedly perform a cesarean. It is thought that a labor lasting longer than 16 to 18 hours may be risky for you or the baby. There may be a halt in the progress of labor for any of the reasons already mentioned— the baby is "hung up" and cannot descend. Fetal distress can be caused by this lack of progress or problems with the umbilical cord. Meconium (a dark, tarry substance from the fetus's large

intestine) may be expelled after your membranes rupture. When a baby is not receiving enough oxygen (is "in distress"), his anal sphincter relaxes and passes meconium, which he can swallow. More meconium will be expelled with each contraction. If you are not yet in the hospital when this happens, wear a sanitary pad or a clean cloth and report it to the doctor *immediately*.

➤ *Gravity is the greatest helper in labor in breech* and posterior presentations. You should be sitting upright as much as possible. If you can do it, sit bolt upright with your knees spread wide and the soles of your feet together to aid in the baby's descent. In home deliveries where vaginal delivery of a breech is attempted (which is not a wise idea), they often use a hands-and-knees position so that gravity helps pull the baby out.

➤ *Piper forceps* are a special kind of gentle forceps used only for delivering breech babies. They are not used to pull the baby out but only to keep his head flexed down.

➤ *It's possible to turn the baby out of a breech position before labor.* If it is successful, you will be able to have a normal delivery rather than a C-section or a high-risk vaginal delivery.

➤ *The doctor can try to rotate* the baby from the outside. During late pregnancy or early labor a doctor can try to convert a breech to a head presentation by grasping the fetus externally through your abdominal wall and turning her 180 degrees by gradually pushing the buttocks to one side with one hand and the head and shoulders to the opposite side. Although this external manipulation can turn the baby, she will often revert right back to the breech position as soon as the doctor releases her!

➤ *The tilt posture* has been successful for some women with breech babies. It is an exercise you can start around the thirtieth week of pregnancy and continue for at least four to six weeks. If you know in advance that your baby is breech, you lie on your back on the floor with your pelvis raised to a level 9 to 12 inches off the floor. Put three large pillows under your buttocks. Your knees should be bent and your feet flat on the floor—the position is awkward. If it's not very comfortable, you're doing it right! Do this twice a day on an empty stomach; stay in the position for 10 minutes each time. Many babies have been encouraged to shift to a head presentation by this method.

Twins

Multiple births, of which twins are the most common, are included as a "complication of pregnancy" because they pose increased risks.

➤ **Identical twins (monozygotic)** are the result of one egg being fertilized by one sperm. The germ plasm of the two offspring is identical: they are of the same sex and exactly alike in skin, hair, and eye color. Identical twins are much less common.

➤ **Fraternal twins (dizygotic)** are the result of two different eggs fertilized by two different spermatozoa. The eggs may be from the same ovary or opposite ovaries. If twins are a boy and a girl, if their blood groups differ even slightly, and/or if they are nonidentical, they must be from two different eggs. Fraternal twins each have a separate placenta, or there are three or four membranes in the partition wall of a single placenta rather than the usual two membranes. Even if twins are the same sex, they are most likely fraternal and bear no greater resemblance to each other than regular siblings.

➤ **There's a greater chance of premature labor** with twins, and all premature babies are at greater risk for a variety of complications. If you are carrying twins, you should avoid physical strain and if possible stop working at 24 weeks instead of the usual 34 weeks. You should also give up traveling at around 24 weeks, to be on the safe side. Some doctors recommend giving up sexual intercourse during the last three months of pregnancy because of the possibility of a prematurely dilated cervix or the early onset of labor.

➤ **There is an increased risk of toxemia** in a multiple pregnancy. Be sure you eat extremely well with a lot of high-quality protein, take long afternoon rest periods, and increase the number of prenatal visits to the doctor or midwife.

➤ **There's a greater risk of losing twins** because so often they weigh less than 4½ pounds—any baby with low birth weight has a higher mortality rate and possibility of complications. Twin babies are sharing nutrition, oxygen, and uterine space, so they're often premature or low birth weight.

➤ **A greater proportion of sluggish labors** occurs with twins than with single births. There is an increased incidence of uterine inertia and poor, inadequate contractions. These problems are all probably due to the uterus being overdistended during pregnancy. The labor and delivery for twins is usually shorter than for single births because the cervix is often partially dilated before labor begins and the babies are usually smaller.

➤ **Spontaneous labor is preferable with twins**. Medications are especially dangerous to multiple births, as they are a risk to any fetus. This decreases the chance of blood loss and the babies, which are usually smaller than average, are safer without chemicals that can interfere with their breathing. It is important that you know how to push effectively because the uterine walls have been stretched thinner so the contractions may not be as effective. Pushing properly will make the births easier on you and the babies.

➤ *It is common to have a cord prolapse* with multiple births—the cord descends before anything else, potentially cutting off the babies' blood supply. This makes a cesarean necessary.

➤ *Unusual presentations* of the babies are common. There are many combinations of fetal positions. One baby vertex (head first) and the second baby breech is the most common presentation, followed by both babies in a head-first position. Five to ten minutes are allowed to elapse before delivery of the second twin. The membranes usually have to be ruptured around the second baby, which is usually smaller. The doctor determines the presenting part and, if necessary, manipulates him to a better position by reaching up into your uterus and turning the baby.

➤ *The discomforts of pregnancy are doubled*. Breathlessness, varicose veins, hemorrhoids, insomnia, and edema can all be twice as bad as in a single pregnancy. The twins take up more room and demand more from your circulatory system, which can increase minor discomforts.

➤ *The likelihood of producing twins* is a hereditary tendency. If multiple births are passed on in a family, it affects both men and women, and such families have several instances of twins on almost every branch of their family trees, not just an occasional pair. This tendency to twinning does not skip generations—if it is true of your family, then it will be expressed in succeeding generations.

Twins happen one in 86 births. Women over 35 are three times more likely to have twins than a woman under 20. Black women are more likely to produce them than Caucasians, and Caucasians are more likely to have twins than Asians. A woman who has already had a pair of twins is more likely to have twins again than a woman who has had a single birth. It should also be noted that even with all the sophisticated tests available it is not uncommon for twins to remain undiagnosed and come as a surprise to everyone!

More twins will be born in the U.S. than ever before: more women are having babies at a later age, when the odds of giving birth to twins rises. The increased use of fertility drugs and in-vitro fertilization also increases the chances of multiple births. Women who become pregnant soon after going off birth-control pills also have a higher chance of bearing twins.

➤ *Twins can present health problems*. Half of all twins arrive prematurely (on the average four weeks early) and the greatest risk for these children is underdeveloped lungs. They may also have less mature nervous systems and be more likely to have ruptured blood vessels in the brain. The risk to the mother carrying twins is increased incidence of anemia, high blood pressure, and hemorrhage after delivery. Birth itself can be more complicated, and as a result, about half of all twins are delivered by cesarean section (as compared to 20% of all births).

Twins may not reach all the developmental stages "on time" because they are premature, but this is ordinarily only a temporary delay. By the time they are three years old, premature babies have generally caught up with other children in physical and mental development.

➤ **Twins can cause stress in a relationship** because of the added pressure they put on a marriage. There is the financial burden of having to provide two of everything at once. This stress on the family puts twins at greater risk of being abused children. There is also a higher rate of postpartum depression in the mothers of twins because of the exhaustion. However, if a couple is aware of these potential problems it can go a long way toward lessening the stress on the marriage.

Polyhydramnios

This is a complication of pregnancy in which you have too much amniotic fluid. Normally there is approximately one liter (slightly over one quart) of fluid—if there is more than about two quarts it is considered polyhydramnios. The condition is often associated with diabetes, toxemia, or multiple births, but the cause is not known for sure. In 20% of pregnancies with polyhydramnios there is a congenital malformation of the baby, especially of the nervous system and gastrointestinal tract. A normal baby swallows amniotic fluid—which may be one way that the amount of fluid is controlled—but a baby with an intestinal obstruction, for instance, cannot swallow.

During pregnancy polyhydramnios can cause greater than normal edema (swelling) of the legs and vulva, difficulty breathing and sleeping, indigestion, heartburn, and constipation, all because of the extra pressure the additional fluid places on your system. The condition also affects labor: the cord is more likely to prolapse. Premature labor can occur because your uterus is overstretched. Unusual presentations are more common because the baby can float around. Labor may also be slower because the uterine muscles are stretched out and the baby's presenting part may float around in the excess fluid rather than engage in your pelvis, which would help to dilate the cervix. The overstretched uterus may also result in postpartum hemorrhage.

There is a relatively high prenatal mortality rate associated with polyhydramnios; the rate increases as the amount of fluid increases. If you have a severe form of this condition, you should see an obstetrician who specializes in high-risk pregnancies.

Placenta Previa

In this complication of pregnancy the placenta is situated low down in the uterus instead of at the top of it and blocks the cervix so the baby cannot exit. It occurs in one in 200 births and is rare in a first pregnancy. The risks increase with subsequent births. The major symptom is vaginal bleeding during the last trimester.

Blood transfusions can protect the mother but are risky for the baby, especially when he must be delivered prematurely. The mother is hospitalized, transfused as necessary, and observed until tests show that the baby is judged to be 5½ pounds. Then the mother is taken to the operating room. If the doctor can feel a lot of placenta blocking the cervix she or he will perform a cesarean. If the doctor cannot feel any placenta or only a small sliver of it then the membranes will be ruptured and labor induced.

Placenta Abruptio

Placenta abruptio is the premature separation of part or all of the placenta from the uterine wall—normally it would separate from the uterus after the birth of the baby. It is a rare occurrence, most likely in women who have had 5 to 6 babies (grand multiparas). It is three times as common for them as women having a first baby. This complication has a tendency to recur in subsequent pregnancies.

The symptoms are the same as for placenta previa: vaginal bleeding accompanied by abdominal pain in the last weeks of pregnancy before labor begins. As with placenta previa it can cause premature delivery. Although the mother is likely to survive the possible hemorrhage with blood transfusions, there's danger to the baby in placenta abruptio because his oxygen supply is cut off. A cesarean delivery may be indicated.

Cephalopelvic Disproportion (CPD)

Cephalopelvic disproportion (CPD) means that the fetus's head is larger than your pelvic opening and therefore the baby cannot fit through and be born vaginally. Between 25% and 40% of first-time cesareans are done because of CPD, or "failure to progress." However, there is a misunderstanding about CPD: some doctors may tell a woman before she has gone into labor that she has a "definite" cephalopelvic disproportion and must have a cesarean. The truth is that CPD is *not* a condition that can be determined absolutely before labor begins, because in theory, *any fetal head can fit through any pelvis.*

During pregnancy your body produces hormones, progestins, which allow your pelvic structure to expand. This is why walking may be difficult or you may be ungainly as your pregnancy advances. It is said that the female body is built to be able to delivery up to a 15-pound baby.

Of course, in reality there aren't many babies that big, and some women's pelvises will not expand enough to allow passage of a baby even half that size. The point is that it is incorrect to tell you that you have *definite* cephalopelvic disproportion *before* you go into labor. Ultasound makes it possible to get a good estimate before labor of the proportion of your pelvis compared to the size of the baby's head. However, there is no way of knowing for certain until you are in labor whether there will be room for the baby's head to exit. Your muscles and joints have to expand in order for the baby to fit through; the size of your pelvic opening is not fixed—it will enlarge. It is a question of whether it will increase enough to allow the baby to exit vaginally.

The decision to perform a cesarean should be based on your progress in labor as well as the baby's position and size. Question a doctor who tells you ahead of time that you *must* have a cesarean because of cephalopelvic disproportion. Once you are in labor, the effect of the hormone relaxin on your connective tissue may allow your joints to expand enough to permit the baby to pass through. If a doctor tells you before your due date that a C-section is necessary, seek a second opinion and *keep on practicing your prepared childbirth techniques*. Inform yourself about cesareans (see the section "Cesarean Birth" on pages 430–450), but don't give up hope of a vaginal delivery until it is clear *during labor* that a C-section is necessary.

Forceps Delivery

Forceps are large, curved metal tongs. The two sides of the tongs are put into your vagina separately and slipped up inside on either side of the baby's head. The tongs are then locked together outside, something like a one-piece salad server, and the doctor pulls the baby out by her head. Some doctors use forceps routinely on women having their first baby—be sure to ask ahead of time whether your doctor practices this way. There *is* a use for forceps, but *not* as a routine procedure. Forceps can save a baby's life in a complicated birth, but no other country uses them for as many normal births as in the United States. Judgment, caution, and skill are required.

The Three Kinds of Forceps Delivery

➤ *High-forceps* is done very rarely nowadays. The cesarean section has replaced the high-forceps method as a way to deliver a baby that will not descend.
➤ *Mid- or low-forceps* is used only when absolutely necessary because it involves inserting the forceps quite high and exerting a lot of pull on the baby. Low-forceps delivery is defined as

intervening when the baby's head has descended below your ischial spines. A low-forceps delivery may be necessary if anesthesia has made it impossible for you to push the baby out.

➤ *Outlet or perineal forceps* is quite common and is used when the baby's head is visible at the perineum, or the scalp can be clearly seen if the lips of your vagina are spread open. The forceps are used to lift the baby out of the vagina.

Usual Reasons for a Forceps Delivery

- To speed up second-stage labor if there is severe fetal distress.
- If the cord is wrapped tightly around the baby's neck, which occurs in approximately 25% of deliveries, or cord prolapses.
- In case of unusual presentations.
- To shorten a very long second stage labor.
- If regional anesthesia doesn't allow you to push the baby out.

Complications of Forceps

Complications of forceps delivery are rare—the common problem is that the forceps can bruise the baby's head, but the bruises disappear in a few days. The rare occurrence is that the pressure of the forceps can cause intracranial hemorrhage and damage the infant's facial nerves. The effects may not manifest themselves until early adulthood. Grand mal seizures in young adults may be the result of this interference with the normal functioning of the brain.

Congenital Malformations

Something is wrong with a baby in two out of every hundred births. Depending on how severe the defect is, the usual joyous reactions to birth will be suppressed. You can be reluctant to name the child and send birth announcements. People may be at a loss about the appropriate way to respond: they may not send flowers or telephone you. It can be lonely and confusing.

There are reactions which parents usually go through and which you can expect to experience if your baby is born with a congenital malformation.

Five Stages of Reactions

1) *Shock*: You will feel helpless, cry, and perhaps have an urge to run away.
2) *Disbelief (denial)*: You cannot believe that it has happened to you.

3) **_Sadness, anger, and anxiety_**: These stages of feelings are the same as for grief: You'll direct them toward yourself, the doctor or midwife, the hospital, and fate or God. Do not intellectualize the grief—do not put up a defensive wall and think, "Aha, this is the third stage and it is predictable that I will feel angry and sad." If your baby has a defect, you and your mate will be mourning the loss of the "perfect" dreamed-of infant. You should allow yourselves to feel the strength and depth of that grieving.

4) **_Equilibrium_**: Within a few weeks or months you will reach a more even keel. However, this adaptation can be incomplete and you may find yourself in tears years after the baby's birth.

5) **_Reorganization_**: You accept the situation and go on with your lives.

These stages are something that you and your mate both have to go through—the danger is that this process can create a problem in you relationship. If you both don't go through the states of adaptation at the same speed it can isolate you from each other. And if you do not keep the lines of communication open it can split you apart. A trauma like this can magnify the weaknesses in a partnership, whereas the birth of a normal child more often highlights the strengths in a relationship. It is important for both of you to recognize the potential problems a malformed baby can cause to your union. For example, either one of you may start drinking heavily to escape the situation, or you may have an affair for the same reason. (The sequel to this book, _Childbirth & Marriage_, covers this topic in depth.)

➤ **_Take things day by day_**. Try not to worry excessively. Tranquilizers are often prescribed which for some women will only blunt their natural responses and delay their adaptation to the problem. If you cannot sleep at night, you may want to seek medical help for temporary relief.

➤ **_Have rooming-in_** even if your impulse is to never want to see the child or to hope she dies. The sooner you adjust to the reality, the better off you'll be. The sooner your maternal feelings develop, the easier it will become. Spending time with the baby will facilitate this process.

➤ **_Talk to the pediatrician_** and elicit his or her support and advice. If you had already selected a doctor before the baby was born, avoid the temptation now to "doctor shop." Sometimes parents will go in search of other diagnoses as to the reason for the child's defect. It may come from a sense of guilt on their part; this kind of quest will only delay their ability to face the situation and cope with it.

➤ **_"Chronic sorrow"_** is experienced by some parents of malformed children. They are not able—or it takes them a long time—to overcome their grief about the baby's condition. Chronic sorrow may to some degree affect all parents of congenitally deformed children; it may be unreasonable to expect the painful impact on a family simply to disappear.

Fetal Surgery

This is a new science with thrilling possibilities for the future, although at present its applications are controversial and limited. It has been found that, while still inside the uterus, the fetus can tolerate corrective surgery, done either by opening the womb or not. However, the method is so new that the risks—and benefits—are still being weighed. There are only a few medical centers around the country equipped to perform prenatal intervention, and so far only a few fetuses have been treated.

With the aid of sophisticated prenatal diagnosis, obstetricians are able to detect serious conditions in the fetus early enough to treat some of them before irreparable damage is done. At the moment there are only four conditions that are considered correctable by experts. One is hydrocephalus, an accumulation of fluid under pressure in the brain that causes brain damage. A second is a urinary-tract obstruction called hydronephrosis, a blockage in the urethra. The third condition is diaphragmatic hernia, a hole in the diaphragm that allows the intestines to be pressed up against the lungs. Surgeons are able to drain excess fluid from fetal cavities and leave behind tiny draining tubes, called catheters, that stay in place until birth. Experts can also use fetal surgery to correct some of the heart defects that impair thousands of newborns every year.

However, there are many cautionary voices in the field. For one thing, it is known that an affected fetus often has a cluster of defects that may have damaged several organ systems. Doctors agree that it may not be wise to correct a heart defect, for instance, only to find out at birth that the fetus's brain is also severely damaged. And in the case of hydrocephalus, many times it is due to problems that may not be corrected simply by unplugging an obstruction—yet one cannot tell in advance. Also, no one yet knows whether relieving the fluid pressure actually prevents brain damage. In addition, even in the correctable form, hydrocephalus is often accompanied by other brain-development problems that may be beyond repair.

It is important for parents to realize how many unanswered questions there are in this field. If a couple is told that their baby is affected, they may be overly eager to accept these still-experimental procedures—without recognizing that their baby may still be very sick when he is born. Another issue rarely raised is the cost of fetal surgery. Even when fetal surgeons do not charge for their services, the corollary costs before, during, and after the surgery can easily run into tens of thousands of dollars, much of which an insurance company may not be willing to pay since these procedures are experimental.

Doctors are still wrestling with the complicated questions of exactly which fetuses to treat and when. They do not yet know whether they are salvaging fetuses that will become profoundly retarded or otherwise handicapped children. They don't know whether they are operating on fetuses who would have survived intact without their help, or whether they are achieving their hoped-for goal of producing healthy, normal children who might otherwise have died.

Death of a Baby

The tragedy of a baby dying at birth or soon thereafter is an unlikely occurrence. There is the same lack of faith in a couple's ability to cope with death as there has been about their ability to cope with birth. This attitude—on the part of the medical community—is changing. The most responsive caregivers are aware that if a couple's baby does die, there are certain stages they will necessarily go through and certain steps they can take to cope most effectively.

Death is difficult for hospital personnel. You need help to confront and resolve your grief, but they rarely can offer it. Even though you might think that caregivers have seen enough death to be able to deal with it, the truth is that it frightens, overwhelms, and saddens them— and they often withdraw from you because they don't know what to do.

Doctors also have trouble acknowledging death. Most doctors have had some special training in helping people with the grieving process. Doctors used to prescribe sedatives for a woman whose baby died even though this can actively interfere with the healthy resolution of grief. Some doctors did this routinely because they didn't know what else to do. Regardless of the cause of the baby's death it can make a doctor feel guilty and inadequate—and your emotions afterward increase that feeling for the doctor. Early discharge from the hospital is just one of the ways that caregivers protect themselves from sadness about death. If you and your mate are aware that you cannot realistically expect support and advice, then you will depend more on each other to get through this difficult time.

> ➤ *The stages of your psychological reaction* to your baby's death are fairly predictable. One thing you may feel is *somatic distress:* a feeling of tightness in your throat and a shortness of breath. These are ways that your body expresses the anxiety and sadness you feel. You may have a *preoccupation* with the image of the dead baby—it may "haunt" you when you are awake or asleep. You will probably also feel *guilt* and *hostility.* You will probably experience a *loss of the usual patterns of conduct*—you may feel disoriented, confused, and out of control of your life. These are the normal processes that people go through after a death.

> ➤ *Grieving is a natural and normal process.* You have to go through it one way or another. It will be better if you accept that

grieving is something you must *do* rather than something that has happened to you. You and your mate have to talk, share tears, and not deny your own *or* other people's feelings.

A man's feelings might be ignored because men are not raised to show their emotions. They often don't know how and others don't expect them to. A man may take on extra work in his business or increase other tasks so that he is constantly busy. A woman should try to draw out her mate—for her good as well as his. Feelings that are denied can surface in unexpected ways. A couple can find new strength together if they can face and fully experience the tragedy that has befallen them.

➤ *Explain to siblings* why you are crying or are moody. It is good for both of you to express your feelings as openly as you can, and it is important to explain this to young children who see the world as revolving around them. Children may think you are upset and angry at them. They also may worry that they are responsible for the baby's death. It is not uncommon for siblings to have bad thoughts about an impending baby and they may be afraid they caused her death unless you explain what happened and why you are feeling sad.

➤ *When a dead baby is seen by both parents it facilitates the grieving process.* You can move forward from the same frame of reference to an eventual resolution of your feelings. If you wish, you should visit a seriously ill infant in the intensive care nursery. Seeing him can help you deal with the reality. If you wish to see or touch the baby when he has died, do so. If you have that inclination, be sure to act on it—it can help make the death a reality. Even seeing a photograph of the baby after death can be beneficial to you and your mate. Holding the baby can help you accept the reality of death and thus allows you to begin the growing process of resolving your grief.

➤ *Have a simple funeral.* The traditional rituals promote grieving and make the death real. Although you may fear that it will only make you feel worse, it can release and relieve many emotions. However, it should be a simple ceremony with *only family present*. For some couples the presence of friends may add to the already heavy emotional burden.

➤ *People's comments* when they learn that your baby has died can be disturbing. People don't intend to upset you, but everyone feels helpless and ill at ease when there is a death and they say whatever they can. One comment you can depend on hearing is "You can have another." Although that probably is true, it is quite beside the point when you are trying to cope with your feelings about the baby you have been awaiting for so long who has just left you. "The baby is better off dead" is often said if there was something wrong with the baby. As far as you're concerned, the baby—and you—would be much better off if the baby were well and alive. "You must pull out of this and get involved in life again" may be some people's way of giving "constructive" advice. Unfortunately they don't necessarily know that death and the grief it produces are something you must experience in order to go on with your life. The worst thing you can do for yourselves in the beginning is to throw yourselves into work or play as a way of "forgetting" about the tragedy. There's no way to forget it, only the possibility of denying it for a while.

People's comments may make you angry; they may also make you feel lonely because there is no one to turn to who really understands. You have each other—take advantage of that. Realize that people mean well and thank them for their concern however inappropriately they may express it.

➤ *It is recommended not to conceive again* until the mourning period is complete. This can take 6 to 12 months, even though there may be times when you feel you are "over it" sooner. Grief takes quite a long time to work itself out, and you'll be cheating yourselves and another baby if you don't allow at least that long. The processes of attachment and detachment cannot easily occur simultaneously. While you are grieving it isn't possible to care fully for a new baby. Give yourselves at least 6 months to emotionally give up the baby who has died. Only then should you attempt to replace her.

➤ *Fetal death in utero* is defined as a fetus over 500 grams or more than 20 weeks gestation. If this happens to you, you'll probably be aware that the baby hasn't moved during a 24-hour period. You should be examined: an absence of fetal heartbeat and an ultrasound test which confirms that growth has stopped both determine whether the baby has died inside you.

Perhaps the hardest part of a fetal death in utero is that it is best to await spontaneous labor. This means that you have to walk around with the dead baby inside you, which can be a grotesque thought for some women. If labor is induced it may cause contractions but no cervical dilation—this means your cervix can tear, causing problems in subsequent pregnancies.

The wait for labor to begin can be several weeks. It is thought that labor may start naturally by a hormonal process triggered by the lack of fetal growth. Blood tests are necessary twice weekly until labor begins. After a 6-week wait it is best to induce labor because the products of conception, the fetus, placenta, and amniotic fluid, are reabsorbed into your body and can cause blood clots. It may be best not to have natural childbirth, but to be sedated. Some people feel that if this is your first pregnancy that it's better not to associate this experience with labor. However, some women may want their mates with them for this difficult labor and delivery and they may want to be awake. As mentioned, seeing and perhaps touching the baby can facilitate your grieving process.

Guilt is something women often feel about a baby that dies inside them. It is similar to the emotional experience of a miscarriage, particularly a second-trimester one. This guilt comes in part because we all believe to some degree in our own potency— that we are in control of what happens in our lives. If we are in control it is something we did—or did not do—that caused this baby to die. Thus we feel guilty. In order to get rid of that feeling we have to accept that there are things we have no power over; for many people, giving up the belief that they are in control means that they have to accept the terror of "the unknown." The death of a baby can force people to see that.

Losing a Twin (or Triplet)

If you lose one of the twins you've been expecting, it can be hard having to mourn for your lost baby at the same time that you're celebrating the birth of the twin. You need time to grieve, but you also need a chance to rejoice: these conflicted feelings can keep you from doing either one unless you understand the dynamics of what you're going through.

➤ Follow the advice about grieving on page 410 so that you can come to terms with the death of the baby you've lost.

➤ Consider having a small memorial service or for the lost baby. This will start clearing the way for emotional attachment to the living baby, who deserves a christening, circumcision, or just plain welcome-to-the-family get-together.

➤ You may feel disappointed that you have lost the specialness of being the parents of twins, which may be something you've been planning for months. It's understandable that you feel cheated at having to give up this dream, but you need to let it go so you can come back down to earth with your living baby.

➤ It may feel unfair to the baby who died to enjoy the one who survived, or you may feel it's disloyal to the baby you lost if you love the living one. These are normal feelings, but don't indulge them and give them substance: tell yourself it doesn't make sense and isn't fair to the baby who is alive.

➤ If you're self-conscious about having to tell the sad news to relatives or friends who've been waiting for the twins, then ask a relative or close friend to get in touch with the people you care about and let them know about your loss. If you feel uneasy going in public with the surviving twin, for fear of people asking about the other baby, then have a friend or relative keep you company and be there to gently explain to people.

➤ Don't let people's insensitivity or thoughtlessness in their comments get to you: they mean well, but you have to expect well-meaning but upsetting remarks from people in such an awkward position.

➤ You may feel you've been punished because of negative feelings you may have had about the prospect of twins. You may also have had self-doubts about whether you were going to be an adequate mother. In all these cases you might subconsciously wonder if you've been punished.

➤ If you were infertile and your twins were conceived through hormone treatments, in vitro fertilization or GIFT, you may feel the loss of the twin is somehow your fault. Get reassurance by talking to your infertility specialist.

➤ You may worry whether the surviving twin is going to suffer from the loss after all those months of sharing a womb. You may wonder whether that child will be troubled as he goes through life knowing he lived and his twin died. Your child will only be as upset as you allow: if you don't make a big deal about it, then it won't be a big deal.

➤ Don't worry now about how it will feel to be reminded of your lost child as your baby reaches the milestones like eating solid food and walking. Yes, it will probably be sad, but you'll deal with it, don't worry.

➤ You may have fears of how this loss will affect your marriage. If you keep open to each other and share feelings instead of bottling them up, you'll pull together and be closer because you have survived a tragedy together.

➤ Don't rush yourself. Let the sadness pass out of you and allow the new baby to let the light in. It is a process which takes time: respect the fact that it cannot be rushed.

Emergency Childbirth

This is not intended as a do-it-yourself guide to birth. These are tips on what to do if the baby wants to be born before you reach the hospital or in a home birth, before the attendant gets there.

If You Get the Urge to Push

➤ Stay calm. Use your breathing techniques to avoid pushing.
➤ If you're at home call the paramedics. They may not get there in time for the birth, but they can take you and the newborn to the hospital afterward to be examined.
➤ If you're driving to the hospital:

— Remind each other not to panic. Babies have been born for centuries without professional help!
— Assess the situation with your partner (or whoever is driving you) to decide if you can make it to the hospital.
— If the urge to push is too strong for you to control, have him pull the car over to the side of the road and stop. If there's nowhere to stop, at least slow down.

— If you have a cellular phone, call 911 or the local emergency number.
— If possible, cover the backseat and car floor with a thick layer of newspapers (which provide a more sterile environment).
— If your partner has stopped the car, you can slump down and deliver the baby over the edge of the backseat into his hands. Otherwise you can lie across the seat.

A Loop of Umbilical Cord Is Visible

➤ When the membranes rupture, a part of the umbilical cord may wash out. This means that the cord is "prolapsed" and has come down before the baby. This is potentially fatal to the baby: the cord is compressed and the baby's oxygen supply is cut off.
➤ If you can see a piece of gray-blue shiny cord bulging out of your vagina, get into a knee-chest position immediately. Get down on your knees with your head down and your buttocks up in the air.
➤ Call the paramedics immediately: tell them you have a prolapsed cord and will require an emergency cesarean delivery (they should know that a cesarean is required with a prolapsed cord).
➤ If the cord is still protruding when you are in a knee-chest position, then cover it with warm, wet sterile gauze pads or a very clean towel.
➤ Do not put any pressure on the cord. It is still your baby's lifeline.
➤ Stay in the knee-chest position all the way to the hospital to reduce pressure on the cord.

Put Fresh Towels or Newspapers Under You

➤ Create a clean place for the baby to be born.
➤ This reduces the chance of infection for you and the newborn.

Never Hold Your Legs Together to Delay the Birth

➤ Under no circumstances should you ever try to "cross your legs" and keep the baby from being born.
➤ Do not allow anyone else to hold your legs together.
➤ This would be dangerous for the baby because it can cause brain damage.

Ease the Baby Out Along with Contractions

➤ Do not think about doing the pushing that you learned in child-birth classes—a baby coming this fast doesn't need pushing help.
➤ Pant lightly with each contraction.
➤ If you push along with the force of your uterus, there is a greater chance that your vagina and perineum will tear.

Deliver the Head Slowly

➤ It is best if you push the head out *between* contractions.
➤ If there is time, your partner should support your perineum to avoid tearing from the rapid birth.
➤ He should use warm, wet compresses or a very clean towel to put the heel of his hand over the area between your vagina and anus.
➤ He can then apply counter-pressure against the pressure coming from inside.

Never Pull on the Baby's Head to Get it Out

➤ Pulling on the head may permanently injure the spinal cord, the nerves of the arms, and the baby's breathing apparatus.
➤ Your partner should support the baby's head as it is born.

If There Are Still Membranes Covering the Head

➤ It's unlikely that the membranes wouldn't have ruptured by now, but if they haven't, then they must be torn off.
➤ The membranes have to be removed in order for the baby to breathe.
➤ Your partner can use his fingernails, a pin, or any clean sharp instrument to get the membranes open.
➤ If there is time, dip the pin (or other tool) into rubbing alcohol before using it.
➤ Be very careful of the baby's head!

Once the Head Is Out

➤ The head is the first part of the baby's body to be born.
➤ Your partner should check around the baby's neck with his fingers to be sure the cord is not wrapped around it.
➤ If there is a loop of cord around the neck, you have to loosen it or it can be fatal to the baby.

➤ Release the cord so that the body can deliver through the loop.
➤ You can also gently release the wrapped cord and pull it over the baby's head.

The Head Turns Naturally to One Side

➤ The head turns so that the shoulders can rotate to be born.
➤ When the baby first comes out, her head will probably be facing down.
➤ Gently wipe off her face with a very clean cloth.
➤ After her head has turned to the left or right, you should push with the next contraction to deliver the shoulders.

Do Not Pull on the Baby

➤ Your partner should support the baby's whole body as she is born.
➤ You can also reach down and help hold the newborn as she exits: she could be injured without that support.

Dry the Baby Thoroughly

➤ Wrap the newborn in a clean receiving blanket.
➤ Keeping the baby warm is extremely important.
➤ Make sure the baby's head is well covered to guard against heat loss.

Hold the Baby with His Head Lower than His Body

➤ The newborn's face should be down or to the side because the mucus in his nose and lungs has to drain out.
➤ This position shouldn't be exaggerated: the head just needs to be slightly lower.
➤ Do not attempt to wipe out the inside of the baby's mouth.

Leave the Umbilical Cord Alone

➤ Do not pull on the cord.
➤ Do not cut the cord.

Put the Baby to Your Breast

➤ Place the baby's mouth at your nipple if the umbilical cord is long enough to reach without pulling on the baby's navel.
➤ The baby's sucking will stimulate oxytocin in your system, which contracts your uterus and helps expel the placenta.
➤ Even if the baby does not want to suck, she will still be warmed and comforted by being at your breast.
➤ Be sure to keep her carefully covered during this, especially her head (which is where the most heat loss occurs).

If the Placenta Is Born

➤ If this happens before you reach the hospital (or in a home birth before the attendant arrives), then gently wrap it up with the baby.
➤ You may feel squeamish about this, but the placenta can provide much-needed extra warmth for the newborn and needs to be kept for inspection by the doctor later.

After the Placenta Is Born

➤ Your partner should massage your uterus firmly with a deep, circular motion.
➤ He has to be firm, but it should not be painful—the pressure should be within the limits of your comfort.
➤ The point where he should push down and rub in a circle is 2 to 3 inches below your navel.
➤ This is extremely important: it assures that your uterus contracts after delivery and stays hard after the birth so there is no hemorrhage.

If There Is Bleeding

➤ Some blood is expected during childbirth.
➤ It is normal to have less than 2 cups of blood when the placenta delivers and for a few minutes afterward.
➤ Getting the baby to nurse immediately after birth can help contract the uterus because of hormones your body produces.
➤ Massaging your nipples gently can be a substitute way of releasing the oxytocin into your system.

The Baby's Color at Birth Is Blue

➤ It is normal for a baby to be bluish when he first comes out and hasn't breathed air yet.
➤ In the first minute the baby "pinks up" as oxygen enters his body.
➤ The hands and feet take longer to lose that blue tinge.

IF YOU'RE ALONE AND THE BABY IS COMING

— Stay calm. Take a deep breath and collect your thoughts.
— Call 911, or the local emergency number; ask them to send paramedics because you're in labor and can't make it to the hospital.
— Call your partner or someone close to you and give them the phone number to contact your doctor.
— If you have a neighbor or friend who lives nearby, ask them to come assist you.
— If you feel the urge to bear down, try to pant to keep yourself from pushing.
— If possible, wash your hands and the vaginal area.
— Lie down on a clean area to wait for help to come. Spread out a thick layer of newspaper (which is sterile) or very clean towels or sheets on your bed or the floor. Put a couple of very clean towels (or anything that has been recently been ironed or been in a hot dryer, which helps sterilize it) on the side to wrap the baby in later.
— The urge to push may become very strong. Don't fight nature: each time you feel the urge, pant lightly with each contraction. In a fast labor like this the uterus doesn't need much help.
— Reach down with your hands and catch the baby as she emerges, putting a little pressure on her head if you can to keep her from popping out.
— Don't pull on the baby or the cord. If you can feel or see the umbilical cord wrapped around the baby's neck, you must gently get it free as quickly as possible. Slip your fingers under the loop of cord by carefully working it over the baby's head.
— Once the baby is out, you don't want her to catch a chill: wrap her carefully in the cleanest coverings you found and set aside.
— If the cord is long enough, put her to your breast in case she will suck. This will help create natural contractions to avoid unnecessary bleeding. Some bleeding is normal.
— If the placenta delivers before help gets there, wrap it in newspaper or towels and place it higher than the baby if possible. Don't think about cutting the cord.
— As long as you and the baby are both warm and comfortable, you should stay still until help arrives.

❧ ❦

CHAPTER FOURTEEN

Taking Care of Yourself and Your Partner Postpartum

There is a wide range of possible physical and emotional feelings you may have in the postpartum (after birth) period. You may feel a few or many of these bodily discomforts and mental upheavals, but if you know ahead of time what to expect it can make it easier. Forewarned is forearmed when you have to face the enormous adjustment of your body and mind postpregnancy as well as a new baby.

Childbirth & Marriage **is a sequel to this book** that focuses on what to expect after the birth of your child. I wrote the second book because I heard from so many couples who were struggling with the "transition to parenthood." That book goes into much more depth about how a baby affects your life. If you are interested in the issues that can affect your marriage after the birth of your child, have a look at that book, too.

IN THE HOSPITAL

➤ *Nurses and doctors may not have much time for you.* They may be very busy because hospitals are often under-

staffed. Do not let negative attitudes of hospital personnel get to
you, particularly where breast-feeding is concerned (see pages
310–311, "Breast-Feeding and the Hospital").

➤ *The food may be bland and unappetizing*, as most institutional food is. Have "care packages" brought in or ask a friend
to visit you around mealtime and bring food of your choice to
you. For instance, if you ordinarily eat health foods, you are
going to be unhappy with the processed, refined-sugar, white-
flour meals served at most hospitals.

➤ *Visitors will tire you out more than you imagine*. You
should try to limit each visitor to a half-hour stay. The other
problem may be that the hospital restricts you to only one visitor
during each visiting period. This means that you have to make
the choice between your mate, your mother, or perhaps a sister
or close friend. These kinds of hospital rules are a terrible way
to separate families right from the start, but it is a policy you
may have to contend with.

CHANGES IN YOUR BODY AFTER BIRTH

Physical changes are the first thing you'll have to cope with after
childbirth. Your body has to go through an enormous adjustment because of hormonal changes, tender and engorged breasts, and the processes of repair taking place in your uterus and vagina.

VAGINAL DISCHARGE (LOCHIA)

➤ *You will have a vaginal discharge* of blood, mucus, and
tissue following the birth of your baby. This is called "lochia"
and occurs because the site in your uterus where the placenta
was attached has to heal. This process takes anywhere from one
to six weeks after birth. Breast-feeding reduces the bleeding
more rapidly. First the lochia is a menstrual-like red flow, which
gradually turns pale pink or brown and then yellow-white or
colorless.

➤ *Use only sanitary napkins for the first two weeks*. The
hospital will charge you a steep fee for each and every napkin
they dispense to you while you're there, so you might want to
bring a box with you to the hospital. The larger hospital-size
napkins available at many drugstores can be helpful in the beginning. Many women find sanitary napkins awkward and irritating. Self-adhesive sanitary napkins that adhere to your
underpants may be less uncomfortable: they are most suitable
when the flow of lochia has decreased somewhat.

> *After the second week postpartum you can use tampons*, as long as your doctor approves. Tampons may help you feel that your vagina is returning to normal. However, many physicians feel that tampons increase the likelihood of infection if used during the first weeks after birth, so this should be discussed. Putting a small amount of some kind of lubricating jelly, such as K-Y, on the tip of the tampon may make insertion easier.
> *If the flow becomes bright red* any time after the first week, especially if it has turned brown and is suddenly red again, *notify your doctor*. It probably means you aren't giving the placental site enough chance to mend. If so, your doctor will most likely tell you to slow down, go to bed for a day, and get more rest.
> *A continuing vaginal discharge* or an unpleasant vaginal odor may indicate incomplete healing of the cervix, or vaginal infection. You should let your doctor know about this so she or he can recommend treatment. *Do not use* feminine hygiene deodorant products, nylon underpants, or panty hose, all of which tend to aggravate the problem. Cotton underpants, which stay drier and allow oxygen to pass through, can help discourage persistent itching and infection.
> *If you soak 2 pads in half an hour* call your doctor or midwife at once. Passing clots in the lochia is normal, but if you are bleeding enough to soak two pads in 30 minutes at any point during the healing process, you should be examined.

Changes in the Vagina and Cervix

> *There may be changes in the size of your vagina* that may be disquieting. It is normal for the vagina to feel slack during the first couple of weeks after giving birth. One of the amazing things about a woman's birth canal is that it can expand dramatically to let the baby pass through, and then resume its usual size and shape. However, this doesn't happen overnight; for some women their vaginas never return to precisely their prepregnant size. By doing the Kegel exercise described on page 161, you will be able to tighten your vagina considerably.
> *Your cervix is contracting, too*. After expanding enough to allow your baby to pass into the birth canal, the cervix returns to its normal size in several weeks. However, once you have given birth you will need a larger size diaphragm. See page 487.

Recovering from the Episiotomy

➤ ***The episiotomy that was cut in your perineum*** to make more room for the baby's head at birth can be sore and itchy afterwards. How big the incision is, and the skill with which your doctor made it, affect how much discomfort you feel. The soreness you feel is a result of the tissues swelling and pulling against the stitches. The swelling is usually worse the first 3 days after delivery and then lessens.

Some women find that recovering from the episiotomy is the most painful part of childbirth. For some women the soreness lasts for 2 to 3 weeks; for others it's gone within a week. There are several things you can try to ease the discomfort; however, *be sure not to use any ice or heat treatment if your genitals are numb from an anesthetic spray or cream*. If you are anesthetized, you won't be able to feel the burning sensation that would warn you if the temperature becomes too extreme.

— *Put an ice pack* on the area around your vagina as soon as possible after the birth. Ice is the most soothing treatment to reduce swelling and discomfort. Ask a nurse for a sterile glove and fill it with crushed ice, then apply this ice pack on your episiotomy wound. You may also find this helpful after you return home.

— *Do the Kegel exercise* immediately after the baby is born and continue to do it often during the postpartum period. It will pull the stitches together and begin the process of mending and strengthening the affected muscles.

— *Local anesthetic creams and sprays* can be helpful, so ask your doctor if she or he recommends them, perhaps along with some aspirin. These products will cost much more if the hospital issues them, so you might want someone to buy them for you in an outside drugstore.

— *Keep your genital area dry and clean* by bathing and changing sanitary napkins frequently. Notify the doctor immediately if you think the area is infected so that scar tissue is not allowed to develop.

— *Perineal pads* (a brand such as Tucks) can be put between your sanitary pad and the stitches to relieve itching and soreness.

— *Put a bottle of witch hazel* in the refrigerator or in an ice bucket. Dip a sterile gauze pad in the cold witch hazel, then apply it to the wound.

— *Some doctors recommend the use of alcohol swabs* after urination and bowel movements to prevent infection and speed healing.

— *Wipe from the front to the back* when you have a bowel movement and then drop the paper in the toilet. Fecal matter can cause an infection if it enters the vagina or urethra.

— *Warm baths or showers* can soothe the healing perineum, although it may be best to wait until the swelling around the wound has subsided before you expose the area to heat. Use plain water only: bath additives can be irritating to a wound.

— *Sitting can be painful*. Putting a soft pillow underneath you, especially on hard chairs, can ease the pain. You might also try a "donut cushion," intended for people with hemorrhoids.

Urination and Urinary Tract Infections

➤ **Birth is a trauma** to your entire pelvic floor, which includes the muscles and tissues surrounding your urethra, vagina, and rectum. Your body may feel different and uncomfortable when you have to perform such simple functions as urinating. In the process of being born, the baby was pressing on your bladder as he descended through your vagina. It will take some time before this area recovers from the trauma of childbirth.

➤ **Difficulty in passing urine** is not uncommon after childbirth. It may be the result of swelling in your perineum, which may close the urethra. If you had a spinal anesthetic, it may have made your bladder less sensitive to how full it is and made it temporarily unable to empty completely. Women who are unable to urinate within 6 to 8 hours after delivery are usually catheterized to allow the urine to pass out of their bladder.

➤ **An increased need to urinate** is not uncommon during the first week after delivery. The extra fluid you retained during pregnancy is being eliminated.

➤ **Leaking urine** (incontinence) after birth is quite common. When you laugh or cough, your bladder may leak until your muscles return to normal.

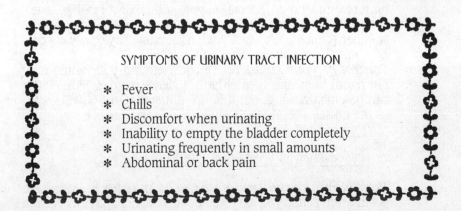

SYMPTOMS OF URINARY TRACT INFECTION

* Fever
* Chills
* Discomfort when urinating
* Inability to empty the bladder completely
* Urinating frequently in small amounts
* Abdominal or back pain

➤ *Postpartum urinary tract infections* are fairly common. Notify your physician promptly if you think you have an infection so you can take care of it before it becomes more serious. There are several signs that you might be developing such an infection, although you probably will not experience all of them.

Bowel Movements and Hemorrhoids

➤ *Giving birth affects your intestines and rectum* because of the pressure exerted on that area during delivery. Your bowels may be sluggish after childbirth and you may not feel able to have a bowel movement. You may also develop swollen, tender lumps in your anus. These dilated veins are hemorrhoids, which can make bowel movements uncomfortable.

➤ *If the pain and swelling of hemorrhoids* are bothering you, try sitting in a shallow tub of warm water. Your doctor can also recommend local anesthetic creams or compresses. Tucking hemorrhoids back in after a bowel movement can be helpful, although be careful that your fingernails aren't long or sharp.

➤ *You may be worried about being constipated* after giving birth, especially if the hospital staff keeps asking whether you've had a bowel movement. Don't strain to move your bowels, just relax and allow your body to find its way back to normal.

➤ *How to deal with constipation* during pregnancy is discussed on page 127, but there are several things it's important to do postpartum. The first is to get up and walk as soon as possible after the birth, which gets your system going. Drink plenty of fluids and eat a lot of fresh fruit, vegetables, whole-grain cereals, and bread to help keep your stool soft.

➤ *Prunes or prune juice* in the morning, followed by coffee or any other hot liquid, works for some people.

➤ *A mild laxative* may be necessary if everything else you try doesn't work, although you should check with your doctor, who may recommend an enema, suppositories, or a stool softener, instead. *For nursing mothers*: If you are breast-feeding, a stool softener (which does exactly what its name says), *not a laxative*, may help without affecting your milk.

➤ *Control of your sphincter* (muscle around your anus) may not return immediately after birth. Release of some fecal matter can be embarrassing, but it is not unusual. Control will return as the muscles regain their tone.

Miscellaneous Postpartum Physical Changes

➤ *Your hair may thin out after the baby is born*. During the postpartum period you may lose 50 to 100 more hairs daily than before your pregnancy. You can see the evidence of this not only in your hairbrush but also on your pillow and clothing. Your placenta and the rich proteins in it were responsible for your hair being thick and shiny during your pregnancy. Without the placenta, you no longer have adequate protein in your system to sustain the previously rapid hair growth. Other reasons for thinning hair can be postpartum stress or a hormonal imbalance. But take heart: there is a remedy! Hair is composed almost entirely of protein, so concentrate on getting a lot of protein in your diet.

➤ *Your hair may be dry and brittle* after your pregnancy. If so, check your shampoo: detergent-based shampoos can strip your hair of vital oils and cause the scalp glands to have to work harder to replace these valuable natural oils. Switch to a cream-based shampoo made of natural proteins and such vegetable oils as wheat germ oil. Use a good conditioner, too.

If your hair is dry postpartum, don't wash it every day. Give it a rest and wash it only 3 to 4 times a week. Don't use rubber bands or sleep in curlers, both of which can break hair. Avoid dying your hair, getting permanents, or using a hair dryer frequently.

➤ *Dry skin is a common problem* postpartum, although a few women may find that their skin becomes more oily. After birth, the fluid balance in your body is disturbed by hormone production. Breast-feeding women are even more susceptible to dry skin: your body is using all available fluids to produce milk.

There are remedies for dry skin problems. Try to drink a lot of fluids, at least 2 quarts a day, preferably in the form of water and juice. Drinking liquids will help replenish the moisture lost to hormone imbalance and milk production. However, drinking will probably not be enough; you'll also need to treat the surface of your skin with moisturizers. Although it's good to take steamy hot baths, do not use bubble baths, which often contain detergents and perfumes that can further dry your skin. Any product you use in your bath should be oil-based.

➤ *Your teeth and gums may have problems postpartum*. Since pregnancy depletes your body's natural supply of calcium, you may find that your gums are inflamed, or that there is grayness at the gum line of your lower teeth. Bonemeal, other calcium supplements, or foods high in calcium are just as important for your health after delivery as they were for the baby's growth during pregnancy. Vitamin C is also helpful for gum problems. When you brush twice a day, use a soft-bristle toothbrush to massage your gums in a circular motion.

➤ *Your uterus should feel firm*, like a grapefruit in the middle of your stomach. Immediately after birth the nurse or midwife will knead your uterus every 15 minutes for the first hour to help the involution process, so the uterine muscles stay firm. They may show you how to knead the uterus yourself. Especially if you are leaving the hospital on early discharge, or if you've given birth at home, it is important for you to know if your uterus remains hard. Postpartum hemorrhage can be very dangerous, but if the uterus remains firm, everything is okay.

Just after the birth your uterus is about 3 finger-widths below your belly button. After 24 hours it will have risen to the level of your umbilicus and then it continues to shrink, until by the end of the first week you probably won't be able to feel it when you press on your belly. By 6 weeks postpartum the uterus should be back to its prepregnancy size.

➤ *Your breasts may feel congested.* If you are breast-feeding you can hand-express milk and wear a firm supportive bra day and night to help relieve congestion. Applying very hot washcloths or an ice pack may also help. If you are not breast-feeding and lactation has been suppressed with medication, do *not* hand-express milk and do limit your fluid intake. A feeling of feverishness can also accompany breast congestion.

➤ *There are controversial drugs* available to stop maternal milk production. A Food and Drug Administration advisory panel called for an end to this practice long ago. Consumer advocate groups have been petitioning the FDA to ban the use of hormones and drugs to stop milk production and breast engorgement. These drugs are only marginally effective and can cause serious side effects such as sharp drops in blood pressure, as well as nausea and dizziness. The manufacturer of the drug, which is marketed under the name Parlodel, still has it on the market for infertility, but the FDA withdrew it for antilactation.

➤ *Chills and hot flashes can occur simultaneously* and can be frightening if you aren't aware that this is a common occurrence. As with many of the physical reactions after birth, it is one of the body's ways of readjusting to the powerful hormonal changes going on.

➤ *Profuse sweating is the body's way of ridding itself* of the excess fluids accumulated in your body during pregnancy. It can be especially bothersome at night, so put a towel on your pillow.

➤ *Thirst can be quite marked postpartum* because your body is losing fluid. Drink plenty of liquids. This thirstiness will pass as soon as your body has recovered its normal balance.

➤ *Weight loss postpartum* is something most women welcome. It is normal to lose between 10 and 20 pounds immediately at birth, depending on how much weight you gained and how much of it was water weight. Although you will undoubtedly have more weight to lose, *do not go on a severe diet right away*, regardless of whether you are breast-feeding. Your body is recovering from the stress of birth in the first month or so and it requires a nutritious, well-balanced diet to do this.

➤ *Menstruation recurs anywhere from 2 months to 4 months* postpartum. There is some variation, but it is usually 8 weeks after the birth if you are not breast-feeding. For several months the interval between periods and the amount of bleeding may be unusual. Painful periods (dysmenorrhea) are almost always improved by pregnancy—for many women who had incapacitating pain before, it never returns after birth. Most women do not ovulate when they are nursing, *but some do*.

➤ ***Birth control is necessary as soon as you're ready*** to have sexual intercourse. *Do not rely on breast-feeding or the lack of menstruation* to protect you against conceiving. You can get pregnant the first time you ovulate, which will be before you have a period. Your old diaphragm will not fit—you will have to be refitted with a larger size by the doctor or midwife about four weeks postpartum. *This is true even if you had a cesarean*. Many doctors will want you to return four weeks after that to check the fit again. *Do not use the birth-control pill while breast-feeding*. Your mate can use condoms with lots of spermicidal foam or jelly.

GETTING PREGNANT AGAIN TOO SOON

It's not advisable to get pregnant again within three months of giving birth, but if it should happen to you, there's no point worrying about it! However, because your body hasn't had a chance to fully recover from the previous pregnancy, you are now considered to be in the "high-risk" category. What this means is that it's important to take especially good care of yourself and follow a few extra precautions.

➤ ***Get early prenatal care*** from the moment you find out you're pregnant again.

➤ ***Wean your baby immediately*** if you're breast-feeding. Your body cannot take the strain of forming a new life and also providing nutrition for the baby who's already here. Just becoming pregnant again is a big challenge to your body. Don't worry about your newborn because she will have already gotten many of the benefits of breast milk by now.

➤ ***Get lots of rest*** because your body has a big challenge: forming a new life while still recuperating from the previous pregnancy and birth. Make sure that your partner and the other people close to you understand how important it is for you to conserve your strength right now.

➤ ***Concentrate on eating well and gaining enough weight***. Even though you probably haven't lost the extra pounds from the first pregnancy, you can't sacrifice the 25 to 35 pounds you need to gain for a healthy baby this time around. In fact, good nutrition is even more important for you than it was before because it's one of the few ways you have to make up for the strain on your body.

FATIGUE

➤ *Total exhaustion is common after childbirth*, but many women are surprised by just how fatigued they feel in the first weeks. The drastic reduction in your blood volume (it decreases by 30 percent) can be felt as exhaustion, although some women experience it as exhilarating. In either case it is *important to continue taking your iron pills for 6 weeks postpartum*. If you feel unusually weak or tired during the first 2 weeks after birth, it may be from anemia.

➤ *Fatigue is the most common complaint* of new mothers. The newborn baby has no conception of day and night. The average newborn eats every 2 hours if breast-fed and every 4 hours if bottle-fed. Although the period of sleeplessness for the new mother is usually greatest in the first 6 weeks to 2 months after birth, *you should expect to be up at least once a night for the first year of the baby's life*. Some women find it is many months, even a full year, before they sleep well again after the arrival of their child.

➤ *There is a fatigue cycle that can be self-perpetuating*. Once you are tired, you get more irritated by chores and the things you do not have time to accomplish. You may feel inadequate and overcompensate by trying to do more, which only tires you out further. Here are some suggestions on ways to avoid creating a fatigue cycle:

- Good nutrition helps fatigue, so be sure to eat properly.
- If you are unable to sleep at night because you are overtired, try to make sure that the hour before bedtime is peaceful.
- Half an hour before bedtime, get into bed with warm milk and read, watch TV, or listen to music.
- Don't eat heavily or drink caffeine or other stimulating drinks before bed.

➤ *Do not ignore the signs of fatigue*. Tune into the signs that your body gives you about being tired or having little energy. Take a nap when the baby naps—don't do chores in that time. For the first week try to limit stair-climbing to once a day and avoid heavy lifting. Visitors can be very tiring—if you want company do not try to be super-hostess. People can take care of themselves—they can go get a drink for themselves from the kitchen, and there's no reason for them not to get one for *you* while they're up! If you do not want visitors and want to be alone, just tell people that your doctor or midwife has forbidden you to have guests for the first week.

➤ *Sleep is essential in the immediate postpartum period*. Studies show that in the last weeks of pregnancy women have a loss of REM (rapid eye movement) sleep. Rapid eye movements are associated with dreaming, which occurs in the deepest sleep. REM sleep is necessary for both physical and psychological replenishment. The loss of REM sleep and the associated disturbance in dream patterns may be related to the impending crisis of childbirth.

This loss of sleep can and must be made up. If you continue to lose sleep after the baby is born, it can lead to physical and emotional disturbances. You *may* feel fine even though your usual sleep pattern is interrupted. However, you may be someone who sleeps the most soundly in the sixth or seventh hour of sleep—if you feel sleepy during the day then you probably are. In this case you should have someone else give the baby a bottle during the early morning feeding so that you can get the sleep you need. Another alternative is to have someone give the baby a bottle while you take an afternoon nap—either way, the intention is to give you more than a 3- to 4-hour stretch of sleep between feedings so that you can get that deep sleep necessary to your well-being.

SIGNS OF POSTPARTUM PROBLEMS (NOTIFY DOCTOR AT ONCE)

— Unusually heavy bleeding on any day, more than a menstrual period, or if you soak more than 2 sanitary napkins in half an hour.
— Vaginal discharge with a strongly unpleasant odor.
— A temperature of 101° or higher. If you develop a rise of temperature to 100.4° F. (38° C.) or higher on any 2 of the first 10 postpartum days, exclusive of the first 24 hours, the assumption is that you have puerperal fever, unless there is an obvious other source like an inflamed breast or bronchitis. Bacterial cultures are taken of the interior of the uterus, your blood, and urine, and wide-spectrum antibiotics are begun immediately.
— Breasts are red, feel hot or painful.

➢ *If you are not feeling well, call the doctor.* Do not wait for the 6-week postpartum visit. Although it is common to feel tired, you should not feel poorly after birth. If you have *pain* anywhere call the doctor right away—it may be a sign of infection, which can occur postpartum. If you have a loss of appetite for an extended period, call the doctor. If there is a sudden increase in vaginal bleeding—if you are passing large clots in the lochia or it turns a sudden bright red color—these may be signs of problems.

➤ *Your mate may not understand* the changes your body has to go through. He has nothing in his own experience which can correspond to pregnancy and postpartum. He may not understand that you look healthy and beautiful and can receive visitors but just don't have the energy to cook or do things around the house. If you are a first-time mother, unsure of yourself, you may feel silly not pitching right in with chores. A skeptical partner can make this worse.

The fact is that it takes a full 6 weeks for your body to return to its prepregnancy condition. No matter how good you feel, you should still be kind to your body and take it easy. Your mate has to protect you, rather than question why you have less energy.

GETTING HOUSEHOLD HELP POSTPARTUM

It is important that you have a good chance to rest after the baby is born: it can affect your early relationship with the child and will also mean that you will recover *fully* from the birth as soon as possible. The kind of help you get will depend on what you can afford and who is available. The essential thing is for you to recognize that although it is humanly possible for you to handle everything alone it will be a great deal more pleasant to have an extra pair of hands around.

You don't actually need help for the baby—the first postpartum week is a special time for you and the baby to spend time together, particularly if you are breast-feeding. Household help is the most useful: to cook, clean, answer the phone, fend off visitors, and run errands. It isn't going to be a big help if you have someone to tend to the baby, whose needs are basically to be fed and changed, leaving *you* to run the house.

➤ *Paid help is preferable if there is room for it in your budget* because when you are paying someone it's a lot easier to ask them to do things. With a friend or relative it can feel awkward to ask them to go to the post office or prepare dinner while you lie in bed with the baby. Two weeks of help would be ideal, but if you can afford only 4 to 5 days, that's certainly better than none at all. It will give you a chance to get your bearings as a new mother.

➤ *Interview possible candidates before the baby is born*. It will be too hectic—and too unpredictable—afterward. If you are going to get professional help it is a good idea to contact an employment agency that specializes in domestic help or baby care. You might also ask women who have had babies in the past few years whether they used anyone they would recommend.

➤ *A trained baby nurse is good if you feel ill at ease* taking care of a newborn and don't think you'll gain enough confidence through the infant-care classes offered by the hospital or the American Red Cross in your community. A trained nurse can show you how everything should be done—but beware of a domineering, bossy woman who seems as if she'll want to take complete charge of the baby and have rigid, set ideas about the "right" way to do things. Also remember that unless you have other help in the house, a trained nurse will do no housework or cooking—she may even expect to have meals prepared for *her*. Professional nannies are scarce and in demand, so they can pretty much "write their own ticket"!

➤ *A CNA or professional baby-sitter* can also be located through an employment agency. These women will usually be willing to do light housework, some cooking, and can also look after the baby and show you the ropes. In the case of these women or trained baby nurses, you should check out their references and find out about them from mothers who have used them recently.

➤ *A student can be less expensive*—although perhaps also less efficient. You should call the local high school and college and see if they have any young women available for light housework or baby care. Some of these students may have cared for younger brothers or sisters at home and may have as much practical experience as professionals. It may also make for a more informal arrangement, which might suit you best if you are not comfortable with the idea of having an older woman around who may have an authoritarian air.

➤ *Grandmothers can be wonderfully helpful* with a new baby. They can also be a pain in the neck. It depends partly on your relationship with your mother or mother-in-law, as well as her attitude about a newborn. She may have been unhappy or dissatisfied with her own birth experience and may try to work out her feelings by participating in yours. Or she can be rigid in her ideas about baby care, which will put pressure on you to give in to avoid a confrontation or to contradict her and start arguments.

If you have a less-than-terrific relationship with your mother—or if you fear she might be more domineering than you'd like—make other plans for postpartum care ahead of time. You can keep her at a distance if you have specific plans already set up and tell her tactfully. If you happen to have a close, easy relationship with your mother-in-law and would like her to be with you after the baby is born, you have to weigh that choice against the insult your own mother may feel. You may be able to finesse it—with reasons of geographic distances or economics—but it can cause hurt feelings. In either case, if you don't want to have your mother or mother-in-law in residence, it may be easier on you if you can delay her arrival until the baby is 2 or 3 months old. By then you will have settled in, gained confidence, and won't be as vulnerable to being dominated—something many women worry about.

➤ *Neighbors and friends can do you a great favor* by bringing over a cooked meal. If anyone asks what they can do for you, say that a casserole you can freeze would be a wonderful gift. This way you can count on having a few meals taken care of, which takes pressure off you. If any of these women are familiar with babies they also might be willing (or even eager) to stay with the baby for a few hours if you want to do things out of the house and don't want to take the newborn along.

➤ *Stock up on disposable plates and napkins*, even if you don't ordinarily use them for aesthetic or ecological reasons. You can also use frozen foods, takeout food, and any other possible shortcut in the postpartum period. You should not feel guilty about this legitimate use of convenience products. You deserve all the help you can get!

THE EMOTIONAL ADJUSTMENT AFTER BIRTH

The birth of a child is one of the more stressful events in a person's life. One study showed that a death in the family was the most stressful life event and that childbirth was the second most. Regardless of how much you may have wanted the baby, how ready you are for it, and how positive your birth experience may have been, it is still an enormous upheaval of your life.

In the immediate postpartum period you may feel exhilarated by the baby's birth and then perhaps experience some "blues" (see "Postpartum Depression," page 496). The second stage of postpartum adjustment is the reality of actually coping. There is the incredible fatigue from the lack of uninterrupted sleep, the stress of incorporating the new little person into your life, your changing role with your mate, and the baby's constant needs.

New motherhood can create a conflict nowadays. Our society makes it difficult for women to pursue their own goals while providing good care for their children at the same time. A woman may want to get out and work, or do something more with her life than housewifery—but there are still the dishes to do, the baby to feed, and no easy solutions for how to incorporate both. You may feel caught between the heavy responsibility of your child and your personal interests and drives. These are all problems you have to begin to face and solve in the postpartum period.

➤ *Do not try to be Supermom.* If you try to live up to whatever idea you have of a "perfect mother," you are bound to feel inadequate. There are aspects of caring for a baby that may bore or annoy you. *Accept yourself* and what you do and do not like about baby-tending. If you can do that, then others—the baby included—will accept it, too. It is not "bad" to dislike constantly changing a baby's diapers.

Don't trap yourself with some image of Supermom, who enjoys the endless tasks of baby care, can give a splendid dinner party, and is also a well-organized interior decorator. For instance, you may enjoy breast-feeding but be annoyed that you have to get up twice in the night to do it. This is a legitimate reaction but may be more honest than those around you are used to.

➤ *Differentiate between your "fantasy" mother and reality.* A fantasy mother is what you're "supposed" to be like. You form your ideas about a fantasy mother from the fairy tales you heard as a child, from television and movies, and from books and magazines. Everybody's fantasy mother is some form of Supermom, but what they all have in common is that they are unrealistic—no woman can live up to those expectations. If you have a demanding fantasy mother, always "telling" you how you should be doing things, you won't ever do things "right." It doesn't give you a chance to be kind to yourself—to give yourself strokes for the things you *have* done "right"—to let yourself off the hook from unnecessary and unrealistic demands.

Try to recognize the fantasy mother within yourself and *listen only to the good messages.* For instance, if your fantasy mother says you should always look lovely, no matter what, then *do* set time aside for a hot bath, a nap in the shade, or a pedicure. It is important for your sense of well-being to pamper yourself at times. But if your fantasy mother says that your *house* should always look lovely, so that if anyone were to drop in everything would be tidy, tell her to buzz off! Decide for yourself which messages are good and then disregard the ones that don't make sense or have any real value.

➤ *Tune out everybody else's theories* about caring for a newborn and parenting. If you get into discussions with people—about breast-feeding, about when to introduce solid foods, about whether a baby should wear shoes or not—everyone knows what is "right." It is not unlike childbirth itself, when everyone knew the Right Way and tried to convince you of it. If you disagree with any of these well-meaning advice-givers, they may make you feel like a "bad mother." Get all the facts you need and then trust your own instincts and judgment.

➤ *Criticism of any kind may be very hard to take* in the postpartum period. You may be hypersensitive to any critical comments. This is part of the adjustment period, and although it helps to know that it is not uncommon, understanding it intellectually may not lessen your feelings of anger and defensiveness.

➤ *A feeling of motherhood* is something you may not experience right away. It has to grow on some women, and that takes time. However, there is a social image that says a woman is automatically infused with a joyous desire to love and nurture a new baby. You *might* feel that way, but you also may be slow to warm up to this new role. Do not feel guilty or as if something is wrong with you. It takes time for you and the baby to get to know each other. Motherhood is not unlike an old-fashioned prearranged marriage: you've never met each other, but all of a sudden you're "stuck" with each other for the rest of your lives! It's understandable that you might want to ease into it slowly; feelings of loving warmth, protectiveness, and involvement in the baby's development will grow eventually.

➤ *A fear of incompetence is perfectly normal.* In America, most girls and women are isolated from birth and babies—they don't have a chance to learn baby care by watching. Just because you are a woman does not mean that you instinctively know how to care for a baby. Experience is essential—seeing someone else do it, or doing it ourselves, is how we learn.

You do not have to perform perfectly. Tell yourself this when you start to get anxious or feel inept. Everyone feels uneasy at first. A newborn is tiny and fragile and mysterious, but if you are reasonably intelligent there's very little you can do to harm him. By trial and error you'll figure things out. The important thing is to ease up if you're making unrealistic demands on yourself. It is really okay not to know how to handle a new baby. Call someone and ask for help. Read a baby-care book. One thing's for sure: before long it will be second nature to you.

➤ *Allow yourself to have negative feelings about the baby.* There will be ways in which you feel put-upon by the burdens of baby care. It's all right not only to have those feelings but to voice them. A baby turns your life upside down and you're more than entitled to resent that. It is okay to feel jealous that your mate may come home and go directly to the baby instead of to you. Just as it is normal and healthy to have ambivalent feelings about getting pregnant, it is equally healthy to have misgivings about motherhood. It's not all fun or exciting—there's a lot of drudgery. It is fine to feel negative at times and it's good for you to admit that. If you try to swallow these feelings they will undoubtedly surface in your relationship with the baby. It would be much better to get it off your chest by talking about it—or by rearranging your schedules or priorities—than to be a martyr with bottled-up resentment.

Isolation

➤ *You may feel horribly isolated after the baby is born.* A new mother needs support and guidance in learning baby care and also holding on to her identity. You may find yourself home alone for eight hours or more. You will be deprived of adult recognition and the strokes and interchange that take place during an intelligent adult conversation. It can be depressing if you are stuck at home all day without any support and only a tiny baby for company.

➤ *Loving helpers, guidance from experienced women*, and the exchange of affection are all as important as good food and rest in the postpartum period. A woman can feel cut off from other adults, which can lead to apathy. Many women feel sad in the immediate postpartum period, but if they have close contact and support, the stroking they receive can end the sadness that could progress to depression. The hormonal imbalance and physical adjustments after birth can affect your emotions—you have to work to overcome that.

➤ *Before the baby is born, you should seek out friends* who have had experience with babies. If you don't know any, then you should try to find an organization of parents. Some childbirth instructors hold postpartum classes and the La Leche League and others have parent "rap sessions." You can also arrange to visit women from your childbirth class after birth. You are all going through the same stage of adjustment together and just knowing you aren't alone is a big help.

➤ *For those women who have or want their mother around,* she can be a wonderful source of love and encouragement.

➤ *It is important to get away from your house,* either with or without the baby, for a short or long outing every day. It helps you maintain a sense of identity—that you still interact with the outside world even though the main focus of your life right now is at home with the baby. Get used to using baby-sitters early on—it's good for you to have the independence and it's good for the baby to get accustomed to not having you around constantly.

TAKE CARE OF YOURSELF

➤ *Nurture yourself*—it is too easy to fall into the trap of feeling that everything is more important than your own "selfish" needs. "Selfish" is *not* a bad word. In fact, it's important for your own well-being and that of your family that you are selfish at times. If you are not rested and satisfied with your life, everyone will be cheated. You will have less patience, feel resentful, and it will come out in the way you deal with the baby and other children, your mate, and your career if you're working. Everyone loses out if you aren't good to yourself.

➤ *Be a baby yourself* when you feel like it. Especially in the beginning you may feel overwhelmed by the responsibilities and constant demands of a newborn. It may all seem like too much for one person to handle and still keep her sanity and sense of humor. Listen to those feelings. Turn to your mother or your mate or a close friend and let them baby you a little. It's important to get your perspective on this new role of motherhood and realize that it does not mean you have to be on top of things all the time: caring for the baby, running the house and perhaps also a business. There are people to take care of you, too, if you let them.

➤ *Set aside time for yourself and no one else.* Use it however you want to—and don't feel it has to be practical or constructive. Use your private time to write letters or in a journal, to do exercises, to read a great novel or a trashy magazine, to make yourself a dress, or to take a walk. Or just to nap. You may be amazed at how all-consuming a new baby can seem—unless you make a point of protecting a certain piece of each day for yourself. Ask yourself, "What can I do for fun every day?" Listen to music, read while you nurse the baby, dance in front of the mirror—whatever gives you pleasure.

➤ *Set up priorities for yourself.* Unless you have help, it is not going to be possible to run an organized household with everything tidy, washing and ironing done, great meals, a well-loved baby, and time for yourself. Something has to give. Decide what you will give up: it might be ironing. It might be that you used to cook elaborate meals and now will simplify cooking. You might give up the idea that it's necessary to have a kitchen floor that is always spotless. Something has to go: you have to make a purposeful decision what it will be and then really let it go. Do not be a slave to your house or baby—skip certain chores. Leave things until "tomorrow." You'll drive yourself nuts otherwise.

Now decide what you will *not* give up. There may be activities in your life that are not essential, but in determining your priorities there will be things to protect. It might be playing the piano; it might be planting a flower or vegetable garden; it might be going to an exercise class; it might be cooking a fancy dish. Whatever nurtures you is what you should be determined not to lose in the midst of the new responsibilities a baby brings.

POSTPARTUM DEPRESSION

"Baby blues," or postpartum depression, affects anywhere from 15 to 80% of women. It usually lasts one to seven days and is marked by tearfulness, anxiety, depression, restlessness, and irritability.

➤ *Hormones are a major reason for this emotional unpleasantness.* It is caused by the precipitous drop in the amount of estrogen and progesterone in your system after delivery or by an imbalance in the two hormones. Women who have difficulty adjusting to changing hormone levels in the premenstrual period tend to have greater difficulty adjusting to hormone levels postpartum, meaning that they are more sensitive to hormonal fluctuations.

➤ *Lowered thyroid function may be related to postpartum depression.* The psychosomatic nature of pregnancy (the way in which your body affects your emotions) should not be ignored. If you're feeling low for quite a while after the baby's birth, you should have your thyroid levels checked. There may be a relation between low thyroid and emotional/social stress, which childbirth certainly is. In one study it was found that third-time mothers had lower thyroid levels in their blood than first-time mothers, indicating that pregnancy may inhibit thyroid activity, which in turn is linked to how you feel.

➤ *A woman's psychological makeup influences postpartum blues*. The way that you deal with new situations in general and the way that you feel about yourself will be reflected in how you handle a new baby. The inability to master and control a new event in your life can bring on a depression. If you are a very dependent person, or are preoccupied with meeting your own dependency needs, or if your sense of identity is not clear, you may have difficulty adjusting to maternal responsibilities. If you are a chronically anxious person you are more likely to have anxiety-stress reaction in the postpartum period. If you have ambivalent feelings about femininity or mothering, you may get depressed. And a woman who has had many life adjustments will deal differently with postpartum problems than a woman for whom this is the first major stress in her life.

➤ *It is difficult to predict postpartum adjustment by the way that you adjusted psychologically during pregnancy.* Sometimes a serene pregnancy can lead to a rough postpartum. This can be true of a woman who hasn't fully faced what is happening—she may admit she is pregnant but deep down refuses to believe that she'll actually have a child. Perhaps she hasn't prepared herself for motherhood but has sailed through pregnancy as if she didn't have a worry. A postpartum disturbance may reflect her inability to accept the new situation.

Some women have negative or ambivalent feelings during pregnancy but don't seek help, hoping that childbirth will solve everything. It is safe to say that for women like this the arrival of the baby just makes things more complicated. And if these women finally face their problems once the baby is born, they may feel it's "too late" to do anything about it, which can then lead to depression unless they get help sorting out their feelings.

➤ *A lack of support for new mothers can lead to depression.* In "the old days" a woman was surrounded by helpful kinfolk and neighbors when she had a new baby. In our society today a new mother often has no actual support and is also cut off from the mainstream of life when she is alone at home with the baby.

Postpartum blues may also come from the loss of the supportive relationship with her doctor or midwife. During pregnancy a woman may have turned to them for support—in fact, a woman might have been using complaints of physical symptoms to mask emotional problems—and now that support system has ended.

THE "MISSING PIECES" SYNDROME

"Missing pieces" is a psychological syndrome which affects some women after birth. They repress or forget aspects of their labor and delivery and experience frustration, anger, and tears when they try to remember and are unable to.

SIGNS OF "MISSING PIECES" SYNDROME

* *You are obsessive:* talking and asking about your birth experience over and over. Other people may make fun of you or become annoyed.

* *You may have dreams* with a recurrent theme and hope that the missing components will come to you this way.

* *You may feel you haven't slept well*, feel fatigued when you wake up, and feel lethargic during the day.

* *You may be unable to focus* on the present situation and be preoccupied with finding the missing links in your birth experience. You may have little or no interest in the baby.

The reasons for "missing pieces" are:
A long labor, which may result in confusion and a loss of a sense of how events took place.

A rapid labor, which makes it hard to put sequences in a logical order or understand what is happening at the time: a sensory overload. Because labor was going so fast, you may have gotten less information from your attendants about your progress at the time.

Any high-risk condition during labor causes stress and anxiety so that you do not hear what's said to you or may forget it later. Especially when there is an unexpected cesarean, a woman is vulnerable to forgetting important areas of the experience.

Unfulfilled expectations which don't integrate with the actual outcome of the birth may mean that your energies were directed to coping with your grief over your unmet expectations rather than focusing on the events of the birth.

Medications which are administered can affect your alertness and sense of the passage of time. Also the conditions requiring the use of drugs—complications or a lengthy labor—may cause you anxiety. You also may have been upset because you felt strongly about avoiding drugs, but you accepted them because you couldn't cope with the contractions.

> ➤ *There are several ways to deal with the "missing pieces" syndrome.* Get information from your mate and the medical personnel. Do not accept the attitude that your requests are silly, stupid, or unimportant. Fill in the gaps you can't remember by talking to those who shared the event with you. The important thing is to integrate the birth experience for yourself so that you are satisfied.

> ➤ *Get professional help with any postpartum disturbance that lasts longer than one to two weeks.* "Baby blues" are caused by any or all of the reasons listed (pages 496–498), but do not normally last longer than a week or two. If you find yourself depressed or unable to cope with your life after the baby is born, seek outside help. If you don't do this, problems can become magnified and your depression can deepen and damage your physical health, as well as the health of your relationship with the baby and your partner.

THE MAN'S POSTPARTUM REACTIONS

The father's adjustment postpartum has many of the same elements as your adjustment, although in most cases a man will be away at work all day whereas you'll be home with the child at least in the first weeks. Perhaps the most common feeling a man has is that the baby comes first and gets all the attention—in some relationships the man may have had that position with his wife and now feels displaced by the baby. The truth is that the baby *is* getting most of your time and attention, especially at first; then you may be so tired by the time your mate gets home that you just want to lie down. There are several ways to insure that your mate doesn't feel slighted and to make time for yourselves apart from the baby. It's as important for you as it is for the man.

Ways to Stay Close as a Couple

> ➤ *If you find you're exhausted* by the end of the day (which is when your mate probably comes home from a fairly demanding

day himself), why not take a nap together? It can give you a lovely sense of closeness and intimacy while replenishing your energy.

➢ *Set aside certain special time together*—it may seem a little contrived, but it also may be the only way you're sure to protect your need to have time alone. A new baby can turn your lives so topsy-turvy that it *seems* as if it just isn't possible anymore for you two to go off together. It is possible—it just takes some planning.

➢ *Nothing can be as easy and spontaneous as it was* before the baby was born. Everything you do now has to take the baby into account. Either you have to take the baby along, or you have to arrange for someone else to look after her. Do not make the mistake of feeling that it's more effort than it's worth—it is extremely important for you and your mate to have time to yourselves. A baby puts a big strain on a relationship and you can't just sit back and expect that everything will fall into place on its own. Making time for yourselves doesn't necessarily mean elaborate planning—once you are committed to the idea it can be quite simple.

➢ *Decide what you most enjoyed doing together* pre-baby or what you would like to start doing now. It might just mean setting aside the forty-five minutes when your mate comes home as a time to put your feet up, have a drink, and talk about the day or play cards. Maybe you'd like to go out to the movies once a week. Perhaps it means going for a drive on Saturday afternoon and having an ice-cream soda. If you play tennis together, make a permanent "date" to have two hours to do it on Sundays. It really isn't important what you do—all that matters is that you recognize the health of your relationship depends on sustaining some of the intimacy and closeness that a new baby can disrupt *if you let him.*

➢ *Two is company, three's a crowd.* Think of that cliché as it applies to you and your mate and the baby. It's fine to take the baby along on certain outings, and it's nice if you want to include him. But there is a difference between just the two of you window-shopping and what it's like with a baby and all the paraphernalia along. Having a baby in your lives changes the way you feel about yourselves individually and how you relate to each other—welcome the change, but also hold on to the way you were beforehand. Many marriages suffer soon after a baby is born because the partners are not aware that the need for *twoness* continues.

Five Factors Which Influence a Father's Adjustment

1. *Preparation for parenting can make a man more relaxed and confident* about the new baby and able to enjoy her more.

If at all possible you and your mate should see infant-care demonstrations either at a hospital, through the American Red Cross, or wherever they are offered in your community. Most men feel shut out of their baby's early months because they don't know how to do anything and are afraid to make mistakes. Men can feel inadequate because they don't know how to feed, bathe, or diaper a baby—they're afraid the baby will cry because they aren't doing something right and then they won't know how to stop it.

A terrible mistake made by many new mothers, who are anxious themselves, is to give all sorts of instructions to their mate when he's got the baby and then to criticize the way he's doing it. If you watch a new mother and father, you're apt to hear her saying, "No, you're squeezing her leg, hold her head up," or: "Hold her higher up to burp her." It's no wonder that fathers feel so inept and fearful—how would you feel if every time you went to pick up your baby or feed him there was someone giving you orders ahead of time about how to do it and then giving you negative feedback?

Keep in mind that it is the man's baby, too. The implied message of the way many women treat their mates is "Okay, you can have my baby for a little while, but you better not mess up . . . Oh no, you messed up, I was afraid of that." Keep your mouth shut. Your mate isn't going to harm the baby—he's as protective of her as you are and is reasonably intelligent. He is not going to choke the baby or drop her on her head. So what if he doesn't keep the bottle of juice at the exact angle *you* think is best? He'll work it out by trial and error if you leave him alone and let him pick up the cues from the baby.

If you find you simply cannot button your lip—that you just *have* to butt in with some important tidbit of advice—then leave the room while he's with the baby. It's quite common for women to cluck and complain that the baby's father doesn't share care, yet those women will not recognize that they have driven the men away. The most important reason to let a man get used to his baby is *not* so that he can change a diaper or play patty-cake when you want to take a bath. The more essential reason is that a man deserves the opportunity to be intimate with his child. *If you badger him you are depriving him of his rights.*

It is lovely for the baby to receive care from her father and that nurturing can be wonderful for the man, too. He will be able to experience himself in a new way—expand the ways in which he gives and receives love, setting the foundation for the kind of parenting that men have often been excluded from. Given a choice, most fathers would want to have greater involvement with their child than bouncing her on their knee for 10 minutes at the end of the day. When a man learns that he can "mother" too—that this enriching experience is not the private territory of women—it can give him much pleasure and satisfaction. It is within your power to give your mate that chance—the same chance you have.

2. ***Agreement about roles is another aspect of a man's adjustment.*** Couples who discuss and agree on the ways to share and divide basic family tasks have an easier time. Couples who don't make an agreement usually fall into the pattern of woman-does-everything-in-the-house-and-for-the-baby, man-does-his-thing-outside-the-home. More often than not this unplanned arrangement makes the woman feel resentful—which she lets the man know in both subtle and overt ways—and makes him defensive or guilt-ridden in return. It also can make the man feel excluded from the baby's care yet burdened with the responsibilities of his work, which may pressure him more with the added expense of the child.

    Men tend to adopt either the Breadwinner role or the Equal Parent role, in which infant care is shared, although usually not 50–50, since he's not home during the day. Both are effective patterns to cope with the stresses and strains *as long as both partners feel comfortable.* That is at the heart of the matter—and you won't straighten it out unless you both discuss how you feel, what you'd ideally like, and what can realistically be done.

3. ***Support from his workplace is important to a man's adjustment.*** For instance, the option of flexible-hour scheduling, so that a man can come home early to give the new mother a break, can mean the difference between success and failure at creating a situation that works well for all three of you. A man should talk to his employers before the baby is born and try to get some flexibility from them, at least in the early postpartum period.

4. ***Support from families is important to good beginnings for a new family.*** If the baby's grandparents have respect for the new parents' wishes to be alone—yet also visit, bring gifts, and give steady encouragement—it can be an important support structure. Nowadays people live so cut off from each other and the nuclear family is so isolating that to have the support of one's family and extended family can be a great comfort. It can give you the feeling that you aren't out there all alone, struggling to make order out of the instant chaos that a baby creates.

5. ***The health of the baby and his disposition can be an important factor in*** the ease with which a father adjusts. A baby who isn't healthy can cause feelings of rage, guilt, desperation, exhaustion, and helplessness. A fussy baby who cries often can create these feelings on a smaller scale. There really isn't much you can do to improve these situations except hope that a sickly baby will gain his health and a less-than-sweet-tempered one will grow more mellow.

CHAPTER FIFTEEN

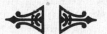

Taking Care of Baby

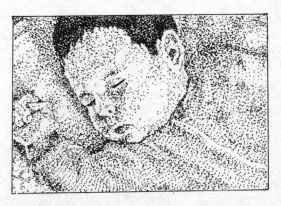

Most pregnancy and childbirth books end right at the birth of the baby—which is sort of like leading you down a road and stopping at the edge of a cliff! Although this chapter is by no means a complete guide to newborn baby care, it is an attempt to present some aspects which may involve consumer decisions on your part: choosing a pediatrician, circumcision, buying baby things, diet after weaning, etc. There is also a section on "what to expect"—bringing a newborn home is a thrilling, exhausting, and sometimes overwhelming experience. Many new parents in America have never been around little babies until they have their own: this chapter lets you know which "strange" aspects are actually normal and also how to recognize symptoms that require a doctor's care.

CHOOSING A PEDIATRICIAN

This is something you should do before the baby is born. Some pediatricians will meet with you and your partner without charge when you are pregnant. If you have chosen a doctor beforehand, it can be a relief not to have to scramble around for professional advice if questions or problems arise in the early postpartum weeks.

Also, if there are nonroutine procedures that you want in the hospital you can ask your pediatrician to make requests before the birth. If you want to nurse on the delivery table, want your baby with you in the recovery area or released from the stabilization nursery quickly, or if you don't want the baby to receive any artificial nipples, you have a better chance of a positive reaction from the hospital staff if arrangements have been made through a medical channel. If you choose a pediatrician ahead of time, the hospital notifies the doctor as soon as the baby is born and she or he will come to do the first examination rather than a hospital staff pediatrician. The doctor may submit a separate bill for this or it may be part of the total fee for first-year baby-care visits.

Factors to Consider

- ➤ *The office location can be important* if transportation is a problem. It helps not to have to go far if you have to bring a sick child to the doctor.
- ➤ *What is the waiting room like?* Is it cozy? Is it geared to children, with small chairs and toys and books? Just as you can tell quite a bit about people from their living rooms, you can tell something about a pediatrician from his waiting room. If the waiting room has a formal adult-oriented decor, this can tell you about the pediatrician's attitude toward children.
- ➤ *House calls are a fast-disappearing luxury*, but pediatricians are just about the only doctors who will sometimes make them. If you have a feverish baby and it is wintertime, it is preferable not to have to take her outdoors. Ask whether the doctor will make house calls and, if so, under what circumstances.
- ➤ *How busy is the practice?* You shouldn't have to call too far ahead for an appointment and you should be able to come in quickly in an emergency.
- ➤ *Does he or she have a group practice?* If the pediatrician shares the practice with one or more doctors, will your child see a different doctor each time? A child feels more secure with continuity and stability, and it is preferable for you and the child to develop a relationship with the pediatrician you choose—rather than having to try to relate to the doctor(s) he or she has chosen to practice with. It is understandable if the other doctors handle telephone calls or emergencies in the evenings or on weekends, for example, but you should find out ahead of time.
- ➤ *Personality is the first important criterion* in choosing a pediatrician. Does she or he seem warm toward children? Do you and your mate feel at ease with the doctor, comfortable

asking questions, and satisfied with the replies? Does the doctor treat you as equals or is she or he patronizing?

➤ *The doctor's style of child rearing* will affect you even if you view a pediatrician as there only for medical problems. In the areas of health and nutrition, for example, a doctor's attitudes about how to raise a child are tied up with decisions about when and what to feed. Does the doctor prefer a rigid style of raising children? For instance, does he or she have an automatic date for the introduction of solid foods, as opposed to introducing them when the baby is ready? There is no "right" way—whatever makes you more comfortable is best. Precise instructions make some parents feel more secure; they make some parents, who might prefer things more loose and unstructured, feel hemmed in.

➤ *Breast-feeding is an area in* which there will be problems if you don't share the same views as a pediatrician. If you choose *not* to breast-feed and a doctor strongly recommends nursing for all patients, then you may feel pressured and judged if you bottle-feed. And if you *want* to breast-feed, you may have a tough time unless a pediatrician is actively supportive. It is not enough for a doctor's attitude to be, "Sure, breast-feeding is fine with me." Especially if you are a first-taking mother, you are going to need encouragement and help from everyone around you.

For example: a doctor is *not* supportive if his or her response to problems you have is to suggest supplementing breast-feeding with formula. And a doctor who recommends the early introduction of solids is not actively supporting breast-feeding. Discuss nursing with a pediatrician ahead of time and make sure that your beliefs are compatible.

➤ *A good attitude toward a working mother* is essential in a pediatrician. If you are going to work when your baby is small, you're going to have to contend with a negative response from various people—there's no sense in adding to your burden by paying a professional to add to the negativism! A doctor's disapproval can undermine your confidence in your mothering. His or her attitude may come out in subtle ways—small comments about you being gone all day when the baby is sick, for instance—and can make you uncomfortable. The problems will only be greater if you are breast-feeding and working. It is important to find a pediatrician who respects your personal goals independent of your child. The baby is the patient, so the child's welfare will be the primary concern—if he or she feels that a mother who works is "cheating" her child, then isn't the doctor for you.

➤ *Circumcision is a decision* you should make before the baby is born and discuss with a pediatrician. A doctor can give you his opinion about the pros and cons, but the decision ultimately rests with you: the section on circumcision that follows should help you decide. If you have a strong opinion either way, you should find a pediatrician who is either noncommittal or agrees with you.

> *Be sure to contact any doctors* you meet if you decide not to choose them. This is an important courtesy, especially if they did not charge you for the interview.

> *Once you have chosen a pediatrician* it's good to know when you should call. Many new parents worry about calling a doctor too much for seemingly unimportant matters that nevertheless concern them. On the other hand, there are times a doctor should be contacted because the baby's symptom *may* be a signal of a problem.

WARNING SIGNS! CALL DOCTOR IF BABY HAS THESE SYMPTOMS

* EXCESSIVE CRYING and unusual irritability
* EXCESSIVE DROWSINESS; sleeping at times when he/she usually plays
* POOR SLEEP with frequent waking, restlessness, and crying
* FEVER with a rectal thermometer; flushed face, hot and dry skin
* SEVERE LOSS OF APPETITE; refusal to take familiar foods
* REPEATED VOMITING; throwing up most of a feeding more than once
* BOWEL MOVEMENTS WITH BLOOD or pus, mucus, a green color, or unusually loose or frequent stools
* COUGH OR SEVERE RUNNY NOSE
* INFLAMMATION OR DISCHARGE FROM EYES
* RASH that covers a large portion of the body or persists after changing laundry habits
* TWITCHING, CONVULSIONS, INABILITY TO MOVE
* PAIN

CIRCUMCISION

Circumcision has been a routine procedure in this country for many years. It is now being questioned by health professionals and parents who are unsure of the medical advantages of circumcision. Also, people have begun to worry about the pain and trauma to newborn babies from this surgical procedure.

The practice of circumcision came from ancient Semitic cultures, when there were months of traveling across deserts without water to bathe in. This is obviously not applicable to life in modern society, although Jewish parents usually want to continue to have their baby boys circumcised for reasons of religious tradition.

The American Academy of Pediatrics, in contradiction to its earlier recommendation against routine circumcision, suggests that newborn circumcision has potential medical benefits and advantages. The AAP recommends discussion between parents and pediatricians of the disadvantages and risks.

Recent evidence has shown that uncircumcised newborn males are 10 to 15 times more likely to have a urinary tract infection (UTI) than circumcised infants. Because of these findings, the AAP formed a new task force on circumcision and released a report in April of 1989, modifying its firm stance opposing routine neonatal circumcision. The report stated that "circumcision may result in a decreased incidence of urinary tract infections" and that "evidence concerning the association of sexually transmitted disease and circumcision is conflicting." Further studies are needed about this controversial subject before the final word is written.

Sixty percent of American boys are circumcised, but some parents are rebelling against surgically altering the natural design of the body, particularly when it means causing their babies unnecessary pain. Although expectant couples usually try to learn everything they can about pregnancy, birth, and infant care, it is rare for them to question circumcision. Couples learn about nutrition, drugs, prepared-childbirth techniques, and breast-feeding, but often the only thing they know about circumcision is that it's done because "that's the way a penis is supposed to look and it's cleaner."

Those parents who have had their babies circumcised and regret it recommend that a couple attend a circumcision before deciding to have it done to their son. They believe that few parents would consent if they had to be present at their baby's circumcision and saw what is involved.

> *A description of circumcision*. The baby is placed on his back in a "circumstraint," a plastic tray in which his arms and legs are strapped down. Sterile drapes are placed over him with a hole through which his penis is exposed. A hemostat is applied to the tip of the foreskin to crush it and a slit is made to enlarge the tip. A small instrument is then used to reach inside the tip of the penis to separate the foreskin from the glans, two layers of skin which normally adhere to each other.

There are several different methods of circumcision. In one method a metal clamp is placed over the foreskin for about five minutes to control postoperative bleeding. Then the foreskin is cut off and the clamp removed. Alternatively, a small protective bell is placed over the glans and under the foreskin. In this method a string is tied tightly over the foreskin and the plastic bell. Some of the foreskin in front of the string is trimmed away and then a plastic ring is left around the end of the penis. The remaining foreskin atrophies (dries up) in about a week and the plastic ring then falls off. Yet another method is for the foreskin to be cut off with a knife or scissors; then stitches are put in to control the bleeding or sometimes a cauterizing needle is used.

➤ *No anesthetic is used*. This is tied to a belief that newborns' nervous systems are not yet fully developed so they do not feel as much pain as later on. The degree to which the baby suffers is not known, although there has never been a scientific study which could support the theory that babies have little or no feelings. But when a circumcision is performed on an older child or man, it is considered painful enough to use anesthesia.

The American Academy of Pediatrics notes that circumcision has "inherent disadvantages and risks"; the academy acknowledges that the baby experiences pain in the procedure and for a few hours afterward. There is a new local anesthesia technique called a dorsal penile block that can eliminate the newborn's pain and reduce his distress during circumcision. However, the academy cautions that there is only limited experience with the technique. Instead of generally recommending local anesthesia for newborn circumcision, the academy has recommended waiting for the results of large, scientific studies on the possible risks of this procedure.

➤ *Misinformation about circumcision is rampant*. Despite what was believed at one time, circumcision does not reduce the occurrence of cancers. It was previously thought that there was less penile and prostate cancer and less cervical cancer in women who had intercourse with circumcised men. It has been found that venereal disease and a lack of good hygiene in uncircumcised men was the cause of the higher cancer rate, not the lack of circumcision itself.

➤ *It has never been proven that circumcised men* can hold an erection for longer. It has also never been proven that uncircumcised men have greater sexual pleasure.

➤ *Good hygiene is a viable alternative to circumcision*, but many people seem misinformed about it. They are concerned when they are told that smegma collects under the foreskin and must be washed away. However, smegma is the same substance that collects on female genitals and is regularly washed away. Children are taught to wash behind their ears and to brush their teeth, so there is reason why a boy cannot be taught to wash his penis.

The general belief is that circumcision is "cleaner" and that care of a child's intact (uncircumcised) penis is difficult. A doctor may forcibly retract the infant's foreskin in the hospital or when the baby comes into the office for a visit. Sometimes parents are instructed to retract and clean under the baby's foreskin every day. Manipulating the foreskin forcefully is not a good idea. It can be more traumatic for the baby than circumcision, since that happens only one time. The normally tight and nonretractable foreskin of the infant should be left alone until it gradually loosens on its own, which can take up to 3 or 4 years. Ninety-five percent of infants have a nonretractable foreskin at birth. Eighty-five percent are nonretractable at 6 months, and 50% remain so at one year of age. This is normal. The foreskin is not expected to retract easily until 2 years or older. In some boys the foreskin is not fully retractable until late puberty.

Hygienic Care of Uncircumcised Infants

➤ The newborn's foreskin should not be manipulated in the first days of life.
➤ Parents should not retract the foreskin for cleaning. Some doctors may recommend doing this, but it can cause unnecessary problems.
➤ A parent should show the son how to retract his foreskin and wash his penis when he is four years old. He should be supervised for a while and then expected to care for himself.

Sex identification with the father, male siblings, and other boys later on in school is often a reason for circumcision. Some psychologists believe that a boy has an easier time making a sex identification with his father and other close male figures if his penis looks the same as theirs. Also, a boy who has a foreskin may suffer some social stigma when he goes to school and most of the other boys have been circumcised. However, with 40% of American boys now uncircumcised, chances of being the "only one" are unlikely. The locker rooms of the twenty-first century will have boys with both kinds of penises.

As for a boy's identification with his father, there are other significant differences between the adult and child penis, besides the foreskin or lack of it (size, pubic hair, testicles, etc.). Those who favor leaving boys intact also suggest that parents can help children learn to respect differences with other people, whether it's the other person's penis, nose, or other personal aspects.

If you decide to circumcise your child, there are several pointers to keep in mind:
— The procedure should not be performed right after birth in the delivery room. At some hospitals this is done for the doctor's convenience. It is unfair to the newborn baby, who is coping with the difficult adjustment to life outside the womb (leaving aside the issue of how much pain the baby does or does not feel at this stage).
— Circumcision should be delayed at least until 12 to 24 hours after birth.
— The baby's weight must be considered. If he weighs less

than 6 pounds, the doctor may want to delay the operation until the baby is larger.

— The mother or father may want to hold the baby for the procedure, as this might lessen the trauma for the infant.

— Care of the penis after circumcision involves applying petroleum jelly to help protect it until it has healed.

Immunization of the baby is usually begun at 2 months of age. Most pediatricians believe that the medications should be begun at this early age because they prevent diseases which can take a child's life. However, some doctors are questioning whether exposure to these powerful medications could be safely delayed until the child is a bit older. If you have questions about the timing of immunization, take it up with your doctor, although most doctors do adhere to the immunization schedule on the chart below.

Free immunization is available through many health departments. Contact your local county health department for information.

IMMUNIZATION CALENDAR

2 months:	DTP 3-in-1 shot (Diphtheria, Tetanus, Pertussis)
	Sabin Oral live polio vaccine
4 months:	DTP booster
	Polio booster
6 months:	DTP booster
1 year:	Tuberculin test
15 months:	Measles/rubella vaccine
	Mumps vaccine
	Hepatitis now recommended
18 months:	DTP booster
2 years:	Polio booster
	HIB vaccine (hemophilus influenza type B)
4 to 6 years:	DTP booster
	Polio booster

PKU TEST

This test is done to screen all babies after birth. Some hospitals administer this screening test between the second and fourth day of life, others wait until the sixth or fourteenth day. PKU is a rare metabolic disorder (occurring one in 10,000 births) that causes mental retardation. There is no cure, but the disease can be controlled through diet, which is why all babies are tested. If both parents have PKU, then all offspring will inherit it. If another family member already has PKU, then a baby with a negative PKU test should be retested at one, 2, and 6 weeks of life to be absolutely sure. A small blood sample is obtained by pricking the baby's heel.

If a baby has PKU she lacks the ability to metabolize an amino acid called phenylalanine. All natural proteins contain an average of 5% of this amino acid. Excessive amounts of phenylalanine build up in the bloodstream and cause severe mental retardation and/or brain damage. The untreated symptoms of PKU are irritability, hyperactivity, vomiting, convulsions, skin rashes or severe eczema, a musty barnlike odor with urine or sweat. Treatment involves excluding milk, meat, eggs, and cheese from the diet and substituting specially formulated Lofenalac milk for as long as the major portion of brain growth occurs, or several years.

NAMING THE BABY

This may pose a problem for couples who are not married or who are married but each use their own last names.

> *It is only custom which dictates that a baby take his father's surname*. If parents, married or not, use different surnames, a child can be given either one's surname on a birth certificate.
>
> There are other alternatives for naming a baby when a couple wants to exercise their freedom in choosing a name. You can hyphenate last names, use one last name as a middle name, use one first name as a middle name and one last name as the baby's surname. There is also the possibility of combining both parents last names (without a hyphen) into a whole new name (a recent example of this would be one of Robert Kennedy's daughters, who named her child [by Governor Cuomo's son] Kennedy-Cuomo).

> *State laws differ and can be challenged in court*. Find out the laws in your state. Do not accept what is told you by a clerk. People who stand behind counters and work for the government have an unpleasant way of "laying down the law." They may not know any better, but they accept "common practice" (i.e., what most people do) as law—which it is not. Do not allow an officious clerk to intimidate you.

> *In Massachusetts, Virginia, Florida and other states*, married couples have given the mother's birth-given surname to their children.

> *In common law, a child born to a married couple* does not automatically assume the *father's* surname. In common law, a child born to an unmarried couple does not automatically assume the *mother's* surname. This is also true for marriage: al-

though the custom is for women to give up their surnames and take their husbands', common law does not automatically dictate this.

➤ **The law allows you** to name your children as you please, but social habits are hard to break. You may encounter such resistance to children from a marriage being given the mother's surname that you may have to take legal action to enforce your rights. The social expectation is that the children from an *unmarried* couple will be given the mother's surname; there may be resistance if you want to give the baby the father's surname.

PREPARATION AND SUPPLIES FOR THE BABY

➤ **The baby's room should be painted** with nontoxic, non-yellowing paint. You should not repaint over old paint, because babies can get lead poisoning from flakes of old paint, and as they get older, babies put *everything* in their mouths.
➤ **A bassinet or cradle** is cute, but the baby will outgrow it quickly. Don't buy one, but if someone gives or lends you a cradle, you can use it until the baby gets bigger.

Requirements for a Crib

• Only borrow a crib if it meets these important safety factors:
• Bars no farther apart than 2⅜ inches, or the baby's head can get stuck between them.
• A railing 26 inches higher than the lowest level of the mattress support, so the baby can't climb over easily.
• A mattress that fits snugly, or a baby can get her head stuck between the mattress and crib.
• Smooth surfaces, safe and sturdy hardware, and a secure teething rail all the way around.
• A crib with one side-drop is more stable and less expensive than one in which both rails can be lowered.
• Crib guards make it safer and softer for the baby. *Never use pillows for this purpose*: they can smother the baby and are bad for posture.

WARNING: *Mesh-sided cribs and playpens can be dangerous if the sides are left down.* Children have suffocated when they rolled into the space between the mat and the loose mesh siding, when the sides were down. The government has sued nine manufacturers that make mesh-sided cribs and playpens; as a result there are now warning labels on the products. However, there are an estimated 6.5 million people with unlabeled products whose babies are in danger. When buying, look for a product with no gap at all between the mattress and sides. A child can become caught in a gap of as little as two inches. *Never, ever* leave a child in one of these cribs with the side down—always lock the hinges.

➤ ***Basic bedding needs:*** a waterproof mattress; 2 to 3 waterproof mattress pads; 2 quilted crib pads; 4 to 6 crib sheets; crib bumpers; 2 crib blankets or bag-type sleepers.

Miscellaneous

- A rectal thermometer.
- Blunt baby nail scissors, which are easiest to use when the baby is asleep.
- Premoistened wipe cloths, if there is no water nearby.
- Rubbing alcohol the for the umbilical cord until it falls off.
- Baby soap and mild, "no tears" shampoo.
- Diaper rash ointment (Desitin, Diaparene, Peri-anal; more economical is a one-pound plastic jar of zinc oxide from a pharmacy).
- CONTROVERSIAL: Some people say that oils and powders are bad for a baby's skin, but you'll have to judge for yourself. Talcum powder is ground rock. Alternatively you can use cornstarch; put it in a large salt shaker for convenience.
- DO NOT USE: Cotton swabs in either ears or nose—they can cause damage.
- Avoid mineral oil, which absorbs all the oil-soluble vitamins through the skin.
- A strap on the changing table is essential. If you're going to use a bureau top for changing, be sure to make a secure strap; babies can fall off easily in the time it takes you to turn around.
- A pacifier can be useful at times when the baby won't quiet down, or has the need to suck but you are not able to feed him right then, or has been fed but his sucking needs are not satisfied. Even parents with an adamant prejudice against pacifiers are usually won over by their usefulness. NUK brand—or another orthodontic model—is the most humanlike nipple; it is curved so that it doesn't harm the developing palate.

What About Diapers?

➤ ***Diapers*** are a decision you have to make for yourself, although most parents choose disposable diapers. Disposables are more expensive and add a lot of waste ecologically, but they are less trouble. They also protect better against leaks and reduce the chance of diaper rash.

Since most everyone leans toward using disposable diapers, here is some information about cloth diapers to balance out the scales. This is not an endorsement of one kind over the other, just an attempt to let you see both sides before you decide. You might consider trying a diaper service for a few weeks and comparing the two.

— **EVEN WITH A DIAPER SERVICE**, cloth diapers are less costly. *With a service*, you'll need 80 to 100 diapers a week.

— **IF YOU'RE GOING TO WASH THEM YOURSELF** every day, you need 2 dozen. If you're going to wash them every other day, you need 3 to 4 dozen. This staggering amount is an indication of why mothers have turned to disposable.

— **YOU'LL NEED 3 TO 6 PAIR OF WATERPROOF PANTS** to go over cloth diapers. You can also use diaper liners once the child has a schedule of bowel movements. That way you can lift the liner out and flush it away.

— **CLOTH DIAPERS WITH RUBBER PANTS OVER DO NOT LEAK** through the leg openings any more than disposable diapers.

— **IF YOU USE CLOTH DIAPERS** you may still want to use disposables when you travel. You can also use a disposable diaper opened up underneath the baby so that you don't make a mess if you're changing the baby at someone's house.

Baby Clothes

➢ *Hand-me-downs are sometimes softer* than newly purchased clothes because they are often made of 100% cotton instead of the fire-retardant synthetics used now.

➢ *Don't be bashful about accepting* other people's baby clothes—the child will grow out of them so quickly and it's wasteful to spend and accumulate your own basic clothing if there's someone willing to give (lend) you theirs.

➢ *The fire-retardant chemical TRIS* has been banned from use in sleepwear. Government tests showed that it can cause cancer and was absorbed through the baby's skin or ingested orally by sucking on pajama sleeves. Many of these products were on the market but not labeled as containing TRIS. Be very careful about sleepwear you buy.

➢ *Get the 6-month size* in any clothes for a newborn.

➢ *You will need 6 to 10 T-shirts*. Some mothers favor the over-the-head style of T-shirts, while others find it hard to push and pull the baby's head and arms through the small openings. Those mothers prefer the snap-across or other wraparound styles. Try one of each kind for yourself before deciding.

➢ *Other basic needs:* 4 to 6 stretch coveralls, 2 to 4 gowns (kimonos or sacques), and 4 to 6 receiving blankets. If you aren't using cloth diapers, you'll want to have a dozen around for general nursery use: wiping up, over your shoulder for burping, etc. "Onesies," or one-piece underwear that snaps between the baby's legs, are very convenient.

➤ *If the baby develops a rash*, it may be from clothes washed with detergent containing phosphates or from fabric softener. If the rash is on the baby's face it may be from sheets and blankets. Change your washing habits to eliminate this possible cause of rash.

Exercise Equipment for Baby

➤ *Jumpers* are not recommended by some doctors, who contend that they force physical development ahead of natural timing.

➤ *Bouncers and walkers* can be hazardous if the "X" part of the supporting frame does not have a plastic cover. Babies' fingers have been amputated when the design of the bouncer did not provide for the "X" being covered. Springs should stretch no more than ⅛-inch apart for the same reason: a baby's fingers could get caught and chopped off. Walkers should not tip if the child bumps into another object.

➤ *These devices should not be used too much* or they may impair development of reflexes when the child learns to fall naturally.

Travel Equipment

➤ *The stroller should be tested with the baby in it*—it should not tip if the child reaches out. It should have no sharp edges and no scissor-type action parts, which can harm fingers. Umbrella-type strollers can be rickety, but they are popular because they fold up for getting in and out of buses and cars and are no storage problem. Strollers can also be used inside the house as a chair for the baby.

➤ *Infant car seats are an absolute must if you own a car*. Nearly 1,000 children under 5 years of age die every year in car accidents. There are significant injuries yearly to another 60,000 who weren't in car seats. If you always use a car seat you can prevent such a tragedy. Most states require the use of car seats and seat belts for all passengers under the age of 12.

➤ *You have to develop the strict habit* of *always* using the car seat for *any* length trip. Even if a baby gets active or vocal you should not remove him from the carrier while the car is moving—instead, take a rest stop.

➤ *Car seats for small babies* are designed so that the infant rides backward with his entire head and body cushioned by impact-absorbing materials. A built-in harness holds the baby

RULES ABOUT CAR SEATS

* FASTEN THE HARNESS OR ANCHOR STRAPS *TIGHTLY*. This allows the child to sustain a very severe jolt during a collision because harness webbing is not stretched to absorb impact.
* ALWAYS PLACE THE BABY FACING *BACKWARD*. No child should be placed sitting forward until he weighs 17–20 pounds and can sit up well.
* CHECK INSTRUCTIONS FOR SAFE DEGREE OF TILT. Some infant seats can be reclined with an adjustable tilt feature. Never set the seat farther down than the instructions indicate; doing so could permit the child to be forced out head-first in an accident. And do not recline a forward-facing car seat. Child car seats are safer when used in the upright position. Children learn easily how to sleep sitting up.
* ALWAYS SECURE THE SEAT WITH THE AUTO SEAT BELT. If the lap belt does not fit around the car seat or through its frame, try another seating position in the car or get a seat-belt extender.
* ALWAYS USE THE HARNESS. If you don't do up the harness, the child can be thrown out of the car seat.
* DO NOT MISTAKE THE PADDED ARMREST FOR PROTECTION. Always use the harness in any car seat. The armrest on pre-1981 models is a cosmetic feature and will not protect the child in any way. In fact, it is a hazardous object for an unharnessed child to be thrown against.
* DO NOT BUNDLE THE INFANT IN BLANKETS. The shoulder harness can't be correctly positioned if the infant is heavily bundled before being placed in the seat. In cold weather you can cut holes in one blanket you'll use only for the car: pull the straps through the holes, buckle the harness, then fold the blanket over.
* FOR THE BABY'S COMFORT use clothing with legs for a snug fit of the harness between his legs. Do not use papoose bunting or a sack sleeper.
* THE BABY'S POSITION IN THE SEAT should be with her back flat against the back of the seat, not curved. You should support a small infant's head and body with rolled diapers or thin blankets placed in the small of her back and on either side of her body.
* ALWAYS FASTEN THE TOP ANCHOR STRAP. If you forget to do this, the car seat can pivot forward in a frontal crash.
* BE SURE TO DOUBLE STRAPS BACK THROUGH BUCKLES. If strap buckles of the harness and anchor straps are incompletely threaded, they can pull out unnoticed. This defeats the entire safety system.
* NEVER LET THE CHILDREN RIDE LOOSE. If you allow your child to ride without the car seat a few times, it will only make buckling up more difficult the next time. Do not give in, even if the child complains or manages to climb out of the car seat. You can keep your restless passenger happy with frequent stops, music, or games. Don't make any exceptions to the rule about using a car seat.

firmly in place. *Always use a car seat exactly as the instructions read*. Some brands convert to a forward-riding seat.

— *Check the length of your car's seat belts*. Infant car seats are attached with the car's seat belt—some car dealers can supply a belt extender if yours are too short to accommodate the infant seat. Also, measure the space where you are going to put the seat to be sure it will fit.

— *Some models require a top anchor strap* which has to be bolted to the rear window-ledge of the car. If you have a sedan-type car this will work, but installation may be difficult in the cargo area of a station wagon or with a fast-back car, so make sure you are able to install this style of seat.

— *There are carriers which are found safe* in tests that were sanctioned by the group Action for Child Transportation Safety. If you want more information, you can contact this organization at 400 Central Park West, #15P, New York, NY 10025.

— *Infant car seats can be quite costly*, so watch want ads and garage sales for used models.

Bathing the Baby

A daily bath is not necessary for a baby, although some grandmothers may disagree! Every 2 or 3 days is plenty for a full bath, since the only part of the baby that gets dirty is washed with every diaper change. Also, soap and shampoo are not necessary on newborn skin—and some people say should *not* be used at all in the early period of a baby's life.

➤ *You can bathe a baby in the kitchen sink*, which saves you from having to bend over.

➤ *Sponge-bathe a baby until the umbilical cord falls off* about a week after birth. You can dab the stump with cotton dipped in alcohol or just leave it alone. After that you can get the baby wet all over.

➤ *The temperature of the water should not be too hot*; it should feel just warm to *your elbow*, not to your hands. Also, be careful that the baby does not get chilled because a newborn's temperature-regulating mechanism is not yet efficient. Be sure the room where you bathe him is not chilly or drafty and dry the baby off right away.

➤ *Most babies love the water* and enjoy moving around in it. Some children, however, scream when they are bathed—if yours does this, don't worry: she will soon learn to enjoy the water.

➤ *Basic supplies* for bathing are 3 to 4 towels and 3 to 4 washcloths made of soft terrycloth. *Do not use cotton swabs in the nose or ears*—they can easily hurt the baby.

➤ *Try going into the bathtub* with the baby. Hold him securely (it's slippery!) and you'll find the baby will play, move his muscles, and make swimming motions. You can also breast-feed in the tub, which is relaxing and enjoyable for both of you.

WHAT TO EXPECT IN A NEWBORN

Most parents have never even seen a newborn baby before. There are certain "oddities" you should be prepared for so that they don't surprise or concern you. Most newborns do not look like cherubs; some parents are so disappointed by this that they have a hard time accepting their baby's looks. Try to see some pictures of newborns so that your expectations are realistic. The parent-child bond can be hindered if you are displeased with how your baby appears.

General "Odd" Normal Traits of Newborns

➤ *All new babies sound like they have a cold*—they sniffle and sneeze. This is because their breathing organs are new and have to adjust.
➤ *The "startle reflex"* is normal and something a baby grows out of. A newborn tends to jump at noises and may tremble. You may worry that the baby is nervous, but this is just a sign of her system adjusting.
➤ *The rooting reflex causes the baby to turn her head* toward anything that touches her cheek. This is an instinctive mechanism that helps the baby find food. You need only touch the baby's cheek with the nipple. Do not touch both the baby's cheeks at the same time or hold her by both cheeks to guide her head toward the nipple—this will just confuse her.
➤ *A wobbly head occurs because a baby's head is large* and her neck muscles are not developed. The head always needs support for the first few months.
➤ *Hearing is impaired during the first few days* after birth because the middle part of the baby's ear behind the eardrum is still full of amniotic fluid. Gradually it gets absorbed and evaporates, but until then, sounds reaching the baby's ears are muffled.
➤ *Smells and textures all interest the newborn*. You can wear different fabrics when holding the baby to give him varying sensory stimulation. The baby may be excited by crinkly, colorful paper that makes a noise when the infant touches it.
➤ *The umbilical cord should be kept dry*. You can cleanse it with alcohol on a piece of cotton or just leave it alone. Keep the cord stump protected and above the diaper. Notify the doctor if it bleeds, gets red, or has an unusual odor, all signs of infection.

Most stumps take about 6 or 7 days to drop off and there may be a slight amount of bloody drainage when this happens.

➤ *The external genitals are often swollen at birth.* The maternal hormones of pregnancy have passed to the baby; this swelling recedes gradually. The girl's clitoris may be swollen so that it looks like a little penis and she may have vaginal bleeding. This is from the estrogenic hormones that were in the mother's system: it will disappear in a short time.

➤ *Milk in the baby's breasts is fairly common for both* males and females. The same hormones that prepare your breasts to lactate affect the baby, who can have milk in her breasts for a few days after birth.

➤ *The nails may be long at birth*. They will be soft and are easiest to trim when the baby is asleep. If you are nervous at first using even blunt baby scissors, you can just make a small cut on the side of the nail and peel off the rest.

➤ *The baby's temperature* is something you should be aware of because a newborn has an inefficient heating system. If a baby has cool hands and feet but a warm body, that means he is at a good temperature. Feel with your finger along his neck or legs to determine if the body is warm.

The Baby's Skin

➤ *The skin of a newborn is very sensitive.* It is susceptible to infection, so all nursery linens and clothes should be sterilized by washing in hot water in a machine and all attendants should wash their hands carefully.

➤ *Skin color at birth may be a blotchy red* or grayish blue regardless of the baby's race. Some babies start to develop racial color when born and others remain a very light color for at least the first few hours.

➤ *The skin may peel a few days after birth*, like a peeling sunburn. Do not use lotions or pull off the skin—it will come off naturally.

➤ *Lanugo, the downy hair covering the baby's skin* at birth, can be quite heavy and noticeable, especially if it's dark. Lanugo is most abundant over the back, shoulders, forehead, and cheeks. It usually falls out and is rubbed away during the first weeks of life. This does not mean the child will have hairy skin later on—there is no relation between that and lanugo.

➤ *Mottling, or marbleized spots on the skin*, is normal when you are undressing the baby.

➤ *Mongolian spots are irregular, greenish-blue pigmentation* over the lower back that occurs in Negro, Mediterranean, and Asian races. These spots will disappear by school age.

➤ *Prickly heat is clusters of minute pink pimples* surrounded by areas of pink skin. It is due to the overactivity of sweat glands. It can be cured by ventilating the skin using a weak solution of bicarbonate of soda and a bland powder, but be he sure the baby cannot touch the mixture and then put his fingers to his mouth. Most important, put lighter clothes and covers on the baby.

➤ *Milia look like whiteheads.* They are concentrated on the baby's nose, chin, and forehead. These are immature oil glands and will disappear by themselves. Leave them alone—squeezing them can cause infection.

➤ *Diaper rash can be caused by too-strong soap* used on diapers or diapers that haven't been boiled long enough to kill the bacteria. Change your laundry habits and use zinc oxide or a commercial preparation like Desitin, which contains zinc oxide, on the affected area.

The Baby's Eyes

➤ *The baby's eyes are usually blue or slate-gray.* The permanent color comes in between 6 months and one year. The iris flecks with brown about the third month if the eyes are going to be hazel or brown. A blue-eyed child retains the blue shade.

➤ *A newborn's eyes are crossed* because the muscles that keep both eyes pointing in the same direction aren't working yet. In a few weeks they will correct themselves as they develop.

➤ *It has only recently been realized that little babies can see at all.* However, they do have a fairly rigid distance of focus: around 9 inches away from their eyes. If you want the baby to look at something, it is best to show it at this distance. An amazing natural phenomenon is that during breast-feeding this is just about the distance from your face to the baby's. It is evidently a built-in part of the mothering system that a baby's focal distance is correlated to where her mother holds her for nursing.

➤ *Tears usually don't arrive until around the third month.* The tear glands don't function at all for the first weeks, so crying is tearless until then.

➤ *The baby may have a red spot or two* in his eyes postpartum. This is caused by a blood vessel that broke during delivery and will clear up by itself.

Bowel Movements

➤ *The first elimination* will be meconium, the greenish, tarlike substance that is in the baby's intestines at birth. If you are in the hospital and don't have rooming-in you may never even see this dark material, which is eliminated for the first few days. If you are breast-feeding, after your milk comes in, the baby's bowel movements become loose and yellow. At first the meconium is streaked with yellow from the colostrum, and then when your milk comes in, the baby's bowel movements are yellow, watery curds. As the baby gets older, the stools are more the consistency of wet toothpaste.

➤ *A newborn may seem constipated* because he strains when he has his first bowel movements. This is because his organs are new and have to adjust to this new task.

➤ *A breast-feeding baby may not urinate much* for the first day or so because he isn't getting many fluids at first. Eventually he will soak 8 to 10 diapers a day once your milk is in.

➤ *If a baby's urine is dark,* he may be dehydrated. Call your doctor, who may suggest giving some water.

Colic

➤ *Colic can be agonizing for you* and of course, for the baby. A baby with colic has abdominal cramps and her knees draw up from the gas and pain—inevitably she cries a lot. Breast-fed babies tend to have colic less frequently because breast milk is more easily digested.

Colic occurs mostly in the evening; walking and rocking a baby can help. You can try tummy massage or placing the baby on her stomach over your warm hand or knee. A towel or receiving blanket warmed in the dryer and folded under the baby's painful stomach may help soothe her to sleep.

Although colic usually disappears around 3 months of age it can be very hard on new parents. The frequent crying and wakefulness can stretch your physical and mental tolerance to the limit.

Perhaps worse of all is that you know your baby is suffering and you are impotent—your sense of helplessness can frustrate and make you angry. One solution is to have other people around to hold and comfort the baby so that you can at least get out of the house for part of each day to restore your sanity!

Jaundice

Jaundice has three forms: normal (or physiologic) jaundice, abnormal jaundice, and breast-milk jaundice, which is very rare.

➤ *Physiologic jaundice* is normal and has no complicating factors. Babies show signs of it around 3 to 4 days postpartum, but before one to 2 weeks of age. A baby is born pink, regardless of race; with jaundice a baby will show a slight yellowing of the skin—a tinge of yellow almost like a tan. The other characteristics are a whiteness of the eyes, mucous membranes, and body fluids due to excess bilirubin in the blood.

➤ ***The cause of jaundice*** is that in utero the baby has more red blood cells than she needs after birth. During the first week of life the baby must break down the excess red blood cells and discard them through the feces, urine, skin, and lungs. The liver picks up one of these unnecessary substances, bilirubin, an orange or yellow substance in the bile, and converts it to a conjugated bilirubin—a form that can be easily excreted. Sometimes it takes a newborn's liver a week or so to catch up on converting the bilirubin to a nontoxic substance that her body can excrete. This is why jaundice happens, accounting for the yellowish cast to the skin.

➤ ***You should do something*** if the baby is obviously jaundiced— if the yellow color is medium to strong. This may be hard for you to judge, since you probably don't have any experience in gauging a newborn's jaundice! The best way to determine

---

  FACTORS THAT MAY CONTRIBUTE TO JAUNDICE

— The possibility of an ABO blood group incompatibility: if you are O and your baby is A or B, you may have antibodies that will destroy some of the baby's cells.
— The baby is dehydrated: has not had enough fluids, the weather is hot, and/or the baby is not receiving enough colostrum or milk, which is why some doctors recommend giving a newborn water during early feedings.
— The baby is too cool.
— The baby experienced a lot of bruising during birth, which means an excess number of red blood cells must be broken down quickly.
— While pregnant you took aspirin, caffeine, sulfa, Valium, or other drugs which can interfere with the baby's ability to convert bilirubin.
— The baby's liver is immature.
— The baby is premature, making her more susceptible to becoming jaundiced because premies' livers are almost always immature.
— You're an RH-negative mother with an RH-positive baby: occasionally this combination results in the destruction of some of the baby's red blood cells.

whether the baby has normal or abnormal jaundice is to take
him to the pediatrician, who will determine whether he needs a
blood test.

➤ **Treatment of abnormal jaundice** is especially important if
the jaundice occurs in conjunction with fever, lack of meconium
passage, cold, oxygen deprivation in labor, or a diabetic mother.
The dangerous causes of jaundice are a hemolytic disease, or an
infection because of the rapid destruction of red blood cells. Some
doctors will leave the jaundice alone to correct itself, but standard treatment is to admit the baby to a hospital, put him in an
incubator with his eyes covered, and turn on fluorescent lights
("bili lights"). The baby's blood is tested every 12 hours to 24
hours if the level is rising significantly by heel prickings.

➤ **The disadvantages of hospitalization** are that you and the
baby are separated, breast-feeding is limited or often discouraged, and skin-to-skin contact is limited. In some hospitals it is
standard procedure *not* to remove the protective eye coverings
even when the baby is not under the bili lights. You must guard
against this lack of photic (light) stimulation in the first days of
life. If your baby is put in the hospital or kept there, be sure to
read page 323 about the importance of spending time feeding
and holding a baby kept in the nursery.

➤ **Alternative treatment** should be discussed with your pediatrician. Do not attempt these alternatives to hospitalization without your doctor's support. Give the baby a 2- to 3-minute
sunbath in the early morning and late afternoon, protecting the
infant's eyes. Vitamin D—which the sunlight contains—is
known to help jaundice. Extra fluids help "flush out" the system, so you can give plain boiled water in an eye dropper after
breast-feeding or in a bottle if you're bottle-feeding. You will still
have to take the baby twice daily to the hospital for a blood test
to determine the bilirubin count and whether it is rising, falling,
or stable.

➤ **Home phototherapy** is offered by many pediatricians who understand the drawbacks of hospitalizing a newborn. Home therapy for jaundice consists of a nurse who comes out to your
home, sets up the phototherapy unit, and explains the simple
use of it, including putting patches on the baby's eyes. Then the
nurse will return every 24 hours to obtain follow-up bilirubin
tests. This takes place under the supervision of your pediatrician,
who continues to manage the situation with the help of the visiting nurse.

Ask your pediatrician whether home phototherapy is available and if he's comfortable with this alternative to hospitalization. A great deal will depend upon you and whether you are
too anxious or uncomfortable to take on the responsibility of the
extra care involved.

➤ **The dangers of jaundice** are that high levels of unconjugated
(unconverted) bilirubin in the blood can directly damage the ba-

by's nervous system and brain cells. This is particularly true if the infant is immature or under stress. If the jaundice continues to be increasingly severe, the most effective and rapid way to remove dangerous concentrations of bilirubin in the blood is to give the baby an exchange transfusion.

➤ *Breast-milk jaundice* is most unusual. It sometimes occurs 4 days or more postpartum, mostly at the beginning of the second week of life. It is probably caused by a hormone related to progesterone called pregnendiol, which is secreted in the milk. You can continue breast-feeding unless bilirubin levels approach 20 mg/100 ml during the first week of life. If that happens, you have to discontinue nursing temporarily. You can hand-express your milk for 2 to 3 days to allow the bilirubin level to go down. Breast-milk jaundice *does not* cause any harm to the baby.

Crying

Crying is a baby's way of expressing discomfort or hunger, but it may also be a way of "letting off steam." If the baby cries you should check his diaper for wetness and determine how long ago he last ate. Once you've eliminated those two reasons and the baby still cries when you put him back down, you have a couple of options. Some people set a 15-minute limit on crying—they let the baby cry that long before picking him up again. Although it may jangle your nerves, a baby will usually not continue crying that long: 15 minutes can feel like *hours* to you! It may just be that the baby needs to cry as a way of releasing tension.

The important thing to remember is that a tiny baby does not cry as a manipulative way of getting your attention. At such an early stage a baby's mind doesn't work that way. Years ago it was said that you'd "spoil" a baby by picking him up. *You cannot "spoil" a tiny baby.* By picking up a crying baby you are setting up a communication system: you're letting the baby know that his cries are heard and that somebody out there cares. *You can be as responsive and indulgent as you want.* Responding to a crying baby gives him a sense of security early on—this can help a baby develop into a person with more independence later in life.

It is now known that a lack of nurturing as a child can cause unusual behavior and even violence later. If you reply to a baby's only way of communicating with you—by tending to him when he cries—you are laying the foundation for a child's ability to reach out and trust that his needs will be met. A baby who has not had good nurturing may grow up to be a person who is unable to relate one-to-one with another person. The way that you treat a small baby has a lot to do with what kind of person he becomes. For example, if you pick up the baby when he cries and he stops crying, you can view the baby either as "socially responsive" (he made a demand and was satisfied when it was answered), or you can see him as "exploitative and spoiled." There is a tendency to construct a fantasy about a baby's personality from the way that you perceive the crying and then to handle the baby accordingly. If you have the first attitude toward crying, you will give the baby attention; if you choose the second way to look at it, you will leave the baby to cry. In each case your response or lack of it will contribute to the way the child comes to perceive himself and others.

It is possible that overhandling of a baby can tire him out and *cause* crying and fussiness. This can also happen if there are many people around or the baby is going along with you on extended outings, for instance. A baby needs time to sleep peacefully and be left alone. One way to comfort and quiet an overstimulated baby is to swaddle him. Most hospitals swaddle babies in the nursery: they wrap the baby securely in a receiving blanket so that he is snug and cozy. If your baby gets fussy from too much sensory input, you can swaddle him so that he calms down and sleeps.

Sleep Problems

Sleeping through the night is not something that some babies do "naturally" and others "refuse" to do. The way that you organize your baby's environment has a profound effect on whether the child can sleep through the night. Solid sleeping habits should be developed early on. From a very young age, many children resist sleep. As a parent, this can become a test of whether you have the self-confidence to impose limits on your baby's behavior.

The most important thing for new parents to realize is that they should be in control of the baby's sleep and feeding schedule—and not the other way around. Several of the couples interviewed for this book went through hellish months of sleeplessness—needlessly. They did not understand the part they played in having a baby that would not sleep. The loss of sleep for the parents—as a couple and individually—is a heavy burden. A situation like this can also cause you to resent the baby, and the baby to suffer a diminished sense of self-esteem and independence if he continues to depend on you throughout the night.

If you feel that a problem is developing with your baby's sleep habits, nip it in the bud. There is an excellent paperback book that covers the subject with intelligence, humor, and compassion. *Helping Your Baby Sleep Through the Night* is written by Joanne Cuthbertson and Susie Schevill, both of whom are married to pediatricians.

Sudden Infant Death Syndrome (SIDS)

Every new parent worries at some time about babies that die in their sleep. SIDS is a mystery that perplexes the medical community, too: there is still no explanation for this illness, which used to be known as "crib death." Sudden infant death syndrome claims the lives of thousands of babies in America every year, with the age of greatest danger being between two and four months of age. 90% are under six months.

This disease has been around for centuries, but despite years of searching for answers, medical science is stilll baffled. There has been no conclusive explanation of why seemingly healthy infants die in their sleep, although SIDS does seem to be sleep-related, since most incidents occur during normal sleeping periods. Over the years there has been speculation and misinformation about what causes SIDS. There have been theories about a subtle underlying brain abnormality in the infants who die from SIDS, but researchers cannot agree whether the problem might lie in the brain stem, which controls heart rate and breathing, or the areas of the brain that control sleep patterns, or the areas that control specific functions, such as regulation of body heat. But none of these abnormalities has been identified or proven.

There is some encouraging news: from 1992 to 1995 there was 30% decline in the number of babies who died from sudden infant death syndrome. This good news was probably the result of a public service program called "Back to Sleep," which promoted putting infants to sleep on their backs rather than on their stomachs. In fact, most of the recommendations from experts on protecting your baby are related to sleep habits.

Recent research has come up with some clues as to possible causes for SIDS. Instead of just having to worry and wait, new parents can take preventive measures to protect their child.

SAFETY PRECAUTIONS TO PREVENT SIDS

➤ **Put baby to sleep on her back.**
- Begin this healthy sleeping pattern right from the beginning.
- A baby will go to sleep in the position he gets used to from birth.
- Insist that anyone who spends time with your baby follows the "Back to Sleep" rule, no exceptions.
- If your baby will not accept this position, wait beside the crib until she's fallen asleep on her stomach, then turn her over.

➤ **Do not put baby to sleep on his side.**
- Infants sleeping on their sides can roll onto their stomachs, increasing the risk.
- Sleeping face-up is the safest possible position.

➤ **Remove any dangerous sleeping materials.**
- Use only a firm mattress with a fitted sheet.
- Avoid any soft bedding such as sheepskin, comforters, quilts or pillows. 30% of SIDS victims had their mouths and noses covered by soft bedding materials like the above.
- Carbon dioxide from exhaled air can reach high levels if it gets trapped in soft, fluffy bedding where the infant then re-breathes it.

➤ **Don't overheat a sleeping baby.**
- Overheating may put a baby into a deeper level of sleep, lessening his ability to awaken if he experiences breathing problems.

- Check your baby's temperature by feeling her head or the back of her neck, not the feet and hands, which are usually cooler. If she feels hot or damp from sweating, then remove a layer.
- Keep the nursery at a temperature that feels comfortable for you, no warmer.
- Don't bundle a baby so tightly that he can't move freely.
- If you swaddle your baby keep her arms free from the blanket so she can reposition herself.
- Don't cover the baby's head for sleep, which retains too much heat.

➤ **Choose breast-feeding if possible.**
- Bottle-fed babies have a higher risk of SIDS.
- The protective quality of breast milk is not known, but statistics show that breast-feeding lowers your baby's risk.
- Breast-feed for at least the first four months and you'll get your baby past the highest-risk period for SIDS.

➤ **Don't allow any smoking in your home.**
- If you smoke anywhere in your house your baby is two times more likely to die of SIDS.
- If the baby's father smokes (even if you do not) the risk of SIDS is more than three times higher than a smoke-free home.
- The risk for SIDS increases as you increase the number of cigarettes smoked in the home, or the number of smokers.
- Even though breast-feeding lowers the risk of SIDS, if the mother is a smoker she eliminates that advantage for her baby.
- If you smoked during pregnancy your baby's chances of SIDS are higher: double if you stopped in the first trimester and five times higher if you smoked in the last two-thirds of pregnancy.

➤ **Protect your baby's general health.**
- Regular prenatal care gives your baby an advantage against SIDS.
- Keep immunizations up-to-date.
- Go to well-baby checkups so you can catch any possible health problem very early.

➤ **Find out if you have a high-risk baby.**
- Medication can be given preventively to a baby who is known to have breathing difficulties, which may be a cause of SIDS.
- You should talk to your pediatrician about whether your baby may be a candidate for drugs to lower high levels of chemicals in the spinal fluid which interfere with breathing:
  — Does your baby have any known breathing problems?
  — Has your baby had a previous life-threatening event?
  — Did you lose a baby previously to SIDS?
- If the answer is yes to any of the above, talk to your pediatrician.

➤ **What SIDS Is Not**
- SIDS is not contagious.
- SIDS is not caused by child abuse.

- SIDS is not hereditary.
- SIDS is not caused or prevented by baby's sleeping with parents.
- SIDS is not prevented by any product for sale.

If you want more information than what you find here, you can contact The Sudden Infant Death Syndrome Alliance, 1314 Bedford Avenue, Suite 210, Baltimore, Maryland 21208; (410) 653-8226; (800) 221-SIDS; FAX (410) 653-8709.

A Temperamentally Difficult Baby

A very alert, sensitive baby can be difficult. One way she may show fatigue from too much attention is to have intestinal cramps and gas. You should try to make this kind of baby's environment as placid as possible. Don't have the baby around when there are adult arguments going on: even the raised voices of a heated discussion can upset her.

Give the baby enough privacy. This kind of baby needs solitude and a chance to explore her quiet room before catapulting into a house full of people. When you go out with an alert baby who is very sensitive to sensory input and new experiences carry her wrapped in your arms or in a front carrier. Holding her close to your body helps her feel secure in new situations.

Love and Kisses

Loving a baby—in the way you feed and play with him—teaches him the capacity to love. It appears that a child who fails to make the vital human connections in infancy will have varying degrees of difficulty in making them later in childhood. The formation of the love bond takes place during infancy. Later on, his ability to regulate the aggressive drive is largely dependent upon the quality and durability of these bonds. The absence of human bonds or the rupture of them early in life can have permanent effects on the later capacity for human attachment and for the regulation of aggression.

The baby is an active participant in attachment: the baby elicits nurturing and protective behaviors in you, stimulating your maternal instinct. Do not worry, however, if you don't feel this instinct right away. For many women it is a gradual process and takes time. You may feel like a partner in an arranged marriage, expected to instantly love and cherish someone you've never met before. You should not feel there is something wrong with you if you aren't overcome by a wave of emotion for your baby right at the start—give yourself a chance to ease into it. Try to spend as much time with the baby as feels comfortable, so that you get to know each other.

Regardless of what you are feeling, you should know that the baby becomes attached to you very early in his life and with increasing intensity. A baby in the third and fourth weeks of life, for example, will smile selectively in response to his mother's voice. Experiments have demonstrated that no other sounds in the same frequency will elicit the baby's smile. At about 8 months a baby demonstrates a clear discrimination of your face by smiling. By the time your baby is 8 to 12 months old you are discriminated from all other people: the baby will demonstrate his needs and attachment to you by showing distress when you leave and by having grief reactions if the absence is prolonged beyond the baby's endurance.

Studies have shown that accidental or experimental separations of baby and mother lead to panic states in both of them. Infant monkeys, during prolonged separations from their mothers, suffer grief and mourning states that cannot be distinguished from those seen in human infants. Pathological behaviors will occur as the infant settles into a stuporous state. One hears of the babies in orphanages who receive food but become seriously ill and even die because they do not receive sufficient emotional nourishment. This is called "failure to thrive." Never underestimate the importance of your expressions of love to your baby.

Let the baby adjust to your lifestyle. A big mistake new parents make is to readjust their lives and schedules to accommodate a newborn. It will be much better for you and the baby won't know the difference if you just incorporate the child into *your* lifestyle. Let a baby get used to normal household noises—voices, music, machines—and she will accommodate. If you tiptoe around and whisper when the baby is asleep, she will become accustomed to that kind of quiet and will have trouble getting used to normal sounds. There are many ways in which a baby will change your life over which you *cannot* exercise any control, so let your lives continue as normally as possible and the baby will fit in.

Another example is that a baby doesn't have to be put to sleep at any magic hour. A baby's bedtime can be whatever is good for you. If you like to get up late and go to bed late the baby can fit into that pattern as comfortably as if you "get up with the chickens and go to sleep with the cows." There also does not have to be any strict regularity—if you can be flexible, so can the baby. She will be perfectly fine and happy just as long as she gets sleep, has clean diapers, a full tummy, and plenty of hugging.

FEEDING THE BABY

Some Pointers About Feeding

➢ *Begin a feeding in a calm, relaxed atmosphere*. If the baby is hungry and crying do not let yourself get upset so that you rush and get tense. The baby isn't going to starve. All babies cry sometimes—it's nothing to get anxious about. Quiet the baby down before you feed him; sometimes just putting him into a nursing position can do this. But if the baby is tense his stomach will be tight, his breathing will be out of rhythm, and he won't nurse or digest as well.

➤ *When you nurse, hold the baby firmly* so that he knows you are there and feels secure. Hold his foot or bottom with a firm touch and keep his back fairly straight—he can't digest well if he's all hunched over. If you are bottle-feeding there are certain important aspects of nursing you should know that are covered in the section beginning on page 571.

➤ *When you give the baby a night feeding*, change his diaper before you feed him. This way he will be clean and dry and will wake up, which means he will nurse well rather than dozing and reawakening.

➤ *Burping a baby is important after feeding*, depending on the individual. You will learn your baby's patterns: whether he is a quick or slow burper, or whether he needs to burp at all, and which position works best. You can burp a baby over your shoulder or with his face downward on your lap, patting his back in either case. Another position is with the baby sitting up: you support his back and head with one hand, gently moving the baby back and forward as if he was bowing. He is less likely to spit up in this position.

➤ *Choking can happen because there is a delicate balance* between a baby's breathing and swallowing. If the baby spits up, chokes, and gags, *sit him up immediately*. This should be an automatic reflex on your part—you should not worry about the baby making a mess or anything like that. Sit the baby up instantly if he chokes.

➤ *Lay the baby on his side or stomach to sleep*. That way mucus or milk cannot go down the wrong passageway.

➤ *If you are bottle-feeding* it's important to offer the bottle on both sides. If you always hold the baby on your left side and the bottle in your right hand, the baby's eye coordination can suffer. Breast-feeding mothers automatically have to alternate sides so the baby can get both breasts.

BREAST-FEEDING

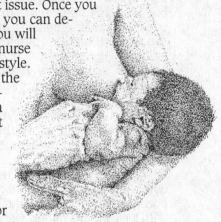

Breast-feeding is an important issue. Once you have all the available information you can decide for yourself whether or not you will breast-feed, and if so, how long to nurse or how to breast-feed in a busy lifestyle. Each set of parents has to weigh the physical, psychological, and emotional factors and come up with a decision about breast-feeding that is right for them.

This section will cover the supportive atmosphere necessary for breast-feeding, general information about how the breasts work and what breast milk does for an infant, a look at both the advantages and drawbacks to breast-feeding, and advice about breast-feeding while working outside your home. There is also a section on diabetes and breast-feeding and a chart indicating which drugs are harmful if used when nursing.

Why Is Breast-Feeding Less Popular than the Bottle?

Since 1950 only 30% of babies have been breast-fed, which has not changed much from year to year. There is a higher level of breast-feeding among college-educated women, but generally it has declined in popularity ever since the the bottle was introduced.

➤ *It is a status symbol.* Originally only upper-income women bottle-fed their babies. This is part of the influence to bottle-feed, even though people may not be consciously aware of it.
➤ *More women are working.* Although it is possible to breast-feed and have a career, it requires an energetic commitment and maneuvering. All the same, many working women do not return to their jobs when the baby is less than six months, so this is not as strong a reason as it might seem.
➤ *Vigorous promotion of infant formula.* Advertisements and free samples to doctors and women leaving the hospital greatly influence the decision not to breast-feed. In fact, this pressure is so potent that the International Pediatric Association recently made recommendations about the commercial promotion of formula: "The dissemination of propaganda about artificial feeding and distribution of samples of artificial baby foods should be banned from all maternity units." This group found that the

promotion of formula undermined breast-feeding, which they recommend.

➤ *The breast as sex symbol.* Some men and women think of breasts only as they relate to sex. They have difficulty acknowledging the milk-producing function of breasts. People can be so conditioned in their attitudes toward bosoms that they are repulsed by the thought of breast-feeding.

➤ *Lack of profit from breast-feeding.* Commercial interests cannot gain by promoting breast-feeding—which is another reason for its decline. Since no money can be made from breast-feeding, there has been no organized effort to educate or encourage women. Since there are comparatively few women breast-feeding, encouragement from other women isn't always possible.

The La Leche League was started in 1956 to fill this gap. Some women complain that the LLL is too gung-ho. It is important to understand that this small, volunteer organization with local groups nationwide is working against a cultural mainstream. They are David fighting Goliath: women who believe that breast-feeding is best for mothers and babies versus huge corporations that make millions of dollars from promoting formula. It is a hard task requiring almost fervent dedication.

La Leche League is the only group that exists for advice and encouragement about breast-feeding, but it is necessary right up front to caution that the ideology of many LLL members is not the "right" point of view. Some of the members are adamant about their philosophy that a mother should have sole responsibility for feeding her child (which means that breast-feeding has to pretty much dominate her life). The league's book, *The Womanly Art of Breastfeeding,* holds this point of view: it does not acknowledge the mother as an independent person with demands which may exclude her baby. This concept of Total Mothering, also referred to as "natural mothering," may seem overwhelming to you—the righteous attitude that often goes with it can also be off-putting. However, if you keep in mind what the La Leche League represents and their uphill battle, perhaps you won't be as critical.

Support Is Essential to Successful Breast-Feeding

We live in a society where the majority of women do not breast-feed. So be aware that other people's attitudes have a direct effect on breast-feeding. Particularly a first-time mother is acutely sensitive to other people's reactions. Verbal, nonverbal, and even unconscious judgments by those around her can influence a mother who is trying to breast-feed. The attitudes of her mate, obstetrician, pediatrician, nurses, mother, immediate or extended family, and friends are all important.

Even subtle criticism—a grandmother's comments or a doctor who mentions that a baby is at the bottom of the weight-gain graph for his height—can inhibit a woman's milk supply for a feeding or two.

Therefore, if you do want to breast-feed you should be aware of the effect of other people's attitudes. Let others know ahead of time that you're going to breast-feed only if you're prepared to hear negative reactions without getting discouraged. You can also protect yourself from problems by talking only to those people you cannot avoid having contact with in the early weeks postpartum. Explain to them that their support is going to be essential to the ease and success of your breast-feeding. If they have questions or are against it, then ask them to read this section or other material so that they are fully informed about the subject.

> ➤ *Your own negative presumptions* and partial information can interfere with breast-feeding. You may be interested in trying it, but you've let yourself be negatively influenced by bits and pieces you've heard. Learn everything you can ahead of time—if you decide to breast-feed, give it your full commitment, or you'll be your own worst enemy. You may say, "I'm too tense a person to breast-feed," or "I doubt I'll have enough milk," both of which are erroneous statements. You may have heard that a friend had trouble breast-feeding and you don't want to have to go through it. That's ridiculous—would you not have had a baby for that reason, too? Someone else's experience has nothing to do with yours.

> ➤ *The first couple of weeks* of breast-feeding are the most frustrating. You are learning a new skill, you may feel insecure, and there is often a lack of knowledgeable people to help you. Your baby may also not be fully cooperative—she may be groggy from drugs you had during delivery, or she may not have had a chance to reinforce the sucking instinct at birth. The important thing is to anticipate that the first couple of weeks are going to be difficult—if they're fairly easy, you have a nice surprise. At least you won't give up because you didn't *expect* to be frustrated.

The Hospital and Breast-Feeding

> ➤ *Choose a hospital* where breast-feeding is encouraged and with a flexible feeding schedule. Try to get a hospital that permits the baby to stay with you immediately from birth, or at least has the shortest possible observation period after birth. Some hospitals will release your baby from the stabilization nursery within 4 hours, but many still have a strict 24-hour observation period.

> Ask the hospital what percentage of mothers breast-feed. If it's at least 40%, they will probably be flexible to your needs. If

it is under 25%, the hospital is not oriented to breast-feeding, which can make it harder for you. It is routine at many hospitals to give a baby glucose and water during the observation period. Your efforts at breast-feeding are undermined from the start with a baby that has sucked from a rubber nipple—it is so much easier that the baby may refuse your breast. Have your pediatrician write on your chart: *No bottles by request* or *No artificial nipples*.

➤ *Schedules, routines, and allegiance to the clock*. Breast milk digests in 2 to 3 hours, yet hospitals have a 4-hour feeding schedule. This means that your baby is going to get hungry and cry in the nursery: he might be given a bottle of glucose and water to quiet him. The rubber nipple undermines breast-feeding; the baby's hunger will be satisfied; he will fall back to sleep and he won't be interested in your breast when he's brought to you. (But if your chart says, *No artificial nipples*, the baby may cry from when he gets hungry until he exhausts himself, falls to sleep, and is too tired to nurse properly when you get him.)

Many hospitals have a policy of not allowing a baby to have anything to eat for the first 12 hours of life. However, the advantages of early sucking are known: a baby whose sucking reflex is reinforced at birth and frequently thereafter is going to learn to nurse well. Also, frequent sucking insures you will have a good milk supply which will come in sooner and helps prevent engorgement of your breasts. The hospital schedule makes frequent sucking difficult, thereby increasing the chance that breast-feeding will be compromised.

➤ *If you cannot get rooming-in*, at least try to get your baby every 3 hours. That extra hour can make a big difference in the success of your breast-feeding, but realize that special requests upset the smooth routine. If you want your baby an hour sooner than all the other babies are brought to their mothers, it means that a nurse has to remember this out-of-the-ordinary request and stop whatever she's doing to bring your baby to you.

Lactation Consultants

A lactation consultant (also known as a lactation educator or specialist) is a new kind of health-care provider. If you are having difficulties breast-feeding, you can get direct care through a private consultation with a specialist.

Lactation consultants can be found through the hospital by contacting the head nurse of the *newborn unit*, usually not through the maternity nursing staff. Your pediatrician can also provide the names of lactation consultants.

A consultation usually runs about an hour and a half, beginning with an extensive questionnaire to fill out. Then the specially trained consultant will check your breasts, evaluate your ejection reflex and milk supply, and examine the baby's position and way of sucking. Then she will suggest techniques to correct your breast-feeding problems or at least reduce them.

A lactation consultant usually rents or sells breast pumps, loans or sells books, and has a doll on which to demonstrate correct and incorrect techniques of nursing. She may also operate a telephone hotline for information and support.

Preparation for Breast-Feeding

In the last weeks of your pregnancy you can prepare your breasts with a *daily routine* to "toughen them" and open the milk ducts.

- ➤ *Rub your nipples* gently with a towel. This friction accustoms your nipples to the stimulation they will get from the baby. Rub them until they are uncomfortable, but never to the point of pain.
- ➤ *Pull out your nipples firmly*, using some kind of oil or cream as lubricant.
- ➤ *Flat or inverted nipples* don't stick out by themselves—they fold back into the breast and need additional preparation. If you aren't sure whether you have inverted nipples, pinch the areola (the darker circle) just behind the base of the nipple. If it comes out, even a little, it is not a true inverted nipple. If your nipples react to pressure by retreating, they are inverted, which is rare. One treatment for bringing out truly inverted nipples is to use breast shields. However, nipples are only guides for the baby— they don't really need to protrude for successful nursing.
- ➤ *"Nipple-rolling"* is a good preparation for both inverted and normal nipples. Pull out the nipple with your fingers and roll it between your thumb and forefinger for a few minutes to make it stand out. Do this when you get dressed and undressed during the final weeks of your pregnancy.
- ➤ *Go without a bra for part of each day*—or wear a nursing bra and open the front of it—so that your nipples get friction against your clothing.
- ➤ *Expose your nipples* to the air and sun.
- ➤ *To open your milk ducts* you can hand-express a few drops of colostrum during the last 6 weeks of the pregnancy. This may reduce engorgement, which sometimes happens when your milk first comes in and can be very uncomfortable.

STEPS TO OPEN MILK DUCTS

— **CUP THE BREAST IN ONE HAND.** Use your other hand to place your thumb above and the forefinger below the nipple on the edge of the areola (the brown or darker area). The milk ducts are under here. Press inward toward the chest wall. Squeeze the thumb and forefinger together gently; release and repeat.

— **DO NOT SLIDE THE THUMB AND FOREFINGER** out toward the nipple or you will cause soreness. Shift your fingers to new positions to reach all of the milk ducts, which radiate out from the nipple in a circle. Alternate where you squeeze every few minutes so that all the ducts get a workout.

— **DO THIS VERY GENTLY** and only once or twice a day. It may take some time to get colostrum and some women never do, but it is still good preparation for breast-feeding.

➤ *Redheads and women with fair complexions* are the most prone to difficulties with soreness and nipple problems because their skin is so tender. They should follow the preparatory steps above to minimize problems during breast-feeding.

➤ *Nursing bras are a good idea during breast-feeding* because they support your breasts and also protect your clothes if you leak. You will need a minimum of 3 bras: one on, one in the laundry, and one in the drawer.

➤ *Smaller-breasted women like stretch bras*, which give enough support and are comfortable and convenient. They can just lift the entire bra up over their breast while they're nursing.

➤ *Disposable nursing pads absorb any leakage* and also protect your breast from any detergent residues which can irritate it. An economical alternative to ready-made pads is to cut a disposable diaper into 9 sections, with the plastic backing removed. *Avoid plastic-coated pads*: they can cause a rash, especially in hot weather.

➤ *Breast shields can be used to catch leaking milk*. *Do not save the milk* that leaks into the shields—it can turn bad very quickly. Also, wash the shields frequently in hot soapy water and dry thoroughly.

➤ *Breast-feeding is not the main cause of sagging breasts*. Sagging breasts are more often caused by not wearing a bra during pregnancy when your breasts are heavy and need support. *You can prevent or minimize sagging* by wear a proper nursing bra, don't nurse for too long a period (more than 6 months), and limit the number of children nursed.

➤ *The size of your breasts has nothing to do* with your ability to produce milk. The amount of milk you make is determined by how much your baby stimulates your breasts: the more sucking, the more milk is produced.

Nutrition When Nursing

Nutrition is very important during breast-feeding. Your diet during pregnancy can affect lactation. If you cut down on salt, calories, and protein during pregnancy, it is unlikely that you will have enough stored fluid, fat, and protein to sustain a good milk flow.

Lactation is a greater nutritional stress on your body than pregnancy was. Progesterone, which is secreted throughout pregnancy, acts as an appetite stimulant. This seems to be the main factor in the additional weight most women gain over and above the "products of conception." If you are breast-feeding *you need this energy reserve*.

> ➤ *You should have no caloric restrictions*. You should use the same daily food guide as when you were pregnant with the addition of one daily serving from the milk or milk products group. When nursing you need an extra 500 calories and extra 20 grams of protein a day.
> ➤ *Continue taking an iron supplement* during breast-feeding: 30 to 60 mg of elemental iron daily.
> ➤ *Do Not take oral contraceptives during breast-feeding*. Consult the chart on pages 564–567 to see which other medications are unsafe during lactation.
> ➤ *You need to drink plenty of fluids to produce milk*. You have to drink 2 to 3 quarts of liquid a day—more if the weather is hot and you're perspiring. One way to meet this need for fluids is to get in the habit of having a large glass of any liquid beside you while you nurse—you can sip on it while the baby drinks. You may be aware that you get thirsty soon after nursing starts—have a glass of milk, juice, water, or beer to replenish what the baby takes out.

How the Breasts Work and the Content of Breast Milk

> ➤ *Colostrum* is a watery or creamy yellow liquid that precedes your milk supply. The colostrum has twice the protein of mature breast milk (which arrives within about 5 days). Colostrum is high in vitamins A and E. A baby is not born hungry; by the time he needs more nourishment than colostrum, your milk will have come in.
>
> Colostrum has an enzymatic effect to break down the mucus in the baby's digestive tract. Once your milk comes in, no mucus remains and the baby's passageways are prepared for milk. The laxative effect of colostrum clears meconium: the dark, tarry substance in the baby's lower intestine at birth. Meconium contains bilirubin, which can be reabsorbed by the baby if the meconium remains in the intestines. Too much bilirubin causes jaundice. The early appearance of milk is also important because it hydrates the baby and helps prevent high-level jaundice.

➤ *Probably the greatest benefit of colostrum and breast milk* is the antibodies it gives the baby. During the first 6 weeks of life a baby is most vulnerable to infection, but she doesn't manufacture many antibodies. Colostrum (and milk, to a lesser extent) contains IgA, a rich source of antibodies that protect against allergy and pathogens and enter through the gastrointestinal tract. Colostrum and mature milk contain maternal antibodies against various bacteria and viruses: protection against anything you have had or have been immunized against is transferred to the baby (such as *E. coli*, polio, mumps, influenza, etc.).

➤ *There are certain antibody protections which human milk provides*. The immunity given by the milk during the first 6 weeks may last beyond that time, so even a short nursing period is advantageous. *Human milk contains: enzymes* (lactoperoxidase, lysozyme), which promote chemical reactions that kill bacteria; *leukocytes*, which are cells that limit or prevent the spread of infection; *lactoferrin*, a milk protein that binds the iron that bacteria need for growth; and *antistaphylococcal* agents that guard against staph infections.

Milk contains living white cells which not only make antibodies but also can actually engulf and destroy disease-causing bacteria and viruses in the infant. A breast-fed baby's intestines are inhabited primarily by *lactobacilli*, "harmless" bacteria, while the intestines of a bottle-fed baby contain high levels of *E. coli*, potentially disease-causing bacteria. There is a lactobacillus-promoting factor in human milk which aids the growth of this kind of bacteria. The bacteria cause an acid environment to develop, which in turn discourages the growth of *E. coli*.

➤ *The fat content of your milk goes through changes*, leading to speculation that it adjusts to the child's needs. The fat content decreases after 5 to 6 months of lactation, which may be what a child requires in the second half of his first year. The evening feeding has an increased fat content, perhaps promoting longer sleep at night. The low milk-fat content in the morning may allow for a more alert baby.

➤ *The "let-down reflex" allows your milk to be released* when the baby sucks. You have no conscious control over the let-down reflex, but it can happen when you hear your baby cry, or even when you're away and *think* of the baby—your milk starts flowing. Tension, distraction, and embarrassment all inhibit this reflex, so try to create a peaceful environment during the first few weeks of nursing.

➤ *You may get strong uterine contractions* when you breast-feed during the first few weeks. This is because the baby's sucking releases the hormone oxytocin into your system, which makes your uterus contract. These contractions can be strong after a first baby; you may need your childbirth breathing techniques to stay comfortable.

➤ *If you are accidentally given medication to dry up your milk* you can still breast-feed. In some hospitals hormone shots are given routinely on the delivery table to inhibit milk production. However, the effects wear off, and although it will *delay* your milk supply coming in, the baby's sucking will bring it back anyway.

CAUTION: One drug used to suppress lactation is the hormone DES (diethylstilbesterol). *This drug is a known human carcinogen and could increase your chances of cancer in later years.* There is also evidence that the risk of blood clots is ten times greater if DES is used to dry up your milk supply. *Even if you don't plan to nurse*, you'd be better off nursing for the first week and then gradually drying up your milk supply to avoid using this potentially dangerous drug.

➤ *The length of a feeding is around one hour.* It takes the baby about 10 minutes to "empty" your breast. He gets the most milk in the first 5 minutes. Then the stored milk is depleted and richer, creamier milk is produced "on the spot." Therefore the last part of the feeding is the most nutritious.

➤ *"Demand feeding" is the most successful.* This means that you let the baby nurse whenever she is hungry. Some doctors prescribe a schedule on which you're supposed to feed the baby, but this may make the baby fretful and diminish your milk supply. The more a baby sucks, the more milk you produce—"demand feeding" stimulates milk production that is appropriate to the baby's needs. It focuses you on the baby instead of on the clock.

However, "demand" and scheduled feedings are not really opposites. A baby fed on demand will settle down to a schedule soon—her own schedule, though, not one predetermined by a doctor.

➤ *You can skip a feeding regularly* and still breast-feed successfully. Many people say that arranging for child care is easier with bottle-feeding, but you might consider an alternative: after a month or two of breast-feeding, alternate with regularly scheduled bottle-feedings. Try not to miss more than one breast-feeding daily in the first two months. *Regularity* (missing the same feeding[s] daily) is the key to successful part-time breast-feeding. This is one way to maintain independence—which may include working—and still nurse.

➤ *There is a nasal spray with oxytocin that can help* if you're having problems with breast-feeding. This spray has no side effects and will help speed up the let-down reflex. If you are still in the hospital, a nurse can phone your doctor's office and get permission to give you the spray. It has been a great help to women having trouble with early nursing. One quick spray into each nostril a few minutes before nursing can make the milk flow easily and alleviate much of the pain from the baby's sucking. You probably won't need the spray after you are fully lactating (your milk has come in), but it can be a great aid during those first few days.

How to Breast-Feed

It will be easiest to have someone show you how to breast-feed and be there with you when you first attempt it; this is a general description of what to do.

— Hold the baby in the crook of your arm. If you're right-handed begin on the left side so that your right hand is free to direct your breast.
— Depress the breast with your index and middle fingers, the nipple protruding between them, so that you give the baby a good place to latch on.
— Touch the baby's lips with the nipple. He will open his mouth. (The baby's natural "rooting" instinct makes him turn when touched on the lips or cheek. You will confuse the baby if you push his opposite cheek toward your nipple or pull both cheeks at once.) Then place the breast as far into his mouth as it will go and the baby will begin sucking. Be sure the areola is in his mouth and not just the nipple or the milk ducts will not be stimulated and your nipples will get sore.
— If you have soft, small nipples, a young baby may open her mouth and shake her head back and forth at your breast, trying to locate the nipple. So that the baby doesn't have this trouble finding the nipple you can put a cold, wet cloth on your nipple for a moment—this will cause the areola to shrivel and the nipple to protrude and become firm.
— For the first feeding stay on the left breast about 10 minutes and then switch to the right breast and let the baby stay there as long as she likes.
— Milk flows in both breasts at every nursing and it is better to use both at each feeding. Start with the heavier of the two breasts; let the baby suck 10 minutes on that side and then switch to the other.
— If your breasts are large you may need to use your index finger to maintain an air hole to the baby's nose until she gets experience and knows how to do it alone.
— To break the suction of a nursing baby, put your finger gently into the corner of her mouth until she releases. Never *pull* a nursing baby off your breast—that hurts!

About Hand-Expressing Milk

Hand-expressing milk is necessary if you have to stop breast-feeding temporarily because you are ill, you have to take medication, if you want to go away, or if you want to breast-feed while working and want to keep a store of your milk at home. You can have a weekend away alone with your partner, for example, and pick up breast-feeding where you left off when you come home if you express a little milk by hand each day to remind the breasts of their function. If you anticipate your departure you can express a couple of ounces in a bottle before each feeding, freeze it, and thus leave food for the baby while you're away.

> *In the back of the nipple* under the areola are the ducts through which the milk flows. To get it flowing, support your breast with one hand and place the thumb and forefinger farther apart, at the same time pushing them gently into your breast. Then squeeze them gently together, pulling the areola out toward the front.
> *Milk should spray out* if you're pressing the right area. If it doesn't, don't worry. Keep trying until you massage the milk ducts correctly toward the nipple.
> *While expressing, shift your fingers* to slightly different locations every couple of squirts. Do not slide your fingers on the skin because that can cause soreness. By changing the area of impact you give all the milk ducts a workout.

Breast-Feeding Outside Your Home

Nursing in public may seem awkward at first. Our culture is hostile to breast-feeding in public. Breasts are connected to sex in most people's minds and seeing them—especially used for a different purpose—can make people uncomfortable. You should take people's discomfort into consideration when you breast-feed in public, but it should not be a deterrent. *Discretion* is all that is necessary. Once you get the hang of it people won't even realize you're nursing. Wear knits or tops that can be unbuttoned from the bottom and lifted up. Wearing a jacket or sweater that partially covers the baby works well, also.

The Advantages of Breast-Feeding

A report from the Rockefeller Foundation suggested four ways in which the food habits of Americans need to be altered: their diets should contain less salt, less sugar, a lower fat content, and there should be a *return to universal breast-feeding of infants*. This impressive recommendation is but one more piece of evidence that breast-feeding is better both physically and emotionally than bottle-feeding. The only *disadvantage* to breast-feeding is the environmental pollutants that can reach your baby through breast milk. This consideration is covered in the section beginning on page 568.

The choice that you make about how to nourish your baby is the first decision you make about parenting (outside of circumcision) that has a long-lasting effect on your child's life. Don't just throw that decision away—you may come to regret it. It is every woman's right to decide how to feed her child, just as it is her right to determine where and how she will give birth. Just as with that decision, it is her duty to herself and the baby to make an informed, thoughtful choice. Please do not decide against breast-feeding or conversely feel you're "morally obligated" to breast-feed until you have all the facts.

The Advantages to the Baby

- ➤ **Breast-fed babies have been shown healthier** in certain studies. One study concluded that there was a three times greater incidence of illness in bottle-fed infants. These infants were compared to an equivalent group of breast-fed babies, and the bottle-fed babies had twice as many episodes of ear infection in the first year; 16 times more acute lower respiratory illness; 2½ times more significant vomiting or diarrhea; 8½ times more hospital admissions. This study also showed that while the average child gets 6 to 8 respiratory infections per year, bottle-fed babies get more seriously ill, because human milk and colostrum supply antibodies to viruses. It was also concluded that the length of time a baby is breast-fed is correlated positively with health. Infants who were breast-fed longer than 4½ months became ill *one-half as often* as those who were breast-fed less than 4½ months and those who were bottle-fed.

    There are certain diseases that are considered problems chiefly for bottle-fed babies. *Many of these diseases can apparently be avoided if the newborn is breast-fed for at least the first 2 weeks of life.*

- ➤ **Human milk is more digestible**. A baby's stomach learns gradually to digest. In the first days after birth the colostrum precedes the true milk, which gives the stomach and digestive juices time to learn how to function. The chemical composition of the colostrum is the same as what the baby was fed before birth because both are derived from the mother's blood. A breast-fed baby usually spits up less and the vomit doesn't have the harsh smell of "spoiled milk" as with bottle-fed babies. Breast milk is the most easily digested and well-balanced food you can give a baby.

- ➤ **Breast-fed babies are rarely constipated** because the curd of breast milk is smaller and more easily digestible than the curd of cow's milk. Breast milk contains enzymes which aid digestion. A breast-fed baby's bowel movements have a less offensive odor and the baby is less likely to have diaper rash.

- ➤ **Human milk has 20 mg of cholesterol per 100 mg.** Most formulas have 1.5 to 3.3 mg per 100. The amount of cholesterol needed by infants has not been established, but animal studies show that low cholesterol in infancy meant *higher* serum cholesterol levels when they got older. The higher cholesterol content of breast milk appears to promote lower serum cholesterol levels in adulthood. The implication is that low-cholesterol formulas may contribute to atherosclerosis in later life, which is a big health problem in the United States.

➢ *The small content of iron* in breast milk is bound to the protein lactoferrin, which enables virtually all of the iron to be absorbed by the baby. Lactoferrin also acts as an antibacterial agent.

➢ *Taurine is a nonprotein nitrogen compound* that is two times more abundant in breast milk than in cow's milk (which is the base for most artificial formulas). The importance of taurine or the harm of a deficiency in bottle-fed infants has not been proven, but it is known that a newborn has only 25% of his mature brain weight at birth. After birth a baby is still in a phase of rapid growth and there is a great demand—which may be critical—for specific essential nutrients.

➢ *The breast milk of mothers of premature babies* has been discovered to differ from that of women with full-term deliveries. The milk of mothers of premies has been found to contain substantially higher concentrations of protein, sodium, and chloride. Studies show that premature babies fed this preterm milk tolerated their diet much better.

These new findings contradict a widely held belief that premature infants fed formula grow more quickly than those fed mother's milk. Premies who breast-feed and get preterm milk grow as well, but most important, they are more apt to avoid the intestinal infections that are associated with some premature babies who take formula.

These findings also call into question the controversial issue of feeding preterm infants. Because they are not developed enough to breast-feed, premature infants who do receive mother's milk normally are fed from a milk bank: human milk pumped from several mothers, all of whom had pregnancies that went a full nine months. It was this milk that was found to be deficient for premature infants. This new research suggests that when premies receive mother's milk, it should be pumped from the natural mother only.

The Problems with Cow's Milk

➢ *Cow's milk has three times the percentage of salts* as breast milk. In the first weeks of life the baby's kidneys are not sufficiently developed to handle this high phosphate content.

Convulsions sometimes occur between 6 to 8 days after birth in children who have been fed cow's milk.

➢ *Cow's milk proteins are foreign* and quite allergenic to babies. During the first 6 weeks of life, the intestine is rather permeable and may allow absorption of foreign proteins. These absorbed proteins may sensitize the infant and lay the foundation for food allergies. (After about 6 weeks the local immune response of the baby helps prevent the absorption.)

➢ *If the baby's immediate family* has a history of allergies, breast milk will reduce the baby's exposure to foreign milk proteins and possible allergy. Allergies seem to be a familial condition. If a parent or sibling has an allergy of any type, the baby is more likely to develop allergies as well. Moreover, once an individual is allergic to one substance other allergies become more common.

A few babies develop an allergy to cow's milk. Symptoms of this allergy include: vomiting; colic; skin irritations such as dermatitis, hives, or eczema; gastrointestinal infections; respiratory illness; stomach bleeding; growth retardation; and central nervous system damage. Allergic reaction to milk can be life-threatening for an infant. Severe vomiting and diarrhea are symptomatic of this allergy: if it is not treated promptly, it can lead to rapid dehydration and death.

When there is a family history of allergy the baby should not be given cow's milk formula from birth. A baby's allergic reaction may be minimized if cow's milk is withheld during the first months of life. Most pediatricians recommend soymilk formula instead, but one study showed that 30 to 50% of children who were allergic to cow's milk developed an allergy to soymilk as well. In such cases you can substitute either a meat-based formula or a predigested milk formula (Nutramigen) if you don't breast-feed.

➢ *There is less likelihood of overfeeding* when you breast-feed. You don't know the amount the baby is getting—he just nurses until satisfied. There is a theory that breast milk is so perfectly suited to a baby's needs that it first satisfies thirst and then gives more substantial nourishment. The milk at the beginning of nursing is more watery; higher-calorie milk comes naturally at the end of the feeding. Cow's milk formulas do not satisfy thirst. A baby's thirst may be misinterpreted as hunger, so he might get more calories than he needs or should have.

A mother's encouragement to a baby to drink the entire contents of a bottle is probably responsible for the higher caloric intake of bottle-fed babies. Research suggests that consuming a large amount of calories early in life can lead to the development of an excessive number of fat cells. Later on these fat cells can be reduced in size—but not in number—by dieting. Bottle-feeding mothers have to be cautioned against pressuring infants into finishing each feeding and to avoid a similar attitude toward their eating throughout childhood.

➤ **Strong sucking develops correct palate** formation. A breast-feeding baby has to suck harder to get milk. A bottle does not require a baby to use the same strength when he sucks. Nursing from the breast also develops muscles that are used later for speaking.

➤ **Breast-feeding is a continuation of the intimate physiological relationship** that began when your baby was in utero. During nursing, bottle-fed babies do not seem to receive the same intimate physical contact—skin-to-skin contact, close holding, eye-to-eye contact—that breast-feeding babies get.

If you watch a woman bottle-feed her baby you'll notice that she often doesn't hold him close to her body with firm contact. Sometimes bottle-feeding mothers even feed a baby while he's in a plastic chair, or they prop him up, encouraging the baby to hold his own bottle. Some parents have the misguided notion this is "progress"—that the sooner a baby is separated from close physical contact, the more quickly he is developing. Regardless of what you feed your baby and what container it comes in, a baby deserves the warm, close, secure feeling of being held in your arms when he eats. All too soon a baby *does* grow up and become increasingly independent. The physical and emotional pleasure of being held next to your body helps a baby develop into a secure, self-reliant person.

There are tangible results of the close contact which breast-feeding babies enjoy. A breast-feeding mother doesn't have to think about how to hold the baby—she has no choice but to snuggle the child against her. Studies have shown that breast-fed babies that were *not separated* from their mothers after birth averaged a half-pound over their birth weight at 6 to 7 days of age. Bottle-fed babies are expected to fall below their birth weight and take 7 to 10 days to regain the weight they had when born.

➤ **It has been said that breast-feeding** is "the first way to tell the truth to a baby and keep a promise." At the breast a child commences to learn how to relate to another person as a warm, loving, caring human being.

The Advantages to the Mother

➤ **Breast-feeding immediately after birth** promotes uterine contractions and reduces the risk of postpartum hemorrhage. Further suckling helps the uterus return quickly to its prepregnancy size.

➤ **Some experts say that there is a decreased incidence of breast cancer** in women who breast-feed.

> *There is a value in being forced to sit or lie still* while breast-feeding. The early weeks postpartum are when the baby makes the heaviest demands to nurse. This corresponds to the time when you should be resting and allowing your body to rebuild. The time that breast-feeding requires protects you from the tendency to overexert yourself in the first weeks after birth.

> *Prolactin is the milk-making hormone.* It is believed to be important in promoting maternal attachment. Some studies have shown that prolactin increases motherliness.

> *Breast-feeding is important for the reciprocal development* of you and your baby. Each time a baby is born a mother is born, too—and your further development is enhanced by close, intimate contact with the baby.

> *Breast-feeding is less expensive* than formulas, which are very costly. The extra 500 calories and extra 20 grams of protein that a breast-feeding mother needs a day can be provided by a peanut-butter sandwich on wheat bread and a glass of milk.

> *Breast-feeding is more convenient.* There are no bottles to clean or formula to worry about. Traveling is much easier; when the baby is hungry you just put her to your breast. There is none of the hassle of trying to sterilize bottles and have enough formula while traveling.

> *Breast-feeding requires only one arm*, so it leaves you freer to do other things simultaneously. You can hold a book, write a letter, or talk on the telephone while nursing.

Complications of the Breasts and Nipples from Breast-Feeding

If a baby is not allowed to breast-feed immediately at birth, it can cause complications. Babies not allowed to suck at the breast when they first have the need tend to forget the sucking instinct in the hours of frustration that follow. There can be a deep psychological trauma to you when the baby is finally brought to you and won't take your breast.

However, if you were heavily medicated during labor and delivery you may not be able to hold the baby. Also, the medication is secreted into the colostrum and it may be better not to add it to the system of a baby already struggling with the labor medication you took.

If your baby has been given a bottle before he breast-feeds, he will not know how to nurse at your breast, which requires stronger sucking. First of all, make sure the baby gets no more bottles. And don't feel rejected. You'll just have to show the baby how to do it. If your breasts are still soft enough to put way into the back of his mouth, prop the baby on a pillow in your lap under your left breast, if you're right-handed. Express some milk into the baby's mouth. Compress your breast between your fingers, put it as far back into the baby's mouth as it will go and express more milk. Eventually the baby will coordinate the right movements to latch onto your breast.

If the baby gets upset, comfort him over your shoulder, and when he's quiet, try again. You can alternately put some breast milk on your knuckle and when the baby sucks well on that, transfer him to your breast. Or you can use a breast pump and have the baby drink directly from it like a cup. It is messy but preferable to an artificial nipple, which miseducates the baby's sucking technique.

Engorgement of Your Breasts

➤ **Engorgement** of your breasts can happen on the third or fourth day postpartum with the onset of lactation. Your breasts will feel hard and tender.

➤ **One cause of this can be** that the baby did not start nursing from birth. If you don't get the colostrum flowing before your milk supply comes in, this can result in hard, painful breasts.

➤ **Make sure that your bra is supportive** but isn't too tight; 15 minutes before you put the baby to your breast take an aspirin or a glass of wine or beer to lessen the pain.

➤ **Ice packs or heat can help lessen the discomfort;** alternate the two, depending on which feels best.

➤ **A warm shower is good,** or applying a washcloth that is as hot as you can stand.

➤ **Once your milk starts flowing the engorgement will pass**.

What to Do About It

➤ **One remedy is to get in the shower** and turn a gentle stream of water warmer and warmer until it's as hot as you can stand. Once the blood is circulating well, massage your breasts gently one at a time. Have one palm underneath supporting the breast and working upward toward the nipples. The other palm should start at your collarbone and work down toward the nipple. Then your upper hand should massage the side of the breast, working from your armpit in toward the nipple, then from your breastbone toward the nipple. The lower hand should massage on the opposite side of the breast. The object of this massaging is to get the milk flowing and to continue working the lumps caused by backed-up milk down toward the nipple.

➤ **There are several preventive steps you can take** to avoid painful breast engorgement. The first is that the baby should be nursed soon after birth to facilitate lactation. The wait of 6 to 12 hours in some hospitals is too long a fasting period for successful breast-feeding.

➤ **No bottle should be given to the baby**, of either water or formula. It will interfere with the natural establishment of lactation. It is easier for the baby to nurse from a bottle: some may simply wait for the post-breast-feeding bottle, which sabotages nursing. The mother's milk will collect in her breast, so there will be diminished milk production, which depends greatly on emptying the breast.

Preventing Engorgement

➢ *To help prevent engorgement*, become aware of how the breast works and fit your nursing schedule around that. In the first 2 hours after nursing, the breast produces most of the milk for the next feeding.

➢ *Breast engorgement will be more likely to occur* if the breast is kept from the baby for longer than 2 hours.

➢ *One hour after a woman's breast is emptied,* it has already produced 40% of the supply for the next feeding. Two hours afterward she may have as much as 75%. Although it might seem sensible to wait until a higher percent of her milk capacity has been regained, that kind of schedule can lead to breast soreness.

➢ *Because breast milk is quickly digested* (maybe in 2 hours, but certainly sooner than the 4-hour interval for breast-feeding that is often recommended), the baby becomes overly hungry. A very hungry baby is going to suck more vigorously. Also, if the mother has waited the extra hour for her breasts to fill "to capacity," congestion of the areola becomes a problem. The baby cannot put the nipple and areola into the back of his mouth and his abnormally vigorous, hungry sucking will cause pain.

➢ *A good way to facilitate nursing if your breasts are engorged*, or even if they aren't, is to express a little milk at the beginning of each feeding. This will soften the areola, allowing the baby to get the nipple to the back of his mouth easily. With two fingers placed around the areola, you can gently press against your chest, emptying the sinuses and making the areola soft. This will be a great help for the first couple of weeks of breast-feeding.

Mastitis (Breast Infection)

➢ *Mastitis is an infection of the breast caused* by a clogged milk duct or a staphylococcal infection. It is not to be confused with engorgement, which occurs on the third or fourth day postpartum.

➢ *True mastitis rarely occurs before the end of the first postpartum week* and usually not until the end of the third or fourth week. It is believed that the infant harbors the bacteria (*Staphylococcus aureus*) in her nose and throat and the organism enters the breast at the time of feeding through the nipple, via a fissure or abrasion which may be quite small. The baby may have gotten the bacteria in the hospital from the partially washed hands of one of the staff, but there are many other ways it could have been picked up.

➤ *The symptoms of mastitis are sudden:* you will feel poorly, have a fever, headache, and engorged breasts that feel warm. The tender area will be hard and red. If you contact the doctor promptly, the condition won't become serious. A drop of your milk is sent for bacterial culture and penicillin G or another antibiotic is given in the meantime. If your temperature and inflammation don't subside within 48 hours, an abscess usually forms, but this is quite uncommon. In this case the baby must be completely weaned from your breasts and the doctor has to drain the abscess.

➤ *It is not necessary to stop breast-feeding* if you get mastitis. If your doctor says to stop, call the La Leche League, which will give you information about nursing and mastitis. They usually recommend that you continue nursing from the affected breast, that it will heal more quickly. The baby will not get sick, as was once thought.

➤ *Stay off your feet* as much as possible and apply heat to the breast with wet washcloths.

➤ *Offer the sore breast first* at each feeding—that way it will probably be emptied and the clogged duct will unclog.

➤ *The other alternative is to breast-feed only from your healthy breast* and express enough milk from the infected side to relieve pressure. You can then supplement your breast milk with a bottle, being careful to use only "premie" nipples, which have small holes. This way your baby cannot get milk too easily from the bottle and learn to prefer it over your breast.

Sore Nipples

➤ *Sore nipples can occur even if you prepared your breasts* before nursing. Be sure to let your nipples air-dry and never keep on a wet bra or a wet pad. *No nursing bra should ever have waterproof backing*: tear it out or get rid of the bra. This is a cause of sore nipples. Also, make sure the baby has the whole areola in her mouth when sucking.

➤ *Do not use soap, alcohol, tincture of benzoin, or petroleum jelly* on your nipples. If you choose to use an ointment, do so sparingly: these substances can keep out the light and sunlight, which are important to healing.

➤ *There are several substances which are commonly recommended* to minimize nipple discomfort: vitamins A and D cream or concentrate, oils, aloe vera, and expressed breast milk or colostrum. Massé breast cream is also commonly used—although based on new information about the danger of lanolin (see below), you should check the ingredients to see if a product contains lanolin.

➤ *Pure lanolin may be contaminated with pesticide residuals*. Lanolin has been recommended for years as a natural remedy for nipple pain; however, some samples showed contamination. The tests were done by the Division of Colors and Cosmetics of the Food and Drug Administration (FDA) and the Environmental Protection Agency (EPA) National Toxicological Program. Although the reports stated that "the levels of pesticides did not present an immediate toxic hazard," breast-feeding mothers who apply lanolin to their breasts may be unnecessarily exposing their babies to toxic chemicals. We do not know the potential effects on a newborn who ingests lanolin products, so why run the risk?

➤ *Warm, dry heat is the best cure for sore nipples.* Leave your breasts exposed to the air as much as possible. To make an ultraviolet lamp just buy an ultraviolet bulb and put it in any light socket. Sit 3 feet from the lamp: expose your nipples a half-minute the first day, one minute the second and third days, and 2 minutes the fourth and fifth days. If your skin does not redden, you can increase to 3 minutes on the sixth day and maintain that level until the soreness is gone. If there *is* redness at the 2-minute level, cut back to one minute for several days and increase by a half-minute if possible. Be sure to use a towel or other cover for your eyes. The bulb gets *very* hot after use. Time yourself carefully with a kitchen timer.

➤ *Do not curtail nursing*—this will just prolong the problem. In fact, continuing to nurse frequently is the best solution. Leisurely nursing every 2 or 3 hours is easier on tender nipples. This way your breasts don't get overfull and the baby doesn't get ravenous. Give the least-sore breast first because the baby sucks hardest when she is hungry. You may limit nursing to 8 to 10 minutes on the sore side, but no less than that. Change nursing positions at each feeding. If your nipples are very sore and you limit sucking time to 10 minutes on each side, the baby's sucking needs may not be satisfied and you may have to offer a pacifier.

➤ *A mother who has a great deal of pain* from a sore nipple may have to limit nursing to only 5 minutes on that side. Actually, the first 5 minutes empties most of the milk from the breast and 10 minutes will empty it completely. You have to decide for yourself how bad the pain is and whether it's better to have the baby suck for more than 5 minutes even if the nipple is very sore, because you get the benefit of emptying the breast completely.

➤ *If the baby seems satisfied,* she can certainly manage for 5 or 6 days while the nipple is sore with only 5 minutes of nursing time. Remember to put the baby first on the breast that is not sore, or less sore. The baby is more likely to take the sore one gently in her mouth because she's less hungry by then. A good rule of thumb is to nurse a sore nipple second, but to nurse a sore breast first, to empty it.

➤ *Apprehension* may be related to sore nipples. Slightly tender nipples may cause enough tension to hold back the let-down reflex. This delay in the milk may make the baby angry so that he pulls and tugs on the nipple. This makes it even sorer and causes you greater concern. Try to make a conscious effort to relax before nursing.

To ease the discomfort while nursing take an aspirin or glass of wine or beer 15 minutes beforehand. This will help relax you and encourage the let-down reflex. If you're having a problem with the let-down reflex, you can hand-express some milk before the baby starts nursing. If you're having real difficulty with your let-down reflex when your nipples are sore, talk to your doctor about prescribing some oxytocin.

➤ *Ice water or ice eases the pain* of sore nipples immediately. Crush the ice, wrap it in a washcloth, and apply it to the nipple area.

➤ *A fungus infection can cause sore nipples*. The baby may have thrush, which is common and bothersome, but not serious. If the nipple soreness persists and there are white spots inside the baby's mouth, or if the baby has persistent diaper rash or you have vaginitis, or if you have been fine and suddenly develop sore nipples again—call the doctor for treatment.

➤ *Cracked nipples can be caused by anything* that keeps the baby from getting his jaws on the areola. Most hair around the nipple doesn't bother a baby, but sometimes he will react by pulling back and chewing on the nipple. Trim the hairs if this happens. Treatment is the same as for sore nipples, but more so. Sit in the sunshine by an open window, letting the sun bake your breasts—but not burn them, obviously. In the winter the sun coming through the glass is helpful. For some women, a sunlamp is too strong: in this case the heat of an ordinary naked lightbulb is good.

➤ *A blood blister on the tip of your nipple* is caused by vigorous sucking. It is not significant and you should just leave it alone when it is in the blister and scab stages. It will go away by itself.

➤ *Hematoma (bruising) in and around the nipple* during breast-feeding is often found as a result of abnormal sucking with painfully engorged breasts. This bruising is often caused by the mother waiting too long between feedings, allowing the breasts to get engorged and the baby to become so hungry that he sucks abnormally vigorously.

Hematoma into the nipple is caused by palate sucking. There is rarely a problem on the sides of the nipples, because the sides of the baby's mouth are more gentle on the nipple than the upper or lower portions of the mouth. The top part of the baby's mouth sucks with the greatest force. Sometimes the bruising appears right on the edge of the nipple, a clear indication that the baby is not getting the nipple to the back of his mouth. Be sure that the whole areola goes into the baby's mouth when nursing.

Problems with the Baby and Nursing

➤ *Afternoon fussiness and hunger* are a common complaint in the first month of breast-feeding. The baby nurses well in the morning and sleeps 3 or 4 hours between feedings; in the afternoon she cries and wants to be fed nearly every hour. The reason this happens is that as the mother goes through the day she tires, and milk production suffers as she runs around. One way to overcome this problem is to do most of your chores and errands in the morning, and by early afternoon relax, preferably with the baby near you.

➤ *Strenuous exercise can create difficulties* in nursing. If a breast-feeding mother does intense exercise it can result in higher lactic acid levels in her milk, which may influence its taste and quality. If your baby is having difficulties related to nursing, you can experiment for a few days and see if less exertion on your part results in the baby feeding more easily.

➤ *Insufficient milk supply* is a common complaint during the first postpartum days. A major cause for this is a delay in starting breast-feeding postdelivery or infrequent feedings afterward. The breast has to be stimulated by the baby nursing often, more than the every-4-hour schedule at some hospitals. The baby has to nurse several times from each breast in every 24-hour period; if the breasts are not emptied frequently, milk production will suffer. Supplementary formula feedings will reduce the milk supply because they reduce breast stimulation.

Another reason for a low milk yield is the emotional factor of a new mother being told her milk supply is poor or that her baby is hungry. This can make a woman feel guilty and anxious, which will lead to reduced milk production and a poor let-down reflex. If you are aware of these potential problems, you can avoid them. You might want to try the oxytocin nasal spray described on page 539 to help your let-down reflex.

➤ *If you're worried about your milk supply*, there are a couple of things you should know about breast-feeding babies. Generally speaking, a baby who is breast-feeding will eat every 2 to 3 hours. She should gain one-half to one ounce a day in the first six months of her life. Babies tend to lose a little weight after birth, but by the time she is 2 weeks old she should be at least back to her birth weight.

If you feel your baby is constantly wanting to eat—she's still hungry after feeding and a pacifier doesn't satisfy her—you may suspect your milk supply is low. Have a breast-feeding consultation with your pediatrician or, better yet, a lactation specialist.

➢ **The baby may refuse to nurse**. A baby may be sensitive to your diet and can be fussy about particular foods which impart a flavor to your breast milk. Some foods to avoid or eat sparingly if your baby is fussy include: onions, garlic, cabbage, Brussels sprouts, and chocolate. When you're menstruating your milk may be offensive to the baby. If so, you can cut down the nursing time until your period is over.

➢ **A teething baby can refuse to nurse**. Rub teething gel on her gums. If your let-down reflex requires vigorous sucking, which may be hard for a teething baby, you can use a nasal-spray oxytocin before difficult feedings, or hand-express some milk first so the baby doesn't have to suck so hard.

➢ **The baby may bite when nursing**. This usually doesn't happen until around 3 months and ordinarily occurs at the end of a feeding. Say "NO!" loudly and suddenly; terminate the feeding right then. At the next feeding don't continue nursing after the baby begins to play around, and she will learn soon enough.

➢ **You cannot see how much the baby is eating**. This may bother some women who feel the need to know the quantity that the baby consumes. Don't worry about it. The beauty of breast-feeding is that it is a supply and demand system: you produce milk in response to how much the baby sucks. A breast-fed baby eats until satisfied. As long as the baby has frequent wet diapers, is alert, and looks healthy, she's getting enough. You can always check intake by output: except in very hot weather a baby will wet a lot of diapers. This is one way to verify that the baby is getting enough.

➢ **The baby will be hungry sooner** than if you feed her formula. Breast milk digests more quickly—cow's milk is hard for a baby to digest and the large curds stay in her stomach longer. If your baby won't sleep through the night once you've got a good milk supply, after the early postpartum period, you might consider giving some formula before bed.

➢ **Breast-feeding takes longer than bottle-feeding**, which some women consider a disadvantage to nursing. You can give a baby a bottle in about 10 minutes, but breast-feeding realistically takes about an hour. However, with a bottle you and the baby may miss out on that contact with each other which is so important for both of you. Breast-feeding forces you to sit still and enjoy. If you are accustomed to having a superefficient, rushed, very organized rhythm, you may have to change it temporarily. It may be good for you to have a change of pace—and you shouldn't undervalue the time you spend in an intimate embrace with your baby. All too soon your baby will be changing and growing—try to make whatever adjustments you can

YOU SHOULD NOT BREAST-FEED IF YOU HAVE

— *AIDS* (transmitted via body fluids, including breast milk)
— *Drug addiction* (cocaine, tranquilizers, heroin, methadone, marijuana, heavy use of alcohol)
— *Heavy smoking habit* (nicotine is passed to the baby)
— *Serious infection* (such as tuberculosis)
— *Chronic health problems* (heart or kidney impairment; diabetes [see pages 555–556])
— *Extreme underweight or serious anemia*
— *Conditions requiring certain medications* (see page 561)
— *A powerful aversion to nursing* (this means a strong revulsion you can't overcome, not the normal doubts and worries)

NOTE: A history of breast cancer is not a reason to avoid breast-feeding. There is no proof of any "virus passed through breast milk" in families with a history of premenopausal breast cancer. It is also considered safe for a mother who has had cancer in one breast to breast-feed, and nursing is can be especially wonderful for a mother who has had to confront this illness.

in your life so you can enjoy every stage of the baby's life without thinking of it as "wasted" time.

Psychological Problems with Breast-Feeding

Some women just aren't comfortable with either the idea or the physical reality of breast-feeding. There can be a vast number of reasons for this. For example, a woman who can't stand the idea of breast-feeding may have been rejected as a child and is now afraid of warm, close relationships. Some women cannot nurse because unconsciously they identify with their own mother, who was cold and rejecting. One often learns to be a good mother from having had one.

If you are unhappy or tense breast-feeding you shouldn't bang your head against a wall. You will probably be able to relax, cuddle, and enjoy your baby more with a bottle. There are many people who believe that *how* a baby is fed is as important as *what* he is fed. A baby gets two things in his mother's arms: he gets food and love (and develops the capacity to love). If you can give that to your baby more freely and easily by *not* breast-feeding, then a bottle will be better for you both.

Diabetes and Breast-Feeding

➤ **Breast-feeding is usually advised against** for diabetic mothers. Initially, breast-feeding may be associated with hypoglycemic episodes; milk production is often deficient and nursing is rarely successful. However, breast-feeding can help offset the high-risk atmosphere associated with diabetic pregnancy, as well as giving a diabetic mother the pleasure of nursing and of knowing her body can do it. Some of the possible complications follow.

➤ **Hypoglycemia can be expected between 5 and 7 hours postpartum**. Immediately after delivery there is an increased risk of hypoglycemia while your body makes diet/insulin/exercise adjustments, whether you are breast-feeding or not. The loss of human placental lactogen is accompanied by an increased insulin sensitivity. IV glucose and insulin are monitored until stabilization is reached at about 18 to 24 hours postpartum. Then you can take daily insulin again by injection.

Your daily insulin requirement will probably be only 60% of the dose you were taking before you became pregnant. The requirement will gradually increase for 4 to 6 weeks postpartum. Breast-feeding may reduce your insulin requirement beyond this 4- to 6-week period. Nursing may reduce it due to a prolonged attenuation of growth hormone secretion. Insulin need declines in women who rigidly control their diets and increase their activity postpartum, independent of the effect of breast-feeding.

Hypoglycemic reactions (insulin reactions) are associated with rapid falls in your glucose levels. The symptoms are: visual disturbances, headache, sweating, shaking, loss of coordination, and finally loss of consciousness. Hypoglycemia triggers the release of epinephrine, which inhibits oxytocin, the hormone that mediates the let-down reflex. Thus, high levels of epinephrine can inhibit your let-down reflex and interfere with breast-feeding. Trace amounts of insulin and epinephrine reach the breast milk, but the infant's digestive enzymes deactivate the hormones.

➤ **Hyperglycemia: occasional high blood sugar** may occur as diet/insulin/exercise adjustments are being made throughout the breast-feeding period. Any infection, illness, or even emotional upset can cause an increase in your blood glucose and glycosuria. You can test your urine 3 or 4 times daily for sugar, and periodic fasting and random blood sugar tests (under a doctor's care) can be made to assess diabetic control.

➤ **Acetonuria may accompany high blood sugar**. Acetones are detected in your urine by Ketodiastix or Acetest tablets. The usual treatment for ketosis is increased insulin, increased carbohydrates, and bed rest. If you are breast-feeding you have to be particularly concerned about avoiding acetonuria. Ketones can enter the breast milk but are not harmful. They are ingested by the infant and utilized along with other dietary substances.

➤ *Lactose may be found in your urine* during late pregnancy and lactation. You will have to use urine-testing materials which will not react positively to lactose but are specific for glucose. TesTape, unlike most others, is specific for glucose.

➤ *Infections must be treated aggressively* with a nursing diabetic mother. If you develop an infection, antibiotics are usually prescribed, but many of them are detrimental to the nursing baby and enter your breast milk in high concentrations (see page 564). *Antibiotics to avoid are*: erythromycin, Estolate, Symmetrel, tetracycline, streptomycin, and doxycycline, to name a few. Alternatives can usually be prescribed and many antibiotics (including erythromycin) do not necessitate weaning, just a temporary interruption in breast-feeding.

➤ *Treat plugged milk ducts promptly* because they can quickly develop into an infection. Clogged ducts often result from wearing a too-tight bra or wearing a nursing bra while you sleep. If an infection does develop, keep the breast emptied, apply heat, and stay in bed. Allowing milk to stay in your breast will result in painful engorgement and further obstruction of an already plugged duct.

➤ *Abrupt weaning should be avoided*: it may cause an emotional upset for you and the baby and will make diabetic control difficult.

➤ *Monilial infections of the vagina* are common in diabetic women, especially if their glucose control is poor. When you are breast-feeding, monilia can infect the nipple. The prevention is to keep nipples dry between feedings or the infection will return despite treatment. The doctor may prescribe Lotrimin cream or suppositories, or Monistat ointment. Mycostatin was popular at one time, but it has only a 3- to 4-week shelf life. Be sure to wash these ointments off the breast before nursing.

➤ *Infant teething or illness in you or the baby* may mean you have to decrease nursing for a while (weaning) and then nurse more frequently. This may cause mysteriously high urine or blood sugar, followed by unexpectedly low test values. You can usually compensate for this by eating less, exercising more, or adjusting your insulin.

Working and Breast-Feeding

There are two contemporary trends at odds with each other which meet head-on when a working woman decides to breast-feed. On the one hand there is increased employment and more substantial careers for women, but this conflicts with a trend toward increased breast-feeding and what is referred to as "natural mothering." This is a philosophy that a mother should have constant contact with her child, including breast-feeding on demand, for the first one or two years of his life—a belief system that is incompatible with employment outside the home.

A working mother also has a twofold problem in juggling her commitment to her job and her child. At work she must almost pretend that her child does not exist, yet she has to arrange her life as much as she can to take the child into consideration. She faces criticism from both sides: if she works she is considered a selfish, "bad" mother by those who favor "natural mothering," and because of her commitment to her child she may be reprimanded by those in the workplace if she rearranges her time on the child's behalf.

The reality is that there are increasing numbers of women who want to have a life outside their home. Many of the women having babies today are doing so after they have firmly established themselves in a career they do not want to relinquish. On top of that, there are women who may wind up forced to work to support their children. More than 50% of all two-parent families have both parents working. Also, statistics show that one-quarter of the children in America do not live with both their natural parents—and the vast majority stay with their mother. A full one-half of black children do not live with both their parents. By the age of eighteen, 35 to 45% of all children in the United States will spend five years or more in a single-parent home. Since most men do not meet child-support payments, the mother usually seeks employment.

Breast-feeding and working outside the home not only are possible but have great benefits if you are willing to make the effort. Working and raising children at the same time can produce a destructive guilt: you feel torn between the two, as if you are cheating the children, have to make it up to them, and so on. Breast-feeding provides an important source of confidence in your mothering ability. The practical aspect is that breast-fed babies are usually healthier. Preventing sickness in your baby is important to your psychological well-being. As hard as it may be to leave a baby to go to work, it creates that much more guilt to leave a *sick* baby. Breast-feeding itself is not a common choice among American women, and working and breast-feeding is even more unusual. It may be difficult, but the rewards are worth the investment of your time and energy if you are interested in pursuing the combination.

➤ ***Certain character traits may hamper you***. For instance, independence and a motivation to succeed, which help in a career, can hinder you with breast-feeding. Nursing is not a rational, predictable process: it cannot be controlled and organized in the way that many jobs can. Breast-feeding is emotional, intuitive, sensual, and enjoyable. Your expectation of accomplishing too much during early breast-feeding—and pride in your independence—may keep you from asking for help. You are going to have to overcome the antidependency sentiments which our society applauds, particularly for people with careers, so that you can reach out for help with breast-feeding if you need it.

➤ *Avoid negative attitudes* to your decision to breast-feed and separate regularly from your baby. Criticism is the last thing you need—it is a stress and can inhibit your let-down reflex during the initiation of lactation and undermine your efforts. Try to find other women who are in your position and even organize a support group among yourselves. You can share mutual problems and solutions—just knowing other women sharing your situation can be a great comfort.

➤ *The initiation of breast-feeding is the foundation* for success when you return to work. It is absolutely essential that you have encouragement from everyone close to you. This is vital for breast-feeding success even for women who are not simultaneously pursuing careers. Especially if you are a first-time mother, you should optimally take off a minimum of 4 weeks from work and preferably 6 weeks. It is rare to be able to establish a good nursing relationship—with a well-conditioned let-down reflex and an adequate milk supply—in less than a month.

➤ *Hand-expression of milk will be necessary* to maintain a milk supply once you are separated from your child. It will also be necessary so you can deal with breast engorgement. Practice the hand-expression of colostrum before the baby is born. If you aren't comfortable using your hands, try a breast pump, because you have to be able to hand-express your milk.

➤ *In the hospital you should realistically expect little or no help* with breast-feeding. Seek out women who have breast-fed before your baby is born so that you have someone to call if you need help. Breast-feeding will go much smoother if you have minimal medication during the birth—that way the baby will be alert and will suck more enthusiastically. An early start to breast-feeding—preferably on the delivery table—will also help establish your relationship with the baby. Be sure to have rooming-in, if possible, and make certain that your baby is given *no bottle supplements,* which sabotage breast-feeding.

➤ *The day a woman comes home from the hospital* is considered the most critical time for problems with her milk. Your let-down reflex is affected by *fatigue, anxiety, insensitive remarks*, and other stressful factors. If these occur in the early days, their impact can interfere with your milk supply.

   You should come home and literally go right to bed, taking the baby with you. Take along your favorite food and drink; wine and beer in moderation are traditional aids to relaxation. Remove yourself from the responsibilities of the house and arrange for help in the beginning, if possible. Household help that contributes to good nursing—by freeing you to relax with your new baby—is a well-deserved indulgence.

➤ *Returning to work and how you handle breast-feeding* is a personal choice. However, it is vital that you maintain a flexible attitude. *There is no absolute definition of success in breast-*

feeding for a working mother. There is no measurement of success as gauged by a number of weeks or any other absolute scale. Remember this: If your nursing relationship brings satisfaction to you and your baby, then you have succeeded.

Every drop of breast milk you give your baby helps him. The longer you nurse, the more protection against disease and allergy you've offered the baby. If you find you go back to work and cannot sustain breast-feeding, you have not failed. If you nurse for six weeks and then discontinue nursing, you can be pleased that you've given your baby the best possible nutrition in the important early weeks.

➤ *You have several options about how to handle breast-feeding* and your return to work. You can take the baby to work, or you can possibly arrange to work at home. A sitter can bring the baby to you at lunch or during coffee breaks, although there is no guarantee that the baby will nurse on your schedule. There is also substitute feeding, which is probably the most practical.

➤ *Substitute feeding is best if your milk is used,* although formula can be substituted. You can begin to collect your milk before you return to work. Express the milk into a container that is cold and sterile: putting it through the dishwasher is sufficient sterilization. Cool it afterward. Cover it securely and label it with the date. It will last up to 2 years in a freezer and up to 6 months in a refrigerator freezer. The antibodies in the milk are stable when frozen, but some other anti-infective properties are not. But having frozen milk gives you security: you won't have to worry about manual expression on a daily basis for the first few weeks, and if you have days when you can't produce fresh milk, the baby will still have some.

It is best to express the next day's milk at work and refrigerate it until use, saving the frozen milk for when fresh is not available. If you express milk at work, do it at the same time and place each day. This conditions your milk to let down to a stimulus other than sucking. You can also collect the leakage from your breasts by wearing a Netsy Milk Cup, which is a plastic dome-shaped cover (from the Netsy Co., 34 Sunrise Avenue, Mill Valley, California 94941).

You have to refrigerate the collected milk right away, as it will spoil rapidly, especially when the weather is warm.

➤ *Introduce the baby to the person who will be giving the substitute feedings* before you return to work. The person should stay for increasingly long periods of time but with *no attempts to feed the child* the first few times. With older babies—past 6 or 7 months—they may already be experiencing separation anxiety, so the introduction should be more gradual for them.

At first you should go out for one to two hours, staying within reach. The substitute should try to feed the baby about half an hour *before* the baby's usual feeding time. Feeding before the baby gets really hungry gives her time to deal with the bottle before acute hunger sets in. This prevents the escalating panic in the infant who has to cope with an unfamiliar way of eating *and* extreme hunger.

The substitute should gently insert the nipple in a back-and-forth manner . . . and stop if the baby gets too upset. The sitter should try again 15 to 20 minutes later. Using Nuk nipples is a good idea, as they are closest to human nipples. If the baby gets really upset, you should return and try again the following day. Don't worry—some babies just take longer to adjust to substitute feeding.

➢ **Rejecting the bottle or breast** is not uncommon. Some babies 6 months and over who are receiving solid foods may choose to wait as long as 6 to 7 hours for you to return. This is okay. Bottle rejection may indicate a loss of the *mothering person:* it is important for the substitute to "mother" the baby, not just feed her. If the baby refuses the bottle, the substitute should cuddle the baby, coo and talk to her, and then attempt the feeding again.

Refusing your breast may mean the baby is refusing you. You have to make an extra attempt at prolonged and continuous contact: stroking, cuddling, holding, and maintaining eye contact. The danger here is that you may withdraw because the baby has rejected you for leaving. A rejection cycle can be established: the infant is suffering most from feelings of separation and loss, yet you withdraw. Signs of your withdrawal are wanting to avoid the infant, not wanting to nurse, the failure of your let-down reflex, and the expectation that the nursing relationship is going to fail. If not stopped in time, this cycle can end your breast-feeding.

➢ **Maintaining milk supply does not just happen by itself**, as is the case with breast-feeding mothers who do not work. Hand-expression of milk stimulates about one-third as much milk as sucking does. You *must* allow the baby to nurse when you are home—roughly 4 feedings a day is usually right.

➢ **Starting the morning right is important**: your breasts are fullest after a night's rest. Each day you should try to get up half an hour early so you can have a relaxed feeding and avoid feeling guilty because you had to rush.

➢ **Coming home at the end of the day** is also very important, because you and the baby have mutual emotional and physiological needs at that time. Your breasts are full and the baby is hungry. You must plan to set aside this home-coming time for the baby. Arrange with your partner and other children that all family business has to be postponed until one hour after you get home and that their needs will be met at that time. Try to get help with the dinner—either paid help, your partner, children, or convenience foods—so that there is one less demand on you.

➤ *Nighttime feedings help to maintain your milk supply.* Most infants will continue to nurse at night. The easiest way is to take the baby to bed with you so that you can roll over and nurse without fully waking up. This gives you extra closeness to the baby, and the extra energy you save by not having to get up is especially important since you have to go to work in the morning.

➤ *The main problem you will encounter* is that some days your milk supply will be low. You should expect this to happen. Some minimal curtailment of activity usually solves the problem. *Stress is the biggest offender*. When signs of stress approach the danger stage, you should try to reduce pressure and demands both at home and in your business life. Some signs are the "it's-too-much-trouble" syndrome, excessive concern about the baby having enough to eat, worry about expressing milk, and a significantly reduced milk supply. *Stress tolerance is reached* when you are no longer able to nurse the baby when he's hungry. Take the day off, go to bed with the baby, drink plenty of fluids, and you should be back on course by the following day.

Medications and Breast-Feeding

Almost any drug you take will appear quickly in your breast milk, in approximately the same concentration as in your blood. The amount of medication in your milk and its effect on the baby varies; consult your doctor as well as the chart that follows, because many drugs will not have an adverse effect. However, there should be a *careful and continuous observation* of a nursing infant for possible unwanted effects from drugs in breast milk.

➤ *Although only trace amounts of a drug may* be found in breast milk, the cumulative effect over a 24-hour period of nursing may equal a full dose for an infant. Within the first postpartum days certain enzyme systems which are normally required to metabolize or detoxify some drugs may not be fully developed in the newborn. Some drugs, such as insulin and corticotropin, are destroyed in the infant's gastrointestinal tract and are therefore unimportant constituents of breast milk.

➤ *Some sulfa drugs prescribed for postpartum urinary tract infections* in the mother will pass into her breast milk, remain active after withstanding the acidity of the infant's stomach and may cause kernicterus or Gray's syndrome (jaundice).

➤ *Several anti-infective agents will cause vomiting* and skin rashes; some of the penicillin compounds may cause sensitization of the infant. Tetracycline may discolor the infant's teeth. Atropine can cause drowsiness, urinary retention, tachycardia, and respiratory symptoms in the baby. Anticoagulants and aspirin taken just before nursing may delay the infant's clotting time. Laxatives, excluding senna derivatives, may cause diarrhea in the baby. Bromides, which are found in Bromo-Seltzer and many over-the-counter sleeping aids, have caused rashes and drowsiness in the nursing baby.

➤ *A number of psychotropic drugs* cause lethargy and weight loss in the baby, including Valium, Lithium, Meprobamate, and Primidone. The effects of barbiturates are controversial, but they probably should be avoided due to their action on the infant's liver enzymes. Ergot preparations for migraine headaches can cause vomiting, diarrhea, weak pulse, and unstable blood pressure in the infant. Some drugs are toxic to the nursing baby if taken over a long period of time and require close monitoring of the infant and determination whether the benefit of taking the drug outweighs the risk. Steroids, diuretics, and oral contraceptives are among these medications.

➤ *Iodides affect the infant's thyroid gland.* Radioactive iodine, sodium, and gallium should be avoided if possible; even mothers who are not breast-feeding should have no contact with the baby for 48 hours afterward.

➤ *If a nursing mother does have to take medication* of any kind it is best to take it right before breast-feeding. If she takes the drug as she is beginning to nurse, by the end of the breast-feeding session the drug will have reached peak serum concentration at a point when there will be very little breast milk left for the drug to pass into. This strategy is not always workable when the infant is nursing 7 or 8 times a day, but as a general rule, try to take medication right when you start to nurse.

➤ *Marijuana is stored in mammalian milk,* and there have been no studies to suggest that it is acceptable for mothers to smoke marijuana while they are nursing. Because the effects on the infant of chronic exposure to THC, the chemical component of marijuana, are unknown, nursing mothers should abstain from using it. Mother's milk (both animal and human) is very high in fat and is therefore a prime place for the deposit and accumulation of the by-products of marijuana. Furthermore, milk is one of the routes through which the female body excretes, or gets rid of, THC.

Animal tests have shown cannabinoid present in all organs of suckling infant rats whose mothers were exposed to THC. When female mice took the drug either just before or just after birth, their male offspring had long-range sexual alterations. This included hormonal imbalances that decreased the size of the testes, as a result of exposure through the placenta and/or breast milk. In addition, when these animals went through puberty there were changes in their sexual behavior and hormone levels that were apparently due to their early exposure to marijuana.

➢ *Cocaine can reach a baby through breast milk,* as confirmed by recent research. Studies have demonstrated that cocaine not only crosses into breast milk, but remains there for over 36 hours. Researchers found that there can be severe damage, even death, if a baby gets a high enough dose of cocaine through breast milk. In one study, the mother was snorting cocaine while breast-feeding: within 3 hours of using half a gram of cocaine her child had become irritable, had vomited, and had developed diarrhea. It took two and a half days for the cocaine to clear from the child's urinary tract, after which the child did well. In another case, a child died and the autopsy showed high levels of cocaine in his blood. The mother admitted to using crack before breast-feeding. It shouldn't be necessary to say anything more: When nursing don't put anything in your body but food.

MEDICATIONS TO AVOID WHEN BREAST-FEEDING

DRUG	EFFECT
Analgesics	
Aspirin, phenacetin, and combinations (Alka-Seltzer, Bufferin, Cope, Excedrin, Rhinex, Vanquish)	Possible bleeding
Ergotamine (antimigraine) *(Cafergot, Ergomar, Gynergan, Migral)	Vomiting, diarrhea, weak pulse, unstable blood pressure, shock in 90% of infants
Antacids (Alka-Seltzer, Gelusil, Maalox)	Possible bleeding
Antibiotics	
*Chloromycetin	Anemia, shock, death
*Erythromycin	Sensitization, allergy to drug
Erythromycin estolate (Ilosone)	Hepatoxic
Symmetrel	Vomiting, rash
Tetracycline	Bone growth retardation
Streptomycin	Nephrotoxicity
*Penicillin	Possible sensitization, allergy
*Antituberculosis (Isoniazid)	Mental retardation
Anticoagulants	
*Dicumarol	Blood-clotting takes longer; hemorrhage in infant
*Heparin	
Anticonvulsants	
Primidone	Mother should not nurse
Dilantin	No acute side effects; occurs in only small amounts in milk
Mysoline	Causes only drowsiness in baby

*Especially harmful.

MEDICATIONS TO AVOID WHEN BREAST-FEEDING (*cont.*)

DRUG	EFFECT
Antineoplastics MAO inhibitors (for high blood pressure)	Nursing should stop
Antispasmodics *Atropine combinations* *(Artane, Arlidin)	Diminished milk secretion; heart irregularities in infant
Barbiturates (Amytal, Luminal, Seconal, Tuinal)	May have inducing effect on baby's liver enzymes; should be avoided
Nembutal	May sedate baby
Hypnotics (Doriden)	Drowsiness
Chloral hydrate and *combinations*	Drowsiness
Bromides and others (Bromural, Equanil, Phenergan, Bromo-Seltzer)	Drowsiness, rash
Cardiovascular preparations *Hypotensives and* *combinations with* *diuretics* Ismelin *Reserpine	 Hazardous to infant Increased respiratory tract secretions, cyanosis, and anorexia in infant; galactorrhea in mother
Cocaine	Mother should not nurse; can lead to infant death
Cough preparations Potassium iodide	Possible thyrotropic effect in infant; skin rash
Diuretics *(Thiazides and* *combinations)* (Diuril, Enduron)	Dehydration possible; may be harmless if taken under supervision (but manufacturers say to avoid if nursing)

*Especially harmful.

MEDICATIONS TO AVOID WHEN BREAST-FEEDING (*cont.*)

DRUG	EFFECT
Hormones	
*Androgen-estrogen combinations (Deladumone, Premarin w/ Methyltestosterone)	All estrogens cause gynecomastia and lower milk production
Estrogen (DES, TACE)	See above
Corticoids and analgesic combinations	All corticosteroids may cause poor growth and development
Glucocorticoid anti-inflammatory combinations (Aristocort, Cetacort lotion)	Poor growth in infant
Progestins (Depo-Provera, Gynorest, Nortulate)	Lower milk production
Progestins and estrogens in combination (Demulen, Enovid, Ortho-Novum, Ovulen)	Lower milk production
Parathyroid-dihydrotachysterol thyroid inhibitors *(Tapazole)	Osteoporosis, bone dysgenesis, reduced thyroid activity, goiter, anemia
Laxatives	
Senokot	Loose stool
*Dorbantyl, Dorbane	Diarrhea
Marijuana	Hazard to infant
Muscle relaxants	
Carosoprodol	Manufacturer suggests avoidance when nursing
Valium—see "Psychotropics"	

*Especially harmful.

MEDICATIONS TO AVOID WHEN BREAST-FEEDING (*cont.*)

DRUG	EFFECT
Psychotropics	
Butyrophenones and combinations (Haldol)	Causes rash, diarrhea
Hydroxyzines (Vistaril, Atarax)	Nursing discouraged; effects unknown
Lithium carbonate	Effects unknown; nursing discouraged
Meprobamate and combinations *(Equanil, Miltown)	Alternate drug advised
Librium	Effects unknown
*Valium	Effects unknown; nursing discouraged
Radioisotopes	
I_{131}	Suppress thyroid gland; all mothers, breast-feeding or not, should not have contact with baby for 48 hours
Urinary anti-infectives	
(Bactrim, Septra)	Sulfanilamides contraindicated if infant less than two months old
(Thiosulfil, nalidixic acid)	May be noxious if taken continuously
Mandelic acid	Photosensitivity, rashes
Vaginals	
AVC creams and other sulfanilamides *Flagyl vaginal insert	Jaundice of newborn (Gray's syndrome or kernicterus)
*Vaginal douches and gels containing povidone-iodine	Possible thyroid problems from high iodine levels

*Especially harmful.

Environmental Contamination of Breast Milk

We are all exposed daily to chemicals through food, air, and water. Some of these environmental contaminants are soluble primarily in water and others are soluble primarily in fat. When we ingest or inhale water-soluble chemicals, our bodies generally metabolize and excrete them. Fat-soluble chemicals are not excreted: they are stored in body fat for many years. As fat-soluble chemicals are accumulated, they reach a steady-state level after which further chemical residues are no longer stored but are directly excreted. There are two ways of mobilizing (getting rid of) these fat stores and the chemicals they contain: weight loss and lactation. Otherwise, the fat stores remain relatively immobile.

The fat-soluble chemicals which affect breast-feeding are called chlorinated hydrocarbons. Human breast milk can be contaminated with this type of chemical from agricultural and industrial sources. These chemicals increase the risk of cancer to the nursing infant and pose a threat of other physiological responses. The average amount of these chemicals in breast milk in the United States exceeds the safety standards proposed by the World Health Organization and the Food and Drug Administration (FDA). The information herein on the dangers of breast milk has been drawn from the excellent report *Birthright Denied* by the Environmental Defense Fund.

Chlorinated hydrocarbons fall into two categories, agricultural and industrial.

AGRICULTURAL CHEMICALS

➤ *The chief ones are pesticides:* DDT, aldrin, dieldrin, chlordane, heptachlor, toxaphene, benzene hexachloride (BHC), etc. They all have similar characteristics: they concentrate in the fat of organisms leading to *bioaccumulation*—for example, the residues of DDT in a fish can be thousands of times greater than the residues of DDT in the water it lives in—and *biomagnification*; persistence in the environment for many years; carcinogenicity, and other chronic and acute toxic effects.

There is global contamination from these long-lived pesticides. They concentrate in the fat of animals. Of all foods tested by the FDA, the categories with the highest residues are meat, fish, and dairy products.

➤ *The Environmental Protection Agency (EPA)* establishes tolerance levels of pesticide residues in food, allowing low levels which they believe are safe for human consumption. These tolerances are often based more on the expected level of the chemical rather than on a current evaluation of toxological data—therefore, we cannot assume that foods will not harm us just because the government says they are safe.

➤ *Pesticide residues occur more frequently* and in higher concentration in human milk than in cow's milk or infant formula. DDE (the form in which DDT is stored in the body) is the most frequently found pesticide in human milk, with dieldrin the second most common. The FDA has not done conclusive testing of formulas. Theoretically the pesticide residues should be much lower in formulas than in cow's milk, because in processing cow's milk which could be contaminated with pesticides, the fat is removed; in most formulas it is replaced with vegetable fat, which is usually less contaminated.

INDUSTRIAL CHEMICALS

➤ *There are many of these, but only two* have been officially reported as appearing in breast milk: PCBs (polychlorinated biphenyls) and their chemical cousins, PBBs (polybrominated biphenyls).

➤ *PCB contamination of food is essentially limited* to fish that spend part or all of their lives in fresh water. PCBs have had a widespread and uncontrolled industrial application for the past several decades. Industrial chemicals are discharged by factories into the air and water. They find their way into the food chain, where they can be concentrated and bioaccumulated. Fish reflect the pollution of water that receives industrial discharges. Because fish can concentrate PCBs in their bodies up to 9-million-fold, the levels of PCBs in the flesh of many fish far exceed the established FDA tolerance level. Fishing has been restricted in several areas of the country—this is not a localized problem, but one with national significance. See page 82 for more information.

➤ *In Michigan PBBs* (used as a flame retardant) accidentally got mixed into livestock feed in 1973 and 1974, causing illness and death to thousands of exposed animals. The contaminated food disappeared from grocery shelves, but it did not disappear from mother's milk ten years later. The Public Health Department in Michigan advised women from contaminated farms to discontinue nursing, although urban consumers of milk and meat were also exposed.

➤ *Currently, PBB contamination is limited to Michigan.* However, millions of pounds of this chemical have been manufactured and distributed throughout the United States in commerce. When these products are disposed of in landfills and dumps, and thereby enter the environment, this problem can become more widespread.

WAYS TO MINIMIZE CONTAMINANTS IN YOUR DIET

➤ *No one knows how long it takes to* cleanse the fat stores of all chemical residues. Some scientists are optimistic and say that being on a chemical-free diet for a few years would assure a woman of minimal residues in her milk; others contend that a woman should start a chemical-free diet as soon as she reaches puberty to prepare for her later childbearing years.

➤ *Fish that have lived in fresh water* for part or all of their lives are the major dietary source of PCBs. *This is one food that should be eliminated from your diet.* In particular, the fish to avoid are bottom-feeding estuarine fish (catfish, flounder, sole), Great Lakes fish (salmon, carp), fatty fish (buffalofish, eel), and fish from the Hudson River. Ocean fish (cod, haddock, halibut) are usually free from PCB residues so you should eat these if you include fish in your diet. See page 82. Many of these fish are now farm-raised and therefore safe—just be sure of their origin.

➤ *Animal origin foods are the major dietary source* of chlorinated hydrocarbon pesticides. In these foods—meat, fish, and dairy products—the pesticide residues are bioaccumulated in the fat over the lifetime of the animals and fish.

➤ *Meat is monitored by the U.S. Department of Agriculture.* The types of meat in which pesticide residues were most frequently found were *beef, veal, chicken, and turkey,* with grass-fed beef having a much lower residue level than the usual grain-fed beef. The meat in which pesticides were least frequently found were *sheep, goats, and swine.*

If you eat meat you should remove the fat and discard the drippings. In general, the better cooked the meat, the lower its fat content. And the fat is where the pesticide residues are stored.

➤ *Dairy products should be only lowfat*: yogurt, skim milk, buttermilk, ice milk, and uncreamed cottage cheese. *Avoid high-fat dairy products*: butter, cream, high-fat cheese. Again: the fat contains the residues.

➤ *Eggs have a surprisingly low residue of most pesticides* (with the exception of DDE) and so can be eaten with relatively low risk. However, the yolks must always be fully cooked to avoid the risk of salmonella.

➤ *Margarine made of corn oil is* least likely to contain pesticide residues, including DDT. Look at labels carefully: many margarines are made with DDT-containing cottonseed oil.

➤ *A lowfat, semivegetarian diet* would seem to be the most residue-free. Such a diet also lowers dietary fats and cholesterol, which is recommended to prevent heart disease and cancer.

➤ *A totally vegetarian diet* may be an excellent way to reduce pesticide residues in your system, if you start it well enough in advance of breast-feeding. A French study published in 1974 sampled the milk of women who were primarily vegetarians.

The results showed that if 70% or more of the diet contained organic food (i.e., grown without synthetic chemical pesticides or fertilizers) the pesticide residues in the breast milk were less than one-half of those in the median French human milk samples. All of the women who had significantly lower pesticide residues in their milk had been on the diet for 6 or more years, while those women whose pesticide residues were higher were generally on the diet for 3 years or less.

➤ *Your drinking water* can be a source of problems. See page 118.

Bottle-Feeding

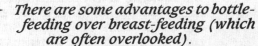

➤ *There are some advantages to bottle-feeding over breast-feeding (which are often overlooked).*

➤ *You have more freedom of movement*: you are not the only person who can supply the baby's food and therefore you aren't restricted by a feeding schedule, since other people can give a bottle. If you have a job, you may be able to return to it sooner.

➤ *You can get more rest* because your partner and others can feed the baby.

➤ *The gratification and closeness associated with feeding* can be shared by all: the father, mother, and grandparents. However, this should be a secondary consideration. Other people can share the care of the baby in many ways: by changing and dressing, bathing, or taking her for a walk.

➤ *You escape the potential discomforts of breast-feeding* (leaky breasts, sore nipples), and not nursing may preserve the shape of your breasts better. Although it is pregnancy itself which softens a firm breast regardless of whether you nurse, breast sagging is more common in those who breast-feed. However, it doesn't occur in all or even most of those who do breast-feed.

➤ *Formula-feeding may fill the baby up more* so she will go longer between feedings.

➤ *There is more certainty for you* because you know exactly how much food the baby is getting. This visible evidence is gratifying to some women who would not know the exact quantity a breast-feeding baby was receiving. This seems a weak rationale that caters to some people's compulsive need to measure and time things strictly. A breast-feeding baby gets just as much as she needs because of the natural supply-and-demand system.

➤ *Your physical condition does not affect the milk*, so if you were ill or taking drugs it would not affect your supply or pass the medication on to the baby.

DISADVANTAGES TO BOTTLE-FEEDING

➤ *The injection given in the hospital* to dry up your milk supply is potentially dangerous. Your milk production will stop by itself if you don't nurse the baby, so why intervene when nature will take care of it? Some hospitals give an injection of testosterone (a male hormone) to prevent lactation. *Many hospitals use the hormone DES (diethylstilbesterol), a known human carcinogen* which could increase your chances of cancer in later years. There is also evidence that the risk of thromboembolism is increased tenfold if DES is used to suppress lactation.

➤ *One option you should consider is* to nurse for the first week and then gradually dry up your milk supply. You will be giving your baby all the benefits of colostrum and you will be avoiding the use of these potentially dangerous drugs.

➤ *Obesity in mother and child* can be greater with bottle-feeding. The 30% increase in your weight during pregnancy prepares your body for the greater nutritional stress of lactation. You lose the opportunity to shed that body fat accumulated during pregnancy, specifically to support breast-feeding. Also, a bottle-fed child gains and grows more rapidly than one that breast-feeds. This creates more fat cells, which may lead to obesity later in life.

➤ *Bottles and nipples require sterilization*—some people say that careful washing or putting them in the dishwasher is sufficient. Ask your doctor his opinion.

➤ *Plastic bottles* are safer than glass.

➤ *Nursers (with a disposable plastic inner lining*) are more expensive, but it means less washing. The liner collapses during drinking so the baby takes in less air.

➤ *Nipples should be discarded* when they become flabby. If the flow is not fast enough you can enlarge the opening with a heated needle; if you make the hole too big you can close it by boiling the nipple for 5 minutes. The Nuk nipple is the most like a human nipple and is orthodontic, enabling the palate to develop more naturally. However, the nipple has an "up" and a "down" side, so you have to explain this to anyone giving the baby the bottle and to the child later on.

THE EMOTIONAL RISK OF BOTTLE-FEEDING

➤ *The psychological aspects of nursing may be lost in bottle-feeding unless you understand them*. It is essential to know what takes place naturally during breast-feeding so that you can re-create it in bottle-feeding. Breast-feeding creates a biological synchrony of suckling, tactile intimacy, cradling, comforting, sensory arousal, and communication through signs. These are all somewhat technical ways of saying that the baby has many needs besides just nourishment that are met during nursing. A breast-feeding mother does not have to premeditate meeting any of these needs.

➤ *If you bottle-feed, you have to make sure you* are meeting these needs. There is the risk that many of these aspects can be sacrificed if you do not know about them. If the bottle is substituted for the breast, the biological necessity for the baby to experience intimacy in a close grasp has to be compensated for by your intelligent knowledge that *the baby receives both food and love in your arms*.

➤ *Most mothers do approximate the breast-feeding position* when they give a bottle. However, there are many who feed their baby by means of a propped bottle in the crib, or who give the bottle while the baby reclines in a plastic seat. *Body intimacy in an embrace is essential for the psychological and physiological growth of the baby.* There are many solitary babies who do not know—or are intermittently deprived of—the sensual delights and comforts of their mother's embrace. The baby of an unknowing mother can be deprived of essential conditions of attachment if she isn't nursed close to her mother's body in a close grasp.

➤ *The breast automatically binds the baby* to a specific person—the bottle does not guarantee this union. The mother who doesn't know any better can easily adopt the attitude that *anyone* can give the baby a bottle. The section on "Love and Kisses," pages 528, makes it clear that a baby needs to make a strong attachment to one person for her development.

➤ *The minimum guarantee for the evolution* of the human bond is for an infant to have prolonged intimacy with a nurturing person, a condition which is biologically insured by breast-feeding. With bottle-feeding the continuity of the nurturing experience becomes dependent on your personality. You may want mobility and freedom and perceive that your baby—particularly the need for you to be the primary person nurturing that baby—as something that ties you down. This is a frequently cited reason for bottle-feeding—thus, a woman who does not recognize the biological necessity for her baby to receive both food and love in her arms may be absent for many feedings.

➤ *The breast was "intended" to bind a baby and her mother* for the first year or two of life. Breast-feeding insures the continuity of mothering as part of the formation of human bonds. The point here is not that everyone "should" breast-feed, or that you are cheating your baby emotionally by bottle-feeding; what is at stake is *how* a baby is fed and by whom. It is in your arms that a baby's ability to relate and to communicate with other people is initiated. A baby who is fed by a variety of caregivers while she sits in a hard plastic seat, a baby who is congratulated for holding her own bottle as soon as possible, is a baby who is deprived of the pleasure and security of her mother's arms, which may have ramifications in later relationships. If you feed your baby with a bottle, it places a responsibility on you that you would not have if you breast-fed. It is now your conscious effort, rather than an automatic corollary, that insures the integrity of the human bond between you and your baby.

INFANT FORMULA

➤ *The alternative to breast-feeding is formula*; in order to decide between these two methods of feeding you need full information about formulas. Although they may not be contaminated with residues of chlorinated hydrocarbons as frequently as human milk, formulas may contain different contaminants. If you decide to bottle-feed your baby or to supplement breast milk, you should know which formulas pose the fewest health problems and are the most balanced nutritionally.

➤ *Infant formulas try to approximate the natural* composition of human milk; although there is no formula that is identical in composition, some come closer than others. The aspects to consider in comparing a formula to breast milk are its protein-to-fat ratio, the amino-acid content, the type of carbohydrate used, and the levels of minerals present. Cow's milk in fluid and evaporated form is significantly different in its protein-to-fat ratio than human milk. Therefore you should not consider feeding these to your baby instead of formula—they are less expensive substitutes for breast milk, but are not good for a growing infant.

➤ *Check with your pediatrician about the formulas which most closely approximate human milk* in their content of protein, fat, amino acids, carbohydrates, and minerals.

➤ *If you have a family history of allergies* and are not going to breast-feed, you should probably avoid milk-based formulas. You can use either a soy-based formula or a predigested cow's milk formula. Although these alternative formulas do not resemble human milk as closely as milk-based ones (there are differences in carbohydrates, protein, and nutrient levels), they can prevent an allergenic response in the baby.

➤ **Corn is also a common allergen**. Therefore, parents concerned about allergies should find a milk-free *and* corn-free formula: one that has no corn syrup, corn oil, etc. Double-check the ingredients listed on any formula before purchasing it.

➤ **Soy milk is not a substitute** for mother's milk or formula. The Food and Drug Administration has warned parents not to use Edensoy or similar soy drinks instead of breast milk or infant formula. Soy drinks, sometimes sold as soy milk, are not the same as soy protein infant formulas. Some health-food stores and older literature from Eden Foods, Inc., may give the false impression that soy drinks are nutritionally comparable to cow's milk. The FDA has stated that this is not true; Eden Foods voluntarily recalled their misleading pamphlets.

➤ **Human milk has a high-fat, low-protein content.** This is believed necessary to provide enough calories and to aid in the absorption of small quantities of iron. Infant formulas approximate this ratio and several come close. However, even when the ratio is similar, the composition of the protein and fat is usually different. The protein in human milk is primarily lactalbumin, which is easily digested by infants. The protein in formula is primarily casein, which is not as easily digested.

➤ **Sugar** is added to formulas to simulate the natural sweetness of breast milk. Most cow's milk formulas add lactose, the natural sugar present in human milk, but all milk-substitute formulas (soy milk) add sucrose. Sucrose is refined white sugar—some formulas contain as much as 40 to 50 percent sucrose by weight.

➤ **The level of cholesterol** in human milk is higher than that in formula. Human milk has 20 mg of cholesterol per 100 mg, while most formulas have between 1.5 and 3.3 mg per 100 mg. The effects of this are not fully known, but it is speculated that exposure to high cholesterol in early life may be necessary to stimulate the metabolic systems which break down cholesterol later on. The amount of cholesterol needed by infants has not been determined, but animal studies show that *low* cholesterol level in infancy led to *higher* serum cholesterol levels when the animals got older, compared to those that had moderate amounts of cholesterol in their infant diets. The implication is that low-cholesterol formulas may contribute to atherosclerosis in later life, a big national health problem in the United States.

➤ **Human milk contains lower levels of minerals**, which minimizes the load on the baby's kidneys. There is also a higher level of sodium (salt) in cow's milk and formula, which can cause water loss from the kidneys. In cases of dehydration from diarrhea or overheating this can lead to hypernatraemia, a condition in which the abnormally high sodium level in the blood may result in brain damage and later intellectual retardation. There are also higher levels of phosphate in cow's milk and formulas—in certain circumstances this can prevent adequate absorption of calcium. This can lead to hypocalcaemia or neonatal tetany, newborn diseases caused by a deficiency of calcium in the blood, which causes convulsions. These diseases are not a problem for most formula-fed infants, but they do occur and therefore must be mentioned.

CONTAMINANTS IN FORMULA

➢ *Lead has been a serious problem in liquid formulas*, where it has been found in a variety of studies over the years. Unfortunately, the results of these studies are contradictory in terms of how much lead was detected and whether there was more in canned or bottled formula. However, just the possible presence of lead is a cause for concern. It can cause neurological disorders ranging from learning disabilities, mental retardation, and hyperactivity to paralysis, convulsions, and coma. The blood system and kidneys can also be adversely affected.

➢ *It is not known what minimal amount of lead is acceptable*. The FDA has a standard for lead intake by infants, but the Environmental Defense Fund, a private organization, states that it is too lenient. Evidently the FDA acceptable levels of lead are based on inaccurate measurements and do not take into account the huge increase in absorption of lead from milk compared to lead in other foods. There is no doubt that infants are particularly susceptible to lead poisoning. Also, children absorb substantially higher amounts of lead from dietary sources than adults do; infants may absorb even higher amounts.

➢ *Experts cannot agree on where the lead* in formulas is coming from, but there is no doubt that it is present in many liquid formulas. Some say that the lead derives from the solder used on the seams of the cans, which does not explain why bottled formula sometimes contains lead. Others speculate that lead could be associated with the food additive carageenan, which is added to stabilize formula.

➢ *There have been two studies of liquid formulas*: One indicates that glass-bottled formula is preferable, but the other study contradicts this. Powdered formula was not tested, and although lead levels might be lower, the tap water added to prepare it has contaminants of its own. This lack of conclusive data makes it even more difficult for you to decide how and what to feed your baby. Although it is necessary to include this information about lead contamination of formula, it is not sufficiently definitive to be used in choosing one formula over another.

➢ *The tap water used to dilute formula can contain contaminants.*

THMs are a group of chemicals formed during the chlorination of water, which kills the bacteria that cause infectious diseases. The chlorine reacts with the organic matter in the water supply to form THMs. Chlorination cannot be stopped because it is the most effective disinfectant method available and the EPA states that it is necessary for public health safety. The irony is that THMs have been shown to cause cancer in test animals, and the EPA says that they *may* pose the same risk to humans. According to the EPA, studies in areas of high cancer rates have suggested a link between cancer and chemical contaminants in drinking water.

➤ *A granulated activated carbon (GAC) filtering system* in a community can safeguard its water. The EPA report showed that *industrial chemicals* discharged into surface waters are not usually removed by current drinking water treatment facilities. Many organic chemicals, some mutagens, and suspected carcinogens are present in drinking water samples from all over the country. These chemicals *could* be removed at the treatment plants by filtration with activated carbon, but this is still rare in most communities. The EPA estimates that a GAC filtering system would cost a community about $10 per family per year.

If a formula manufacturer does not properly treat the water used in preparing formula, then these organic chemicals will be present. If you use concentrated or powdered formula and dilute it with tap water, it will introduce these chemicals. You can find out if your community is one of the few in the country that does filter its drinking water supply with activated carbon, which removes these impurities. Otherwise you can purchase a carbon filter system for your home or buy distilled water. You might consider using such water for yourself and the rest of your family, as well.

➤ *Another problem with tap water in certain parts of the country is high nitrate levels.* Approximately 5% of communities in the United States have high levels in the drinking water, and public health officials recommend that it not be used for infants. Nitrate, when reduced to nitrite in the stomach, can combine with hemoglobin in the blood and prevent oxygen from being adequately distributed throughout the body, causing the baby to turn blue, a disease known as methemoglobinemia. High-nitrate-containing water is a serious health hazard to infants if it is added to their formula.

➤ *In certain parts of the country lead pipes* have been corroded by water and the *lead level* is high—Boston is one such area. If this water is used to dilute concentrated formula or frozen orange juice, or in the preparation of cereals, it poses a health hazard to the baby. Prenatal exposure can also be a problem because lead exposure can cause birth defects in the fetus.

➤ *Improper handling of formula* can lead to bacterial contamination. If there are unsanitary conditions—which often occurs in poor areas—bottles and formulas can be contaminated with bacteria and cause gastrointestinal illness. This can be a life-threatening problem to a baby, who can easily become dehydrated from vomiting and diarrhea.

➤ *The other problem in poor areas* is that formula can be overdiluted in order to cut costs.

Introducing Solid Foods

➤ *The age to introduce solids* should be governed in part by the baby's physical capabilities. The voluntary transfer of food from the front to the back of the mouth is not evident until 3 to 4 months of age.

➤ *Appetite appears to be regulated by the hypothalamic* portion of the brain. Normally, the desire to eat is suppressed when an adequate number of calories has been consumed. It is not known when this appetite-regulating mechanism begins in infants. The use of solid foods in higher caloric density than breast milk or formula during the period when an infant cannot yet regulate her intake by calories may result in excessive energy (calorie) intake. Human milk or formulas have 67 to 77 calories per 100 grams. For an equivalent 100 grams of meat there are 103 calories, for desserts, 96 calories, and for dry cereals with milk, there are 107 calories.

➤ *Parents can overestimate a baby's caloric* need and encourage the baby to finish all the food in the jar or on the plate. To make this potential problem even worse, some companies are now marketing jars that are 11% larger in order to capture a bigger share of customers. This will further encourage overfeeding.

➤ *Some doctors say* that the early introduction of solids predisposes an infant to allergies. They say that delaying the use of the more allergenic foods (egg white, citrus fruit, wheat) until 12 months of age will minimize the likelihood of allergy.

➤ *The early introduction of home-prepared foods* is equally undesirable.

➤ *The early introduction of solids* is not only physiologically unsound, it is also a bad idea economically. Commercially prepared baby foods are more expensive per unit calorie than most milks or formulas.

➤ *There are some doctors who urge deemphasizing* the role of milk in a baby's diet. They feel that lean meat and vegetables provide all the calcium and protein of milk without the saturated fats and cholesterol. These doctors recommend that after 3 months of age you should discontinue formula or breast-feeding and use a maximum of 14 to 18 ounces of lowfat (2% fat) milk daily. This is only one theory—you can discuss it with your pediatrician.

➤ *Human milk or a substitute* supports the normal growth of most infants from 4 to 6 months of age with some vitamin and iron supplementation. Some mothers—particularly those who bottle-feed—are unaware that the American Academy of Pediatrics has urged against the *unnecessary early introduction of solid foods* into a baby's diet. One reason that parents rush to start a baby on solid foods is because it is considered a mark of accomplishment. "My child is already eating cereal," you may hear a woman say with pride.

➤ **Another reason that solids are introduced** quickly is because some people believe it causes the infant to sleep through the night, but this claim has not been substantiated. There is no data to support linking solid foods and better sleeping. Then there is the pressure from advertisements that induce women to start solids.

➤ **According to one study, bottle-feeding** mothers are more likely to introduce solids at a much earlier age than those who breast-feed; those who begin solids before the baby is 3 months old are more likely to use commercially prepared foods rather than home-processed ones.

Diet After Weaning

➤ **Skim milk (nonfat) does not provide enough energy** to sustain an infant's growth during the first year. It doesn't contain enough calories, which are the gauge used to express the fuel or energy value of food. Skim milk is deficient in iron, ascorbic acid, and essential fatty acids. It is also too high in salt and protein (protein provides 40% of the calories in skim milk), which put too much pressure on a baby's kidneys. A baby needs some fat because he has to build up a fat storage in case of serious illness when his food intake might be temporarily interrupted.

➤ **If your family has a history of high cholesterol levels** or premature coronary deaths you should have your child checked. People with this tendency can be singled out before age 3 with a series of blood tests.

➤ **Nitrate-rich foods** can cause a disease which causes a baby to turn blue because oxygen is not adequately distributed throughout the body. Nitrate in the diet can convert to nitrite in the intestines, which then combines with hemoglobin in the blood and prevents oxygen distribution. There is a very small risk of this happening, but *spinach, carrots, and beets* should not be given to a child under 3 months because of susceptibility to this illness. Ideally, these vegetables should be served only after 5 to 7 months of age. They are best served fresh—mashed, boiled, or steamed—rather than kept in the refrigerator several days.

> *Home-prepared foods should not be salted*. The drawbacks to salt in commercial baby foods are discussed below. There are several good books available on home preparation with recipes. Basically, you should feed your baby appropriate family foods minus the seasonings.

> *Commercially prepared baby foods* have drawbacks in the areas of salt, starch, and sugar. Several manufacturers now offer certain items minus the salt or sugar that was once routinely added—read labels carefully. You should also not be misled by certain kinds of advertising: for example, a company can claim that it adds no preservatives, artificial flavors, or colors to its foods but they may add sugar to the majority of its products. Once you read this section, then consider making all or some of your baby's food at home.

> *Never store opened commercial baby food* in the refrigerator for more than 3 days. Take out only the portion your baby will eat.

> *Do not feed the baby directly from the jar* until an age when the baby can eat the entire contents. The enzymes in saliva start breaking down food in the jar and cause the uneaten portion to be "watery" because of this process.

> *You should know what you're paying for* and what you're actually giving your baby: vegetable/meat dinners contain an average of only 9% meat. So-called high meat dinners have around 30% meat.

> *Salt was added to baby foods for* a long time. Manufacturers used to claim that salt helped maintain the sodium/potassium balance, aided in kidney function, and that the iodine in it helped prevent thyroid problems like a simple goiter. The National Academy of Sciences Committee recommends a very low amount of salt but some pediatric nutritionists consider even this an excessive amount. Many baby food companies have eliminated salt entirely from their products.

> *Starch in baby food* is defended by the manufacturers. They claim that modified starches derived from corn or tapioca act as stabilizers, are an energy source, and that they are never more than 6% of the total product. However, modified starch may comprise as much as one-fourth of the total solids. It adds only calories and replaces more expensive, nutritious ingredients that have protein, minerals, and vitamins. Few single-ingredient foods contain modified starch. Combination foods give a manufacturer increased shelf-space in stores, but it is the consumer who pays: larger volumes of few choices would cost the companies less to produce and this saving *could* be passed on to you.

> *Sugar is a real problem in commercial foods.* Studies show that infants can differentiate and will generally eat more of a sweet food. Companies put sugar in more than half their foods, which accustoms children to sweetness and teaches them to ex-

pect it. It is often added to foods that do not naturally contain much sugar. Cereals, especially those in jars, often have sugar added. In desserts, sugar is often the principal ingredient.

Sugar adds only extra calories: no vitamins, minerals, or protein. The regular eating of sweet foods in infancy may stimulate a preference for sweet foods in childhood and adulthood. *Every possible step should be taken to reduce a baby's intake of and taste for sugar.*

➤ **Honey should not be fed to children** under 12 months of age. This recommendation is made by the Centers for Disease Control and by the world's largest honey producer, the Sioux Honey Association of Sioux City, Iowa: Honey poses a threat of botulism if fed to infants. There is a significant link between honey exposure and type-B infant botulism, and many samples of honey were tested and found to be contaminated.

➤ **Sodium nitrite or nitrate** is in some baby foods. Gerber adds it to ham-containing "toddler meals" as a coloring and flavoring. It is not needed as a preservative: all baby food is heat-sterilized, killing all microorganisms and spores. Nitrite may react with other chemicals in the body to form nitrosamines, small amounts of which cause cancer in animals. Infants are the most sensitive segment of the population and should not be exposed to even the tiniest amounts of potential carcinogens.

MISCELLANEOUS DANGERS TO THE BABY

➤ *Infant swim classes have become popular for babies* only a few months old, but they present some dangers. The California Medical Association has issued strong warnings, especially about the dangers of forced infant submersion. Instructors often use this technique to get a child used to getting her face wet: *parents don't know that children have died or been permanently harmed by water intoxication.* This is a condition which occurs when a child ingests too much water: the victim may have convulsions, seizures, go into shock, or even become comatose. *This condition can happen hours or days after the swim class, even if the child did not seem affected at the time of the lesson.*

The most dangerous classes are those aimed at the youngest children, the classes which promise to "waterproof" or "drownproof" children under age 3. Although they can learn to propel themselves, children that age don't understand water safety— and it is the age at which a child is most vulnerable to drowning.

An additional hazard of kiddie swim classes is that there can be bacteria in the water from other children which can result in ear infections, sinus conditions, and ingestion of bacteria into the lungs. The California Medical Association recommends that you avoid submerging any child until she has developed immunities to bacteria, and until other physiological and psychological growth have also taken place.

➢ *The use of vitamins for infants is an area of controversy*. Although vitamin supplements are sometimes routinely prescribed as "nutritional insurance," many knowledgeable pediatricians are opposed. The consensus is that a healthy, full-term baby has no need for vitamin supplementation. A breast-fed baby gets everything he needs from mother's milk, while infant formula already contains vitamins to approximate breast milk.

➢ *Waterbeds are dangerous for babies less than 2 years old*: they cannot turn over on a waterbed and can smother. *Do not leave a young child of any age unattended on a waterbed: if the child is under 2, do not even turn your back on the child.*

➢ *Bath support rings can be lethal for babies*. Never leave a small child alone in one of these "support ring" bathing devices, which usually are constructed with 3 or 4 legs with suction cups. The suction cups can suddenly release from the bottom of the bathtub, allowing the device and the baby to tip over. A baby can also slip between the legs of the device and become trapped under the ring. *An adult should always be present when a bath ring is used.*

➢ *Certain crib toys are hazardous for babies*, some of whom have hung themselves on these devices. Numerous babies, most over 5 months old, have strangled, suffered brain damage, or been narrowly rescued from strangulation due to these playthings. Though some of the stuffed animals, dolls, mirrors, etc., that are strung from mobiles or stretched across the crib are more dangerous than others, the hazard exists with all of them once a baby is able to reach the toys.

➢ **WARNING:** Remove all crib toys strung across the crib or playpen when your child is beginning to push up on hands and knees or is 5 months of age, whichever occurs first. These toys can cause strangulation.

➢ *Structured exercise programs for infants* are not recommended by the American Academy of Pediatrics. These programs, most of which involve massage and passive exercise, have become increasingly popular in the United States. Some of these programs involve purchasing equipment and instructional materials for enhancing a baby's quiet alert states and "learning." Promoters claim that this will improve a baby's physical prowess or intelligence. However, the AAP feels there should not be pressure on parents and infants to accelerate the child's normal development, especially because "the possibility exists that adults may inadvertently exceed the infant's limitations."

The American Academy of Pediatrics emphasized in the policy statement that although it is important to provide a stimulating environment for infants, parents do not need special skills or equipment to do this. "An infant should be provided with opportunities for touching, holding, face-to-face contact, and minimally structured playing with safe toys. If these opportunities occur, an infant's intrinsic motivation will guide his or her individual development. . . .'' The point here is to avoid getting caught up in the Super Baby syndrome and allow your child to blossom naturally.

Household Pets and the New Baby

Household pets may have had a central part in your life before the birth of your baby. In some ways pets may even have been surrogate children and received a great deal of loving from you. It is inevitable that when you bring a newborn home it will change the kind of attention your pets now receive. This can create jealousy in the animal and set up a rivalry between it and the new baby. Make an effort to include your pet as much as you can when the baby joins the household. New parents have a tendency to push the pet away—both because they haven't got as much time for it and because they want to protect the baby. This will only increase the animal's feeling of rivalry.

Make a careful observation of the animal when it is around the baby—some dogs become protective and nurturant of a baby, others may feel antagonistic. When you aren't there, it may be a good idea to close the nursery door, at least in the early postpartum period. There is an old wive's tale (untrue) that a cat can jump into a crib and smother a baby. However, household pets do pick up dirt and germs, and it's best not to have them in nose-to-nose contact with a newborn.

ANIMALS ARE GOING TO FEEL JEALOUS

➢ Your pets may have been like children for you.
  • Many couples ''practice parenting'' on their pet(s).
  • Be compassionate about how displaced your animal(s) must feel to be ''thrown over'' for a noisy, strange-smelling intruder.
  • Take the pet's perspective of the new arrival: you're fussing over a little bundle in the same tone of voice you probably used for the pet(s).
➢ You're going to have less time and affection for pet(s) now.
  • Your pets may have had a central place in your life before the baby was born.
  • It's inevitable that once your baby arrives your pets are going to get less of your emotions.
  • This is going to make the animal(s) jealous and set up rivalry with the baby for your affection.

➤ Encourage the pet to make friends with the baby.
  • Being overprotective will only increase a pet's feeling of jealousy because he's being pushed aside.
  • When bringing the baby close to the pet, pat the animal and use an encouraging, gentle tone of voice.
  • If the animal sniffs or licks, these are natural reactions: control your knee-jerk reactions to shoo the pet away in protection of the baby.
  • Don't reprimand the animal with a harsh tone or strike it.
  • Try to see the situation from the animal's point of view: he's confused and displaced.
  • Take advantage of the fact that pets generally want to please you.
  • Encourage a friendship with the baby with positive reinforcement.

PREPARING A PET FOR THE NEW ARRIVAL

➤ Get obedience training if your dog doesn't already follow commands.
  • You'll need to be able to control and direct your dog when the baby is around.
  • You are going to need basic commands such as "Sit," "Stay," "Down," "Leave it," "Off," etc.
  • You may not feel you have the time or energy to train the dog during pregnancy, but having control may be what allows your dog to make a smooth transition with the baby.
➤ Expose your pet(s) to children, especially infants.
  • Encourage people to bring babies to the house: this will familiarize your cat or dog with having an infant on the animal's home turf.
  • Don't worry if your dog is agitated by young children: this doesn't mean there will be a problem with a baby.
  • Youngsters are quite a different adjustment for a pet than an infant. Small children move quickly, talk loudly, and can make motions and sounds that are threatening and startling to pets.
➤ Bring a baby doll home and pretend it's real.
  • Put a baby doll in the crib, hold it in your arms, and talk to it as you would a real baby.
  • This will accustom your pet to what's ahead. (Don't let any friends see you doing this or they'll think you're off your rocker!)

ONCE THE BABY COMES HOME

➤ Acquaint the dog or cat with your baby's scent.
  • Bring home a receiving blanker or piece of clothing that has been used on your newborn baby.
  • Sense of smell is vital to a dog; this is an important "first introduction."
➤ Make an effort to include the pet as much as possible once the baby joins the family.
  • New parents have a tendency to push a pet away.
  • You haven't got as much time for the animal now and you're feeling protective toward the baby.
  • Spurning the pet only increases the animal's feeling of being displaced or rejected.
➤ Get new toys or chew bones for a dog and catnip for a kitty.
  • Give the dog a treat in the beginning when he's around the baby.
  • Consider it a bribe, or a positive reinforcement; the dog will associate the baby with something he likes!
➤ Observe the pet around the baby.
  • Some pets become protective and nurturant of the newborn.
  • Other pets may feel antagonistic.
  • If the animal seems hostile, be wary: look for a tail that is held down and doesn't wag, flattened ears, or more overt hostility such as growling or bristling hair.
  • To be safe, at least in the early weeks, don't leave any pet alone with the newborn: close the nursery door and/or always have a person around.
  • There are some pets, particularly older ones, that may not be able to welcome the baby and make accommodation, but give the animal every opportunity first.

ARE PETS UNHEALTHY FOR BABIES?

➤ Household pets do pick up dirt and germs from the ground.
  • It's best not to have them in nose-to-nose contact with the infant.
➤ Cats often like to make a nest in the crib or bassinet.
  • You probably don't want your baby to sleep on a blanket of cat hairs!
  • You can close the cat out of the room with the baby's things in it.
  • You can also cover the baby's bed with anti-insect gauzy netting sold for cribs or a similar mesh netting made especially to keep cats out.

SOME FINAL THOUGHTS

I'm glad to say that I am still passionate about childbirth even after nearly twenty years of being immersed in the subject. If anything, the healthcare, social, and personal issues surrounding pregnancy and birth seem more important than ever. Women have told me that because of this book they came to view me as a friend during their childbearing experience. I am honored. And I don't take that trust lightly: I want to do everything possible to make pregnancy and childbirth safe and beautiful for parents and babies; therefore, here is an entirely new edition of the one book I hope has everything you need. So if you have questions this book doesn't answer, or you can't get what you want from your healthcare providers, or you just need some reassurance, get in touch with me. I learn something from everyone who contacts me, and I can pass it on to others.

I still get crazy when I hear bad hospital stories; I still get frustrated when I meet couples who complain about the system and are doing nothing to take responsibility for their own health care; I am still in awe of the miracles of medicine; I still get all choked up when I see a baby coming into this world. It seems as though the world has another chance every time a baby is born; we all have to make sure that birth is the very best it can be.

I still have an urge to stop pregnant women in the street and ask if they're okay. "Is everything all right?" I want to ask. "Are you satisfied with your doctor? Are you eating enough protein? How about breast-feeding? How's your relationship doing?"

I also still weep inside when I learn of couples with tiny children whose marriages are suffering—sometimes to the point of separation or divorce. It is vital that you find your strength together as a couple during pregnancy so that childbirth and raising a family together can be a powerfully positive time in your lives.

In fact, I was so concerned about the effect of a new baby on a couple's relationship that I wrote a whole book about it! I wrote *Childbirth & Marriage* for parents-to-be and new parents because I could see that new parents need all the help they can get if they're going to have a mutually satisfying marriage while raising a child. Until *Childbirth & Marriage* there was nowhere to turn for support and information about that transition to parenthood and the effect it has on your relationship. I hope that the two books together will help you get the full measure of joy and fulfillment from giving birth and raising a child together.

Index

AND BABY MAKES THREE...
COMPREHENSIVE GUIDES BY
TRACIE HOTCHNER

PREGNANCY PURE&SIMPLE

77434-8/$11.00 US/$15.00 CAN

PREGNANCY & CHILDBIRTH

Revised Edition
78039-9/$12.50 US/$16.50 CAN

THE PREGNANCY DIARY

76543-8/$12.00 US/$16.00 CAN